Textbook of
Pediatric Gastroenterology, Hepatology and Nutrition

Textbook of Pediatric Gastroenterology, Hepatology and Nutrition

Editors

Anupam Sibal
MD FIMSA FIAP FRCP (Glasg) FRCP (Lon) FRCPCH FAAP
Group Medical Director, Apollo Hospitals Group
Adjunct Professor, Department of Pediatrics
School of Medicine, University of Queensland
Brisbane, Australia
Member, Institute Body
Postgraduate Institute of Medical Education and Research
Chandigarh, India
Senior Consultant Pediatric Gastroenterologist and
Hepatologist
Indraprastha Apollo Hospitals
New Delhi, India

Sarath Gopalan
MD (PGIMER, Chandigarh), Fellowship in Pediatric
Gastroenterology and Clinical Nutrition (UK), MAMS
Senior Consultant Pediatric Gastroenterologist and
Hepatologist
Indraprastha Apollo Hospitals
Executive Director
Centre for Research on Nutrition Support Systems
New Delhi, India

Co-editors

Akshay Kapoor MD
Consultant Pediatric Gastroenterologist and Hepatologist
Indraprastha Apollo Hospitals
New Delhi, India

Vidyut Bhatia MD
Consultant Pediatric Gastroenterologist and Hepatologist
Indraprastha Apollo Hospitals
New Delhi, India

Foreword
John Walker-Smith

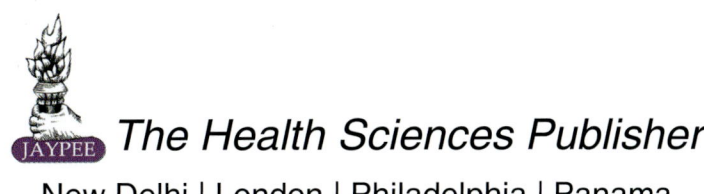

The Health Sciences Publisher
New Delhi | London | Philadelphia | Panama

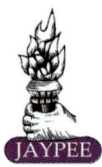

Jaypee Brothers Medical Publishers (P) Ltd

Headquarters

Jaypee Brothers Medical Publishers (P) Ltd
4838/24, Ansari Road, Daryaganj
New Delhi 110 002, India
Phone: +91-11-43574357
Fax: +91-11-43574314
Email: jaypee@jaypeebrothers.com

Overseas Offices

J.P. Medical Ltd
83, Victoria Street, London
SW1H 0HW (UK)
Phone: +44 20 3170 8910
Fax: +44 (0)20 3008 6180
Email: info@jpmedpub.com

Jaypee Medical Inc
The Bourse
111 South Independence Mall East
Suite 835, Philadelphia, PA 19106, USA
Phone: +1 267-519-9789
Email: jpmed.us@gmail.com

Jaypee Brothers Medical Publishers (P) Ltd
Bhotahity, Kathmandu
Nepal
Phone: +977-9741283608
Email: kathmandu@jaypeebrothers.com

Jaypee-Highlights Medical Publishers Inc
City of Knowledge, Bld. 237, Clayton
Panama City, Panama
Phone: +1 507-301-0496
Fax: +1 507-301-0499
Email: cservice@jphmedical.com

Jaypee Brothers Medical Publishers (P) Ltd
17/1-B Babar Road, Block-B, Shaymali
Mohammadpur, Dhaka-1207
Bangladesh
Mobile: +08801912003485
Email: jaypeedhaka@gmail.com

Website: www.jaypeebrothers.com
Website: www.jaypeedigital.com

Textbook of Pediatric Gastroenterology, Hepatology and Nutrition

First Edition: **2015**

ISBN 978-93-5152-740-4

Printed at: Ajanta Offset & Packagings Ltd., New Delhi

CONTRIBUTORS

A Riyaz
MD DCH DNB DM (Gastroenterology)
Pediatric Gastroenterologist
Professor and Head, Department of Pediatrics
Goverment Medical College
Calicut, Kerala, India

AK Patwari
MD DCH MNAMS FIAP FAMS
Head, Department of Pediatrics
Hamdard Institute of Medical Sciences and Research
Associated HAH Centenary Hospital
Hamdard University
New Delhi, India

Akshay Kapoor
MD
Consultant Pediatric Gastroenterologist and Hepatologist
Indraprastha Apollo Hospitals
New Delhi, India

Amita Mahajan
MD MRCP (UK) CCST (Ped Oncol, UK)
Pediatric Hematology and Oncology Unit
Apollo Center for Advanced Pediatrics
Indraprastha Apollo Hospitals
New Delhi, India

Anupam Sibal
MD FIMSA FIAP FRCP (Glasg) FRCP (Lon) FRCPCH FAAP
Group Medical Director, Apollo Hospitals Group
Adjunct Professor, Department of Pediatrics
School of Medicine, University of Queensland
Brisbane, Australia
Member, Institute Body
Postgraduate Institute of Medical Education and Research
Chandigarh, India
Senior Consultant Pediatric Gastroenterologist and
Hepatologist
Indraprastha Apollo Hospitals
New Delhi, India

B Sumathi
MD (Ped) DCH DM (Gastro)
Assistant Professor
Department of Pediatric Gastroenterology
Institute of Child Health
Chennai, Tamil Nadu, India

Bhupinder K Sandhu
OBE DSc MD FRCP FRCPCH
Consultant Pediatric Gastroenterologist
Bristol Royal Hospital for Children
Honorary Professor
Centre for Child and Adolescent Health
University of The West of England and
University of Bristol
United Kingdom

Boosba Vivatvakin
MD DTM&H (Hon)
Consultant Pediatric Gastroenterologist
Pediatric Gastrointestinal Unit
Chulalongkorn University
Bangkok, Thailand

BR Thapa
MD
Professor and Head
Division of Pediatric Gastroenterology, Hepatology and
Nutrition
Postgraduate Institute of Medical Education and Research
Chandigarh, India

Deepak Goyal
MD PDCC (Ped Gastro)
Associate Consultant
Department of Pediatric Gastroenterology,
Hepatology and Liver Transplantation
Medanta – The Medicity
Gurgaon, Haryana, India

Deirdre Kelly
MD
Professor
Department of Pediatric Hepatology, The Liver Unit
Birmingham Children's Hospital HNS Trust and
University of Birmingham
Steelhouse Lane
Birmingham
Past President
British Society of Paediatric Gastroenterology,
Hepatology and Nutrition
European Society for Paediatric Gastroenterology,
Hepatology and Nutrition

Dhanasekhar Kesavelu
MBBS MRCPCH (UK) FRCPCH (UK) CCT (UK)
Consultant Pediatric Gastroenterologist
Apollo Children's Hospital
Chennai, Tamil Nadu, India

Dinesh Banur
MBBS DCH MRCPCH (UK) FRCPCH (UK) CCT
Consultant Pediatric Gastroenterologist
Columbia Asia Hospital
Bengaluru, Karnataka, India

Efstratios Saliakellis
MD PhD
Clinical Fellow
Department of Pediatric Gastroenterology and Nutrition
4th Pediatric Department
Aristotle University of Thessaloniki
Greece
Division of Neurogastroenterology and Motility
Department of Gastroenterology
Great Ormond Street Hospital
London, United Kingdom

Garima Garg
MD
Junior Consultant
Pediatric Intensive Care Unit
Fortis Escorts Heart Institute
New Delhi, India

Hanifah Oswari
MD PhD
Gastrohepatology Division
Department of Child Health
University of Indonesia
Indonesia

Huma Cheema
MRCP (UK) DPGN (London University)
Professor Head
Department of Gastroenterology, Hepatology and Nutrition
The Children's Hospital and The Institute of Child Health
Lahore, Pakistan

James Huang
MBBS (Hons, S'pore) MRCPCH (Paeds, UK)
Registrar
Division of Gastroenterology, Hepatology and Nutrition
Department of Pediatrics
KTP-National University Children's Medical Institute
National University Hospital
Singapore

John Matthai
MD (Ped) DCH FAB (Ped Gastro) FIAP
Head, Neonatology Division
Professor, Department of Pediatrics
PSG Institute of Medical Sciences
Peelamedu, Coimbatore, Tamil Nadu, India

Juliet Sio Aguilar
MD MSc
Professor and Chair
Department of Pediatrics
Attending Pediatrician and Pediatric Gastroenterologist
University of the Philippines, Manila
College of Medicine–Philippine General Hospital
Philippines

K Vijayaraghavan
MD MSc (Community Health) MSc (Applied Nutrition)
Former Senior Deputy Director
National Institute of Nutrition
Hyderabad, Telangana, India

Kathleen B Schwarz
MD
Professor, Department of Pediatrics
Director, Pediatric Liver Center
President, Federation of International Societies of
Pediatric Gastroenterology, Hepatology and
Nutrition (FISPGHAN)
Division of Pediatric Gastroenterology, Hepatology and
Nutrition
Department of Pediatrics
Johns Hopkins University School of Medicine
Baltimore, USA

M Geetha
MD (Ped) DNB (Ped) DM
Gastroenterologist
Amrita Institute of Medical Sciences and Research Center
Kochi, Kerala, India

Malathi Sathiyasekaran
MBBS MD DCH DM
Senior Consultant Pediatric Gastroenterologist
Kanchi Kamakoti Childs Trust Hospital and
The Childs Trust Medical Research Foundation
Chennai, Tamil Nadu, India

Manas Kalra
MD DNB (Ped Hemato-oncology) FNB
Pediatric Hematology and Oncology Unit
Apollo Center for Advanced Pediatrics
Indraprastha Apollo Hospitals
New Delhi, India

Manav Wadhawan
DM (Gastroenterology)
Senior Consultant Hepatologist
Indraprastha Apollo Hospitals
New Delhi, India

Marion M Aw
MBBS MMed (Ped) MRCP (UK) FRCPCH (UK) FAMS
Pediatric Gastroenterologist and Hepatologist
National University Children's Medical Institute
Singapore

Md Iqbal Hossain
MBBS DCH PhD
Senior Scientist
Centre for Nutrition and Food Security, icddr, b
Clinical Lead, Nutrition Unit
Dhaka Hospital, icddr, b
Adjunct Associate Professor
School of Public Health, BRAC University
Bangladesh

Mohammad Nurul Akhtar Hasan
MD
Fellow
Pediatric Intensive Care Unit
Fortis Escorts Heart Institute
New Delhi, India

Neelam Mohan
DNB (Ped) FIAP FIMSA FACG
Director
Department of Pediatric Gastroenterology,
Hepatology and Liver Transplantation
Medanta – The Medicity
Gurgaon, Haryana, India

Neerav Goyal
DNB (GI Surgery)
Senior Consultant GI and Liver Transplant Surgeon
Indraprastha Apollo Hospitals
New Delhi, India

Nikhil Thapar
BM MRCPCH PhD
Senior Lecturer and Honorary Consultant
Division of Neurogastroenterology and Motility
Department of Gastroenterology
Great Ormond Street Hospital
London, United Kingdom
Stem Cells and Regenerative Medicine
UCL Institute of Child Health
London, United Kingdom

Nkem Onyeador
MBBS MRCPCH Specialist
Registrar in Pediatric Gastroenterology
Bristol Royal Hospital for Children
United Kingdom

Olivier Goulet
MD PhD
Professor Department of Pediatrics
Head, Department of Pediatric Gastroenterology,
Hepatology and Nutrition
Chair, National Reference Center for Rare Digestive Diseases
Necker-Enfants Malades Hospital
University of Paris-Descartes
Paris, France

Osvaldo Borrelli
MD PhD
Consultant and Honorary Senior Lecturer
Division of Neurogastroenterology and Motility
Department of Gastroenterology
Great Ormond Street Hospital
London, United Kingdom

Palittiya Sintusek
MD
Consultant Pediatric Gastroenterologist and Hepatologist
Chulalongkorn University
Bangkok, Thailand

Paolo Quitadamo
MD
Endoscopy and Digestive Motility Unit
University of Naples "Federico II", Italy
Clinical Fellow
Division of Neurogastroenterology and Motility
Department of Gastroenterology
Great Ormond Street Hospital
London, United Kingdom

Parag Karkera
MCh (Pediatric Surgery) MS (General Surgery)
Assistant Professor
Department of Pediatric Surgery
BJ Wadia Hospital for Children
Mumbai, Maharashtra, India

Parvathi U Iyer
MBBS MD
Associate Director
Pediatric Cardiothoracic Surgeon
Fortis Escorts Heart Institute
New Delhi, India

Rajeev Redkar
MCh (Pediatric Surgery) MS (General surgery) FRCS (Ped)
FRCS (Ed) FRCS (G) FCPS DNB IAS
Consultant Pediatric Surgeon
Lilavati Hospital and Research Centre
Shushrusha Citezen's Co-operative Hospital
BJ Wadia Hospital for Children
Mumbai, Maharashtra, India

Ramaswamy Ganesh
MBBS DNB MNAMS
Consultant Pediatrician
Kanchi Kamakoti Childs Trust Hospital and
The Childs Trust Medical Research Foundation
Chennai, Tamil Nadu, India

Ravinder Goyal
MD DM
Assistant Professor
Division of Pediatric Gastroenterology, Hepatology and
Nutrition
Postgraduate Institute of Medical Education and
Research
Chandigarh, India

Rimjhim Shrivastava
MD
Short Term Trainee
Division of Pediatric Gastroenterology, Hepatology and
Nutrition
Postgraduate Institute of Medical Education and Research
Chandigarh, India

Sandipan Sarkar
MD
Senior Resident
Pediatric Intensive Care Unit
Fortis Escorts Heart Institute
New Delhi, India

Sanjiv Verma
MD
Senior Resident
Department of Pediatric Hepatology
Institute of Liver and Biliary Sciences
New Delhi, India

Sankaranarayanan VS
MD (Ped) DM (Gastro)
Professor and Head
Department of Pediatric Gastroenterology
Madras Medical College
Retd Professor and Head
Institute of Child Health and Hospital for Children
Consultant Gastroenterologist
Kanchi Kamakoti Childs Trust Hospital
Chennai, Tamil Nadu, India

Sarah Paul
DCH MD
Head, Neonatology Division
Professor, Department of Pediatrics
PSG Institute of Medical Sciences
Coimbatore, Tamil Nadu, India

Sarath Gopalan
MD (PGIMER, Chandigarh), Fellowship in Pediatric
Gastroenterology and Clinical Nutrition (UK), MAMS
Senior Consultant Pediatric Gastroenterologist and
Hepatologist
Indraprastha Apollo Hospitals
Executive Director
Centre for Research on Nutrition Support Systems
New Delhi, India

Seema Alam
MD
Additional Professor
Department of Pediatric Hepatology
Institute of Liver and Biliary Sciences
New Delhi, India

Siham Al Sinani
MD FAAP FRCPC
Senior Consultant
Department of Pediatric Gastroenterology, Hepatology and
Nutrition
Child Health Department
Sultan Qaboos University Hospital
Muscat Oman

SK Mittal
MD (Ped) FIAP
Pediatric Gastroenterologist
Chairman
Centre for Comprehensive Child Health
Ghaziabad, Uttar Pradesh, India
Visiting Professor
Chacha Nehru Bal Chikisalya
New Delhi, India

Srikanth KP
MD
Senior Resident
Division of Pediatric Gastroenterology, Hepatology and
Nutrition
Postgraduate Institute of Medical Education and Research
Chandigarh, India

S Srinivas
MD DM
Consultant Pediatric Gastroenterologist and
Hepatologist
Apollo Children's Hospital
Chennai, Tamil Nadu, India

Subash Gupta
MS FRCSEd
Chief Liver Transplant Surgeon
Indraprastha Apollo Hospitals
New Delhi, India

Sujit Chowdhary
MBBS MCh FRCS FACS
Senior Consultant
Department of Pediatric Urology and Pediatric Surgery
Indraprastha Apollo Hospitals
New Delhi, India

Suresh Vijay
MD RCPCH
Consultant
Inherited Metabolic Disease (IMD)
Birmingham Children's Hospital
United Kingdom

Tahmeed Ahmed
MBBS PhD
Director
Centre for Nutrition and Food Security, icddr, b
Professor, Public Health Nutrition
James P Grant School of Public Health
BRAC University
Dhaka, Bangladesh

Vidyut Bhatia
MD
Consultant Pediatric Gastroenterologist and
Hepatologist
Indraprastha Apollo Hospitals
New Delhi, India

Wafa'a Al-Qabandi
BM BCh DCH MRCP
Department of Pediatrics
Faculty of Medicine
Kuwait University
Kuwait

Wikrom Karnsakul
MD
Assistant Professor
Department of Pediatrics
Johns Hopkins University School of Medicine
Baltimore, USA

Yogesh Waikar
MBBS MD DNB Fellow in Pediatric Gastroenterology and Liver
Transplant MNAMS PGCC
Consultant Pediatric Gastroenterologist and
Hepatologist
Care Hospital
Nagpur, Maharashtra, India

FOREWORD

This textbook is a landmark in the history of pediatric gastroenterology and hepatology. It demonstrates the coming of age of this discipline in much of the developing world. The authors are a talented group of leaders in their fields of interest. The technological advances in recent years within this field are quite remarkable. Perhaps, the most dramatic and complex in practice, is the development of pediatric liver transplantation with immense advantages for children who would otherwise have died, in past years. At another level, it is important to appreciate that much simpler therapeutic techniques, also based upon scientific research, such as the development of oral rehydration therapy (ORT), have had dramatic beneficial effects for much larger numbers of sick children with dehydrating diarrhea due to infection. Across the world, there has been a dramatic fall in diarrheal disease mortality, especially in infancy, chiefly related to development (public health measures of particular importance) but in part, especially in developing communities to the use of ORT. Whilst the contents of this book may have the greatest appeal in the countries of the contributors, it has international appeal as a state-of-the-art text across the world.

I have visited relevant centers in Asia since the 1980s up to Sri Lanka in 2013. The changes have been dramatic. Outside help and advice from experts in the United States and Commonwealth countries, especially Australia, Canada and the United Kingdom have played an important role. However, great success has come from the "home teams". This has been assisted by the provision of training opportunities in the nations mentioned, with very positive outcomes. The Commonwealth Association of Paediatric Gastroenterology, Hepatology and Nutrition (CAPGAN) has contributed. This began in Asia in 1991 with a conference in New Delhi on Diarrhea and Malnutrition in Children and most recently in 2013 in Colombo.

The field of medicine described in this text is one where immense benefits occur by multiple interactions between a wide range of medical disciplines and contact between countries, developed and developing. Clinical problems evolve and change over the years, in part related to development per se. In my own professional experience from the 1960s till now, within developed communities in Australia and the United Kingdom, I have seen a remarkable decline in infection-related disorders, especially in infants and young children and a remarkable rise in inflammatory bowel disease in older children, in recent years. This continuing change in the pattern of disease provides a great challenge and also opportunity to those concerned with the clinical care of children with this group of disorders and to scientists investigating these disorders. These disciplines are fields where research and improved service go hand in hand, for the benefit of individual children. Much more research is required across the world, with international collaboration of key importance.

It must always be remembered that all these endeavors are directed towards improving the care of children with gastrointestinal and liver problems and indeed to prevent these disorders, in the long term. Huge advances have been made during my own clinical experience over the past 50 years, but there are still fearsome challenges ahead.

John Walker-Smith
MD BS (Sydney) FRCP (London & Edinburgh)
FRACP FRCPCH MA (King's College, London)
Emeritus Professor
Department of Pediatric Gastroenterology
University College London
United Kingdom

PREFACE

The last few decades have witnessed an exponential growth of knowledge in pediatric gastroenterology, hepatology and nutrition. The understanding of the pathophysiology of several disorders has improved while newer disorders have been described. Newer genetic, metabolic and biochemical tests have become available.

Novel therapies for treatment of diseases, such as tyrosinemia and neonatal hemochromatosis, have evolved over the last decade. Treatment for hepatitis B and C has improved. Especially impressive has been the transfer of liver transplantation from the realms of fantasy to becoming a routine procedure for many centers across the world. Techniques such as gene transfer and hepatocyte transplantation are likely to see the end of the tunnel in the coming years.

Advancements in the field of luminal gastroenterology have been no less remarkable. Newer modalities in endoscopy, such as endoscopic ultrasound and capsule endoscopy, have revolutionized assessment of gastrointestinal disorders. We now have newer therapy in the form of biologicals for management of inflammatory bowel disease. The field of enteral and parenteral nutrition continues to evolve. Fecal microbiota transplantation is being explored as therapy for several conditions. Intestinal transplantation is now established therapy.

This book specifically looks at disorders of the gut and liver from a developing country's perspective. This book is meant to be used by postgraduates, pediatric gastroenterologists as well as pediatricians with an interest in gastroenterology. While this book features topics that are relevant and necessary for postgraduate teaching, updates on latest developments have also been included. The authors have been chosen carefully based on their expertise. Many contributors are internationally recognized experts. We would like to thank all the contributors, for their contribution. We hope that this book will serve as a valuable clinical resource.

Anupam Sibal
Sarath Gopalan
Akshay Kapoor
Vidyut Bhatia

ACKNOWLEDGMENTS

We would like to express our gratitude to Dr Prathap C Reddy (Founder Chairman), Apollo Hospitals Group, for his guidance and encouragement. We would also like to thank Dr Preetha Reddy (Executive Vice-Chairperson), Ms Suneeta Reddy (Managing Director), Ms Shobana Kamineni (Executive Vice-Chairperson) and Ms Sangita Reddy (Joint Managing Director), Apollo Hospitals Group, for their constant support.

A big thank to Mr Jaideep Gupta, Mr P Shivakumar, Mr AK Singhal, Gen LR Sharma, Ms Anjali Kapoor, Ms Usha Banerjee, Ms Raji Chandru, Mr Rohit Kapur, Mr CP Tyagi, Dr Ritu Rawat, Mr Raj Raina and Mr Sachin Patidar, for providing an environment that encourages academics and research.

No words will suffice to acknowledge the untiring efforts of Ms Neha Kapoor, Ms Harsimran, Dr Smita Malhotra, Dr Rajesh Kumar, Dr Karunesh Kumar and Dr Hasnain Hussain, in getting this textbook published.

We thank Shri Jitendar P Vij (Group Chairman), Mr Ankit Vij (Group President) and Mr Tarun Duneja (Director–Publishing) of M/s Jaypee Brothers Medical Publishers (P) Ltd, New Delhi, India, for undertaking the task of publishing this book. A special word of praise for Ms Shivangi Pramanik from the publishing house, for her efficient coordination.

CONTENTS

SECTION 2:   Nutrition

SECTION 3: Hepatology

Section 1

Gastroenterology

Chapter

1

Developmental Anatomy and Physiology of the Digestive Tract

Yogesh Waikar

The digestive system comprises of the salivary gland, esophagus, stomach, duodenum, jejunum, ileum, colon with an accessory connecting hepatobiliary pancreatic system. It is important to keep in mind developmental, anatomical as well as physiological aspects of gastrointestinal tract, which forms the basis of clinical gastroenterology.

APPLIED DEVELOPMENTAL ANATOMY AND PHYSIOLOGY OF ESOPHAGUS

The human esophagus develops from foregut by four weeks of age. Incomplete division of trachea and esophagus between the fourth and fifth week of life can lead to developmental abnormalities like tracheo-esophageal fistula, duplication cyst and esophageal atresia. Lengthening of the esophagus is achieved primarily by ascent of the pharynx rather than descent of the stomach in the seventh week.[1] Various genes and molecular pathways are involved in the development of the esophagus. Defects or mutation can lead to aberrations and congenital structural abnormalities. The esophagus starts at the lower border of cricoid, passing through the mediastinum thereby providing a convenient access for transesophageal biopsies of lymph nodes and mediastinal masses with the help of endoscopic ultrasound (EUS) and even transesophageal echocardiography.[2] Narrowed portions of the esophagus that are easily negotiated using the endoscope are at the start at the oropharyngeal junction, aortic arch, the left main bronchus, and the diaphragm. A shorter intra-abdominal portion of the esophagus is one of the responsible factors for gastroesophageal reflux (GER) in infants.

The parasympathetic supply is from the vagal and the sympathetic supply to esophagus is from the cervical and thoracic sympathetic trunks and greater splanchnic nerves. The upper one-third of esophagus has predominantly striated muscle. The epithelium of the esophagus is non-keratinized squamous.

Various calculations are used to determine length of esophagus in children. The commonly used are Song et al.[11] [Esophageal Length = 0.242 × (height) + 0.2078 cm], Strobel et al.[12] [Esophageal Length = 0.226 × (height) + 6.7 cm] and Jolley et al.[13] [length = 0.207 × (height) + 4.61] the esophageal length, defined as the length from the incisors to the gastroesophageal junction. Knowledge regarding esophageal length is important to calculate placement of esophageal probes for pH studies in children.

At 20 weeks of gestation, the fetus can swallow about 15 mL/day of secretions. The full-term neonate can swallow about 450 mL/day.[14] At 34 weeks, 30-seconds of sucking at 2-minute intervals develop, coordinated with swallowing.[15] The pressure difference between that at the fundus of the stomach and at the lower end of esophagus rises proportionately with postconceptional age.[16] At 28 weeks of gestation, lower esophageal pressure is about 4 mm Hg and by term, it is 18 mm Hg.[22]

APPLIED DEVELOPMENTAL ANATOMY AND PHYSIOLOGY OF STOMACH

In the fifth week of gestation, the stomach appears fusiform in shape and dilated in the median plane. The rotation and growth of stomach in abdominal cavity is responsible for its innervation pattern.[17] Gastric volvulus results due to abnormal rotation of one part of the stomach around another part which may be organoaxial, mesenteroaxial or combined.

The columnar epithelium of stomach is established by seventeenth week of gestation. The mucus-producing pit cells can be visualized proximally towards the gastric lumen and acid-secreting parietal cells are visualized more distally towards the middle and lower regions of the gastric gland. Chief cells secrete pepsinogen and predominate at the base of glands. Neuroendocrine cells, including enterochromaffin cells, enterochromaffin-like (ECL) cells, and D cells (somatostatin), are seen at the base of the gastric gland. The proximal stomach is responsible for the storage of food and receptive relaxation.[18] The distal stomach, the antrum and pylorus, is responsible for grinding and emptying solid food. The gastric emptying rate is dependent on many factors like osmolality, consistency, temperature, pH, size of food particles, antral distention, concentration of lipid, protein, and acid in the duodenum, and colonic distention.[19] Gastric motor activity appears between 14 and 24 weeks, starting at the gastric pacemaker (on greater curvature of the stomach).[20] The normal frequency of gastric slow waves is 3 cycles per minute (CPM). Gastric slow-wave activity can be measured noninvasively using the electrogastrography.[21] Migrating motor complexes (MMC), a propagated sequence of contractions that migrates from the stomach into the intestine and toward the ileum every 90 to 120 min consists of 3 phases. Phase 1 is a pattern of quiescence that always follows phase 3. Phase 2 is a period of irregular contractions. Phase 3 is a distinctive pattern of regular high-amplitude contractions repeating at a maximal rate for 3 to 10/min. MMC begins in the esophagus or stomach. Motilin is responsible for initiating phase 3 contractions that begin in the stomach and are observed by 32 weeks of gestation.

Water, electrolytes, hydrochloric acid, and glycoproteins, mucin, intrinsic factor, and enzymes are secreted by stomach (Table 1.1). Central cephalic, local enteric exocrine epithelial cells and endocrine-like neural regulatory cells regulate gastric secretions. In newborns, gastric pH ranges from 6.0 to 8.0. On day 2 to 3 pH reduces to 1 to 3 slowing stabilizing by 2 years.[22]

Table 1.1: Common secretions in stomach and their corresponding cells
Gastrin → Antral G cell
Histamine → ECL cell
Adolescents somatostatin → D cell
Gastric lipase → Chief cell
HCl and intrinsic factor → Parietal cell
Gherlin → Gr cells in the basal part of oxyntic gastric gland

APPLIED DEVELOPMENTAL ANATOMY AND PHYSIOLOGY OF INTESTINES

Small intestine starts from the pylorus to the ileocecal valve, occupying the central and lower parts of the abdominal cavity consisting of duodenum, jejunum, and ileum. The average length of the small intestine is 250 to 300 cm in the newborn.[26] The caliber of the small intestine gradually diminishes from its origin to its termination. The duodenum constitutes approximately the first 25 cm of the small intestine in adults; the remaining length is arbitrarily divided into the proximal two-fifths, designated as the jejunum, and the distal three-fifths, designated as the ileum.

The first portion of the duodenum begins at the pylorus and ends at the neck of the gallbladder, the second portion, descends from the neck of the gallbladder along the right side of the vertebral column to the level of the third lumbar vertebra. The third portion, courses over to the third lumbar vertebra, passing from right to left, with inclination upward, lying inferior to the origin of the superior mesenteric artery in front of the aorta. Fourth portion ascends immediately to the left of the aorta, up to the level of the second lumbar vertebra, where it makes a ventral turn to unite with jejunum.

The jejunum is thicker and more vascular than the ileum, diminishing in size with distal progression. The intestinal luminal diameter is also greatest in the jejunum, shrinking in diameter as it progresses distally. The plicae circulare are crescentic luminal protrusions of submucosa covered by mucosa, running circumferentially along the inside diameter of the intestinal wall, are most prominent in the distal duodenum and proximal jejunum, decreasing in number and size towards the ileum and do not smooth out when the intestine is distended.[27] The Peyer's patches are more prominent during childhood and regress in size and number with advancing age are predominantly seen in ileum.

The mesentery begins as an anterior reflection of the posterior peritoneum, attached to the posterior abdominal wall along a line extending from the left side of the body of the lumbar vertebra to the right sacroiliac joint.

The ileocecal valve opens when a peristaltic wave overcomes the resting resistance at the terminal ileum.

The colon is approximately 60 cm long in the newborn, increasing to approximately 150 cm in the adult. The caliber of the large intestine is greatest at the cecum and gradually diminishes as it approaches the rectum. The colonic wall remains fairly constant in thickness throughout its entire length and lacks the villi. Small intestinal villi are formed by 16 weeks.[26] Colonic villi presist in fetal life disappears by 29 weeks. Colon is larger in caliber as compared to small intestine. Large intestine is mostly retroperitoneal and fixed. Its outer longitudinal muscular layer is in form of three distinct longitudinal bands, teniae coli, extending from the cecum to the rectum. Colon has a characteristic sacculated haustra. The luminal surface of colon is interrupted by plicae semilunares. Appendices epiploicae are fatty projections found scattered over the free surface of the entire large intestine, with the exception of the cecum, vermiform appendix, and rectum. The anal canal is about 2 cm long in the infant, increasing to about 4.5 cm in the adult.[27]

Appendix measures between 2 and 20 cm long, with length longest in childhood.[28] It generally shrinks during further development in adult life.

Intestinal motility is well established by 32 weeks of gestation.[26]

Anal canal are the vertical projections bounded below by anal valves at the level of pectinate line. The depression between anal canals is called as anal fold. The pectinate line represents the junction between endodermal (columnar epithelium) and ectodermal (squamous) portions of anal canal.[27] The contraction of puborectalis muscle pulls the rectum forward to retain stool, and the relaxation straightens the anal canal, allowing defecation. This is important to understand in normal defecography. The anal canal is surrounded by complex muscle fibers under voluntary control called as external anal sphincter and under involuntary control called as internal anal sphincter.

Interstitial cells of Cajal are present within the myenteric plexus between the circular muscle and the submucosa and are responsible for intestinal contractile activity and regulation of intestinal tone.

Brunner's gland secret mucus in the duodenum. They contribute to a protective alkaline pH and promote gallbladder contractility. They also help in promoting pancreatic secretions. Crypts of intestinal villi are lined by undifferentiated columnar epithelial cells, goblet cells, Paneth cells, tuft cells, cup-like cells, and enteroendocrine cells. The villous also contain similar columnar cells. Cells overlying Peyer's patches in ileum are M cells which act as antigen presenting cells. The apical surfaces of the intestinal epithelial cells carry multiple brush-border transporters important for absorption of nutrients. Similar to the enterocytes, surface epithelial cells of colon are called as colonocytes. Paneth cells secrete a wide spectrum of antimicrobial peptides (AMPs) against gram-negative and gram-positive bacteria, fungi, protozoa, and viruses.[26] The junctions between enterocytes allow for physiologic passage of fluids, electrolytes, and small macromolecules comprising up to 11 amino acids.[28] Pathologic insult to enterocytes may loosen up these junctions thereby increasing permeability of particles.

APPLIED DEVELOPMENTAL ANATOMY OF PANCREAS

The pancreas forms as a result of fusion of dorsal and ventral pancreatic buds of the foregut. The ventral pancreas rotates clockwise around the duodenal axis. The dorsal pancreatic bud forms the anterior part of the head of the pancreas, the body, and the tail of the pancreas.

The ventral pancreatic bud forms the posterior part of the head of the pancreas and the posterior part of the uncinate process. Abnormalities in development or in rotation of these buds lead to development of structural congenital abnormalities of pancreas.

The dorsal and ventral duct systems fuse resulting in the longer dorsal duct draining into the proximal part of the ventral duct to form the main pancreatic duct of Wirsung. The proximal portion of the dorsal duct forms an accessory of Santorini.[29]

REFERENCES

1. Gray S, Skanadalakis J. Embryology for Surgeons. The Embryological Basis for the Treatment of Congenital Defects. Philadelphia, WB Saunders, 1972;63-281.
2. Ingram M, Arregui M. Endoscopic ultrasonography. Surg Clin North Am. 2004;84:1035-59.
3. Bax K, Gupta S. Allergic eosinophilic esophagitis. Indian Journal of Pediatrics. 2006;73:919-25.
4. Vandenplas Y. Reflux esophagitis in infants and children: a report from the working group on gastro-oesophageal reflux disease of the European Society of Paediatric Gastroenterology and Nutrition. J Pediatr Gastroenterol Nutr. 1994;18:413-22.
5. Cucchiara S, D'Armiento F, Alfieri E, et al. Intraepithelial cells with irregular nuclear contours as a marker of esophagitis in children with gastroesophageal reflux disease. Dig Dis Sci. 1995;40:2305-11.
6. Fox VL, Nurko S, Teitelbaum JE, et al. High-resolution EUS in children with eosinophilic "allergic" esophagitis. Gastrointest Endosc. 2003;57:30-6.
7. Bajpai M, Mathur M. Duplications of the alimentary tract: clues to the missing links. J Pediatr Surg. 1994;29:1361-5.
8. Carachi R, Azmy A. Foregut duplications. Pediatr Surg Int. 2002;18:371-4.
9. Ramesh J, Ramanujam T, Jayaram G. Congenital esophageal stenosis: report of three cases, literature review, and proposed classification. Pediatr Surg Int. 2001;17:188-92.
10. Towbin AJ, Diniz LO. Pediatr Radiol. 2012;42(12):1437-40. doi: 10.1007/s00247-012-2482-3. Epub 2012 Aug 11.
11. Song TJ, Kim YH, Ryu HS, Hyun JH. Correlation of esophageal lenghts with measurable external parameters. Korean J Int Med. 1991;6:16-20.
12. Strobel CT, Bryne WJ, Ament M, Euler AR. Correlation of esophageal lengths in children with height: application to the Tuttle test without prior esophageal manometry. J Pediatr. 1979;94:81-4.
13. Jolley SG, Tunell WP, Carson JA, Smith EI, Grunow J. The accuracy of abbreviated eosphageal pH monitoring in children. J Ped Surg. 1984;19:848-53.
14. Pritchard J. Fetal swallowing and amniotic fluid volume. Obstet Gynecol. 1966;28:606-10.
15. Crump EP, Gore PM, Horton CP. The sucking behavior in premature infants. Hum Biol. 1958;30:128-41.

16. Newell S, Sarkar P, Booth I, McNeish A. Maturation of the lower oesophageal sphincter in the preterm neonate. Pediatr Res. 1986;20:692.

17. Moore KL. The Developing Human. 6th edn. Philadelphia, Elsevier Science, 1998;271-8.

18. Read NW, Houghton LA. Physiology of gastric emptying and pathophysiology of gastroparesis. Gastroenterol Clin North Am. 1989;18:359-73.

19. Lu YX, Owyang C. Duodenal acid-induced gastric relaxation is mediated by multiple pathways. Am J Physiol. 1999;276:G1501-6.

20. Sase M, Tamura H, Ueda K, Kato H. Sonographic evaluation of antepartum development of fetal gastric motility. Ultrasound Obstet Gynecol. 1999;13:323-6.

21. Stern RM, Koch KL, Stewart WR, Vasey MW. Electrogastrography: current issues in validation and methodology. Psychophysiology. 1987;24:55-64.

22. Schubert ML. Gastric exocrine and endocrine secretion. Curr Opin Gastroentrol. 2009;25:529-36.

23. Reiquam CW, Allen RP, Akers DR. Normal and abnormal small bowel lengths: an analysis of 389 autopsy cases in infants and children. Am J Dis Child. 1965;109:447-51.

24. Williams PL, Warwick R (Ed). Gray's Anatomy, 36th edn. Philadelphia: Saunders; 1980.

25. Sanders KM. A case for interstitial cells of Cajal as pacemakers and mediators of neurotransmission in the gastrointestinal tract. Gastroenterology. 1996;111:492-515.

26. Duggan C, et al. Nutrition in Pediatrics. 4th edn. Hamilton, Ontario, Canada: BC Decker Inc; 2008;21:241-9.

27. Jadcherla SR. Gastroesophageal reflux in the neonate. Clin Perinatol. 2002;29:135-58.

28. Atsook K, Madara JL. An oligopeptide permeates intestinal tight junctions at glucose-elicited dilatations: Implications for oligopeptide absorption. Gastroenterology. 1991;100:719-24.

29. Uchid T, Takada T, Ammori BJ, et al. Three-dimensional reconstruction of the ventral and dorsal pancreas: a new insight into anatomy and embryonic development. J Hepatobil Pancreat Surg. 1999;6:176-80.

Chapter 2

Common Gastrointestinal Symptoms

Wafa'a Al-Qabandi

▌VOMITING

Vomiting is a common and nonspecific symptom that can be due to multiple disorders ranging from mild to severe and serious conditions (Box 2.1).

BOX 2.1: Important definitions

Definitions

Vomiting: Forceful oral expulsion of gastric contents associated with contraction of abdominal and chest wall musculature.

Nausea: The unpleasant sensation of the need to vomit, which may or may not lead to the act of vomiting.

Regurgitation: Expulsion of gastric contents back into the mouth without the contraction of abdominal and diaphragmatic musculature that characterizes vomiting.

Rumination: Chewing and swallowing of regurgitated food.

Nausea and vomiting can often present together but in many occasions they can occur independently.

Pathophysiology

The vomiting center is located in the brainstem. It receives impulses from four other centers (Fig. 2.1):[1]

- Higher cortical centers: This is involved in the nonorganic causes of vomiting such as the psychological and behavioral factors. It is not well understood.
- Chemoreceptor zone (Area Postrema): Located in the caudal part of the forth ventricle and is affected by chemical triggers in the blood or cerebrospinal fluid. It contains dopamine 2 receptors, muscarinic 1 and histamine 1 receptors.
- Vagal afferent system: This system receives impulses from the GI tract following distension or irritation caused by many factors. It is mediated by serotonin receptors.
- Vestibular system: This system is involved in the emetic response to motion. It is usually induced in cases of labyrinthine disorders and motion sickness. The system is mediated by muscarinic 1 and histamin 1 receptors.

Phases of Vomiting

- *Pre-ejection:* Stomach relaxation and retroperistalsis.
- *Retching:* Contractions of respiratory, intercostal, diaphragm and abdominal wall muscles occur against a closed glottis.
- *Ejection:* Strong contractions of abdominal muscles with relaxation of the upper esophageal sphincter leading to extraction of stomach contents. This phase can occur suddenly and forcefully without the previous 2 phases such as what occurs in projectile vomiting).

Causes of Vomiting in Children

- Vomiting is a symptom with a wide variety of causes. Diagnosing the cause of vomiting depends on history and physical examination.
- There are many ways to differentiate multiple disorders causing vomiting.
- Emergency causes should initially be ruled out versus nonemergency conditions.
- Surgical disorders should also be sought versus non-surgical (medical) problems.
- The type of vomiting whether projectile (forceful) or nonprojectile (Fig. 2.2) might aid in the differential diagnosis.
- The color of vomitus (Fig. 2.3) can help in establishing the site of the lesion inducing vomiting.
- The etiology usually depends on the age of the patient since some causes are more common in a particular age group (Table 2.1).

Evaluation

Evaluation of a child presenting with vomiting could be achieved by a focused history and thorough physical examination. The approach depends on the age of the patient; however, in all ages the priority is to exclude life-threatening problems.[3] Therefore, the initial evaluation should be focused on the following essential points:

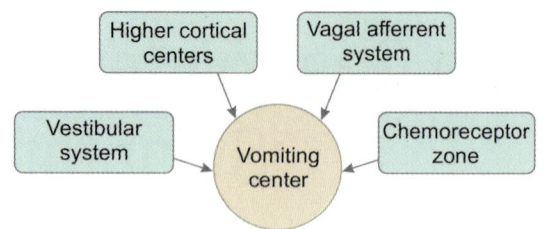

Fig. 2.1: Pathophysiology of vomiting. The vomiting center located in the brainstem receives impulses from four different systems

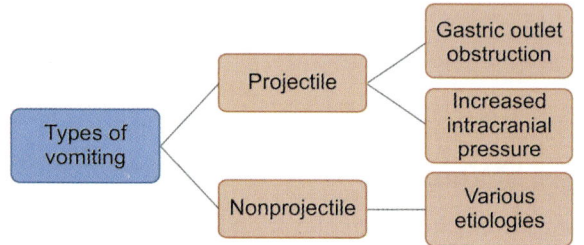

Fig. 2.2: Types of vomiting
Note: The parents might not be able to differentiate between projectile and nonprojectile vomiting

❑ Assessment of the severity of vomiting (level of dehydration and status of consciousness).
❑ Assessment for life-threatening conditions (surgical causes, medical and endocrine emergencies).
❑ Assessment of color and contents of the vomitus (bilious, nonbilious, bloody).
❑ Assessment of the interval of vomiting whether acute or chronic (Box 2.2).

BOX 2.2: Acute versus chronic vomiting

• *Acute vomiting*: A sudden onset of vomiting in a previously healthy child.
• *Chronic vomiting*: Recurrent attacks of vomiting of at least 2 episodes/week in the past 3 months.

History

Table 2.2 lists some of the important information about attacks of vomiting such as timing, relation to food and associated gastrointestinal (GI) and nongastrointestinal (non-GI) factors. History of drug ingestion that can trigger vomiting should be verified. Vomiting in other family members may indicate food poisoning or gastroenteritis.[4] In addition, families with inherited inborn errors of metabolism, other affected individuals might experience vomiting as well.

Age of the Child

❑ As listed in Table 2.1, causes vary in different age groups.
❑ In neonates congenital anomalies of the gastrointestinal tract (GIT) such as atresias or stenoses are more common causing intestinal obstruction. Premature infants are liable to get necrotizing enterocolitis leading to vomiting. Systemic infection is also common in this age group. Obstructive uropathy, hydrocephalus, congenital adrenal hyperplasia and inborn errors of metabolism can cause persistent vomiting at this age.
❑ Infants are liable to develop intussusception, which usually presents with irritability and constipation but can also present with vomiting in this age group. In addition, systemic infection and severe gastroenteritis can occur at this age. Vomiting in infants can also be associated with any mild illness such as upper respiratory tract infection and otitis media.
❑ In older children, appendicitis, meningitis, diabetic ketoacidosis and toxin ingestion are common causes to consider.

Color of Vomitus

❑ *Bilious:* It indicates intestinal obstruction until proven otherwise.

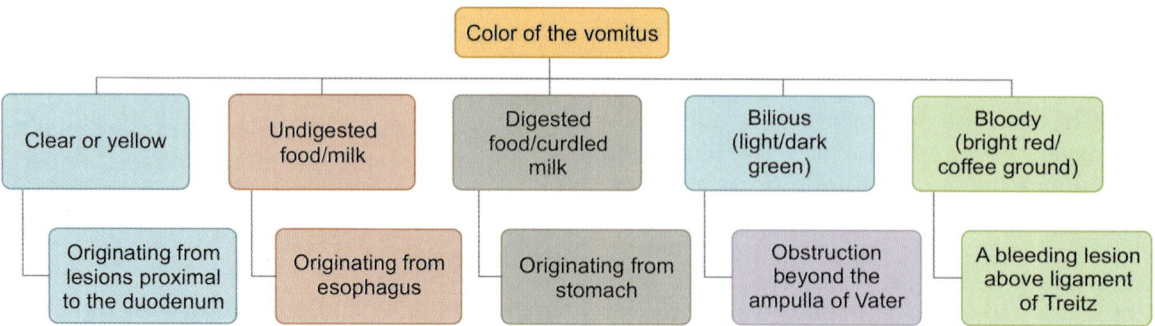

Fig. 2.3: Color of the vomitus. The vomitus color can aid in diagnosing the cause of vomiting

Table 2.1: Differential diagnosis of vomiting in children[2]

Neonates <1 month	Infants >1–12 months	Toddlers >1–4 years	Children >4–12 years	Adolescents >12–18 years
Esophageal atresia	GERD	Gastroenteritis	Gastroenteritis	Gastroenteritis
GERD	Gastroenteritis	Infection (UTI, pharyngitis, otitis media, respiratory, CNS)	Infection (pharyngitis, CNS, respiratory)	Peptic ulcer disease
Feeding intolerance	Infection (UTI, CNS, respiratory, otitis media)	GERD	Poisoning	Drug abuse
Infection (UTI, meningitis, sepsis)	Pyloric stenosis	Poisoning	DKA	DKA
Meconium ileus	Protein intolerance	Eosinophilic esophagitis	IBD	Migraine
Congenital intestinal atresia/webs	Inborn errors of metabolism	DKA	Eosinophilic esophagitis	Appendicitis
Malrotation with midgut volvulus	Intussusception	Malrotation	Appendicitis	Pancreatitis
Pyloric stenosis	Adrenal insufficiency	Celiac disease	Peptic ulcer disease	Gallstones
Hirschsprung's disease	Malrotation with midgut volvulus	Appendicitis	Pancreatitis	IBD
NEC	Hirschsprung's disease	Pancreatitis	Intracranial lesion	Eosinophilic esophagitis
Intracranial lesion	Intracranial lesion	Intracranial lesion	Celiac disease	Middle ear disease
Congenital adrenal hyperplasia	Renal insufficiency	Hepatitis	Hepatitis	Intracranial lesion
Inborn errors of metabolism	Munchausen by proxy syndrome		Migraine	Hepatitis
	Child abuse		Cyclical vomiting	Cyclical vomiting
				Bulimia
				Pregnancy

Abbreviations: NEC, necrotizing enterocolitis; DKA, diabetic ketoacidosis; GERD, gastroesophageal reflux disease; IBD, inflammatory bowel disease.

Table 2.2: Important clues in the history

Time of the day	Relation to food	Associated symptoms		History of drugs/toxins	Family history
		GI	Non-GI		
Early morning vomiting suggests a raised intracranial pressure	Vomiting triggered by food suggests gastritis, pancreatitis and food allergy	Diarrhea: suggests GE, IBD Abdominal pain: the site of pain might suggest the cause	Headache: migraine Ear pain: OM Sore throat: pharyngitis Dysuria: UTI Dizziness/vertigo: Middle ear disease	Paracetamol Salicylates Chemotherapeutic drugs	GE Jaundice Food poisoning

Abbreviations: GI, gastrointestinal; GE, gastroenteritis; IBD, inflammatory bowel disease; OM, Otitis media; UTI, urinary tract infection.

□ *Blood (coffee ground or fresh bright blood):* Upper gastrointestinal bleeding lesion proximal to the ligament of Treitz.

□ *Yellow:* This is from stomach secretion and occurs in most nonobstructive disorders. If the lesion is localized in the GIT then it is proximal to the ampulla of Vater. Yellow vomiting, however, does not exclude gut obstruction. Obstructive lesions proximal to the ampulla of Vater such as pyloric stenosis and gastric volvulus may present with this type of vomiting.[5,6]

- ❏ *Undigested food:* The lesion is usually esophageal.
- ❏ *Curdled milk:* Arises from the stomach proximal to the pylorus.
- ❏ *Bad odor (smell of feces):* Intestinal obstruction.

When Does Vomiting Occur?

Early morning vomiting should raise the suspicion of raised intracranial pressure.

Relation to Food

- ❏ Vomiting following food intake is suggestive of gastritis, pancreatitis or cholecystitis.
- ❏ Infants with gastroesophageal reflux can present with vomiting after feeds.

Associated Gastrointestinal Symptoms

- ❏ *Abdominal pain*: Location and severity of the pain can aid in the diagnosis. Irritability in infants may suggest abdominal pain.
- ❏ *Diarrhea*: Onset of diarrhea, consistency of stool, frequency and presence of blood or mucus in the stool may help in the differential diagnosis. Gastroenteritis is often the cause of vomiting associated with diarrhea but other disorders such as food allergy, appendicitis and inborn errors of metabolism can present with diarrhea and vomiting.

Systemic Review

- ❏ A thorough review of all systems is important since vomiting is a nonspecific symptom in children. In many occasions, the defect lies in another system and not the GIT.
- ❏ Enquire about urine output, stream of urine, dysuria or irritability during urination in young infants.
- ❏ Earache, runny nose and sore throat can lead to vomiting in children.
- ❏ Ask about headache and relation to vomiting in older children because patients with migraine and chronic sinusitis often present with vomiting.
- ❏ Rash can occur in patients with food allergy associated with vomiting.

Pattern of Vomiting

- ❏ Is it persistent or episodic and cyclical such as that occurs in cyclical vomiting?

Physical Examination

- ❏ Physical examination should be directed towards assessment of the general well being of the child, vital signs and signs/degree of dehydration.

- ❏ This will be followed by a thorough clinical examination to detect the possible etiology of vomiting (Table 2.3).
- ❏ It is crucial to look for signs of serious illnesses that require immediate attention such as meningitis, intestinal obstruction and metabolic emergency.
- ❏ Look for pallor, jaundice and rash especially petechiae or purpura that might suggest meningitis. Remember that food allergy might present with rash also.
- ❏ Examine for signs of trauma and injuries.
- ❏ Examine the throat and ears for signs of infection.
- ❏ Suspect inborn errors of metabolism in case of a strange smell.
- ❏ Chest examination may reveal adventitious sounds suggestive of wheezing or pneumonia.
- ❏ The abdomen should be inspected for abdominal distension, peristalsis and a bulging mass. Palpate the abdomen for tenderness, organomegaly and masses. Listen to the bowel sounds, loud sounds may suggest intestinal obstruction.
- ❏ Examine the genitalia for obstructed/incarcerated hernia, testicular torsion and ambiguous genitalia.
- ❏ Examine the central nervous system and specifically for signs of meningitis and raised intracranial pressure (ICP). Remember that a bulging anterior fontanel in an infant is suspicious of raised ICP.

Table 2.3: Clues on physical examination	
Clinical examination	*Etiology*
Irritability	Intussusception/meningitis
Lethargy	Meningitis/sepsis/severe dehydration
Bulging anterior fontanel	Meningitis/raised intracranial pressure
Jaundiced sclera	Hepatitis
Bulging eardrum	OM
Inflamed throat	Pharyngitis/tonsillitis
Neck stiffness	Meningitis
Chest examination Wheezing/cripitations/ reduced air entry	Bronchial asthma/pneumonia
Abdominal distension	Suggests intestinal obstruction
Abdominal tenderness	Site of tenderness can help in defining the etiology
Abdominal mass • During a test feed • Right upper quadrant	 • Pyloric stenosis • Intussusception
Swelling in the hernial orifices	Inguinal hernia
Blood on rectal examination	Intussusception/IBD

Abbreviations: OM, otitis media; IBD, inflammatory bowel disease.

- Rectal examination can be performed if intestinal obstruction such as intussusception is suspected.
- Examine the eye with a fundoscope looking for papilledema as a sign of raised ICP.

Red Flags in a Vomiting Child

Certain points in history and physical examination might suggest serious underlying conditions and hence considered as red flags in a vomiting child (Table 2.4):
- Bilious vomiting is a sign of intestinal obstruction until proven otherwise.
- Hematemesis indicates an upper GI bleeding and requires especial investigations.
- Vomiting associated with irritability in an infant suggests intestinal obstruction or CNS infection.
- Presence of signs of dehydration indicates a significant attack of vomiting.
- Maintaining a specific posture is probably due to peritoneal irritation.

Investigations

In many children presenting with vomiting no investigations are required. The work up should be guided by history and physical examination.[7-9] If any of the red flags listed in Table 2.4 is present then the patient should be investigated.

The following tests can be performed (Table 2.5):

Blood Work Up
- Serum electrolytes and blood gases should be done in a dehydrated child. In an infant suspected of pyloric stenosis this test can be helpful in diagnosing the problem when hypochloremic, hypokalemic metabolic alkalosis is present. Hyperkalemia and hyponatremia can be seen in a case of congenital adrenal hyperplasia. Also hyperkalemia can be seen in renal failure. An infant with inborn errors of metabolism, acidosis with even minimal dehydration can be detected.

- Renal function is indicated in a dehydrated child as prerenal failure can complicate dehydration. Also an intrinsic renal defect with deranged renal function can present with vomiting.
- Liver function is indicated when a liver disease is suspected.
- Serum amylase and lipase are performed if vomiting was associated with severe agonizing abdominal pain suspicious of pancreatitis.
- Blood gases, serum ammonia and lactate are performed if inborn errors of metabolism are suspected.

Urine Tests
- Urine analysis and culture should be performed in young infants with fever and vomiting since urinary tract infection is subtle in this young age.

Table 2.4: Red flags in a vomiting child

Abnormal symptom/sign	Possible problem
Lethargy	Moderate-severe dehydration/CNS infection
Irritability	Intestinal obstruction/CNS infection
Bilious vomitus	Intestinal obstruction
Blood/hematemesis	Upper GI bleed
Signs of dehydration	Significant vomiting
A specific posture	Peritoneal irritation/pancreatitis

Table 2.5: Investigative work up of a child presenting with vomiting

Blood work up	Urine testing	Radiologic work up	Endoscopy
Electrolytes Renal function	Urinalysis	Plain X-ray abdomen (suspected bowel obstruction)	Upper GI endoscopy (esophagitis and persistent GERD, peptic ulcer disease)
Blood sugar	Urine culture	Ultrasound abdomen (pyloric stenosis, intussusception, appendicitis)	Treatment of esophageal and pyloric strictures
CBC	Urine amino acids and organic acids	GI contrast study (malrotation, IBD)	Extraction of an upper GI foreign body
LFT/RFT		CT abdomen (pancreatitis, liver problems and intra-abdominal masses)	
Blood gases • Amylase/lipase • Ammonia • Lactate • Amino acids			

Abbreviations: CBC, complete blood count; LFT, liver function test; RFT, renal function test; IBD, inflammatory bowel disease; GI, gastrointestinal; GERD, gastroesophageal reflux.

❑ Also urine can be examined for red blood cells, protein and casts that occur in intrinsic renal problems.

❑ Glucose and ketones in urine are suggestive of diabetic ketoacidosis.

❑ Urine can be tested for amino and organic acids in suspected cases of inborn errors of metabolism.

Imaging Studies

❑ Plain X-ray: It is helpful in suspected cases of intestinal obstruction.

❑ Ultrasound abdomen: This is required if pyloric stenosis, intussusception or appendicitis is suspected. It can also be helpful in case of biliary problems, intra-abdominal abscesses, renal anomalies or stones and ovarian cysts in older females.

❑ Contrast studies: It can be performed if malrotation is suspected. This test can also be useful to visualize inflammatory bowel disease involved small intestine. Rectal enemas using air is helpful in diagnosing and treating intussusception.

❑ Nuclear imaging: It can be helpful in the diagnosis of gastroparesis.

❑ CT abdomen is helpful in cases of liver disease, pancreatitis, abdominal and pelvic masses.

Endoscopy

This is indicated in suspected peptic ulcer disease, uncontrolled gastroesophageal reflux, dysphagia, history suspicious of foreign body impaction and suspected inflammatory bowel disease.

Management

Management should be directed to the defined etiology. However, there are essential points to consider in the initial management (Table 2.6).[10,11]

❑ The most important step in the management is to rehydrate the child either by the enteral route or intravenously. This depends on the degree of dehydration and the ability to use the GIT for fluid replacement.

❑ Correct electrolyte and metabolic abnormalities.

❑ Patients with bilious vomiting and hematemesis should be kept nil per oral (NPO).

❑ A nasogastric tube is to be inserted in a patient with bilious vomiting to decompress the stomach.

❑ Consult a pediatric surgeon in a case of bilious vomiting since intestinal obstruction is highly likely.

❑ In a case of hematemesis, deal with the patient as a case of upper GI bleeding.

Table 2.6: Management of a child presenting with vomiting
Essential points in managing a child with vomiting
• Manage dehydration regardless of the cause
• Discontinue oral fluids/feeds (NPO*) in case of bilious vomiting or hematemesis
• Start intravenous fluids in cases of bilious vomiting/ hematemesis and in a moderately dehydrated child
• Insert a nasogastric tube in case of bilious vomiting
• Consult the pediatric surgeons in case of bilious vomiting
• Start antacids/proton pump inhibitors (PPI) if vomiting was persistent
• Treat the causative problem
• Antiemetics are not routinely prescribed but can be used specially ondansetron (serotonin antagonist) in patients with persistent vomiting either oral or intravenously
• Continue feeding the child if no surgical problem detected to avoid malnutrition

*NPO: Nil per oral

Pharmacotherapy

Antiemetics

❑ Multiple antiemetic drugs have been used. Drugs such as promethazine, prochlorperazine, and metoclopramide are known to have serious and unpleasant side effects such as irritability, somnolence and extrapyramidal signs; therefore, they are currently not widely used.

❑ Ondansetron: This is a serotonin antagonist that is relatively safe with no sedative effect. A cochrane review supported the use of ondansetron based on several randomized controlled studies in children. The drug is recommended in cases of acute gastroenteritis as an adjunct to oral rehydration therapy in children. It can be used as an oral or intravenous dose. The dose of ondansetron: Oral dose: 0.1–0.2 mg/kg, intravenous dose: 0.13–0.26 mg/kg (maximum: 4 mg).

❑ Antiemetics should not be used in cases of vomiting of undefined etiology and cases of intestinal obstruction before surgical evaluation. However, they can be used in acute gastroenteritis with rehydration therapy, post-operative cases, chemotherapy induced vomiting, motion sickness and cyclical vomiting.[12]

❑ Gastroesophageal reflux can be managed with H_2 blockers or proton pump inhibitors.[13]

❑ Gastroparesis can be managed with domperidone (dopamine antagonist) and erythromycin (macrolide antibiotic).[14]

❑ Cases suggestive of peptic ulcer disease or gastritis can be managed with H_2 blockers or proton pump inhibitors (PPI) either orally or intravenously.

Table 2.7: Nonpharmacological management of chronic vomiting

Nonpharmacological management of chronic vomiting

- Listening to music during meal times
- Hypnosis
- Muscle relaxation exercises
- Small frequent meals
- Encourage the child to eat slowly
- Eliminate emotionally stressful stimuli during feeds (bad odor)

❑ Cyclical vomiting can be treated with ondansetron and antidepressants or anticonvulsants.

Nonpharmacological Therapy

❑ Alternative and complementary modes of therapy are used in cases of chronic and recurrent attacks of vomiting (Table 2.7).[15]

❑ Distraction and relaxation measures may be helpful in improving the anxiety associated with chronic and recurrent vomiting especially in cancer patients and cyclic vomiting. Music therapy, listening to a story, watching a video game, relaxation exercises and hypnosis are examples of nonpharmacological therapy used in children with vomiting.

❑ Modification of diet and mealtime may be helpful. Provide small and frequent meals and advice the child to chew the food appropriately then slowly swallow it. Avoid fatty foods that may delay gastric emptying. Also, during mealtime, avoid unpleasant sights or bad odors that can stimulate the vomiting center through the limbic system and cerebrum.

❑ Many individuals with abdominal pain and vomiting have used Ginger. It has some prokinetic and antispasmodic effects.[16]

❑ Behavioral therapy can be helpful in children with chronic and recurrent attacks of vomiting and should be tried in refractory cases.

Regurgitation

❑ It is the involuntary movement of swallowed food from the stomach into the mouth. This is different from vomiting in that there is no forceful expulsion of food involving the movement of small intestine, stomach, esophagus and diaphragm.

❑ Regurgitation is common in healthy young infants and usually associated with gastroesophageal reflux.

❑ The diagnostic criteria of regurgitation in infants was best described by Rome III committee report of functional gastrointestinal disorders in infants and toddlers (Box 2.3).[17]

❑ Regurgitation decreases with age in normal infants. If persisted after the first year of life then, it should be evaluated for structural anomalies in the GIT.

❑ Associated hematemesis, irritability with feeds, swallowing difficulties, respiratory problems and failure to thrive should prompt immediate investigations for gastroesophageal reflux disease.

❑ This problem is benign and self-limiting. Therefore, no treatment is required. Parents have to be reassured and advised how to deal with this problem until it resolves. The infant can be given thickened feeds if regurgitation is excessive and nursed on left lateral position.

BOX 2.3: Diagnostic criteria of regurgitation in infants

It must include all the following in healthy infants 3 weeks to 12 months of age:
- Regurgitation 2 or more times for 3 or more weeks
- No retching, hematemesis, aspiration, apnea, failure to thrive, feeding or swallowing difficulties or abnormal posture.

Rumination

Rumination is regurgitation of swallowed food into the mouth, chewing it then either reswallowing or spitting it out. The diagnostic criteria of rumination in infants are described in Box 2.4.[17]

Rumination is considered a psychological problem caused by a disturbed mother-infant relationship. The problem can lead to serious sequel especially if the child spits the food and does not reswallow it. Evaluating such a child needs close observation of his/her behavior. If the child felt he was observed he/she would not perform it. There is no need for over investigations since this is most likely a functional problem. Treatment involves improving mother-infant interaction and providing the infant a better emotional care.

BOX 2.4: Diagnostic criteria for rumination in infants[17]

Diagnostic criteria for infant rumination syndrome
It must include all of the following for at least 3 months:
- Repetitive contractions of the abdominal muscles, diaphragm and tongue.
- Regurgitation of gastric content into the mouth, which is either expectorated or re-chewed and reswallowed.
- Three or more of the following:
  - Onset between 3–8 months.
  - Does not respond to management of gastroesophageal reflux disease or anticholinergic drugs, hand restraints, formula changes and gavage or gastrostomy feedings.
  - Unaccompanied by signs of nausea or distress.
  - Does not occur during sleep and when the infant is interacting with individuals in the environment.

Rumination in Older Children and Adolescents

It is basically the same mechanism of that in infants occurring few minutes after a meal. Box 2.5 lists Rome III committee criteria of rumination in older children and adolescents.[18,19] The problem is more prevalent in adolescent girls. Handicapped children also can suffer from this problem.

This is not a serious problem but if treatment is delayed can lead to nutritional deficiencies. Extensive work up is not indicated, however, few conditions should be excluded such as gastroesophgeal reflux disease, gastroparesis and achalasia. The condition is best managed with behavioral therapy and the prognosis is usually favorable. Some patients will require antidepressant medications.

BOX 2.5: Diagnostic criteria of adolescent rumination syndrome

It must include all of the following:
- Repeated painless regurgitation and rechewing or expulsion of food that:
  – Begin soon after ingestion of a meal.
  – Do not occur during sleep.
  – Do not respond to standard treatment for gastroesophageal reflux.
- No retching.
- No evidence of an inflammatory, anatomic, metabolic or neoplastic process that explains the subject's symptoms.

Criteria fulfilled at least once per week for at least 2 months before diagnosis.

■ DIARRHEA

Diarrhea is one of the most common causes of morbidity and mortality in childhood, besides, it a frequent cause of hospital admissions worldwide. The term was derived from the Greek word "diarrhoia" which means flowing through.

Definition

Diarrhea can be defined as a decrease in consistency or increase in liquidity of stool. It is the passage of 3 or more loose or liquid stools per day or more frequently than is normal for the individual.[20]

Based on stool volume or weight, diarrhea can be defined as stool weight >10 g/kg per day in infants and >200 g/day in older children. Nevertheless, diarrhea should not be defined based on stool volume or weight only. This definition may be used in clinical research and in hospitals but of limited value in clinical practice.[21]

Another way of defining diarrhea is by the duration of symptoms:
- ❏ Acute diarrhea: Diarrhea lasting less than 2 weeks.
- ❏ Persistent diarrhea: Diarrhea existing from 2–4 weeks with usually an abrupt onset.
- ❏ Chronic diarrhea: Diarrhea longer than 2 weeks but with gradual onset and can persist more than one month.

Absorption of Fluid and Electrolytes Through the Gastrointestinal Tract (GIT)

The daily fluid intake in older children and adults consists of 1 to 2 liters of liquid (Fig. 2.4).[22] The GIT secretes around 7 liters of endogenous gastrointestinal (GI) fluid. This makes the total amount of liquid reaching the small intestine approximately 9 liters. 7–8 liters are absorbed from the small intestine and 1–2 liters from the colon; therefore, almost 99% of this liquid is absorbed through the small

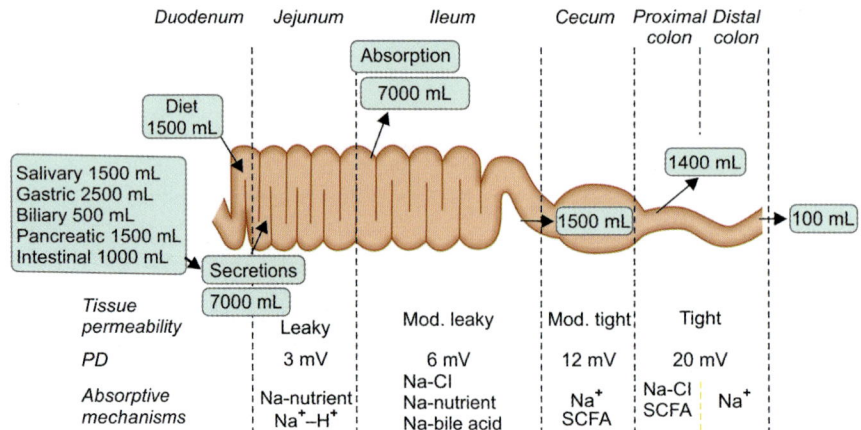

Fig. 2.4: Absorption of fluids through the GIT

Source: Adopted from Venkatasubramanian J, Rao MC, Sellin JH. Intestinal Electrolyte Absorption and Secretion. In: Mark Feldman, Lawrence S Friedman, Lawrence J Brandt (Ed). Sleisenger and Fordtran's Gastrointestinal and Liver Disease, 9th edition. Saunders: Elsevier Inc. 2010.pp.1675-94.

and large bowel leaving a minimal amount only (100–150 mL) to be excreted in the stool.

The GIT has two functions in regards to fluid and electrolytes:

❑ Absorption: Performed in the small intestine and colon.
❑ Secretion: Performed in the small intestine.

The absorption process in the small intestine occurs through the epithelial cells (enterocytes) covering small intestinal villi. There are two surfaces in the cell through which absorption occurs, the apical membrane surface (the cellular path or luminal surface) and the basolateral membrane surface (the paracellular path or vascular surface). The tight junctions between epithelial cells allow or obstruct the passage of fluid and electrolytes across both surfaces. Those tight junctions act as barriers to the flow of luminal contents to the blood. They are leaky with low resistance in the small intestinal epithelium permitting most of the fluid to be absorbed while they are tighter in the colon allowing only minimal fluid absorption.

Absorption

The first step in the absorption is absorption of solute followed by water. Solute and fluid absorption occur in proportion to each other. This means that the intestinal contents and absorbed fluid have the same osmolality as that of plasma. The mechanism of electrolyte absorption via the small intestine is similar to that across the proximal renal tubules in the kidney.

❑ *In the jejunum*: The sodium (Na⁺) gradient is the driving force for other solute and fluid absorption. Na⁺ enters the apical membrane of epithelial cells via Na⁺ dependent coupled transporters. There are Na⁺-sugar (glucose/galactose) cotransporters, Na⁺-amino acid cotransporters and Na⁺-H⁺ exchanger. As those sugars and amino acids are absorbed, Na⁺ is then absorbed and water will follow based on the increased osmotic gradient. Na⁺ leaves the cell into the paracellular space and blood through the basolateral membrane of the epithelial cell via Na⁺-K⁺ ATPase. The action of carbonic anhydrase enzyme inside the epithelial cell on water (H_2O) and carbone dioxide (CO_2) leads to the production of hydrogen (H^+) and bicarbonate (HCO_3^-). H^+ will leave the cell to the lumen as an exchange with Na⁺ via the Na⁺-H⁺ exchanger and HCO_3^- will be absorbed into the blood (Figs 2.5A and B).[23]

❑ *In the ileum:*
  • The same mechanism of absorption occurs using the effect of Na⁺ dependent coupled transporters but there are also other exchangers such as Cl⁻-HCO₃⁻ exchanger. When H^+ and HCO_3^- are produced inside the ileal epithelial cell, both will be secreted into

the lumen as an exchange with Na⁺ and Cl⁻ will be absorbed into the blood not HCO_3^- as in the jejunum. This means that there is a net absorption of $NaHCO_3$ in the jejunum and a net absorption of NaCl in the ileum.

  • Sugars and amino acids with organic solutes are only absorbed through the intestine coupled with Na⁺ and this constitutes the basis of oral rehydration solution therapy in diarrhea.

❑ *In the colon:* The absorption is similar to that of the distal tubules and collecting ducts of the kidney, which is under the effect of aldosterone. This will lead to more

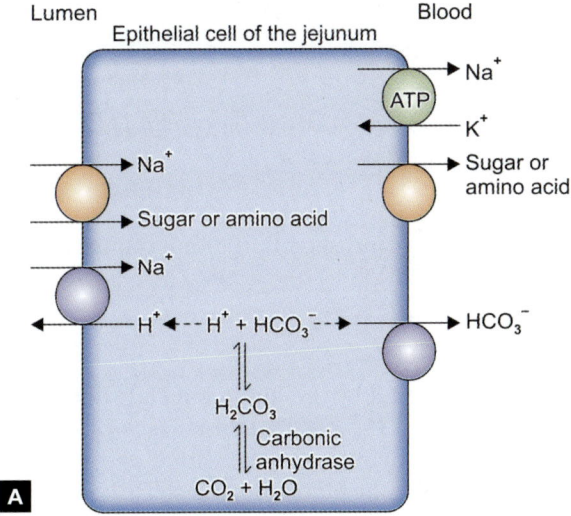

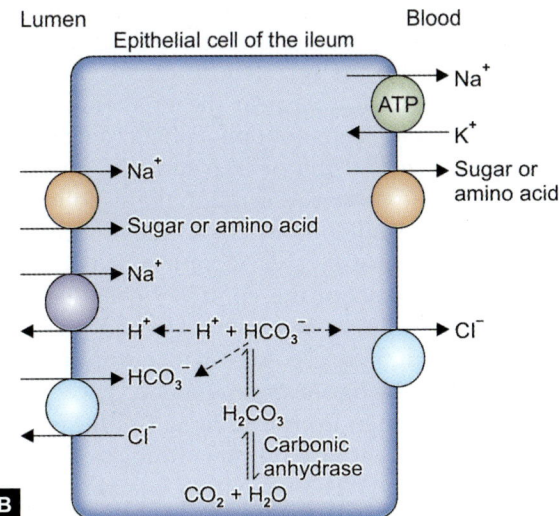

Figs 2.5A and B: Electrolyte transport in the small intestine: (A) Jejunum; (B) Ileum
Source: Adopted from Costanzo LS. A gastrointestinal physiology. In: Physiology, 5th edition. Sunders: Elsevier Inc. 2013.pp. 329-82.

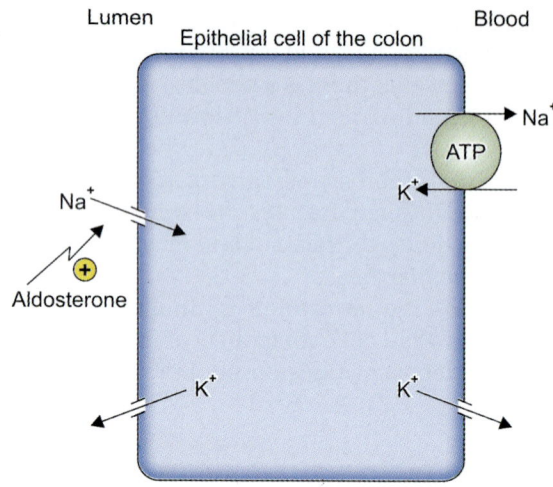

Fig. 2.6: Electrolyte transport in the colon
(*Source:* Adopted from Costanzo LS. Gastrointestinal physiology. In: Physiology, 5th edition. Sunders: Elsevier Inc. 2013.pp. 329-82.)

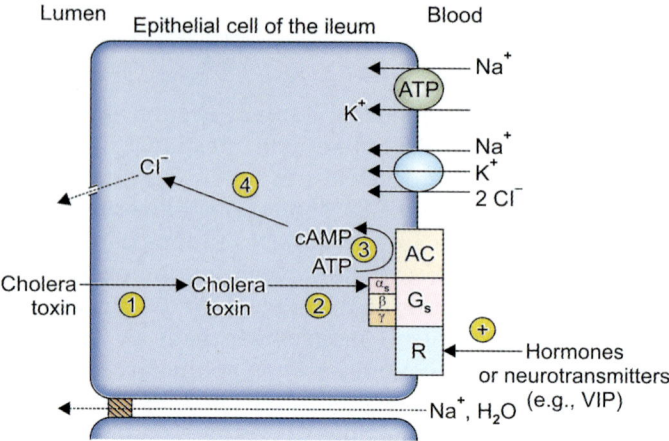

Fig. 2.7: Chloride secretion in the intestine
(*Source:* Adopted from Costanzo LS. Gastrointestinal physiology. In: Physiology, 5th edition. Sunders: Elsevier Inc. 2013.pp.329-82.)

absorption of Na^+ and secretion of potassium (K^+) into the lumen (Fig. 2.6).[23]

Secretion

Secretion is performed by the epithelial cells of the small intestinal crypts. On the basolateral surface of the crypt cell, there is a 3-ion cotransporter, which carries Na^+, K^+ and Cl^- together from the blood into the cell. Cl^- moves into the lumen via Cl^- channels on the apical (luminal surface). Na^+ follows Cl^- and then water flows into the lumen. In the normal situation the epithelial cells covering the villi usually reabsorb the secreted fluid and electrolytes. Activation of adenylyl cyclase in the epithelial cell will generate cyclic adenosine monophosphate (cAMP) at the basolateral surface and this will eventually activate Cl^- channels leading to more Cl^- secretion that is followed by Na and water. In conditions where stimulation of cAMP occurs, the resultant excessive secretion of Cl^- exceeds the absorptive capacity of the epithelial cells leading to secretory diarrhea. This phenomenon occurs in cholera infection and when there are excessive neurotransmitters or hormones stimulating cAMP production (Fig. 2.7).[23]

Diarrhea can range from a mild self-limiting illness to a serious and lethal disease. According to the World Health Organization (WHO) resources, diarrheal disease is the second leading cause of death in children under five years old following pneumonia. Each year, an estimated 2.5 billion cases of diarrhea occur in children with 1.5 million deaths in less than 5 years.[24] It varies with the season and child's age with the highest incidence in the first 2 years of life.

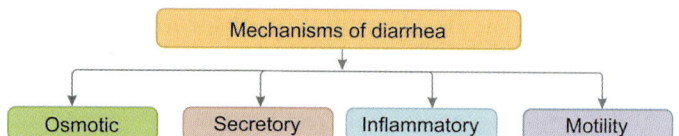

Fig. 2.8: Mechanisms of diarrhea. Most diarrheal disorders have more than one active mechanism responsible for the symptoms

Pathophysiology

Diarrhea can be divided based on the mechanism by which it was induced (Fig. 2.8).[25] Overlap between different mechanisms can occur.

Osmotic

Osmotic diarrhea occurs when a concentrated solute is present in the gut lumen because of defective absorption. This attracts fluid into the intestinal lumen leading to diarrhea. Gastrointestinal infections such as rotavirus and some pathogenic bacteria can damage the intestinal epithelium causing malabsorption of lactose and subsequently osmotic diarrhea.

Secretory

Secretory diarrhea occurs when there is excessive secretion of water into the intestinal lumen more than the capacity of absorption. This can be caused by infections such as cholera and enterotoxin producing bacteria such as *Clostridium difficile* and *Shigella*. Other noninfectious causes such as vasoactive secreting peptide tumors, congenital transport defects (chloride losing diarrhea) and laxative abuse can result in this type of mechanism.

Inflammation

The inflammatory process that damages the intestinal epithelium leads to destruction of the villi and malfunction of the active transporters causing impairment of fluid and electrolyte absorption. Examples of this mechanism are infection with pathogenic organisms, celiac and inflammatory bowel diseases.

Motility-related

Increased gut motility can induce diarrhea as a consequence to inadequate time of absorption. This can be seen in patients with irritable bowel syndrome. On the other hand, gut hypomotility with inadequate peristalsis causes stasis with subsequent bacterial overgrowth and malabsorption leading to secondary osmotic diarrhea.

Causes of Diarrhea

Acute Diarrhea

Acute infectious castroenteritis: The most common cause of acute diarrhea is infection of a pathogenic organism or effect of a toxin produced by the organism. Infection can be viral, bacterial or protozoal (Table 2.8).[26]

Food-borne diarrhea: It is also known as food poisoning and can be caused by either toxin producing organisms or the organism itself colonizing the gut (Table 2.9). Symptoms of vomiting and diarrhea can occur one hour up to few days following ingestion of contaminated food.

Antibiotics-induced diarrhea: This diarrhea is encountered with the use of antibiotics. It is caused by *Clostridium defficile* (*C. defficile*), a gram-positive anaerobic bacteria via a toxin production.

Traveler's diarrhea: It occurs in individuals traveling to a developing country with poor socioeconomic status and sanitation. The most frequently identified pathogen causing traveller's diarrhea was enterotoxigenic *E. coli* (ETEC).

Drugs: Acute diarrhea is a side effect of many drugs including broad-spectrum antibiotics, antacids, prokinetics, antidepressants and antihypertensives.

Chronic Diarrhea

Diarrhea persistent more than 2 weeks is the widely accepted definition of chronic diarrhea (Table 2.10). The terms persistent and protracted diarrhea are not globally used. They usually describe diarrhea that had an acute onset but developed a longer course.[27,28]

Pathophysiology of chronic diarrhea: The same mechanisms causing diarrhea described earlier are also applied in chronic diarrhea. However, to understand the different causes of chronic diarrhea we can describe the pathophysiology as follows:

- ❑ **Infection:**
  - Persistent infection: In immunocompromised patients some bacteria can cause chronic diarrhea. This is unusual in immunocompetent children.
  - Antibiotics-induced diarrhea occurs when *C. difficile* bacteria causes colitis with pseudomembrane formation. This is induced by toxin A and B produced by the bacteria in a recently treated patient with antibiotics. This diarrhea can persists for more than 2 weeks if not diagnosed and properly treated.
  - Parasitic infestation such as *Giardia lamblia* commonly infects infants and toddlers in nurseries. Other parasitic infestations are uncommon in immunocompetent children but can infect immunocompromised patients.
- ❑ **Post-gastroenteritis syndrome:** In some children the enteric organisms responsible for a recent attack of gastroenteritis can damage the intestinal epithelium leading to secondary diasaccharidase deficiency specially lactase with consequent osmotic and persistent diarrhea.

Table 2.8: Causes of acute infectious diarrhea		
Viruses	*Bacteria*	*Protozoa*
• Rotavirus	• *Vibrio cholerae*	• *Giardia intestinalis*
• Norovirus	• *E. coli*	• *Cryptosporidium*
• Adenovirus	• *Salmonella*	• *Entamoeba histolytica*
• Calcivirus	• *Shigella*	
• Astrovirus	• *Campylobacter*	
• Cytomegalovirus	• *Yersinia*	
	• *Clostridium difficile*	

Table 2.9: Causes of food-borne acute diarrhea
Toxin-induced:
• *Staphylococcus aureus*
• *Bacillus cereus*
• *Clostridium botulinum*
Gut colonization:
• *Salmonella*
• *Clostridium perfringens*
• *Vibrio parahemolyticus*
• *Enterohemorrhagic E. coli*
• *Yersinia enterocolitica*

Table 2.10: Causes of chronic diarrhea

Neonates	Infants/toddlers	Children
• Congenital chloride diarrhea	• Post-gastroenteritis syndrome	• Post-gastroenteritis syndrome
• Congenital sodium diarrhea	• Chronic nonspecific diarrhea	• Irritable bowel syndrome
• Glucose-galactose malabsorption	• Food allergy	• Inflammatory bowel disease
• Congenital lactase deficiency	• Giardiasis	• Celiac disease
• Hirschsprung's disease	• Celiac disease	• Lactose intolerance
• Microvillous inclusion disease	• Cystic fibrosis	• Cystic fibrosis
• Tufting enteropathy	• Eosinophilic gastroenteritis	• Bacterial overgrowth
• Autoimmune enteropathy	• Immunodeficiency syndromes	• Factitious diarrhea
• Acrodermatitis enteropathica	• Short gut syndrome	• (Laxative abuse)
• Abetalipoproteinemia	• Bacterial overgrowth	
• Neonatal lymphangiectasia	• Lymphangiectasia	
• Intestinal pseudo-obstruction		
• Short gut syndrome		

☐ **Chronic nonspecific diarrhea**: Toddler's diarrhea, functional diarrhea (Table 2.11),[17] irritable bowel syndrome.

☐ **Excessive intake of osmotic substances:** Carbonated fluids, foods containing sorbitol and manitol, tea, coffee, laxative abuse.

☐ **Inflammatory and immune diseases:** Inflammatory bowel disease (IBD), celiac disease, food allergy, eosinophilic gastroenteritis, immunodeficiency, autoimmune enteropathy.

☐ **Defective digestion:** Cystic fibrosis, chronic pancreatitis, Shwachman–Diamond syndrome, Pearson syndrome, chronic cholestasis, terminal ileum resection.

☐ **Small bowel resection:** Short gut syndrome

☐ **Bacterial overgrowth:** Following any stasis of luminal contents that occur after gastrojejunostomy, GI strictures or fistulas and ineffective peristalsis.

☐ **Structural defects:** Microvillus inclusion disease, tufting enteropathy, phenotypic diarrhea, lymphangiectasia.

☐ **Defects in electrolyte transport:** Congenital chloride diarrhea, congenital sodium diarrhea, acrodermatitis enteropathica, abetalipoproteinemia.

☐ **Enzyme deficiency leading to malabsorption of a nutrient:** Sucrase-isomaltase deficiency; congenital or acquired lactase deficiency; glucose-galactose malabsorption; fructose malabsorption.

☐ **Neuroendocrine hormone-secreting tumors:** VIPoma (vasoactive intestinal polypeptide), Zollinger-Ellison syndrome and mastocytosis.

☐ **Motility disorders:** Hirschsprung's disease, chronic intestinal pseudo-obstruction, thyrotoxicosis and factitious diarrhea due to laxative abuse.

Evaluation of Diarrhea

A detailed history (Table 2.12) is the cornerstone of evaluating a child with diarrhea. Initially, it is important to define:

1. Age of the patient.
2. Duration of diarrhea (acute/chronic).
3. Risk group (immunocompromised, traveler to a developing country).

   • Enquire about the onset of diarrhea and verify whether it is acute or chronic.

   • Ask about stool frequency, consistency and estimate volume.

   • Description of stool characteristics is important (blood, mucus, grease).

   • Diurnal variation of bowel movement may help in the diagnosis since functional diarrhea in childhood occurs only during daytime while IBD diarrhea can awaken the child from sleep.

   • Verify the effect of fasting on stool output. Osmotic diarrhea decreases following a period of fasting while secretory diarrhea is not affected by fasting.

   • Ask about associated GI symptoms such as vomiting, abdominal pain and distension. Also, non-GI symptoms are important to verify such as fever, fatigue, rash, joint pain and weight loss. Recurrent respiratory symptoms and chest infections may suggest cystic fibrosis.

Table 2.11: Diagnostic criteria for functional or nonspecific diarrhea of infants and toddlers

Diagnostic criteria for functional diarrhea

It must include all of the following:
• Daily painless recurrent passage of 3 or larger unformed stools
• Symptoms that last more than 4 weeks
• Onset of symptoms that begins between 6 and 36 months of age
• Passage of stools that occurs during waking hours
• There is no failure to thrive if caloric intake is adequate

Table 2.12: History in a patient with diarrhea

- Onset (abrupt/gradual)
- Duration
- Frequency
- Consistency (watery/loose/soft)
- Volume (approximate estimation)
- Tenesmus
- Characteristics of stool: Blood, mucus, pus, greasy, offensive
- Relation to meals or fasting
- Diurnal variation (nocturnal diarrhea)
- Associated symptoms:
    - Fever
    - Vomiting
    - Abdominal pain
    - Bloating
    - Fatigue
    - Weight loss
    - Respiratory symptoms
    - Rash
    - Joint pain
- Diet
    - Changes in diet/milk
    - Introduction of a new food item
    - Water and food sources
- Recent antibiotic prescription
- Recent travel
- Contact with a sick patient
- Day care center attendance (infants/toddlers)
- Family history
    - Similar illness
    - IBD/CF/congenital diarrhea
- Social history/living conditions
- Past history of bowel resection

Abbreviations: IBD: inflammatory bowel disease; CF, cystic fibrosis.

- History of tenesmus and perianal pain can point to the diagnosis of IBD. Also patients with acute diarrhea can develop perianal excoriation due to acidic stool causing perianal pain especially in infants and young children.
- Symptoms suggestive of recurrent infections such as otitis media, skin infection, urinary tract infection and osteomyelitis may suggest immunodeficiency.
- Dietary history is important to verify:
    - Type of food: Bottle (what formula)/breast milk/solids (type, cooked or raw food).
    - Excessive juices or other hyperosmolar liquids like soft drinks.
    - Source of food and water.
    - How and who is preparing food?
    - Introduction of new item of food to the child's diet.
    - Relation of food items to type and consistency of stool.

- History of recent travel and the place visited is important to know.
- History of recent or prolonged antibiotic ingestion suggests *C. difficile* infection.
- History of previous bowel resection.
- Family history:
    - Acute diarrhea in a family member.
    - Congenital diarrhea/IBD/cystic fibrosis/celiac disease.
    - Sick contact in the family.
- Day care center attendance in infants may suggest giardiasis as a cause of chronic diarrhea.
- Social history is important since living conditions and social status may give a clue to the source and type of food available.

Physical Examination

- ❑ The most important step in physical examination of a patient with diarrhea is assessment of the hydration status (mild, moderate, severe) and the general well being of the child. Dry mucus membranes, fever, sunken eyes, tachycardia, and hypotension indicate dehydration. Signs of dehydration occur more frequently in cases with acute diarrhea because of the rapid loss of body water.
- ❑ A patient who looks ill without clear signs of dehydration may be septic.
- ❑ Plot the child's anthropometric measurements on a growth chart appropriate for his age and verify if he/she suffer from failure to thrive.
- ❑ Assess the nutritional status of the child and look for signs of vitamin and trace element deficiencies such as pallor suggestive of anemia, perianal dermatitis suggesting zinc deficiency and signs of rickets indicative of vitamin D deficiency.
- ❑ Look for clubbing in a patient with chronic diarrhea and examine the chest for signs of chronic lung disease.
- ❑ Look for generalized lymphadenopathy in a case of chronic infection with immune-deficiency.
- ❑ Examine the respiratory system looking for signs of distress and abnormal chest signs indicative of chronic lung disease.
- ❑ Examine the abdomen for distension suggestive of malabsorption disorders or motility problems. Palpate the abdomen for tenderness, palpable masses, guarding and bowel sounds.
- ❑ Look for skin rash.
- ❑ Examine for infection in other sites such as skin, ear, joints and bones.
- ❑ Inspect the perianal area looking for fissures, fistulae or abscesses. A digital rectal examination may also help

in examining the rectum, anal sphincter and assessing presence of blood in the stool.

Investigations

Acute Diarrhea

❑ No tests are required in cases of mild acute diarrhea. In the presence of dehydration serum electrolytes, bicarbonates, urea, creatinine and glucose are essential to evaluate the metabolic needs. Complete blood count as well as blood culture are required if the patient looks septic.

❑ Stool examination: It is not required in case of a healthy and immunocompetent patient. Stool examination consists of microscopy looking for blood/pus cells, ova and parasites and stool culture. This is usually performed in cases of:
  • Bloody diarrhea.
  • Toxic and febrile patients
  • Immunocompromised individuals.
  • Epidemic outbreaks of a specific organism.
  • Persistent diarrhea.

❑ ELISA test performed on stool for rotavirus detection is rapid, sensitive and specific but not available in many laboratories especially in the developing countries.

❑ Stool for *C. defficile* toxin is ordered if there is a positive history of antibiotics intake in the past 3 months. *C. defficile* antigen and PCR on the stool are more sensitive but are not available in many laboratories.[29]

Chronic Diarrhea

❑ Children with persistent and chronic diarrhea need to be investigated in order to define the possible cause and hence provide the best management. Choosing the proper tests is guided by history and physical examination. Table 2.13 lists some of the work up that can be done in a child with chronic diarrhea.

❑ During the evaluation of a patient with chronic diarrhea, one should start with noninvasive tests first such as stool examination and simple blood tests. This is followed by imaging studies (upper/lower series) and endoscopic evaluation.

❑ Blood work up:
  • Complete blood count should be done looking for anemia that may occur in malabsorption states and other chronic disorders. Look for thrombocytosis, which indicates an inflammatory process.
  • Urea and electrolytes are to be done especially in a case of high output watery diarrhea suggestive of a secretory type.
  • Serum albumin is performed in chronic diarrhea looking for evidence of hypoalbuminemia suggestive of malabsorption.
  • Elevated sedimentation rate or C-reactive protein can occur in active inflammatory disorders such as IBD or chronic infections.
  • Celiac serology is indicated in a case of chronic diarrhea regardless of abdominal distension.

Table 2.13: Investigations of chronic diarrhea				
Blood tests	Stool examination	Endoscopy	Imaging	Other tests
CBC/differential	Microscopy for RBC/WBC/ova and parasites	Upper GI endoscopy with biopsy of duodenum/jejunum	Small bowel follow through	Sweat test
C-reactive protein/ESR	Culture	Colonoscopy/ileoscopy with biopsies	MRI enterolysis	Breath hydrogen test after lactose ingestion for carbohydrate malabsorption
Electrolytes	pH	Capsule endoscopy if no lesion detected on conventional endoscopy	Barium enema in suspected Hirschsprung's disease	Breath hydrogen test after lactulose ingestion for bacterial overgrowth
Urea/creatinine	Electrolytes and osmolality			
Serum albumin				
Celiac serology	Reducing substances			
Immunoglobulin levels	Fecal calprotectin			
Serum VIP/serum gastrin	Fecal elastase			

Abbreviations: CBC, complete blood count; RBC, red blood cells; WBC, white blood cells; ESR, erythrocyte sedimentation rate; MRI, magnetic resonance imaging; VIP, vasoactive intestinal polypepetide.

- Presence of recurrent attacks of respiratory symptoms supports a sweat chloride test looking for cystic fibrosis.
- History of recurrent infections is suspicious of immunodeficiency state and hence immunoglobulin levels and white blood cell function is indicated.
- Vitamin B$_{12}$ and folate will be low in malnutrition.
- Fat-soluble vitamins (D, A, E) will decrease in malabsorption disorders. Prothrombin time and INR reflect vitamin K level.
- Stool testing:
  - Stool microscopy looking for red blood cells, white blood cells, ova and parasites.
  - Stool culture.
  - Stool antigen for *Giardia* and *Cryptosporidium*.
  - Stool for *C. defficille* toxin, antigen or PCR.
  - Stool electrolytes and osmolality if the stool is watery. It helps in distinguishing osmotic from secretory type of diarrhea.[30]
  - Stool pH looking for acids that suggest osmotic diarrhea and carbohydrate malabsorption.
  - Reducing sugars in the stool can be helpful in cases of carbohydrate malabsorption.
  - Fecal elastase can be done if pancreatic disease is suspected.
  - Fecal calprotectin can be performed in cases of inflammatory processes.
- Other tests:
  - Hydrogen breath test using lactose as a substrate: In a patient with abdominal distension looking for evidence of lactose intolerance.
  - Hydrogen breath test following lactulose ingestion: In patients with GI stasis due to anatomical problems or short bowel syndrome may help in diagnosing bacterial overgrowth.
- Imaging:
  - Plain X-ray is usually not required unless there is a suspicion of intestinal obstruction with complicated enterocolitis leading to diarrhea.
  - Ultrasound abdomen: This is being used in some centers to diagnose bowel thickening in IBD cases.
  - Contrast study: Such as barium follow through can be done to evaluate the small intestine in IBD cases. Dilated and strictured loops with fistulas can be visualized.
  - MRI enterolysis is being used by many specialists to evaluate small intestinal disease especially in cases of IBD.
  - CT abdomen with contrast also can be helpful to study the small intestine in cases of IBD. It can also be useful in cases of anatomical strictures causing bacterial overgrowth. CT can be helpful in evaluating

the pancreas in cases of chronic pancreatitis associated with pancreatic exocrine deficiency. In addition, neuroendocrine hormone secreting tumors can be visualized by this imaging technique.
- Endoscopy/colonoscopy: These are required in cases of congenital diarrhea, malabsorption and inflammatory disorders.

Management

Acute Diarrhea

- The most important aspect in the management of acute diarrhea is replacement of fluid and electrolyte losses. This can be achieved by oral rehydration solution (ORS) in cases of mild-moderate dehydration and intravenous replacement in severe dehydration. The WHO and UNICEF have jointly published guidelines on the management of acute diarrhea.[31] ORS can be given via a nasogastric tube if the child refuses oral intake before using the intravenous route in cases of mild-moderate dehydration.
- Maintaining nutrition during the diarrhea illness is also crucial. Nutrition can be started after 4–6 hours of rehydration therapy. Breastfed infants should continue breast milk and those who are formula fed should also continue their feeds if tolerated (i.e. no vomiting). There is no need to change the formula to lactose free or soya milk during the management of acute diarrhea. Also, formula dilution is not recommended.
- Those who are on solids can have the usual food appropriate for their age. The BRAT diet (banana, rice, applesauce, and toast) was not well studied and is not recommended by the European Society of Pediatric Gastroenterology, Hepatology and Nutrition (ESPGHAN). Soups can be offered together with oral rehydration solution for older children.[32]
- Zinc supplements have been shown to be effective in decreasing the duration and severity of acute diarrhea in children of developing countries. UNICEF and WHO recommend zinc supplementation (10 mg below 6 months of age and 20 mg in older infants and children for 10–14 days) as a universal treatment for children with diarrhea. However, a recent Cochrane review showed that zinc supplements were not effective in infants less than 6 months of age. It is recommended in malnourished children above 6 months of age and in areas where zinc deficiency is common not in all children with acute diarrhea.[33]
- Antibiotics should not be used routinely in acute diarrhea but they are required in certain conditions such as septic patients, immunocompromised and in the presence of certain organisms such as *Salmonella*,

Shigella and *Campylobacter* that cause inflammatory and invasive diarrhea. Also, febrile neonates and young infants less than 3 months of age with bacterial diarrhea should be treated with antibiotics. Healthy children with *Salmonella* GE do not require antibiotic treatment because it may induce a state of healthy carrier. In addition, bloody diarrhea in a well afebrile child does not also require antibiotics. Patients with traveller's diarrhea can benefit form a short course of antibiotics.

❑ Parasitic infections such as *Giardia* and *Entamoeba histolytica* will respond to antibiotics. *Cryptosporidium* in healthy children does not require any treatment but in immunocompromised patients should be treated with nitaxozanide.

❑ Antidiarrheal drugs are not recommended in children.

❑ Probiotics supplemented ORS can be safely used in children. *Lactobacillus* GG and *Saccharomyces boulardii* have been tested in children with acute diarrhea.[34]

❑ Management of acute diarrhea is usually done at home with educating the parents how to provide ORS and maintain the child's feedings. Regular follow ups are recommended to ensure that diarrhea with its complications are under control. However, hospitalization is required if the patient is in severe dehydration/shock, clinically septic, irritable or lethargic, having uncontrolled vomiting, failure of ORS therapy and inability of the caregiver to manage the problem at home.

Chronic Diarrhea

❑ Management can be done in the outpatient clinic with regular follow-up.

❑ Hospitalization is required when there is severe dehydration, signs of severe malnutrition, lethargic or irritable child, associated intractable vomiting, abnormal social background and evidence of child neglect.

❑ This type of diarrhea is commonly associated with impaired nutritional status and growth. Therefore, regardless of the cause treatment should include supportive measures and nutritional rehabilitation.[35]

❑ An experienced dietician should be involved in the care of these patients.

❑ Nutritional therapy:
  • Nutritional supplementation should consist of appropriate and adequate formula. This can be achieved by enteral or parenteral methods of introducing nutrition.
  • Enteral nutrition can be achieved via oral, nasogastric or gastrostomy feeding.

• The caloric needs should be gradually increased to avoid the metabolic problems that can complicate feeding malnourished children.

• Lactose-free formula is recommended by WHO in children with chronic diarrhea.

• Hydrolyzed or amino acid based formulas should be started in patients with cow's protein intolerance.

• Gluten-free diet is needed in children with celiac disease.

• IBD cases specially Crohn's disease can be managed with a polymeric or elemental formula either exclusively during induction or as a supplement during maintenance therapy.

• Zinc was found to be an important trace element in both prevention and treatment of chronic diarrhea. It restores epithelial proliferation and stimulates immune response. Although WHO recommends zinc therapy in acute as well as chronic diarrhea a recent Cochrane review of the studies done on zinc therapy concluded that it is better be used for children above 6 months of age only if they suffer from malnutrition or in areas where zinc is deficient.

• Vitamin and trace element replacement is crucial.

• In case of congenital diarrhea causing intestinal failure, total parenteral nutrition is indicated.

❑ Drug therapy:
  • Antibiotics are required in cases of immunodeficiency states, giardiasis and bacterial overgrowth.
  • In severe and persistent diarrhea induced by rotavirus infection, oral human immunoglobulin can be tried.
  • Pancreatic enzyme replacement is beneficial in patients with cystic fibrosis and chronic pancreatitis.
  • Steroids can be prescribed for patients with autoimmune enteropathy. IBD cases can also be treated with steroids or other immunosuppressive medications.
  • Salt (NaCl and KCl) replacement is given in patients with congenital chloride diarrhea.
  • Octreotide should be tried in patients with severe secretory diarrhea caused by neuroendocrine hormone secreting tumors to suppress fluid loss.

ABDOMINAL PAIN

Abdominal pain is one of the most common causes of emergency room visits in children.[36] It can originate from abdominal organs or referred from extra-abdominal sites. Pain in children can be caused by a mild self-limiting problem or a serious life-threatening disease.[37] Also, it either presents as an acute problem or chronic and recurrent attacks.

Types of Pain

- *Visceral pain:* Generated by stretch receptors located in the visceral peritoneum, within the walls of hollow viscera, within the mesentery and capsules of solid organs. Distension and ischemia of the abdominal organs stimulate these receptors. Visceral pain fibers are bilateral and enter the spinal cord at different levels, therefore, this pain is poorly localized, dull and crampy.
- *Somatic pain:* Generated by pain receptors located in the parietal peritoneum, roots of the mesentery and mucosa of the gastrointestinal tract. Stretch, ischemia and inflammation stimulate the somatic pain receptors on the same side and level of the lesion. Pain is localized and sharp with positive tenderness and possible guarding and rebound.
- *Referred pain:* Pain perceived at a site distant from the lesion. It is poorly localized and dull. The pain is located in the cutaneous dermatomes sharing the same spinal cord level as the affected abdominal organ. This is the same pain experienced in the back or right shoulder in case of biliary tree pathology.

Causes of Abdominal Pain

The causes of abdominal pain are very variable. It varies in different age groups and it also depends on whether the pain is acute or chronic.

Acute Pain

Refer Table 2.14.

Chronic Abdominal Pain

Chronic abdominal pain is defined as pain present for at least 3 months duration. It can either be due to organic or functional disorders. This type of pain is prevalent in school-aged children and adolescents. 10–15% of school-aged children may suffer from recurrent abdominal pain and this figure can be higher in some populations.[38,39]

Generally, chronic abdominal pain is more experienced in girls and tends to increase with age.

Organic causes (Table 2.15): The abdominal pain is due to a structural, infectious, inflammatory or biochemical defect. It can either originate from the gastrointestinal tract or extraintestinal organs.[40]

Table 2.15: Organic causes of chronic abdominal pain in children	
Gastrointestinal disorders	*Extraintestinal disorders*
• Chronic constipation • Reflux esophagitis • Peptic ulcer disease • Gastritis • Lactose intolerance • Inflammatory bowel disease • Gallstone disease • Chronic pancreatitis • Celiac disease • Familial mediterranean fever • Lead poisoning	• Urinary tract infection • Renal stones • Musculoskeletal diseases • Dysmenorrhea • Pelvic inflammatory disease • Endometriosis

Table 2.14: Causes of acute abdominal pain in children			
<1 year	*>1–5 years*	*>5–12 years*	*>12–18 years*
• Colic • Intussusception • Volvulus • Incarcerated hernia • UTI • Constipation • Gastroenteritis • Hirschsprung enterocolitis	• Trauma • Gastroenteritis • UTI • Constipation • Appendicitis • Pharyngitis • Mesenteric lymphadenitis • Intussusception • Henoch-Schonlein purpura • Volvulus • Foreign body ingestion • Renal colic • Hepatitis • Acute peritonitis • Sickle cell crisis	• Trauma • Gastroenteritis • UTI • Pharyngitis • Constipation • Pneumonia • Henoch-Schonlein purpura • Appendicitis • Mesenteric lymphadenitis • Peptic ulcer disease • Pancreatitis • Renal colic • Diabetic ketoacidosis • Hepatitis • Acute peritonitis • Abdominal migraine • Acute porphyria	• Gastroenteritis • UTI • Constipation • Pneumonia • Peptic ulcer disease • Appendicitis • Dysmenorrhea • Pancreatitis • Biliary colic • Renal colic • Diabetic ketoacidosis • Hepatitis • Abdominal migraine • Pelvic inflammatory disease • Ovarian/testicular torsion • Acute porphyria • Ectopic pregnancy

Functional Causes: The pain is not caused by an identified structural, infectious, inflammatory or biochemical abnormality. Basically, there is no identified cause for the chronic pain. The Rome III criteria, published in 2006, characterized and defined chronic functional abdominal pain in children into five major groups listed in Table 2.16.[19]

Evaluation

A thorough history is the cornerstone of evaluating a child with abdominal pain. The physician should initially define the pain characteristics (Table 2.17).

Location

The site of pain aids in defining the organ involved. Young children are not usually able to localize their pain but if this is possible this will be helpful. Pain of esophagitis can be substernal or epigastric. Gastritis, peptic ulcer disease and pancreatitis pain will be experienced in the epigastric region.

Right upper abdominal pain probably caused by biliary colic and pneumonia. Left upper abdominal pain will be caused by gastritis, pancreatitis, pneumonia or splenic pathology.

Right lower abdominal pain might indicate appendicitis, constipation, mesenteric lymphadenitis, inflammatory bowel disease, irritable bowel and inguinal hernia. Left lower quadrant pain may be due to constipation, colitis and irritable bowel syndrome. Diffuse abdominal pain is usually caused by gastroenteritis, irritable bowel, peritonitis and diabetic ketoacidosis.

Table 2.16: Causes of functional abdominal pain in children
• Functional dyspepsia
• Irritable bowel disease
• Functional abdominal pain
• Abdominal migraine
• Aerophagia

Table 2.17: Characteristics of abdominal pain
• Location
• Onset
• Duration
• Frequency
• Quality/nature
• Severity
• Radiation
• Relieving/aggravating factors
• Associated symptoms

Central periumbilical pain is usually the site of functional abdominal pain. In children, the further the pain is from the umbilicus it is more likely of an organic pathology.[41]

Onset

The timing of the first episode of pain and the events surrounding it is important to know. Is the pain of abrupt or gradual onset? The pain of intussusception or intestinal obstruction is usually sudden. In the contrary appendicitis pain is gradual.

Duration

One should define whether the pain is acute or chronic (more than 3 months). This will help in limiting the differential diagnosis.

Quality

Children may not be able to describe the quality of pain, however, with leading questions from the pediatrician they can give a clue to the type of pain they experience. Colicky pain occurs in intestinal obstruction, biliary colic and renal colic. Burning pain is a feature of esophagitis and peptic ulcer disease. Dull aches in the abdomen might be suggestive of functional abdominal pain. It is also helpful to know whether the pain is intermittent or continuous. Infants with intussusception will have a recurrent spasmodic pain when the patient becomes irritable alternating with periods of calmness and probably lethargy. Patients with appendicitis will have continuous pain that can increase in severity with time.

Severity

The severity of pain is also difficult to be described in children. Older children can self report their pain but young children and infants might not be able to do that. There are certain ways that can aid in assessing the severity of pain in young children. The visual pain scales based on a series of faces that show an increasing tendency of distress can help. The child can be offered these faces and asked to point to the face that nearly describes his pain.[42]

In infants or neurologically impaired children, some observational scales have been created to quantify the severity of pain in these children.[43] They depend on scoring facial expressions, limb and trunk motor responses, level of interaction, cry and ability to be consoled.

The parents can be asked in case of a young child whether the child's activity, feeding, sleep are disturbed by the pain. In case of an older child, we can enquire about effect of pain on school attendance.[44] Severe agonizing pain can be encountered in cases with intussusception and other intestinal obstruction, pancreatitis, renal colic and sickle cell crisis.

The threshold for perceiving pain from different stimuli varies among individuals.

Radiation of Pain

The site of referred pain may help in establishing the diagnosis. Pain of pancreatitis may radiate to the back while renal colic pain may be experienced in the groin as well.

Relieving/Aggravating Factors

It is important to enquire about the triggering or relieving factors affecting the pain such as food, exercise, infection, posture, etc. A patient with constipation may have pain aggravated after meals and get the feeling of a bowel movement. This patient will be relieved after defecation. A patient with esophagitis may suffer more after meals while peptic ulcer disease is relieved with eating. Certain posture may also help in relieving the pain such as pancreatitis pain can be a bit relieved by leaning forward and pain of appendicitis is felt better when lying still in bed.

Associated Symptoms

Symptoms that can be associated with pain may give a clue to the pathology of that pain such as nausea, vomiting, diarrhea, constipation, abdominal distension, fever, cough, dysuria, hematuria, weight loss and disturbed growth. Mesenteric adenitis usually occurs in association with a viral illness. Gastroenteritis will be associated with vomiting and diarrhea. Urinary tract infection might be associated with dysuria whereas renal colic with hematuria. History of polyuria and polydipsia suggests diabetic ketoacidosis. Growth failure may suggest inflammatory bowel or celiac disease. Patients with lead poisoning may give a history of pica and constipation.

There are alarming points in history that should be considered as red flags indicating an organic and probably serious pathology responsible for the pain (Table 2.18).

Physical Examination

- ❑ A complete and thorough physical examination is mandatory in the evaluation of a child with abdominal pain.
- ❑ Physical examination should include general well being of the child whether he or she looks unwell and in discomfort.

- ❑ Observe the patient's posture when presented.
- ❑ The vital signs should be recorded.
- ❑ Measurement of the child's growth parameters with plotting them on the growth chart according to the age is crucial.
- ❑ Look for pallor, cervical lymphadenopathy, finger clubbing and lower limb edema on the general examination.
- ❑ Abdominal examination:
  - The abdomen should be inspected for distension, bruises of previous trauma, peristalsis and a visible mass.
  - Palpation for abdominal guarding is important. This can be diffuse in case of peritonitis or focal and localized such as an inflammatory abscess in a case of inflammatory bowel disease or appendicitis.
  - The site of abdominal tenderness can aid in determining the causative organ.
  - A mass felt on the right upper quadrant in a colicky infant suggests intussusception.
  - Detecting fecal masses especially in the left lower quadrant can be common in cases of chronic constipation.
- ❑ Examination of the pelvis and hernial orifices is crucial to exclude incarcerated inguinal hernia. In adolescent girls pelvic examination is also important in cases of ovarian pathology and pelvic inflammatory disease.
- ❑ Perianal and rectal examination should be performed in any patient with abdominal pain specially those with chronic complaints. Patients with inflammatory bowel disease can have perianal fissures, abscesses or fistulas. In a patient with chronic constipation, the rectum will be overloaded with hard stool. Also, in an infant with

Table 2.18: Red flags in the history and physical examination of a child with abdominal pain	
Red flags on history	*Red flags on examination*
• Persistent localized pain	• Failure to thrive
• Heart burn	• Impaired growth velocity
• Dysphagia	• Abdominal distension
• Recurrent vomiting	• Localized abdominal
• Chronic diarrhea	tenderness
• Blood in the stool	• Abdominal guarding
• Fever of unknown origin	• Abdominal mass
• Weight loss	• Organomegaly
• Impaired growth	• Perianal disease
• Delayed puberty	• Arthritis
• Waking up at night by the pain	
• Family history of IBD/celiac disease	

Abbreviation: IBD, inflammatory bowel disease.

intussusception, rectal examination may reveal red current jelly stool typical of intussusception.

❑ Other systems should be examined as well such as the upper respiratory tract, ears, cardiovascular system and chest.

❑ Examination of the musculoskeletal system may help in detecting the cause of abdominal pain. Inflammation of the psoas muscle may be triggered by hyperextension of the hip and pain might be experienced in the lower abdomen.

❑ Alarming findings of the abdominal pain on physical examination are listed in Table 2.18.

Investigations

History and physical examination will guide further testing for the cause of pain. By investigating a child with abdominal pain we have to determine firstly whether it is an organic disease or not and secondly whether it is an emergency condition that requires an immediate attention and management.[45,46] Tests that are usually required in these patients are shown in Table 2.19.

First Line Tests

❑ *Blood work up:*
  • Complete blood count: To check for anemia and elevated platelet count that might suggest an inflammatory process causing the pain. Also, increased white blood cell count can be seen in infectious episodes although normal count does not exclude it.

• Elevated C-reactive protein or erythrocyte sedimentation rate (ESR) may also indicate inflammatory or infectious disorders.

• Serum electrolytes may be deranged in patients with associated vomiting or diarrhea.

• Blood glucose is elevated in diabetic ketoacidosis and reduced in patients with associated vomiting.

• Renal function test may be deranged in patients with dehydration, renal colic and hemolytic uremic syndrome.

• Serum albumin might be reduced in patients with inflammatory bowel disease specially Crohn's disease.

• Liver enzymes are elevated in patients with hepatitis.

❑ *Urine testing:* Urine analysis can show an elevated leukocytes and nitrites in UTI. Hematuria whether microscopic or macroscopic can be seen in UTI, renal stones, Henoch-Schönlein purpura and hemolytic uremic syndrome. Positive glucose and ketones in the urine is seen in diabetic ketoacidosis. Positive urine culture indicates UTI.

❑ *Stool testing:* Stool microscopy looking for RBC and WBC may be positive in gastroenteritis and IBD. Positive stool culture confirms gastroenteritis. Stool for occult blood may suggest inflammatory bowel and sometimes intussusception if gross blood is not clear in the infant's stool. Stool for ova and parasites may help in cases of chronic abdominal pain.[47]

Second Line Tests

❑ *Blood work up:*
  • Serum amylase and lipase are increased in patients with pancreatitis.
  • Blood gas analysis looking for metabolic acidosis can be expected in patients with dehydration and those with diabetic ketoacidosis.

❑ Breath test for lactose intolerance.

❑ *Imaging investigations:*
  • Plain abdominal X-ray: This can be helpful in detecting signs of intestinal obstruction. Patients with constipation, fecal masses may be seen loading the colon. The plain X-ray also may show a foreign body in the GIT specially a button battery or a sharp object stuck in the GIT. In this case the X-ray should include the neck, chest and abdomen since the foreign body can be lodged in the esophagus and will not be shown on abdominal X-ray. Opaque renal stones can be seen on plain X-ray.
  • Ultrasound abdomen: This study should be performed in infants with colicky abdominal pain to rule out intussusception. It can also help in diagnosing appendicitis, biliary colic and pancreatitis

Table 2.19: Investigations of a child with abdominal pain		
First line tests	*Second line tests*	*Third line tests*
• Complete blood count	• Blood gases/serum CO_2	• Celiac serology
• Serum electrolytes	• Serum amylase/lipase	• Breath test for *H. pylori*
• Blood glucose	• Breath hydrogen test for lactose intolerance	• Esophageal pH manometry
• C-reactive protein/ESR	• Plain abdominal X-ray	• Barium follow through
• Serum albumin	• Ultrasound abdomen	• Endoscopy/colonoscopy
• Renal function test		• CT abdomen/pelvis
• Liver function test		• Sickle cell testing
• Urine analysis		• Capsule videoscopy
• Urine culture		• Laparoscopy
• Stool microscopy		
• Stool culture		
• Stool occult blood		

in children. Abscess formation associated with Crohn's disease can be visualized also by ultrasound.

Third Line Tests

❏ Celiac serology for the possibility of celiac disease.
❏ Breath test for *Helicobacter pylori* (Hp) can aid in testing for this organism, which will be responsible for duodenal or gastric ulcerations.
❏ pH manometry can be performed over 24 hours to detect pathological gastroesophageal reflux especially in infants.
❏ Barium follow through in cases of growth failure and hypoalbuminemia.
❏ Endoscopy/colonoscopy can be ordered in patients with growth failure or persistent localized pain in the upper abdomen or chest.
❏ Capsule videoscopy sometimes is required in cases of significant abdominal pain with associated other GI symptoms but without evident pathology.
❏ CT abdomen is ordered in cases of abdominal pain associated with a mass like effect.

Management

Management of abdominal pain depends on the causative disorder that is defined by thorough evaluation. The aim is to maintain the wellbeing of the child and relieve his suffering. Acute abdominal pain is challenging in the pediatric age group and many pediatricians are reluctant to give analgesics for children.[48] The reason for this is to avoid masking the abdominal signs of surgical problems. Several studies in children and adults have revealed that analgesia including opiods does not actually have a negative impact on the management of acute abdominal problems.[49]

The World Health Organization (WHO) supports pain treatment and considers this as a fundamental human right. Inadequate pain management in children can have a longstanding consequences including emotional and stressful suffering. Treatment can be based on a step-wise fashion depending on the severity of the pain. The WHO has established an analgesia ladder, which was initially developed for children with cancer, but it can be followed in other conditions.[50,51]

The WHO guidelines for pain relief that can be used in a child with abdominal pain are as follows:
❏ Regular follow up and assessment of the severity of pain.
❏ Use of nonpharmacologic measures:
 • Physical factors such as applying a warm pad on the site of pain or messaging the abdomen.
 • Behavioral therapy can be helpful such as exercise, play therapy and biofeedback.
 • Cognitive therapy to distract the child's attention from the pain can be tried such as hypnosis and psychotherapy.
❏ Administer analgesia for the pain. The choice of the analgesic depends on the severity of the pain and it is done on a 2-step basis:
 • *Mild pain*: Acetaminophen and or non-steroidal anti-inflammatory drugs (NSAIDs)
 • *Moderate-severe pain*: Opioids should be given (morphine, oxycodone, hydromorphone, fentanyl and methadone).
❏ Analgesia is better given via the oral route. Intravenous, subcutaneous or rectal administration can be used if enteral therapy is not possible.
❏ Analgesia should be given in a regular basis in moderate-severe pain (by the clock and not as needed).
❏ Anticipate and treat the analgesia side effects.
❏ Adjuvant therapy is used when necessary such as antidepressants, anticonvulsants, etc. during all steps of pain severity.

Less severe and chronic abdominal pain might not require any pharmacological therapy. The cause of the complaint should be defined and hence managed appropriately such as using steroids or other immunosuppressive in IBD, antireflux therapy for reflux esophagitis, antacids or proton pump inhibitors for peptic ulcer disease. Gluten-free diet can relieve the symptoms of patients with celiac disease. Laxatives and diet modification in patients with constipation will also help alleviate their symptoms.

Patients with chronic functional abdominal pain do not usually require any drug therapy. Instead, both patient and parents need reassurance of the absence of serious organic illness. Then psychotherapy and behavioral therapy will help in coping with the chronic complaint.

▌CONSTIPATION

Constipation is one of the most common problems referred to general pediatricians and eventually to pediatric gastroenterologists. The term constipation is derived from a Latin word "*constipare*" meaning, "to crowd together". It is generally defined as infrequent bowel movements, large/hard stools and difficult or painful defecation.[52] The problem can be acute which has been there for few days or chronic and persistent for a long period.

Normal Bowel Movements in Children

To accurately define constipation we need to consider the normal variation in children's bowel movements. Stool frequency varies with age and the type of feeds. Babies pass more bowel movements than older children. In a study involving 800 babies during their first week of life, stool frequency was described to be as many as 4 stools per day. Breast milk babies pass more frequent bowel movements than bottle fed ones. Bowel movements in breastfed babies can exceed 10 times per day.[21]

Stool frequency decrease as the child grows older. Children between 1–4 years can have bowel movements alternating between 3 per day to one every alternate day. By 4 years of age most of the normal children are usually toilet trained and they are expected to pass at least one bowel movement per day.[53]

Definition of Constipation

According to ROME III criteria, chronic constipation is defined when 2 or more features listed in Box 20.6 are present in a child of 4 years or older for the past 8 weeks.[17,19] In children less than 4 years those symptoms must be present for at least 1 month.

BOX 2.6: ROME III definition of chronic constipation

ROME III criteria of chronic constipation in children
Symptoms must include at least two of the following for the past 2 months.
- Two or fewer defecations per week .
- At least 1 episode of fecal incontinence per week in a toilet trained child.
- History of excessive stool retention or retentive posturing.
- History of painful or hard bowel movements.
- Presence of a large fecal mass in the rectum .
- History of large diameter stools that may obstruct the toilet.

The Paris Consensus on Childhood Constipation Terminology Group (PACCT) has included a group of children with fecal incontinence but without a history of constipation (nonretentive fecal incontinence).[54]

Other Important Definitions

Soiling

Passage of liquid stool in an inappropriate place.

Encopresis

Passage of normal stool in an inappropriate place.

Soiling and encopresis have been replaced by fecal incontinence.

Fecal Incontinence

Passage of stool in an inappropriate place. It can be divided into two categories:
- ❑ Organic fecal incontinence: Fecal incontinence caused by an organic disease such as an anal sphincter problem or a neurological impairment.

- ❑ Functional fecal incontinence: Fecal incontinence due to a nonorganic disease (functional disorder). This category can be subdivided into:
  - Constipation related fecal incontinence
  - Nonretentive fecal incontinence (nonconstipation related).

When Does Constipation Start?

There are certain stages in the child's development when constipation is relatively common to occur as shown in Box 2.7.

BOX 2.7: The stages of constipation development in children

Timing of constipation in children
- At the time of weaning.
- At the time of toilet training.
- At school entry or school age.

Epidemiology

Constipation is a common problem in childhood. A systematic review has reported constipation in 0.7% to 29.6% of children. Another study has reported that constipation starts in the first year of life in approximately 17–40% of kids.[55-57]

There is a significant rise in physician visits for this problem in the pediatric age group over the years. The problem has got the same frequency in both genders of young children but is reported at a higher rate in older girls. Positive family history of the same problem might be positive in 28–50% of constipated children.[58]

Pathophysiology of Constipation

The pathophysiology of childhood constipation is multifactorial and not completely well understood. The problem can be caused by organic and pathological disease or can be due to a functional disorder. Box 2.8 includes the organic causes of constipation in children.

Functional Constipation

Functional constipation accounts for the majority of cases. Almost 90% of children with this problem suffer from functional constipation. The condition is usually due to withholding of stool after the experience of passing a painful bowel movement. It can also be secondary to refusal of passing stool in a public toilet such as school.[59,60] Voluntary withholding results in accumulation of stool in the colon specially the rectum. Excessive absorption of fluid will eventually occur from the fecal mass in the colon leading to harder stool masses that are difficult to evacuate. This will cause more withholding and commonly

BOX 2.8: Organic causes of constipation in children

Intestinal problems:
- Hirschsprung's disease
- Anorectal malformations
- Neuroenteric dysplasia

Spinal cord problems:
- Spinal cord trauma
- Spinal cord tumor
- Tethered cord
- Myelomeningocele

Metabolic/endocrine:
- Hypothyroidism
- Diabetes mellitus
- Hypercalcemia
- Vitamin D intoxication

Drugs:
- Opioids
- Antihistamines
- Antidepressants
- Anticonvulsants
- Antispasmodics

Other causes:
- Cystic fibrosis
- Celiac disease
- Cow's protein intolerance
- Sexual abuse
- Anorexia nervosa

BOX 2.9: Risk factors for functional chronic constipation
- Low intake of dietary fibers
- Physical stresses
  - Chronic illnesses
- Psychological stresses
  - Social problems at home
  - School bullying
  - Other school factors/examinations
  - Birth of a sibling
  - Loss of a relative/friend
  - Living in a war-affected area
- Living in an urban area
  - Sedimentary life style
  - Junk food (low fibers)
- Prematurity and low birth weight
- Positive family history of constipation

BOX 2.10: History in a child with constipation
- Time of passage of meconium
- Time of onset of constipation
- Duration of constipation
- Frequency of bowel movements
- Stool consistency or caliber
- Child behavior during defecation:
  - Retentive posture
    - Arching of the back
    - Tiptoeing
    - Straightening of the legs
  - Withdrawal behavior
  - Straining
- Associated symptoms:
  - Abdominal pain
  - Nausea/vomiting
  - Appetite
  - Abdominal distension
- Blood in the stool or toilet paper
- Weight loss/growth failure
- Activity
- Urinary retention/UTI/incontinence/enuresis
- History of CNS problems
- Developmental history
- Drug history
- Dietary history
- History of previous management trials of the same problem
- Social history background and family dynamics
- School performance and school atmosphere enquiry in older children
- Other disease conditions
- Risk factors (see Box 2.9)

leads to a retentive posture when the child gets the urge to pass a bowel movement. This creates a vicious circle which if prolonged will be difficult to break. In addition, overstretching the rectum will inhibit the rectal sensation and the urge to pass stool so that a loaded and impacted rectum will not stimulate a bowel movement.[61] This problem will aggravate the involuntary fecal incontinence and hence creating a psychological stress and trauma to both child and parents.

There are certain risk factors for functional constipation (Box 2.9).[60]

Evaluation of a Child with Constipation

A detailed history and thorough physical examination are the cornerstones of evaluating a child with chronic constipation.

History

When interviewing the parents as well as the child, it is important to know how they define constipation. Then a detailed history should include all the important points listed in Box 2.10.

❑ **Timing of meconium passage:** This is crucial information to obtain in history. Neonates usually pass meconium in the first 24-48 hours after birth. Failure of passing meconium during this period is suspicious of Hirschsprung's disease.

❑ **Time of onset of constipation:** Intestinal structural and neuropathic problems usually present earlier in life such as Hirschsprung's disease, anorectal malformations and neuroenteric dysplasia. Functional constipation usually starts at a certain age of development (Box 2.7) mainly, at 2–4 years of age. We have to enquire about the events surrounding the time of onset of the problem (dietary changes, drug intake, social and psychological problems).

❑ **Stool consistency or caliber:** There are different stool scales that the parents or child can be shown and hence describe the child's consistency.[62,63]

❑ **Child's behavior during defecation:** The child's behavior during defecation is important to describe. Retentive posturing as shown in Box 2.10 is an indication of difficulty in passing stool.

❑ **Perianal symptoms:** Anal pain can commonly be experienced in those children and this makes them withhold the stool more. History of blood in the diaper, toilet basin or toilet paper might be associated with the anal pain due to a perianal fissure. This can be a horrible experience for both the child and parents.

❑ **Associated symptoms:** Associated symptoms such as nausea, vomiting, abdominal pain and distension is mandatory to enquire about. Those symptoms might occur even in functional constipation specially if the whole colon was chronically loaded with stool. Weight gain and growth are crucial aspects to verify in the history. Failure to thrive and delayed growth velocity are indications of organic disease.

❑ Dietary history:
  • Changes in the child's diet are crucial aspects to enquire about in the history. The infant's stool consistency commonly increases when milk is changed from breast to formula regardless of cow's protein intolerance. Starting weaning foods also can harden the infant's stool. The most important aspects of diet contributing to constipation are low fiber diet and poor fluid intake which is the usual diet ingested by most children. School aged children prefer junk food that is deficient in fibers.
  • It is also mandatory to enquire about appetite and whether it is affected by constipation. Interestingly, obese children have an increased incidence of chronic constipation, which might be attributed to poor dietary factors and sedimentary nonactive life style.[64]

❑ **Developmental history:** Developmentally delayed children commonly suffer from chronic constipation. This can be attributed to difficulty in introducing high fiber diet to those children, as well as toilet training problems. Also many of those kids have mobility disabilities and hence aggravating colonic motility.

❑ **Social/school/psychological history:** The social background of the family should be discussed with the parents. All the environmental changes surrounding the time of onset of constipation should be defined such as birth of a new baby, separation of the parents, death of a loved friend or family member, change of home or city. In addition, school atmosphere is crucial to enquire about (school performance, school bullying, change of school, etc.). Child abuse can lead to chronic constipation and the physician should have a high index of suspicion in interviewing a child and a parent with this problem.

❑ **History of other system involvement:** Dysuria, urinary incontinence and flank pain might suggest renal system involvement. Chronic constipation can precipitate urinary tract infection via pressure effect on the urinary bladder by the overloaded rectum and sigmoid reducing its capacity. Central nervous system symptoms should be enquired about on history because patients with spastic or myotonic muscle problems can suffer from chronic constipation.

Physical Examination

A thorough physical examination should be performed in a patient with chronic constipation to exclude evidence of organic disease causing the problem.

Generally inspect the patient for coarse facial features suggestive of congenital hypothyroidism. Examine the skin for dryness or eczema. The abdomen should be inspected for distension and visible bulges. Palpate the abdomen for fecal masses. Examine the back specially the lumbosacral region for a nevus, lipoma, sinus, hairy patch, pit or dimple and scoliosis. Examine the lower limbs for deformities, tone, power and reflexes looking for signs of neuromuscular disorder.

Perianal examination is a crucial part of examining a child with chronic constipation. Inspect the perianal area for position of the anus, stool staining around the anus, fissures, ulcerations and scars. Digital rectal examination will assess the perianal sensation, anal tone, contraction and relaxation of the anal sphincter, size of the rectum and rectal stool masses. However, based on the National Institute of Health and Excellence (NICE) guidelines, rectal examination should only be performed by an experienced physician.[65]

Table 2.20 describes the important red flags on history and physical examination of a child with chronic constipation.

Investigations

Constipation is a clinical diagnosis; therefore, most cases do not require any work up. Investigating a child with chronic constipation should be guided by history and physical examination.

Blood Work-up

Usually it is not required but in a case of chronic and persistent constipation refractory to management, hypothyroidism and celiac disease need to be excluded by doing a thyroid function test and celiac serology respectively.

Imaging Studies

❑ Plain abdominal X-ray: This is not required to diagnose constipation. In functional constipation, this test is done in refractory cases only and not in all cases. It is a subjective investigation that differs between several observers.[66] Also, it was proved that this test is not well correlated with clinical symptoms of constipation.
❑ Transit studies: Radiopaque markers can be ingested and then followed by plain abdominal X-ray to measure colonic transit time. Delayed colonic transit time can even be seen in patients with functional constipation. However, this test is also not required in most cases.
❑ Ultrasound abdomen: This can be used to measure the rectal ampulla diameter in patients with overdistended rectum; however, it is only performed in refractory cases.

❑ Barium enema: It is usually performed for diagnosing Hirschsprung's disease in infants. However, most authorities prefer rectal biopsy to confirm the disease over barium enema.

Anorectal Manometry

This is not a pleasant test to do in children. Therefore, it is performed only for those with refractory symptoms to usual treatment. It is not required to diagnose Hirschsprung's disease. The presence of high amplitude propagating contractions (HAPCs) with the presence of gastrocolonic response indicates normal neuromuscular function.[67]

Rectal Biopsy

This test is performed to exclude Hirschsprung's disease in neonates and small infants who present with constipation. Full thickness biopsy from the dentate line to the rectum is recommended.[68] Based on NICE guidelines,[65] rectal biopsy should not be performed except in the following circumstances:
❑ Delayed passage of meconium more than 48 hours after birth in term babies.
❑ Constipation since first few weeks of life.
❑ Chronic abdominal distension plus vomiting.
❑ Family history of Hirschsprung's disease.
❑ Faltering growth in addition to any of the previous features.

Management

The management of a child with chronic constipation depends on the etiology of the problem. In a case of Hirschsprung's disease referral of the patient to a pediatric surgeon for surgical intervention is mandatory. Patients with medical problems such as hypothyroidism, celiac disease and cow's protein intolerance should be managed according to their specific illness.

The management of functional constipation is however challenging. It is a lengthy and sometimes disappointing and a boring process. The aim of management is:
❑ Remove the disimpaction.
❑ Maintain normal bowel habits without any problems.
❑ Enhance passage of stool in the appropriate place.

Management should involve four crucial steps as follows:
❑ Education
❑ Fecal impaction
❑ Maintenance therapy (Prevention of re-accumulation of colonic feces)
  • Laxatives
  • Dietary modifications
❑ Behavioral therapy.

Table 2.20: Red flags on history and examination of a child with constipation	
Red flags on history	Red flags on examination
Delayed passage of meconium	Coarse facial features
Difficulty in passing stool from birth	Lumbosacral area anomalies
Failure to thrive	Abnormal tone and power of lower limbs
Change of bowel habits following cow's protein introduction	Absent or brisk reflexes
Fatigue	Abnormal position of the anus
	Growth failure

Education

Both the child and parents should be informed that constipation is very common in normal children. The physician should explain the pathophysiology of constipation and fecal incontinence. The child should not be blamed for the soiling because this is an involuntary process. Reassure the parents that this problem is manageable but needs patience and cooperation from both parents and child. The parents should understand that in order to maintain normal habits, this may take weeks or even months of treatment. The school nurse as well teachers should be informed about the child's possible need to visit the toilet especially during the disimpaction treatment.

Rectal Disimpaction

Thirty percent of children with chronic constipation have rectal impaction that leads to fecal incontinence in the majority of those cases. This should be properly managed so as to clear the exit pathway of the colon and thus relieving rectal distension and fecal incontinence.[69] The process of disimpaction can be achieved by the following regime:

- ❑ Oral polyethylene glycol 3350 (PEG): PEG has been recommended as the first line therapy even in young children by NICE and North American Society of Pediatric Gastroenterology, Hepatology and Nutrition (NASPGHAN). A dose of 1–1.5 gm/kg/day is safe and effective in the treatment of impaction. The dose of PEG can be escalated over few days. PEG treatment for disimpaction should be given for 3–5 days but can be continued for 2 weeks.[70]
- ❑ If PEG is not tolerated, then a stimulant laxative (e.g. sodium picosulfate or senna) can be used either singly or in combination with an osmotic laxative (e.g. lactulose). Those laxatives can also be added to PEG if it was not effective in disimpacting the rectum after 2 weeks of therapy.[71,72]

Rectal Enema

Rectal enema was frequently used for disimpaction either singly or in combination with oral PEG. Based on the NICE guidelines, rectal enema should not be used to treat children with disimpaction. They should be used only when oral medications have failed. In addition, rectal enemas using sodium citrate or phosphate enemas should be used under medical supervision only. Manual disimpaction of the rectum should be abandoned in children.

The process of disimpaction can take more than 2 weeks. Overflow and soiling may worsen during this process, therefore, both the child and parents should be prepared for this event. It is preferable to start disimpaction treatment in a weekend to avoid the disturbance that might result. The patient should be reviewed after one week of starting treatment. A direct contact between a specialized nurse and the family can be established via phone calls or regular visits to ensure that guidelines have been properly implemented.

Treatment of the Perianal Area

Managing the perianal area is of utmost importance. Rectal disimpaction will be difficult to achieve if there is an existing fissure. Using a rectal enema on such chronically injured anus is an extremely painful and disturbing experience for the child. Therefore, topical lubricants containing an analgesic or local anesthetic plus steroid ointment should be applied to the perianal region during the disimpaction period.

Maintenance Therapy

Maintenance therapy should be started after the disimpaction process. This can also be achieved in the following way:

- ❑ Oral PEG in a smaller dose than the disimpaction treatment (half the dose).
- ❑ If PEG is not tolerated then substitute it with a stimulant laxative (Senna or biscodyl).
- ❑ An osmotic laxative (lactulose) can be added if stool is still hard.

Other Laxatives

Mineral oil and milk of magnesia (magnesium hydroxide) can be used in children for maintenance therapy. However, compared to PEG they are less.[73]

Probiotics

Probiotics was used to treat children with functional constipation but a systematic review reported that no conclusive evidence that it is effective in treating this problem.[74]

Maintenance therapy can take several months or even years. Do not discontinue maintenance therapy abruptly. This should be done gradually when the bowel movements are regular and normal. Continuous follow up and monitoring is mandatory. A specialist nurse can contact the family by phone twice per week at the start of treatment then once a week or biweekly. This process will reassure the parents and make them feel comfortable in dealing with this problem.

Dietary Modification

- A balanced diet and adequate fluids should be provided to the child with chronic constipation.
- High fiber diet is recommended such as fruits, vegetables, wholegrain cereals and high fiber bread. The American Academy of Pediatrics recommends the daily fiber intake in children to be 5 gm/day with maximum 35 gm.[75]
- Adequate fluid ingestion is also essential. The child should receive the recommended amount of fluids for the age.
- Cow's protein: Cow's protein-free diet can be tried in patients who are refractory to the usual management of chronic constipation.
- Give the parents a written recommendation about high fiber diet and excess fluids.

Behavioral Therapy

This can be achieved by:

- Toilet training with encouraging the child to visit the toilet 15–30 minutes following meals and stay for 5–10 minutes in the toilet. Regular toilet visits will eventually train the colon to move and a bowel movement will be passed.
- Use a footstool for younger children in the toilet to support their legs. This will aid in increasing intra-abdominal pressure (Valsalva maneuver) and hence eases defecation.
- A diary of stool frequency is helpful. This can be shown to the health specialist during regular follow-ups and used as a positive reinforcement.
- A reward system can be adopted specially if the child passed a bowel movement in the toilet or if his pants were clear of fecal material.
- Avoid punishing the child for soiling or inability to pass a bowel movement.
- Advice daily activities.

Sacral Neuromodulation

This can be achieved by percutaneous placement of an electrode in the third sacral foramen and implantation of a stimulating device under the skin in the buttocks.[76] This was found to be effective in patients with refractory constipation.

Surgery for Functional Constipation

In few cases, aggressive medical treatment fails hence surgery may be required specially in cases of slow colonic transit time. Anorectal manometry is required prior to subjecting the child to a surgical maneuver.[77] Surgical therapy may include the following:

- Antegrade continence enema through a cecostomy: This procedure can be beneficial but has got some complications such as leakage around the tube, dislodgment of the tube, skin infection and stoma stenosis.[78]
- Botulinum toxin injection: Intrasphincteric botulinum toxin injection has been used in treating patients with internal anal sphincter dysfunction with reported good effect.[79]
- Rectosigmoidectomy: This is performed for patients with dilated and hypomotile rectosigmoid. This procedure is prone for postoperative incontinence.[80]

Recurrence and relapses of constipation are common and can be managed with escalating the dose of laxatives.

Refer the patient with chronic constipation to a specialist or a pediatric gastroenterologist if the patient did not show improvement following three months of treatment.

GASTROINTESTINAL BLEEDING

Bleeding from the gastrointestinal tract (GIT)[81] can be divided into:

- Upper gastrointestinal (UGI) bleeding: Bleeding from a lesion in the GIT proximal to the ligament of Treitz.
- Lower gastrointestinal (LGI) bleeding: Bleeding from a lesion in the GIT distal to the ligament of Treitz.

Presentations of GIT Bleeding

- UGI bleeding:
  - Hematemesis: Vomiting blood that can be:
    - Bright red blood.
    - Coffee ground material indicating a change of blood color by gastric acid.
  - Melena: A dark colored tarry stool due to the effect of intestinal bacteria on the blood leading to oxidizing hemoglobin to hematin.[82,83]
- LGI bleeding:
  Hematochezia: Fresh or bright red blood evacuating from the anus.
  - It can either be mixed with stool or spontaneous and not related to stool.
  - Blood can also be seen on toilet paper.

Other Presentations

- Hematochezia can be a presentation of a massive UGI bleeding.

❑ Occult bleeding:
  • An invisible bleeding that can be detected by a specific test on the stool.
  • It can be a presentation of both UGI and LGI bleeding.
❑ Both UGI and LGI bleeds can either be painless or be associated with abdominal pain.

Causes of GI Bleeding

The etiology of GI bleeding varies with the age of the patient (Table 2.21); however, the causative disorders may overlap between different age groups.

Approach to a Child with GI Bleeding

❑ Determine the hemodynamic stability of the patient: If the bleeding is massive then the patient very likely presents in a state of shock or near shock which needs immediate attention and resuscitation.
❑ Decide if this is a true blood:
  • There are different food items and drugs that can color the vomitus or stool and easily be misinterpreted as blood.[84]
    – Hematemesis: Food coloring, colored gelatin, red candy beats, tomato skins and antibiotic syrup.
    – Melena: Bismuth, iron medicines, blueberries, grapes, spinach and licorice.
  • The guaiac test can detect blood in gastric aspirate, vomitus and stool. This will be described in the investigations section.
❑ Decide whether the child has an upper or a lower GI bleed: This is crucial because the etiology varies according to the presenting type of bleeding and hence the management.
  • UGI bleeding can present with hematemesis of fresh blood or coffee ground material. It can also present with melena and occasionally bright rectal bleeding when the rate of bleeding is massive. This is common to occur in infants and toddlers.
  • Lower GI bleed presents with bright rectal bleeding that can be isolated or mixed with stool. A proximal lower GI bleeding lesion can occasionally present with melena.
❑ Proceed with the following scheme of approach:
  • Obtain a detailed history
  • Perform a thorough physical examination
  • Investigate for the possible cause
  • Manage the bleeding lesion.

Upper GI Bleeding

History

As shown in Table 2.21, the etiology varies with age of the patient. Therefore, in interviewing parents or caregivers we

Table 2.21: Causes of gastrointestinal bleeding in children		
	Upper GI bleeding	*Lower GI bleeding*
Neonates	• Swallowed maternal blood • Gastritis • Vitamin K deficiency • Stress ulcer • Arteriovenous malformation • Sepsis/DIC • Bleeding diathesis	• Anal fissure • Necrotizing enterocolitis • Midgut volvulus • Hirschsprung's disease with enterocolitis • Lymphoid nodular hyperplasia • Vitamin K deficiency
Infants	• Gastritis • Reflux esophagitis • Mallory-Weiss tear • Peptic ulcer disease • Stress ulcer • Arteriovenous malformation	• Anal fissure • Infectious colitis • Intussusception • Cow's protein intolerance • Volvulus • Lymphoid nodular hyperplasia • Meckel's diverticulum • Arteriovenous malformation
Preschool aged children	• Swallowed blood from the nasopharynx • Gastritis • Reflux esophagitis • Mallory-Weiss tear • Stress ulcer • Peptic ulcer disease • Esophageal varices • Foreign body ingestion • Arteriovenous malformation	• Anal fissure • Infectious colitis • Juvenile polyp • Inflammatory bowel disease • NSAIDs • Meckel's diverticulum • Henoch-Schönlein purpura • Volvulus • Rectal prolapse • Solitary rectal ulcer • Hemolytic uremic syndrome • Lymphoid nodular hyperplasia • Arteriovenous malformation
Older children/ adolescents	• Swallowed blood from the nasopharynx • Gastritis • Peptic ulcer disease • Esophageal varices • Reflux esophagitis • Mallory-Weiss tear • Dieulafoy lesion • Hemobilia	• Infectious colitis • Juvenile polyp • Inflammatory bowel disease • NSAIDs • Meckel's diverticulum • Henoch-Schönlein purpura • Hemorrhoids • Solitary rectal ulcer • Intestinal ischemia • Arteriovenous malformation

should consider enquiring about certain problems that are related to the etiology in each particular age. Nevertheless, there are general points in history of a bleeding child that needs to be verified in all age groups.

Box 2.11 lists the essential points in history of a child presenting with UGI bleed.

BOX 2.11: Essential points in history of a child with upper GI bleeding

- Onset of hematemesis or melena
- Duration of bleeding
- Estimated volume of blood loss
- Associated symptoms:
  - Nausea
  - Abdominal pain
  - Heartburn/chest pain
  - Dysphagia
  - Irritability specially in neonates and infants
  - Poor feeding
  - Weight loss
- Bright rectal bleeding (in massive UGI bleed)
- History of previous similar attack
- History of upper respiratory tract infection (tonsillitis/ pharyngitis)
- History of epistaxis, dental work
- History of drug ingestion (NSAIDs, steroids, aspirin, warfarin)
- History of bleeding disorder (bruises)
- History of liver, heart or kidney diseases
- Family history:
  - Bleeding disorders
  - Liver problems

Other specific information on history is based on the etiology in each particular age:

Neonates

- Upper GI bleeding in neonates is uncommon but may occur due to different causes (Table 2.21).
- The most common cause is swallowed maternal blood which may occur at delivery or when the baby is breast fed via cracked mother's nipples. Those particular babies are well and active. By specific testing (Apt-Downey test) the blood can be differentiated between maternal and fetal origin.[85,86]
- Neonates are also liable to get vitamin K deficiency leading to bleeding (hemorrhagic disease of the newborn). This has to be verified on history if the patient has received vitamin K injection after birth or not.
- Sick neonates in the intensive care unit are liable to get stress erosions or ulcers leading to bleeding. Those include asphyxiated or septic newborns and those with multiorgan failures. Therefore, history of recent illnesses prior to the initiation of bleeding is important to verify.

- Bleeding disorders and coagulopathy can present with GI bleeding at any age including neonates. We should enquire about these problems in other family members.
- Vascular malformations of the GIT also, can present at any age including neonates. These can present with upper or lower GI bleeding that is abrupt and spontaneous without any associations.
- Congenital structural anomalies responsible for GI bleeding usually present in the neonatal period such as duplication cysts.

Infants

- Some of the causes in the neonatal period may also be seen in infants.
- Mallory-Weiss esophageal tear commonly occurs after repeated vomiting and this can be experienced in all ages. Therefore, enquire about the attack of hematemesis if was preceded by bouts or a forceful vomiting which may suggest Mallory-Weiss tear.
- History of upper respiratory infection with tonsillitis or pharyngitis can lead to hematemesis from swallowed blood. This also can be seen in all age groups. An attack of epistaxis to whatever reason can lead to swallowed blood.
- Infants are very liable to get gastroesophageal reflux disease complicated with esophagitis. Therefore, history of chronic vomiting after feeds or position is helpful. Irritability after feedings also can give a clue of pain caused by esophagitis.
- An infant with a recent history of viral illness is liable to get viral gastritis.
- History of drug ingestion such as non-steroidal anti-inflammatory drugs (NSAIDs) and steroids can lead to gastritis.
- Sick infants with sepsis, respiratory distress, multiorgan failure or trauma can develop stress erosions or ulcerations. The status and condition of the infant at the time of hematemesis will be verified on history.
- History of recurrent bleeding episodes especially in the mucous membranes and skin may suggest a bleeding disorder that can occur at this age also. Family history of bleeding disorders should be enquired about in these cases.

Preschool-aged Children

- Many of the causes of upper GI bleeding in infants are also seen in preschool-aged children; therefore, the same points in the history of those problems should be verified at this age.
- Foreign body ingestion is common at this age and should be suspected even if it was not witnessed.

❏ Peptic ulcer disease might also be seen at this age, hence associated epigastric pain should be asked about especially prior to meals. Enquire about family history of peptic ulcer disease since *Helicobacter pylori* which is responsible for the majority of those cases can easily be transmitted between family members.

❏ Esophageal varices caused by portal hypertension due to chronic liver disease can be seen in this age group and this problem can cause massive upper GI bleeding. History of liver disease such as jaundice, itching, edema or abdominal distension and surgery to the liver should be clarified. Some cases of esophageal varices can be due to extrahepatic portal hypertension without the existence of liver disease and in those cases history of prematurity with umbilical vein thrombosis should be verified. Also history of other episodes of thrombosis or even family history of thrombotic disorders should be enquired about.

Older Children/Adolescents

❏ Many of the causes in preschool-aged children may be encountered in older children and adolescents but with different frequencies.

❏ Drug intake or abuse is common in this category, therefore, history of drug ingestion is important.

Physical Examination

❏ The initial step in examining a child with UGI bleeding is assessing the hemodynamic stability. Therefore, examining the vital signs including pulse, blood pressure and capillary refill is crucial to determine whether the patient is in a state of shock or not. If the child is hemodynamically unstable then he/she have to be immediately resuscitated before proceeding to other evaluations.

❏ Following the assessment of the general wellbeing and vital signs one can look for the following:
  • Examine the nasopharynx looking for possible extraintestinal cause of bleeding.
  • Examine the skin for bruises, purpura, hemangiomas and telangiectasia.
  • Look for stigmata of chronic liver disease such as jaundice, clubbing, spider nevi and lower limb edema.
  • Examine the abdomen for tenderness, hepatosplenomegaly and ascites.

Investigations of UGI Bleeding

❏ The work up should be guided by findings on history and physical examination.

❏ In neonates, determine if the blood is of fetal or maternal origin by doing the Apt-Downy test. The baby's blood contains a high concentration of fetal hemoglobin that is resistant to alkali. Swallowed maternal blood contains adult hemoglobin that is denatured by alkali to hematin which has a brown-yellow color. If the supernatant remains pink after adding alkali then this confirms baby's blood and not swallowed maternal blood.[85,86]

Other Tests

❏ Blood work up:
  • Complete blood count (hemoglobin, hematocrit, platelet count)
  • Coagulation profile
  • Serum electrolytes
  • Liver function test (transaminases, bilirubin, serum albumin)
  • Renal function test
  • Blood type and cross match

❏ Stool for occult blood: This is done if there is a doubt of presence of blood especially in case of ingestion of drugs or foods that stain the stool. The Guaiac test kits are used to detect blood in stool and vomitus. Guaiac is a phenolic compound that gets oxidized by hydrogen peroxide in hemoglobin to quinine with a change in color. Some fruits and vegetables plus iron preparations give false-positive results with this test but new Guaiac kits use a buffered hydrogen peroxide limiting the false positivity.[87-89]

❏ Imaging tests: This will be guided by history and physical examination.
  • Plain X-ray: Plain X-ray of the neck, chest and abdomen should be done in toddlers who are suspected of ingesting a foreign body. However, radiolucent objects will not show on plain X-ray.
  • Ultrasound abdomen: This is performed when there is splenomegaly, hepatosplenomegaly or clinical evidence of cirrhosis. It will be combined with Doppler study to visualize the portal, intrahepatic, splenic and collateral veins at the portal hepatic suggestive of portal hypertension.
  • Upper GI contrast studies: These are not required in UGI bleeding because it will interfere with endoscopy or possible angiography.
  • Nuclear studies (Red blood cells scan): This procedure is required when UGI bleeding is massive, recurrent or obscure.
  • Angiography: This procedure is required when the bleeding is massive and the lesion could not be defined by endoscopy. Therapeutic intervention to control the bleeding can be performed at the same

setting when the bleeding lesion or vessel is defined. CT angiography is currently being used instead of angiography because it is less invasive although there is a lot of radiation exposure.

❑ Endoscopy: Endoscopy in a bleeding child should be performed after stabilizing the hemodynamic status of the patient. In addition, it should be done under general anesthesia to protect the airways. Therapeutic intervention can be performed at the same setting to manage the bleeding lesion.

Management of UGI Bleeding in Children (Flow chart 2.1)

❑ The first step in managing a child with UGI bleeding is stabilization of his hemodynamic status. Resuscitation may be required if the patient is in a state of shock.[90-92]

❑ Admit the patient to the intensive care unit if he is hemodynamically unstable or in case of massive bleeding. In a stable status admit the patient to the ward for close observation of vital signs.

❑ A large bore intravenous cannula should be inserted for intravenous infusion of colloid or blood. It is preferable to insert 2 intravenous lines in such patients especially if bleeding is massive. A central line access may be needed.

❑ Packed RBCs should be transfused if there was an acute drop of hemoglobin.

❑ If the patient presents with hematemesis and a bright rectal bleeding, this is most likely caused by a massive UGI bleeding lesion specially if there was no associated coagulopathy or a bleeding disorder. This patient should be managed as an UGI bleeding case.[91,92]

❑ The patient should be kept nil by mouth.

❑ Nasogastric tube with gastric lavage is sometimes required in cases of UGI bleeding to confirm that bleeding is from an upper GI lesion. Also to document if the bleeding is still active and persistent. Nevertheless, iced water lavage is no longer recommended.

❑ Acid suppression by using intravenous proton pump inhibitor is recommended.

❑ Patients who are known to have portal hypertension have to be commenced on somatostatin (Octreotide) to control the variceal bleeding. This can also be helpful to control nonvariceal bleeding. A bolus dose is 1 µg/kg intravenously followed by 1 µg/kg/hour intravenous infusion. The duration of therapy is not defined.[93]

❑ Endoscopy should be performed after active bleeding has settled in order to have a clear view of the UGI (within 24–48 hours). However, emergency endoscopy is necessary when the bleeding is persistent and life-threatening. The interventional therapeutic procedure via endoscopy depends on the pathogenic lesion causing the bleeding.[94-98]

Lower GI Bleeding

LGI bleeding presents with:
❑ Bright red rectal bleeding usually originating from the colon but can also be from the terminal ileum.
❑ Melena occasionally can be a presentation of a proximal small bowel bleeding lesion.

Causes of LGI Bleeding

❑ Table 2.22 shows the causes of LGI bleeding based on the age of the patient.[99,100]
❑ Table 2.22 shows causes of LGI bleeding based on the relation to the type of stool.
❑ Remember that a massive bleeding from a lesion in the UGI can lead to bright red rectal bleeding.

Approach to a Child with LGI Bleeding

❑ The first step is to determine whether the patient is hemodynamically stable or not. Does this patient require immediate attention and resuscitation? If the patient is unwell or unstable then he or she should be resuscitated and stabilized before proceeding to any other testing.

❑ The second step is to determine if the red color from the rectum is actually blood or a stained material. The occult blood (Guaiac test) done on the stool can be done at bed side to detect hemoglobin. Guaiac is a phenolic compound that gets oxidized by hydrogen peroxide in hemoglobin to quinine leading to a change in color. Ingestion of red meat, peroxidase-containing vegetables and iron supplements may give false-positive tests. Another test that is not affected by dietary items or drugs is the fecal hemoglobin test but this can be affected by intestinal bacteria and hence not very reliable as the Guaiac test.

❑ Then proceed with the same approach scheme followed in UGI bleeding:
  • Obtain a detailed history
  • Perform a thorough physical examination
  • Investigate for the possible cause
  • Manage the bleeding lesion.

History

A detailed history about the bleeding episode should be enquired about. Box 2.12 lists some of the important points in history of a patient with LGI bleeding.

Specific questions regarding different disorders causing LGI bleeding listed in Table 2.22 should be addressed.

Flow chart 2.1: Schematic approach of management of UGI bleeding

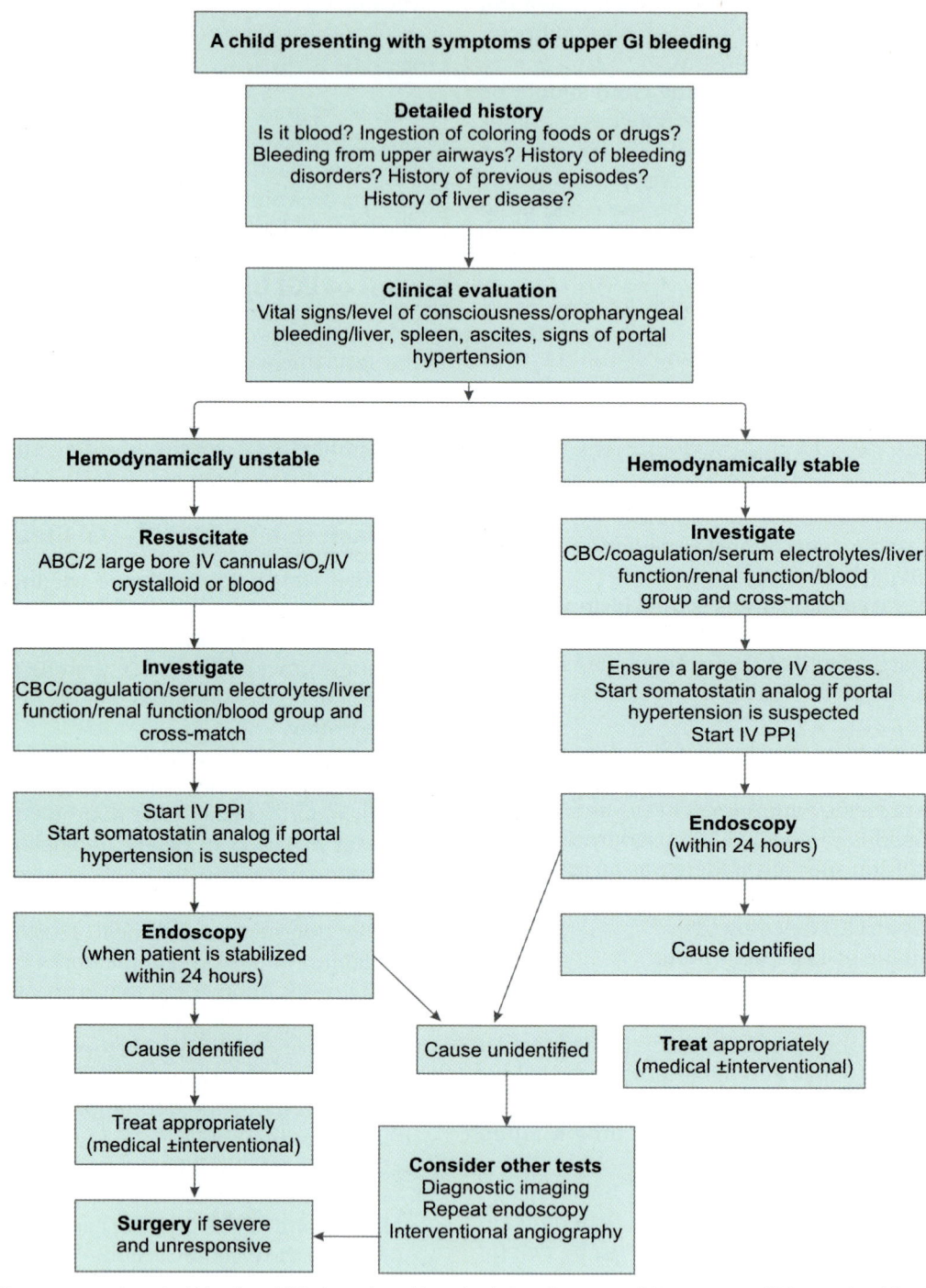

Abbreviations: UGI, upper gastrointestinal bleeding; ABC, airway, breathing, circulation; O₂, oxygen; IV, intravenous; CBC, complete blood count; PPI, proton pump inhibitor.

❑ An ill appearing neonate with LGI bleeding should be suspected to have bowel ischemia due to volvulus. If blood is mixed with loose stool in a premature baby then necrotizing enterocolitis is highly likely. History of delayed passage of meconium associated with abdominal distension and bloody diarrhea is suspicious of Hirschsprung's disease. Neonates can also develop an anal fissure leading to rectal bleeding. Anal fissure is a common cause of LGI bleeding in all age groups.

❑ A sudden attack of LGI bleeding in an infant should alert the physician towards intestinal ischemia associated with intussusception and mid-gut volvulus specially in

Table 2.22: Causes of lower GI bleeding based on the type of stool

Rectal bleeding with normal stool	Rectal bleeding with diarrhea	Rectal bleeding with hard stool
• Juvenile polyp • Vascular malformation • Meckel's diverticulum • Cow's protein intolerance • NSAIDs • Henoch-Schönlein purpura • Nodular lymphoid hyperplasia	• Infectious colitis • Necrotizing enterocolitis • Inflammatory bowel disease • Cow's protein intolerance • Hemolytic uremic syndrome • Hirschsprung's enterocolitis	• Anal fissure • Rectal prolapse • Solitary rectal ulcer • Hemorrhoids

Abbreviation: NSAIDs: nonsteroidal anti-inflammatory drugs.

BOX 2.12: History of a patient with lower GI bleeding

- Onset of bleeding
- Color of blood
- Duration of bleeding
- Estimated amount of blood loss
- Relation of bleeding to stool
  - Mixed with stool
  - On top of stool
  - On toilet paper
  - No relation to stool
- Consistency of stool
- Perianal pain
- Associated symptoms:
  - Abdominal pain
  - Irritability (neonates/infants)
  - Vomiting
  - Fever
  - Weight loss/Growth deceleration
- History of previous episodes
- History of drug ingestion (NSAIDs, anticoagulants)
- History of bleeding disorder
- History of liver, heart disease
- Family history:
  - Bleeding disorder
  - Familial polyposis
  - Liver disease

---

case of an ill looking infant. History of red currant jelly stool in a colicky infant is suggestive of intussusception. History of diarrhea with or without vomiting suspects gastroenteritis and infective colitis. Cow's protein intolerance commonly presents in infants. History of changing the formula from breast milk to formula prior to bleeding is suggestive of this diagnosis.[101] This can be associated with normal or loose stool and usually the infant is well and growing.

- History of spontaneous painless rectal bleeding in a preschool child is most likely due to a juvenile polyp.[102] An acute attack of rectal bleeding associated with diarrhea may be caused by infectious colitis, inflammatory bowel disease and hemolytic uremic syndrome. These may be associated with abdominal pain, fever, vomiting and weight loss. History of tenesmus is suggestive of distal colitis. In cases of hemolytic uremic syndrome there will be associated decreased urine output and anuria.
- Henoch-Schönlein purpura is relatively common in young children and may present with rectal bleeding associated with abdominal pain, purpuric rash and possible hematuria.
- Patients with chronic constipation may present with LGI bleeding caused by anal fissure as well as rectal prolapse that is mistaken for a rectal polyp.
- Lymphoid nodular hyperplasia can be a cause of rectal bleeding in infants and young children with no associated other symptoms.
- Meckel's diverticulum can present with painless rectal bleeding in children. It results from incomplete obliteration of the omphalomesenteric duct. Bleeding results from ulceration of the ectopic gastric mucosa.[103]
- Older children and adolescents who suffer from chronic constipation are liable to get hemorrhoids such as those seen in adults. These can cause painful rectal bleeding with normal or hard bowel movements.

Physical Examination

- The first step is to assess the hemodynamic stability of the patient; therefore, the vital signs have to be assessed.
- Resuscitate the child if he/she is in shock or instability
- Determine if the bleeding is from UGI or LGI especially in a case of massive bright red rectal bleeding by lavaging the stomach through a nasogastric tube. If the lavage was clear then this is most likely a LGI bleeding.
- Assess the growth parameters of the patient.
- Examine the skin for purpura or bruises.
- Asses for signs of liver cirrhosis and portal hypertension (jaundice, clubbing, lower limb edema, spider nevi).
- Examine for signs of atopy (eczema, chest wheezes).
- Examine the abdomen for distension, tenderness, hepatomegaly, splenomegaly, masses, ascites and bowel sounds.
- Examine the perianal area for fissures, fistulas and abscesses.
- Witness the rectal bleed and inspect the color and amount of blood.
- Inspect the stool for consistency and association to rectal bleeding.

Evaluation of LGI Bleeding

Evaluating a child with rectal bleeding should be guided by history and physical examination.[104,106]

- ❏ Blood work up:
  - Complete blood count
  - Coagulation profile
  - Serum electrolytes
  - Liver function test
  - Renal function test
  - Blood type and cross-match
- ❏ Stool work up:
  - Occult blood if blood was not clearly evident.
  - Stool microscopy for white blood cells, red blood cells, ova and parasites.
  - Stool culture in case of bloody diarrhea.
  - Stool for *Clostridium difficle* toxin in case of bloody diarrhea, inflammatory bowel disease or immunosuppressed.[105]
- ❏ Imaging:
  - Plain abdominal X-ray: This is essential in premature babies with abdominal distension, vomiting and rectal bleeding. Plain abdominal X-ray can be diagnostic for necrotizing enterocolitis in these babies. Signs of bowel obstruction can be seen on plain abdominal X-ray in neonates and young infants with volvulus. Those signs may also be seen in infants with intussusception.[107]
  - Ultrasound abdomen: This imaging technique is diagnostic of intussusception in infants presenting with colicky pain and rectal bleeding. It is better than plain X-ray in diagnosing intussusception. Duplication cysts can be visualized by ultrasound. Also, abnormal liver parenchyma suggestive of cirrhosis with visible collateral vessels around the porta hepatis and ciliac axis by ultrasound Doppler can aid in diagnosing portal hypertension. Ultrasound is being used in some centers to help in diagnosing Crohn's small bowel disease by measuring the thickness of the affected small bowel loops.
  - Contrast studies: Some cases of malrotation with volvulus can be diagnosed by a barium study. Intussusception used to be diagnosed by barium enema. This is currently replaced by ultrasound abdomen and air enema which is also used as a therapeutic modality to relieve intussusception. Barium follow through was widely used to study the extent of small bowel disease in Crohn's disease but this is replaced by MRI imaging in many centers.[108]
  - CT abdomen: This is performed in a minority of cases who are suspected to have masses or duplication cysts. CT angiography is currently being used to visualize bleeding vessels.[109]
- MRI: This can be helpful in some cases of inflammatory bowel disease who present with a bleeding inflamed mucosa in the small intestine that is beyond the reach of colonoscopy. MRI enterolysis can detect inflamed thick bowel loops.
- Nuclear scan:
  - ^{99m}technetium isotope scan be performed to diagnose Meckel's diverticulum that can present with rectal bright red bleeding or melena. Meckel's diverticulum bleeds from the ectopic gastric mucosa that uptakes the ^{99m}technetium isotope. Small intestinal duplication cysts can occasionally be diagnosed with the same test because it may also contain ectopic gastric mucosa.
  - Red blood scan can be performed in cases of obscured rectal bleeding but it needs a massive bleeding rate to be positive.
- Angiography: This is an invasive procedure; therefore, it is required in cases of obscure massive bleeding. A therapeutic intervention can also be performed at the same setting to stop the bleeding vessel. CT angiography is currently being adopted because it is less invasive than the usual angiography.
- Sigmoidoscopy/colonoscopy: Lower GI endoscopy is usually recommended in cases of recurrent or persistent bleeding with or without diarrhea. Juvenile polyps are common lesions causing painless rectal bleeding in children. A full colonoscopy is preferred on sigmoidoscopy because in some patients the polyps may be multiple. Colonoscopy is also helpful to diagnose inflammatory bowel disease in a patient with rectal bleeding and diarrhea. Solitary rectal ulcer can be seen on proctoscopy or a short sigmoidoscopy.[110]
- Upper GI endoscopy: This may be required in a case suspected of having massive upper GI bleeding leading to a rectal bleed such as in esophageal varices. Both colonoscopy and endoscopy are used as diagnostic as well as therapeutic modalities.[111]
- Enteroscopy: This kind of endoscopy may be required when the suspected bleeding lesion is within the small intestine and could not be seen on endoscopy and colonoscopy. There are different types of enteroscopy (push, double balloon and helical enteroscopy). This procedure is mainly used in adults but is recently being utilized in children as well.
- Wireless capsule endoscopy: This investigation can be performed in patients with obscured rectal bleeding when other previous scopes failed to reveal the bleeding lesion.[112] However, in case of a defined pathology on this test no therapeutic intervention is possible at the setting.

- Laparoscopy/laparotomy:
  - This is the last procedure to be performed if all other tests failed to show the persistently bleeding lesion.
  - Intraoperative enteroscopy can also be performed when both the surgeon and the gastroenterologist team together to scope and visualize the small intestinal mucosa.

Management of LGI Bleed (Flow chart 2.2)

- ❏ Supportive care:
  - The first step in managing a child with GI bleeding is stabilizing his hemodynamic status regardless of the site of bleeding.
  - Resussuscitate the patient if in shock or near shock by initially infusing a crystalloid (normal saline/

Flow chart 2.2: Schematic approach of management of LGI bleeding

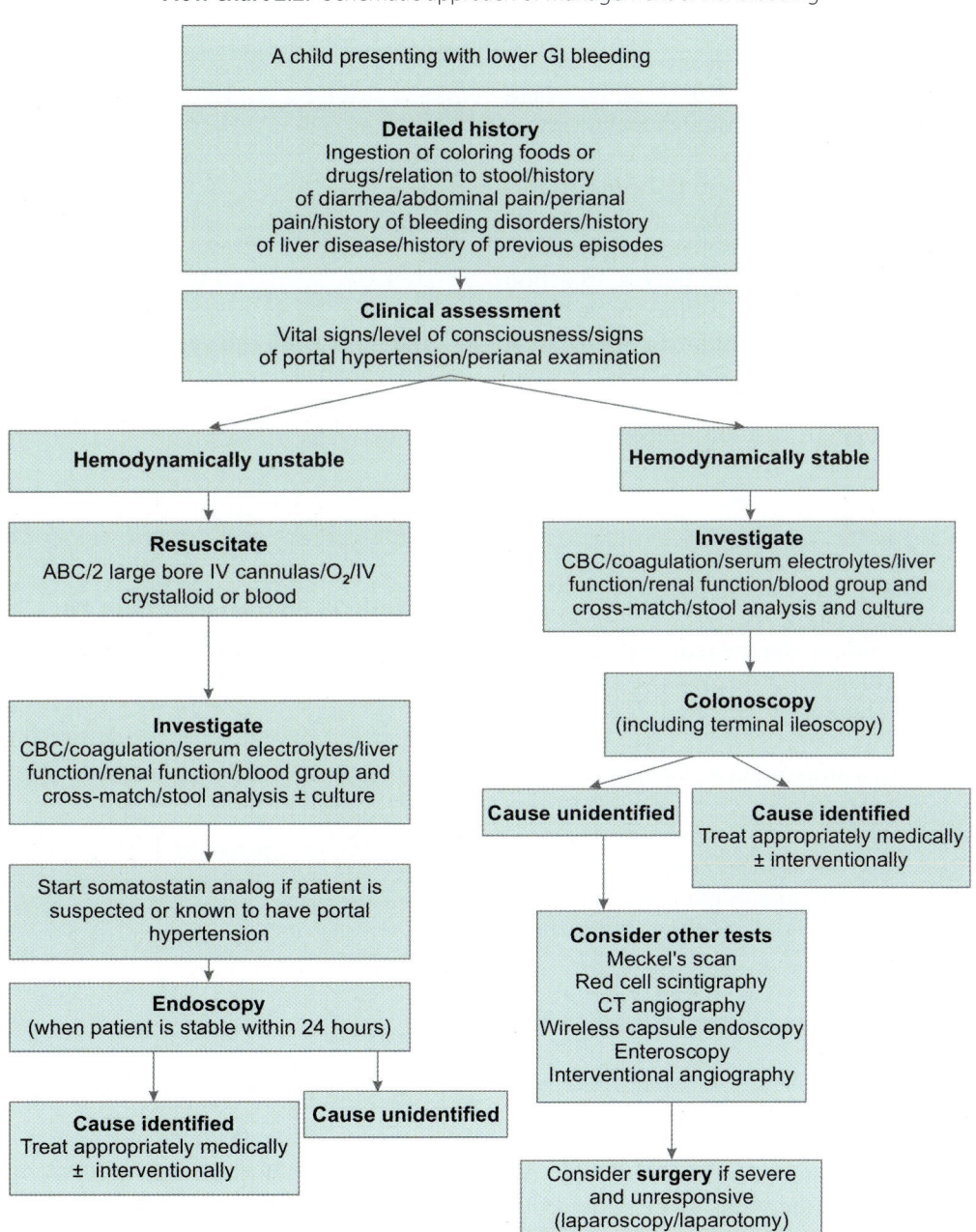

Abbreviations: LGI, lower gastrointestinal bleeding; ABC, airway, breathing, circulation; O₂, Oxygen; IV, intravenous; CBC, complete blood count.

Ringer lactate) then a colloid solution or blood when available.

- Correct coagulopathy if present by transfusing fresh frozen plasma and intravenous vitamin K in a case of liver disease.
- Platelet transfusion can be given if platelet count is low.

❑ Acid suppression: This has been shown to be effective in both adults and children. H_2 receptor antagonists (Ranitidine) or proton pump inhibitor (PPI) can be given intravenously. GI bleeding is a stressful condition that by it may precipitate stress ulcers.

❑ Somatostatin/octreotide: This can be given in a case of portal hypertension who presents with rectal bleeding. Such patients may have small intestinal or rectal varices as well.[93]

❑ Clonoscopic/endoscopy intervention: If the lesion was visualized through colonoscopy then a therapeutic procedure should be intervened based on the pathology found. Polypectomy is performed for polyps. Injection of epinephrine 1:10000 diluted in saline in case of a bleeding ulcer and this may be followed by thermal coagulation. Telengiectatic and angiodysplastic lesions can be managed via colonoscopy as well.[113]

❑ Interventional radiology: In case of a bleeding vessel discovered on angiography, then embolization can be performed.

❑ Surgery:
- This is required for certain pathologies such as some cases of intussusception, malrotation with volvulus and Meckel's diverticulum.
- Resection of a bowel loop may be required in cases of uncontrolled bleeding.

❑ Specific treatment should be directed towards the cause:
- A patient with cow's protein intolerance needs to be put on a hydrolyzed formula.
- Treat the perianal fissure by lubricating the anal mucosa. Also, applying a local topical anesthetic and steroids to the anal area might help. Managing constipation is very crucial during the treatment of anal fissure.
- Rectal prolapse and solitary rectal ulcer should be managed with laxatives and if due to diarrhea then this should be controlled.
- Inflammatory bowel disease is managed with 5-aminosalicylic acid products (5-ASA), local/systemic steroids and possibly antibiotics.
- Treatment of bowel infection depends on the causative organism and the status of the patient.

ABDOMINAL DISTENSION

Definition

❑ Abdominal distension: Visible or measureable increase in abdominal girth.
❑ Abdominal bloating: An individual's sensation of abdominal fullness.

General Causes of Abdominal Distension

Refer Table 2.23.

Table 2.23: General causes of abdominal distension	
Factor	Cause
Fat	Obesity
Flatus	Bloating, intestinal obstruction or pseudo-obstruction
Feces	Chronic constipation
Fluid	Ascites, tumors (especially cystic), distended bladder
Fetus	Pregnancy

The most common causes of abdominal distension in children are listed in Box 2.13.

BOX 2.13: Common causes of abdominal distension in children
• Gaseous distension • Ascites • Organomegaly • Intra-abdominal tumors

Abdominal Distension Due to Gaseous Distension

Composition of Intestinal Gas (Box 2.14)

Nitrogen (N_2), oxygen (O_2), carbon dioxide (CO_2), hydrogen (H_2), and methane (CH_4) account for more that 99% of expelled intestinal gas.[114,115]

BOX 2.14: Sources of intestinal gas
• Swallowed air. • Intraluminal production (chemical reactions and bacterial metabolism). • Diffusion of gases into the lumen from the bloodstream.

Causes of Excessive Gaseous Distension

❑ Excessive air swallowing:
- This is the major cause of stomach air and mostly composed of N_2. Air is introduced into the stomach

with each normal swallow and increases when food is swallowed. Certain items like chewing gum increases air ingestion.

- Crying can also lead to excessive air swallowing which makes abdominal distension more evident.
- Aerophagia is swallowing air but it is usually caused by psychological factors mainly anxiety (Box 2.15).
  - Patients with aerophagia tend to develop belching as a major symptom together with abdominal distension and probably abdominal pain.

BOX 2.15: Diagnosis of aerophagia

Diagnosis of aerophagia based on Rome III criteria
It must include at least two of the following:
- Air swallowing.
- Abdominal distension because of intraluminal air.
- Repetitive belching and/or increased flatus.
Criteria fulfilled at least once per week for at least 2 months before diagnosis.

❑ Excessive intraluminal gas production:
- Three gases are produced in the intestinal lumen, CO_2, H_2 and Methane (CH_4).
- CO_2 is produced in the upper GI from digestion of fat and protein but can be liberated from bacterial fermentation of undigested carbohydrates in the colon.[116]
- H_2 is produced mainly in the colon by the effect of gut flora on carbohydrates. Therefore, it is produced excessively in the following cases:
  - Carbohydrate malabsorption (lactose and fructose). If lactose or fructose was not properly digested they will reach the colon intact and hence get fermented by gut bacteria liberating excessive H_2.[117,118]
  - Excessive intake of high concentrations of some vegetables (legumes and beans), flour made of wheat, oats, potatoes and corn. Those items contain high concentrations of oligosaccharides which are not properly digested by gut enzymes hence become a substrate for the colonic bacterial fermentation.
  - Bacterial overgrowth can lead to excessive gas production due to malabsorption. This occurs in short bowel syndrome and diseased colon.
- CH_4 is produced in the colon as well by the effect of bacteria. Its production is excessive if the colon is diseased like in a case of colonic carcinoma.[119]
❑ Inappropriate gas absorption due to bowel obstruction.
❑ Impaired transit of intestinal gas such as what occurs in irritable bowel disease leading to gas retention and functional bloating.[120]

❑ Expansion of intraluminal gas due to changes in the atmospheric pressure between the blood and intestinal lumen. This means that there will be too much gas in the intestinal lumen that is not effectively absorbed into the bloodstream.

Causes of gaseous distension are described in Table 2.24.

Abdominal Distension Due to Ascites

It is a common cause of abdominal distension in children. There are a variety of causes leading to ascites (Table 2.25).

Abdominal Distension Caused by Organomegaly

❑ Organomegaly is also a common cause of abdominal distension especially in young children when the abdominal musculature is soft and nontense (Table 2.26).

Abdominal Distension Caused by Intra-abdominal Tumors

❑ Intra-abdominal tumors may present with abdominal distension in infants and young children.
❑ Tumors can arise from the abdominal wall, intraperitoneal or extraperitoneal organs.
❑ They can either be cystic or solid masses.
❑ They can be benign or malignant lesions.

Table 2.24: Causes of abdominal distension due to excessive gas	
Intestinal obstruction (partial or complete)	• Hirschsprung's disease • Imperforate anus • Malrotation and volvulus • Intussusception • Intestinal atresia/stenosis • Sigmoid or cecal volvulus • Duplication cysts
Motility disorder	• Intestinal pseudo-obstruction • Diabetes • Drugs • Hypothyroidism • Electrolyte abnormalities (ileus)
Malabsorption	• Celiac disease • Lactose intolerance • Fructose intolerance • Pancreatic insufficiency
Irritable bowel disease	Functional bloating
Infection	• Giardiasis • Bacterial overgrowth • Sepsis associated with ileus
Psychological	Aerophagia

Table 2.25: Causes of abdominal distension due to ascites	
Congenital/ metabolic disease	Nonimmune hydrops fetalis
Liver disease	• Cirrhosis of the liver • Hepatic vein occlusion (Budd-Chiari syndrome)
GI disease	• Protein losing enteropathy • Pancreatitis
Cardiac disease	• Cardiac failure • Right heart obstructive lesions
Kidney disease	• Chronic renal failure • Acute glomerulonephritis • Nephrotic syndrome • Perforation of ureter, renal pelvis or bladder in neonates
Nutritional	Protein deficiency (kwashiorkor)
Lymphatic obstruction (chylous ascites)	• Primary obstruction (lymphangiectasia) • Secondary obstruction (mesenteric cyst) • Surgical ligation of lymphatic ducts
Infection	Acute peritonitis

Table 2.26: Organomegaly causing abdominal distension	
Hepatomegaly	• Cirrhosis of the liver • Malignancy (hepatoblastoma, HCC) • Hemochromatosis • Storage disease (glycogen, lipid, mucoploysaccharidosis)
Splenomegaly	• Chronic hemolytic anemia • Portal hypertension (hepatic/ extrahepatic) • Malignancy (leukemia) • Infection (malaria, viral infections)
Hepatosplenomegaly	• Storage disorders • Liver cirrhosis • Chronic hemolytic anemia • Infection (EBV, HIV) • Connective tissue disorders (Still's disease) • Malignancy (leukemia)
Enlarged kidney	• Hydronephrosis • Malignancy (Wilm's tumor)

Abbreviation: HCC, hepatocellular carcinoma.

❑ Most of the tumors present with a palpable mass on abdominal examination but some can present with abdominal distension especially in young children.
❑ Table 2.27 describes possible intra-abdominal tumors.[121]
❑ Intra-abdominal cystic masses can originate from solid organs such as the liver, spleen, and pancreas and also

Table 2.27: Intra-abdominal solid tumors causing abdominal distension	
Organ/site	Tumor
Stomach	• Teratoma • Lipoma • Adenocarcinoma • Leiomayoma • Leiomyosarcoma • Rabdomyosarcoma
Small intestine	• Lymphoma • Leiomyoma • Leiomyosarcoma
Large intestine	• Colorectal carcinoma • Leiomyoma • Leiomyosarcoma
Pancreas	• Adenoma • Endocrine tumors • Adenocarcinoma • Inflammatory myofibroblastic tumor
Liver	• Hepatoblastoma • Hepatocellular carcinoma
Biliary tree	• Rabdomyosarcoma • Cholangiocarcinoma
Kidney	Wilm's tumor
Adrenal	Neuroblastoma
Ovary	Ovarian germ cell tumor

from the retroperitoneum, omentum, and mesentery (Table 2.28).
❑ They can be classified based on the histopathologic features as: (1) Cysts of lymphatic origin (lymphatic and lymphangiomas). (2) Cysts of mesothelial origin (benign or malignant mesothelial cysts). (3) Enteric cysts. (4) Cysts of urogenital origin. (5) Dermoid cysts. (6) Pseudocysts (infectious or traumatic etiology).[122,123]
❑ Cerebrospinal fluid (CSF) abdominal pseudocyst is an uncommon but important complication of ventriculoperitoneal shunts (VP). It can present with abdominal distension and pain.[124] Infection is most likely the cause. This can be managed with antibiotics; cyst aspiration and a new VP shunt insertion. The retroperitoneal and mesenteric masses are usually benign but can invade other organs when they are very large.

Abdominal Distension Due to Abdominal Wall Problems

❑ Abdominal wall tumors: These are rare in children.
❑ Abdominal wall hernias: These are relatively common especially after a surgical procedure producing a defect

Table 2.28: Cystic masses in children presenting as abdominal distension

Tumor	Organ/site
Hemangioma/Hemangioendothelioma	Liver
Hamartoma (mesenchymal)	Liver
Choledochal cyst	Biliary tree
Lymphangioma	• Mesocolon • Omentum • Retroperitoneum
Duplication cyst	• Duodenum • Ileum
Pseudocyst	Pancreas
Meconium pseudocyst	Small intestine (cystic fibrosis)
Congenital pancreatic cyst	Pancreas
Cystic teratoma	Gonads Sacrococcygeal area
Cystic disease of the kidney	Kidneys
Hydronephrosis	Kidneys
Ovarian cysts	Ovaries
Paraovarian/paratubal cysts	Fallopian tubes
Hematometrocolpos	Uterus
Urachal cyst	Urachus
Hydatid cyst	Liver
Abdominal cerebrospinal pseudocyst	Intraperitoneum (patient with ventriculoperitoneal shunt)

in the abdominal musculature and hence abdominal distension due to bowel protrusion.

Approach to a Child with Abdominal Distension

History and physical examination are important tools in approaching a child with abdominal distension.

History

❑ Age of the child
❑ Time of onset (acute/chronic)
❑ Progressing or stable
❑ Associated symptoms:
  • Breathing problems
  • Vomiting
  • Diarrhea
  • Constipation
  • Abdominal pain
  • Irritability in young infants
  • Loss of appetite
  • Fever
  • GI bleeding
  • Jaundice
  • Failure to thrive
  • Decreased activity
  • Urinary problems
❑ History of known organic disease (liver/kidney/heart/blood disorder/storage disease)
❑ Antenatal history (polyhydramnios/fetal abdominal distension in utero)
❑ Family history of storage disease/blood disorder/liver disease/kidney disease).

Examination

❑ The first step in physical examination is to assess the wellbeing of the child. Decide whether the patient is well or ill. A patient with abdominal distension caused by bowel obstruction is usually unwell, irritable or lethargic.
❑ Examination of the vital signs is crucial including, heart rate, respiratory rate, temperature and blood pressure. Abdominal distension commonly causes respiratory distress by pressure effect on the diaphragm compromising the lung volume. Therefore, the patient might present with tachypnea, tachycardia and even cyanosis.
❑ Check the oxygen saturation.
❑ Check for pallor and jaundice.
❑ Check for signs of dehydration (enteropathy/bowel obstruction).
❑ Measure growth parameters and plot them on the growth chart.
❑ Look for signs of dysmorphism in the face, head, trunk or limbs.
❑ Inspect the skin for signs of chronic liver disease (spider nevi and telengiectasias) and purpuric lesions (liver disease/leukemia).
❑ Look for clubbing (liver disease/malabsorption)
❑ Examine for signs of nutritional deficiencies specially vitamins (A, B, C, D, E) and trace elements (iron, zinc)
❑ Examine the chest for adventitious sounds (cystic fibrosis/immunodeficiency) and check for signs of pleural effusion (anasarca).
❑ Examine the cardiovascular system for heart sounds, murmurs and signs of heart failure.
❑ Abdominal examination: Examination of the abdomen is important to confirm the distension and assess the possible cause. Therefore, the following should be undertaken on examining the abdomen:
  • Measure the abdominal girth
  • Inspect for the degree of distension, surgical scars, symmetry of the flanks, localized bulge, caput medusae, visible dilated veins, protrusion of the umbilicus and erythema of the abdominal wall skin.

- Assess for abdominal wall defects by changing the patient's position and assessing the effect on the distension especially in the presence of a surgical scar. Some infants have got weak or absent abdominal wall musculature leading to abdominal distension from intra-abdominal organs mainly the bowel (Prune-Belly syndrome).
- Palpate the abdomen for tenderness, hepatosplenomegaly, kidneys and other masses.
- Percuss the abdomen to decide whether the distension is due to gas, fluid or masses. Assessing for shifting dullness and fluid thrill is helpful in case of ascites.
- Listen via a stethoscope to the bowel sounds and bruit on the liver (hemangioma/hemangioendothelioma).
- Inspect the inguinal orifices for obstructed hernias leading to bowel obstruction and gaseous distension.
- Examine the scrotum in boys for scrotal edema (hypoalbuminemia/kidney disease).
- Examine the perianal area especially in neonates for imperforate anus and older children for perianal disease associated with inflammatory enteropathy.
- Examine for developmental delay (storage disorders).
- Examine the central nervous system for abnormal movements, cranial nerve abnormalities, tone, power and reflexes.
- Examine the lower limbs for lower limb edema and the back for sacral edema if ascites was suspected.

Investigations

The investigations are usually guided by history, physical examination and type of distension.

In a Case of Ascites

- Check serum albumin and total protein. If serum albumin is low, this means that protein is lost or is not produced.
- Check the urine for protein loss:
  - If protein loss in the urine is excessive then the problem is due to a renal etiology and the patient should be referred to a nephrologist.
  - If urine is negative for protein:
    - Protein is lost through the bowel (protein losing enteropathy).
    - Protein is not produced by the liver (liver cirrhosis).
    - Protein intake is not adequate (nutritional deficiency).

- Check for liver function test including bilirubin, transaminases, serum glucose and coagulation profile (INR).
- Check serum electrolytes and renal profile (urea/creatinine).
- Alpha-fetoprotein in a case of cirrhosis for the possibility of hepatocellular carcinoma.
- Investigate for causes of cirrhosis if liver function is deranged.
- If the patient has got chronic diarrhea without an evidence of liver disease then the ascites is most likely caused by protein-losing enteropathy. In this condition, investigations should be directed towards causes of malabsorption.
  - Elevated fecal alpha-1 antitrypsin in the stool indicates protein loss via the intestine.
- Serum amylase and lipase are indicated if history includes attacks of abdominal pain suggesting the possibility of pancreatitis and pancreatic ascites.
- Reduced fecal elastase can be an indication of pancreatic disease as in cystic fibrosis or chronic pancreatic disease.
- Vitamins and trace elements' levels are indicated if history is suggestive of nutritional deficiency. Those levels are also disturbed in malabsorption and chronic liver disease.
- Blood culture should be collected in a patient with ascites associated with abdominal tenderness and fever since peritonitis is common in these patients.
- Imaging:
  - Ultrasound abdomen:
    - To confirm ascites, assess liver parenchyma, biliary system, spleen, pancreas, kidneys and intra-abdominal masses.
    - Ultrasound Doppler may be required to assess the portal vein flow, collateral veins, hepatic veins and splenic vein in a case of portal hypertension.
  - Computed tomography (CT) or magnetic resonance imaging (MRI):
    - Required if a focal liver mass is seen on ultrasound.
    - If pancreatic disease is suspected.
- Echocardiography:
  - In a patient with cardiac failure.
  - In constrictive pericarditis.
- Tapping the ascitic fluid:
  - This is indicated in the following situations:
    - Suspected peritonitis for culturing the ascetic fluid.
    - Massive abdominal distension to relieve the respiratory compromise.
    - Suspected pancreatic ascites to check ascetic amylase and lipase.

- Suspected chylous ascites especially in a patient with lymphangiectasia or post intra-abdominal surgery.
  - Suspected perforated ureter or renal pelvis in a neonate. This is suspected when ascetic fluid creatinine is elevated.
- The ascetic fluid assessment should include red blood cells, white blood cells, differential white blood cells, glucose, albumin, bilirubin, triglycerides, amylase and lipase. Also ascetic fluid culture is crucial.

Investigations of Abdominal Distension Due to Organomegaly

Investigate for causes of the enlarged organ (hepatosplenomegaly/kidneys).

Investigations of Abdominal Distension Caused by an Intra-abdominal Mass

- Plain abdominal X-ray: Indicated only if there were signs of bowel obstruction.
- Ultrasound abdomen and pelvis:
  - This is the most common imaging modality used in a case of intra-abdominal mass.
  - It is useful to differentiate between solid and cystic masses.
  - Metastatic masses in the liver or other parts of the abdomen could also be visualized.
  - It can visualize minimal ascetic fluid.
  - Intra-abdominal lymph nodes can be seen on ultrasound (para-aortic, mesenteric and porta hepatis).[125]
  - This modality can be affected by bowel gas and it is an operator dependent.
- CT abdomen and pelvis:
  - Should be done with oral and intravenous contrasts.
  - Should be done in arterial, portal venous and delayed phases.
  - Not affected by bowel gas and is not operator dependent.
- MRI:
  - Can be effective in detecting intra-abdominal and pelvic tumors.
  - Contraindicated in patients with magnetic implants.
- Radio-isotope scan:
  - This imaging modality is usually used when other modalities show equivocal results.
  - It can also be useful in detecting metastases.
- Contrast studies: This imaging is not widely used. They can be performed in few cases with gastrointestinal tract involvement using barium follow through and enema.

- Aspiration biopsy for histopathology: This depends on the type and site of the mass.

Investigations of Abdominal Distension Caused by Gaseous Distension

- The initial step in a child with gaseous abdominal distension is to decide whether he/she has got bowel obstruction or not.
- Plain abdominal X-ray:
  - Look for signs of bowel obstruction (dilated bowel loops, paucity of gas in the distal bowel, air fluid levels and free air in the abdomen).
  - In a case of a neonate look for pneumatosis intestinalis (gas in the bowel wall) suggesting enterocolitis.
- Ultrasound abdomen:
  - This is required when intussusception is suspected.
  - It can also show free fluid in the abdomen.
  - This technique can be misled by excessive intraluminal gas.
  - It is observer dependent.
- CT enteroclysis: This modality is helpful in cases with partial or incomplete small bowel obstruction. It involves the utilization of positive (dilute iodinated contrast) or neutral enteric contrast using water or dilute barium in addition to intravenous contrast.[126]
- Barium or water-soluble enema: Required in a suspected case of intussusception or Hirschsprung's disease.
- Suction rectal biopsy: In suspected Hirschsprung's disease.
- Breath test:
  - H_2 that is produced in the gut lumen is partly excreted into stool but mainly is absorbed from the gut into the blood and then excreted via the lungs. This is the rationale behind the breath test.[127]
  - Hydrogen breath test can be used to diagnose gaseous distension caused by lactose intolerance using lactose as a substrate.
  - It can also be used to diagnose cases of bacterial overgrowth using glucose or lactulose.[128]
- Gaseous abdominal distension associated with diarrhea and weight loss requires the work up for malabsorption including testing for celiac disease and cystic fibrosis.

Management of Abdominal Distension

This depends on the pathologic problem causing abdominal distension.
- **Management of abdominal distension caused by ascites:**
  - This depends on the disorder that precipitated the ascites.

- The most important step is comforting the respiratory status.
- Appropriate fluid and electrolyte management is crucial.
- Diuretic intake should be guarded with fluid intake.
- Ascetic tap for draining the fluid is required if the respiratory status is compromised.
❑ **Management of abdominal distension caused by organomegaly:** This will be achieved by managing the disorder causing the organomegaly.
❑ **Management of abdominal distension caused by an abdominal mass:** This is achieved by managing the causative mass. The treatment depends on the type and if applicable, the staging of the mass.
❑ **Management of abdominal distension caused by gaseous distension:**
  - If the distension was due to bowel obstruction whether partial or complete, then this is an emergency situation that requires an immediate action.
  - Stabilize the vital signs including the hydration status since some of those kids become moderately to severely dehydrated.
  - Consult a pediatric surgeon.
  - Manage the patient as a case of bowel obstruction.
  - If the distension is caused by malabsorption, then management of malabsorption should be followed based on the possible cause.
  - If the distension was due to functional constipation, then this problem should be managed appropriately.
  - Young infants with *Giardia* infestation can be given a course of antibiotic.
  - If bacterial overgrowth is highly suspected, then try a course of antibiotics with few diet restrictions (follow the management of bacterial overgrowth).
  - If lactose intolerance was proved on a breath test then avoid lactose ingestion in food or advice the ingestion of synthetic lactase enzyme (lactaid).
  - If the patient has got functional bloating without diarrhea, constipation and weight loss, then dietary modifications may be helpful.
    - Avoid soft drinks containing sorbitol.
    - Avoid chewing gums.
    - Avoid some vegetables (beans and legumes, e.g. cabbage, onions, broccoli and sprouts).
    - Avoid foods containing undigested starch (corn, potato).
    - Avoid flour made of wheat and oats.
    - Decrease the intake of juices (fructose) specially the canned juices containing high sugars.
❑ **Management of aerophagia:**
  - Reassure the parents that this is a benign condition.
  - Stop the use of chewing gums.

- Stop the ingestion of carbonated beverages.
- Psychological referral may be required to manage the underlying anxiety associated with this problem.

▌FAILURE TO THRIVE

Definition

Failure to thrive (FTT) is a descriptive term indicating a sign and not a definite diagnosis. It refers to an inadequate or poor physical growth observed over time on a standard growth chart.[129] There is no consensus, however, regarding a specific definition. In addition, there is no consensus regarding which specific anthropometric criteria should be used to define FTT.

Weight gain is accepted as the predominant indicator of FTT with weight for length/height as the second choice or parameter.[130] The child is said to have FTT if when one of the following is observed over time:

❑ Weight less than 80 percent of ideal weight-for-age, using a standard growth chart.
❑ Decreased weight-for-length.
❑ Decelerating weight that crosses two or more standard percentile lines on a standard growth chart.

However, this is not a good screening tool for FTT. Currently, there is no single measure that adequately identifies the problem in the general infant population. It is also important to note that infants and young children may cross major percentile lines on growth curves during normal growth in the first 60 months. Premature infants will have normal growth parameters when corrected for their gestational age. Large for gestational age babies will regress on the growth chart towards their norm. In addition, children of small parents will eventually grow according to their genetic potential. Therefore, documenting a faltering weight on the growth chart is not by itself a true proof of FTT. Also, children growing on a line parallel to the curve with normal growth rate should not be defined as FTT even if their growth curve is below the 5th percentile (Box 2.16).[129,130] Pediatricians should consider this fact before labeling the child with this term.

BOX 2.16: Common anthropometric criteria for diagnosing FTT

- Body mass index for age less than 5th percentile
- Weight for age less than 5th percentile
- Weight deceleration crossing two major percentile lines
- Weight less than 75% of median weight for age
- Weight less than 75% of median weight for length
- Weight velocity less than 5th percentile

Note: Criteria should be met on multiple occasions

The term is usually used to describe physical growth failure in children younger than 2 years because almost 80% occur in younger than 18 months during the critical period of child growth. Nevertheless, the term can be used in older children as well if they fulfill the above criteria. FTT is applied mostly when there is faltering of weight but with chronicity of the problem both height/linear growth and head circumference will also be affected. FTT reflects undernutrition and it is the end result of inadequate usable calories.

Epidemiology

It is difficult to accurately estimate FTT prevalence because there is no consensus on its definition between differernt authorities. However, it was reported in 1-5% of hospitalized children under 2 years of age. This seems to be an underestimate of the true prevalence since many of the affected children are not referred to hospitals. In the primary care setting, the problem was noted in 10% of infants less than one year of age. The population prevalence has been reported to range from 1.3% to 20.9% depending on the definition used.[131]

Causes of FTT

There are multiple factors leading to FTT but regardless of the cause insufficient nutrition constitutes the major underlying problem.[133-136]
Causes of FTT can be divided into:

- Organic FTT (pathological or medical)
- Non-organic FTT (environmental or psychosocial)
- Mixed/Overlap of organic and non-organic causes
The division of organic and non-organic is not very precise because the cause in many cases is multifactorial involving the interaction of medical and psychosocial factors. All can contribute to the pathology of this problem.

There are 3 basic mechanisms contributing to FTT (Table 2.29):
- Insufficient intake/nutrition
- Inadequate absorption
- Impaired utilization
- Increased metabolic demand
- 80% of children with FTT do not suffer from any medical or organic problem.
- Nonorganic FTT (NOFTT):
  There is no identifiable medical problem responsible for FTT. The causes of NOFTT are multiple (Table 2.30) but how they interact resulting in FTT is not well understood.[137-139]

In many cases there is a mixture of medical and psychosocial factors resulting in FTT. An organic etiology may lead to behavioral problems contributing more to the problem. In addition, presence of a psychosocial variable might make the child more susceptible to physical disorders. Therefore, multiple factors may interact and contribute to FTT in a particular patient. Nevertheless, regardless of the cause, medical or psychosocial, a FTT child is malnourished requiring proper and adequate nutrition to improve his status.

Table 2.29: Mechanisms of FTT

Insufficient intake	Inadequate absorption	Increased metabolic demand	Impaired utilization
Unavailability of food (Starvation)	Food allergy	Chronic systemic diseases (heart, lung, kidney, liver, endocrine)	Genetic disorders (Trisomies, Turner, Russel-Silver)
Breastfeeding difficulties	Celiac disease	Chronic infections	Congenital infections
Diluted formula	Cystic fibrosis	Malignancy	Storage disorders
Mechanical feeding problems: • Congenital orofacial anomalies • Neuromuscular disorders	Inflammatory bowel disease		Inborn errors of metabolism
Chronic vomiting: • GERD • Pyloric obstruction • Malrotation • Increased intracranial pressure	Hepatobiliary disorders		
Developmental delay			
Child neglect			
Psychosocial/family problems			
Behavioral problems (food aversion)			

Table 2.30: Causes of NOFTT

Maternal factors	Infant factors	Mother-infant interaction	Social factors	Others
Depression	Lethargy	Disturbed maladaptive mother-infant interaction	Marital problems	Emotional deprivation
Anxiety	Irritability		Economic problems	Child abuse/neglect
Inability to cope with life stresses	Decreased motor activity		Disturbed family relationships	
Mental subnormality	Passivity			
Emotionless	Behavioral abnormalities			
Other maternal psychological problems	Poor feeding ability			

Approach of a Child with FTT

Evaluating a child with FTT should include a detailed history, a thorough physical examination and observation of the psychosocial environment of the child/family. This will guide proper investigations and plan of management.

History

❑ A detailed history should include medical, nutritional, antenatal, perinatal and postnatal, family and social information.
❑ Onset of the problem: When was weight gain noticed to be faltering?
❑ Medical history:
  • Symptoms of chronic disorders (respiratory, cardio-vascular, hepatobiliary, gastrointestinal, endocrine, neuromuscular, renal).
  • A detailed systemic review will unmask some of the unrecognized problems.
  • Gastrointestinal losses:
    – Chronic vomiting: description of the frequency and amount of vomiting is important.
    – Chronic diarrhea: stool consistency, character as well as frequency should be described. Relation of stool changes to the introduction of different food items should be documented.
  • Renal losses: urine output (polyuria) should be clearly verified (renal tubular acidosis, chronic renal failure).
❑ Prenatal/Perinatal/postnatal history:
  • Pregnancy history and growth in utero should be verified from the mother.
  • Birth weight should be documented in case the child was small for gestation due to intrauterine growth retardation (IUGR).

❑ Developmental history: Enquire about different milestones during the child's development.
❑ Family history:
  • History of GI diseases and malabsorption disorders in the family.
  • Other medical conditions in the family members such as kidney, neuromuscular and endocrine disorders.
  • History of inherited conditions such as inborn errors of metabolism and storage disorders.
  • Family history of food allergy.
  • History of FTT in other siblings.
❑ Medications: This includes current and previous medications ingested.
❑ Allergy: Including allergy to drugs or food items.
❑ Nutritional/feeding history:
  • This is a crucial part in the history of a child with FTT.
  • A dietary history should include a 3-day diary of what the child had ingested. The quantity and type of food accepted by the child varies and therefore a 3-day dietary history is recommended.
  • Enquire about the following:
    – Type of milk intake (breast/formula): In case of breast milk, is it enough and satisfying to the baby? How much time is the baby kept on each breast? How frequent is the baby fed? Does the mother have any problems with her nipples (retracted or sore nipples) or the rest of the breast?[140]
    – In a formula fed baby: What kind of formula? How much milk is provided in each feed? Does the baby adequately ingest the amount of milk offered? How is the feed prepared? Who prepares the feed and is he/she experienced in this task? How frequent is the bottle offered to the child?
    – Does the child cries for feeds or he is forced to ingest them?

19. Rsquin A, Di Lorenzo C, Forbes D, Guiraldes E, Hyams JS, Staiano A, et al. Childhood functional gastrointestinal disorders: child/adolescent. Gastroenterology. 2006;130:1527-37.

20. Wenzl HH, Fine KD, Schiller LR, Fordtran JS. Determinants of decreased fecal consistency in patients with diarrhea. Gastroenterology. 1995;108:1729-38.

21. Nyhan WL. Stool frequency of normal infants in the first week of life. Pediatrics. 1952;10:41-25

22. Venkatasubramanian J, Rao MC, Sellin JH. Intestinal Electrolyte Absorption and Secretion. In: Feldman M, Friedman LS, Brandt LJ (Eds). Sleisenger and Fordtran's Gastrointestinal and Liver Disease, 9th edition. Saunders: Elsevier Inc. 2010.pp.1675-94.

23. Costanzo LS. Gastrointestinal physiology. In: Physiology, 5th edition. Sunders: Elsevier Inc. 2013.pp.329-82.

24. UNICEF/WHO. Diarrhoea: why children are still dying and what can be done. 2009;1-58.

25. Field M. Intestinal ion transport and the pathophysiology of diarrhea. J Clin Invest. 2003; 111(7):931-43.

26. McClarren RL, Lynch B, Nyayapati N. Acute Infectious Diarrhea. Prim Care. 2011;38(3):539-64.

27. Binder HJ. Causes of chronic diarrhea. N Engl J Med. 2006;355(3):236-9.

28. Schiller LR. Chronic diarrhea. Gastroenterology. 2004;127(1):287-93.

29. Swindells J, Brenwald N, Reading N, Oppenheim B. Evaluation of diagnostic tests for Clostridium difficile infection. J Clin Microbiol. 2010;48(2):606-8.

30. Terrin G, Tomaiuolo R, Passariello A, Elce A, Amato F, Di Costanzo M. Congenital diarrheal disorders: an updated diagnostic approach. Int J Mol Sci 2012;13:4168-85.

31. World Health Organization. The treatment of diarrhea. A manual for physicians and other senior health workers. Geneva, 2005.

32. Guarino A, Albano F, Ashkenazi S, Gendrel D, Hoekstra JH, Shamir R, et al. European Society for Paediatric Gastroenterology, Hepatology, and Nutrition/European Society for Paediatric Infectious Diseases evidence-based guidelines for the management of acute gastroenteritis in children in Europe. J Pediatr Gastroenterol Nutr. 2008;46(Suppl 2):S81-122.

33. Lazzerini M, Ronfani L. Oral zinc for treating diarrhea in children. Cochrane Database. Syst Rev. 2013;1:CD005436.

34. Allen SJ, Martinez EG, Gregorio GV, Dans LF. Probiotics for treating acute infectious diarrhea. Cochrane Database. Syst Rev. 2010;11:CD003048.

35. Guarino A, Lo Vecchio A, Canani RB. Chronic diarrhoea in children. Best Pract Res Clin Gastroenterol. 2012;26(5):649-61.

36. McCollough M, Sharieff GQ. Abdominal surgical emergencies in infants and young children. Emerg Med Clin North Am. 2003;21(4):909-35.

37. Marin JR, Alpern ER. Abdominal Pain in Children. Emerg Med Clin N Am. 2011;29:401-28

38. Zackowski SW. Chronic recurrent abdominal pain. Emerg Med Clin North Am. 1998;16(4):877-94.

39. Apley J, Naish N. Recurrent abdominal pain: a field survey of 1000 school children. Arch Dis Child. 1958;33:165-70.

40. King S, Chambers CT, Huguet A, MacNevin RC, McGrath, Parker L, et al. The epidemiology of chronic pain in children and adolescents revisited: a systematic review. Pain. 2011;152:2729-38.

41. Seller RH, Symons AB. Abdominal pain in children. In: Differential Diagnosis of Common Complaints. Saunders, 2012.pp. 20-32.

42. Tomlinson D, von Baeyer CL, Stinson JN, Sung L. A systemic review of faces scales for the self-report of pain intensity in children. Pediatrics. 2010;126(5):e1168-98.

43. Malvia S, Voepel-Lewis T, Burke C, Merkel S, Tait AR. The revised FLACC observational pain tool: improved reliability and validity for pain assessment in children with cognitive impairement. Paediatr Anaesth. 2006;16(3):258-65.

44. McCollough M, Sharieff GS. Abdominal pain in children. Pediatr Clin N Am. 2006;53:107-37.

45. Dhroove G, Chogle A, Saps M. A million-dollar work-up for abdominal pain: is it worth it? J Pediatr Gastroenterol Nutr. 2010:51(5):579-83.

46. Zhou H, Chen YC, Zhang JZ. Abdominal pain among children re-evaluation of a diagnostic algorithm. World J Gastroenterol. 2002;8(5):947-51.

47. Devanarayana NM, Rajindrajith S, De Silva HJ. Recurrent abdominal pain in children. Indian Pediatr. 2009;46:389-99.

48. Green R, Bulloch B, Kabani A, Hancock BJ, Tenenbein M. Early analgesia for children with acute abdominal pain. Pediatrics. 2005;116(4):978-83.

49. Ali S, Ali H. Treating abdominal pain in children: what do we know? Clin Pediatr Emerg Med. 2010;11(3):171-81.

50. McGrath PA. Development of the World Health Organization guidelines on cancer pain relief and palliative care in children J Pain Symptom Manage. 1996;12(2):87-92.

51. WHO guidelines on the pharmacological treatment of persisting pain in children with medical illnesses. Geneva: World Health Organization; 2012.

52. Tabbers MM, Boluyt N, Berger MY, Benninga MA. Clinical practice: diagnosis and treatment of functional constipation. Eur J Pediatr. 2011;170:955-63.

53. Weaver LT, Steiner H. The bowel habit of young children. Arch Dis Child. 1984;59:649-52.

54. Benninga M, Candy DC, Catto-Smith AG, Clayden G, Loening-Baucke V, Lorenzo CD, et al. The Paris consensus on childhood constipation terminology (PACCT) group. J Pediatr Gastroenterolo Nutr. 2005;40:273-5.

55. Vanden Berg MM, Benninga MA, Di Lorenzo C. Epidemiology of childhood constipation: a systematic review. Am J Gastroenterol. 2006;101:2401-9.

56. Loening-Baucke V. Prevalence, symptoms and outcome of constipation in infants and toddlers. J Pediatr. 2005;146:359-63.

57. Ip KS, Lee WT, Chan JS, Young BW. A community-based study of the prevalence of constipation in young children and the role of dietary fiber. Hong Kong Med J. 2005;11:431-6.

58. Morris-Yates A, Talley NJ, Boyce PM, Nandurkar S, Andrews G. Evidence of a genetic contribution to functional bowel disorder. Am J Gastroenterol. 1998;93:1311-7.

59. Hyams JE, Colletti R, Faure C, Gabriel-Martinez E, Maffei HV, Morais MB, et al. Functional gastrointestinal disorders: working group report of the first world congress of paediatric gastroenterology, hepatology and nutrition. J Pediatr Gastroenterol Nutr. 2002;35(suppl 2):S110-7.

60. Borowitz SM, Cox DJ, Tam A, Ritterband LM, Sutphan JL, Penberthy JK. Precipitant of constipation during early childhood. J Am Board Fam Pract. 2003;16:213-8.

61. van der Plas R, Benninga M, Staalman C, Akkermans L, Redekop W, Taminiau J, et al. Megarectum in constipation. Arch Dis Child. 2000;83:52-8.

62. Lewis SJ, Heaton KW. Stool form scale as a useful guide to intestinal transit time. Scandinavian J Gastroenterol. 1997;32:920-4.

63. Bekkali N, Hamers SL, Reitsma JB, Van Toledo L, Benninga MA. Infant stool form scale: development and results. J Pediatr. 2009;154:521-6.

64. Pashankar DS, Loening-Baucke V. Increased prevalence of obesity in children with functional constipation evaluated in a medical center. Pediatrics. 2005;116:e377-80.

65. Bardisa-Ezcurra L, Ullman R, Gordon J. Guideline development group. Diagnosis and management of idiopathic childhood constipation: summary of NICE guidance. BMJ. 2010;340: c2585.

66. van den BM, Graafmans D, Nievelstein R, Beek E. Systematic assessment of constipation on plain abdominal radiographs in children. Pediatr Radiol. 2006;36:224-6.

67. Pensabene L, Youssef NN, Griffiths JM, Di LC. Colonic manometry in children with defecatory disorders: role in diagnosis and management. Am J Gastroenterol. 2003;98:1052-7.

68. Ghosh A, Griffiths DM. Rectal biopsy in the investigation of constipation. Arch Dis Child. 1998;79:266-8.

69. Nurko S, Scott SM. Coexistence of constipation and incontinence in children and adults. Best Pract Res Clin Gastroenterol. 2011;25:29-41.

70. North American Society for Pediatric Gastroenterology, Hepatology and Nutrition. Evaluation and treatment of constipation in children: summary of updated recommendations of the North American Society for Pediatric Gastroenterology, Hepatology and Nutrition. J Pediatr Gastroenterol Nutr. 2006;43:405-7.

71. Bekkali NL, van den Berg MM, Dijkgraaf MG, van Wijk MP, Bongers ME, Liem O. Rectal fecal impaction treatment in childhood constipation: enemas versus high doses oral PEG. Pediatrics. 2009;124:e1108-15.

72. Sondheimer JM, Gervaise EP. Lubricant versus laxative in the treatment of chronic functional constipation of children: a comparative study. J Pediatr Gastroenterol Nutr. 1982;1:223-6.

73. Loening-Baucke V, Pashankar DS. A randomized, prospective, comparison study of polyethylene glycol 3350 without electrolytes and milk of magnesia for children with constipation and fecal incontinence. Pediatrics. 2006;118:528-35.

74. Chmielewska A, Szajewska H. Systematic review of randomized controlled trials: probiotics for functional constipation. World J Gastroenterol. 2010;16:69-75.

75. Carbohydrate and dietary fiber. In: Kleinman RE (Ed). Pediatric Nutrition Handbook, 6th edition, Community on Nutrition. American Academy of Pediatrics. 2009;104.

76. van Wunnik BP, Baeten CG, Southwell BR. Neuromodulation for constipation: sacral and transcutaneous stimulation. Best Pract Res Clin Gastroenterol. 2011;25:181-91.

77. Levitt MA, Pena A. Surgery and constipation: when, how, yes, or no. J Pediatr Gastroenterol Nutr. 2005;41:S58-60.

78. Youssef NN, Barksdale E Jr, Griffiths JM, Flores AF, Di Lorenzo C. Management of intractable constipation with antegrade enemas in neurologically intact children. J Pediatr Gastroenterol Nutr. 2002;34:402-5.

79. Irani K, Rodriguez L, Doody DP, Goldstein AM. Botulinum toxin for the treatment of chronic constipation in children with internal anal sphincter dysfunction. Pediatr Surg Int. 2008;24:779-83.

80. Levitt MA, Martin CA, Falcone RA Jr, Pena A. Transanal rectosigmoid resection for severe intractable idiopathic constipation. J Pediatr Surg. 2009;44:1285-90.

81. Boyle JT. Gastrointestinal bleeding in infant and children. Pediatr Rev. 2008;29(2):39-52.

82. Wyllie R, Hyams JS. Gastrointestinal hemorrhage. In: Pediatric Gastrointestinal and Liver Disease, 4th edition. Saunders, Elsevier. 2011.pp.146-53.

83. Chawla S, Seth D, Mahajan P, Kamat D. Upper Gastrointestinal Bleeding in Children. Clin Pediatr. 2007;46(1):16-21.

84. 84. Flynn DM, Booth IW. Investigation and management of gastrointestinal bleeding in children. Curr Pediatr. 2004;14:576-85.

85. Moustafa MH, Taylor M, Fletcher L. My two-week-old daughter Is throwing up blood. Acad Emerg Med. 2005;12(8):775-7.

86. Rosenthal P, Thompson J, Singh M. Detection of occult blood in gastric juice. J Clin Gastroenterol. 1984;6(2):119-21.

87. Brenner H, Tao S. Superior diagnostic performance of faecal immunochemical tests for haemoglobin in a head-to-head comparison with guaiac-based faecal occult blood test among 2235 participants of screening colonoscopy. Eur J Cancer. 2013;49(14):3049-54.

88. Barber MD, Abraham A, Brydon WG, Waldron BM, Williams AJ. Assessment of faecal occult blood loss by qualitative and quantitative methods. J R Coll Surg Edinb. 2002;47(2):491-4.

89. Moran A, Lawson N, Morrow R, Jones A, Asquith P. Value of faecal alpha-1-antitrypsin, haemoglobin and a chemical occult blood test in the detection of gastrointestinal disease. Clin Chim Acta. 1993;217:153-61.

90. Teach SJ. Gastrointestinal bleeding. In: Fleisher GR, Ludwig S (Eds). Textbook of Pediatric Emergency Medicine, 6th edition. Wolters Kluwer Health/Lippincott Williams & Wilkins. 2010.pp.283-90.

91. Hussey S, Kelleher KT, Ling SC. Emergency management of major upper gastrointestinal hemorrhage in children. Clin Pediatr Emerg Med. 2010;11(3):207-16.

92. Osman D, Djibré M, Da Silva D, Goulenok C. Management by the intensivist of gastrointestinal bleeding in adults and children. Ann Intensive Care. 2012;2(1):46-63.

93. Eroglu Y, Emerick KM, Whitigon PF, Alonso EM. Octreotide therapy for control of acute gastrointestinal bleeding in children. J Pediatr Gastroenterol Nutr. 2004;38:41-7.

94. Qureshi W, Adler DG, Davila R, Egan J, Hirota W, Leighton J, et al. ASGE guideline: the role of endoscopy in the management of variceal hemorrhage, updated July 2005. Gastrointest Endosc 2005;62(5):651-5.

95. Technology Assessment Committee, Croffie J, Somogyi L, Chuttani R, DiSario J, Liu J, et al. Sclerosing agents for use in GI endoscopy. Gastrointest Endosc. 2007;66(1):1-6.

96. Vergara M, Calvet X, Gisbert JP. Epinephrine injection versus epinephrine injection and a second endoscopic method in high-risk bleeding ulcers. Cochrane Database Syst Rev. 2007:CD005584.

97. Barkun AN, Bardou M, Kuipers EJ, Sung J, Hunt RH, Martel M. International consensus recommendations on the management of patients with nonvariceal upper gastrointestinal bleeding. Ann Intern Med. 2010;152(2):101-13.

98. Cappell MS, Friedel D. Acute Nonvariceal Upper Gastrointestinal Bleeding: Endoscopic Diagnosis and Therapy. Med Clin N Am. 2008;92(3):511-50.

99. Teach SJ, Fleisher GR. Rectal bleeding in the pediatric emergency department. Ann Emerg Med. 1994;23(6):1252-8.

100. Arvola T, Ruuska T, Keränen J, Hyöty H, Salminen S, Isolauri E. Rectal bleeding in infancy: clinical, allergological, and microbiological examination. Pediatrics. 2006;117(4):e760-8.

101. Jang HJ, Kim AS, Hwang JB. The etiology of small and fresh rectal bleeding in not-sick neonates: should we initially suspect food protein-induced proctocolitis? Eur J Pediatr. 2012;171(12):1845-9.

102. Durno CA. Colonic polyps in children and adolescents. Can J Gastroenterol. 2007;21(4):233-9.

103. Park JJ, Wolff BG, Tollefson MK, Walsh EE, Larson DR. Meckel diverticulum: the Mayo Clinic experience with 1476 patients (1950–2002). Ann Surg. 2005;241(3):529-33.

104. Lane VA, Sugarman ID. Investigation of rectal bleeding in children. Paediatr Child Health. 2010;20(10):465-72.

105. Huicho L, Campos M, Rivera J, Guerrant RL. Fecal screening tests in the approach to acute infectious diarrhea: a scientific cover review. Pediatr Infect Dis J. 1996;15(6):486-94.

106. Cucchiara S, Guandalini S, Staiano A, Devizia B, Capano G, Romaniello G, et al. Sigmoidoscopy, colonoscopy, and radiology in the evaluation of children with rectal bleeding. J Pediatr Gastroenterol Nutr. 1983;2(4):667-71.

107. Quiroga Gomez S, Perez Lafuente M, Abu-Suboh Abadia M, Castell Conesa J. Gastrointestinal bleeding: the role of radiology. Radiología. 2011;53(5):406-20.

108. Wiarda BM, Kuipers EJ, Heitbrink MA, van Oijen A, Stoker J. MR Enteroclysis of inflammatory small-bowel disease. Am J Roentgenol. 2006;187(2):522-31.

109. Jaeckle T, Stuber G, Hoffmann MH, Freund W, Schmitz BL, Aschoff AJ. Acute gastrointestinal bleeding: value of MDCT. Abdom Imaging. 2008;33:285-93.

110. Balkan E, Kiriştioğlu I, Gürpinar A, Ozel I, Sinmaz K, Doğruyol H. Sigmoidoscopy in minor lower gastrointestinal bleeding. Arch Dis Child. 1998;78(3):267-8.

111. Squires RH Jr, Colletti RB. Indications for pediatric gastrointestinal endoscopy: a medical position statement of the North American Society for Pediatric Gastroen- terology and Nutrition. J Pediatr Gastroenterol Nutr. 1996;23:107-10.

112. Muñoz-Navas MA. Capsule endoscopy in pediatric patients. World J Gastroenterol. 2008;14(26):4152-5.

113. Pai N, Manfredi MA. Endoscopic management of gastrointestinal bleeding in pediatrics. Tech Gastrointest Endosc. 2013;15:18-24.

114. Strocchi A, Levitt MD. Intestinal gas. In: Sleisenger MH, Fordtran JS (Eds). Sleisenger and Fordtran's. Gastrointestinal and Liver Diseases: Pathophysiology/Diagnosis/Management, 5th edn. Philadelphia: WB Sanders Co. 1993.pp.1035-42.

115. Levitt MD. Intestinal gas production. J Am Diet Assoc. 1972;60:487-90

116. Gibson PR, Newnham E, Barrett JS, Shepherd SJ, Muir JG. Review article: fructose malabsorption and the bigger picture. Aliment Pharmacol Ther. 2007;25(4):349-63.

117. Olesen M, Rumessen JJ, Gudmand-Hover E. Intestinal transport and fermentation of resistant starch evaluated by the hydrogen breath test. Eur J Clin Nutr. 1994;48:692-701.

118. Levitt MD, Hirsh P, Fetzer CA, Sheahan M, Levine AS. H2 excretion after ingestion of complex carbohydrates. Gastroenterology. 1987;92(2):383-9.

119. Piqué JM, Pallarés M, Cusó E, Vilar-Bonet J, Gassull MA. Methane production and colon cancer. Gastroenterology. 1984;87:601-5.

120. Salvioli B, Serra J, Azpiroz F, Lorenzo C, Aguade S, Castell J, Malagelada JR. Origin of gas retention and symptoms in patients with bloating. Gastroenterology. 2005;128(3):574-9.

121. Golden CB, Feusner JH. Malignant abdominal masses in children: quick guide to evaluation and diagnosis. Pediatr Clin N Am. 2002;49:1369-92.

122. Onur MR, Bakal U, Kocakoc E, Tartar T, Kazez A. Cystic abdominal masses in children: a pictorial essay. Clin Imaging. 2013;37(1):18-27.

123. Nam SH, Kim DY, Kim SC, Kim IK. The surgical experience for retroperitoneal, mesenteric and omental cyst in children. J Korean Surg Soc. 2012;83:102-6.

124. Pernas JC, Catala J. Case 72: pseudocyst around ventriculoperitoneal shunt. Radiology. 2004;232:239-43.

125. Ullah Q, Nakielny RA. Investigation of abdominal masses. Surgery. 2012;30:306-9.

126. Kohli MD, Maglinte DD. CT enteroclysis in incomplete small bowel obstruction. Abdom Imaging. 2009;34:321-7.

127. Sachdev AH, Pimentel M. Gastrointestinal bacterial overgrowth: pathogenesis and clinical significance. Ther Adv Chronic Dis. 2013;4(5):223-31.

128. Gasbarrini A, Corazza GR, Gasbarrini G, Montalto M, Di Stefano M, Basilisco G, et al. Methodology and indications of H2-breath testing in gastrointestinal diseases: the Rome Consensus Conference. Aliment Pharmacol Ther. 2009;29(Suppl 1):1-49.

129. Perrin EC, Cole CH, Frank DA, Glicken SR, Guerina N, Petit K, et al. Criteria for determining disability in infants and children: failure to thrive. Evid Rep Technol Assess (Summ). 2003;72:1-5.

130. Olsen EM. Failure to thrive: still a problem of definition. Clin Pediatr (Phila). 2006;45(1):1-6.

131. Olsen EM, Petersen J, Skovgaard AM, Weile B, Jørgensen T, Wright CM. Failure to thrive: the prevalence and concurrence of anthropometric criteria in a general infant population. Arch Dis Child. 2007;92:109-14.

132. Sullivan PB. Commentary: The epidemiology of failure-to-thrive in infants. Int J Epidemiol. 2004;33(4):847-8.

133. Olsena EM, Skovgaard AM, Weilec B, Jørgensena T. Risk factors for failure to thrive in infancy depend on the anthropometric definitions used: The Copenhagen County Child Cohort. Paediatr Perinat Epidemiol. 2007;21(5):418-31.

134. Bithoney WG, Dubowitz H, Egan H. Failure-to-thrive/growth deficiency. Pediatr Rev. 1992;13(12):453-60.

135. Gahagan S. Failure-to-thrive: a consequence of undernutrition. Pediatr Rev. 2006;27:e1-11.

136. Casey PH. Failure-to-thrive: transitional perspective. J Dev Behav Pediatr. 1987;8(1):37-8.

137. Heffer RW, Kelley ML. Nonorganic failure-to-thrive developmental outcomes and psychosocial assessment and intervention issues. Res Dev Disabil. 1994;15(4):247-68.

138. Steward DK, Garvin BJ. Nonorganic failure-to-thrive: a theoretical approach. J Pediatr Nurs. 1997;12(6):342-7.

139. Nangia S, Tiwari S. Failure-to-thrive. Indian J Pediatr. 2013;80(7):585-9.

140. Wright CM, Parkinson KN, Drewett RF. The influence of maternal socioeconomic and emotional factors on infant weight gain and weight faltering (failure to thrive): data from a prospective birth cohort. Arch Dis Child. 2006;91:312-7.

141. Skuse DH, Gill D, Reilly S, Wolke D, Lynch MA. Failure to thrive and the risk of child abuse: a prospective population survey. J Med Screen. 1995;2:145-9.

142. Block RW, Krebs NF. Failure-to-thrive as a manifestation of child neglect. Pediatrics. 2005;116:1234-7.

143. Robertson J, Puckering C, Parkinson K, Corlett L, Wright C. Mother-child feeding interactions in children with and without weight faltering; nested case control study. Appetite. 2011;56:753-9.

144. Jaffe AC. Failure-to-thrive: current clinical concepts. Pediatr Rev. 2011;32(3):100-7.

145. Sills RH. Failure-to-thrive: the role of clinical and laboratory evaluation. Am J Dis Child. 1978;132:967-9.

146. Khoshoo V, Reifen R. Use of energy-dense formula for treating infants with non-organic failure-to-thrive. Eur J Clin Nutr. 2002;56:921-4.

147. Clarke SE, Evans S, Macdonald A, Davies P, Booth IW. Randomized comparison of a nutrient-dense formula with an energy-supplemented formula for infants with faltering growth. J Hum Nutr Diet. 2007;20:329-39.

148. Careaga MG, Kerner JA Jr. A gastroenterologist's approach to failure-to-thrive. Pediatr Ann. 2000;29(9):558-67.

149. Black MM, Dubowitz H, Krishnakumar A, Starr RH Jr. Early intervention and recovery among children with failure-to-thrive: follow-up at age 8. Pediatrics. 2007;120:59-69.

150. Mehanna HM, Moledina J, Travis J. Refeeding syndrome: what it is, and how to prevent and treat it. BMJ. 2008;336:1495-8.

151. Holme AR, Blair PS, Emond AM. Psychosocial and educational outcomes of weight faltering in infancy in ALSPAC. BMJ Open. 2013;3(7).pii:e002863.

152. ud Din Z, Emmett P, Steer C, Edmond A. Growth outcomes of weight faltering in infancy in ALSPAC. Pediatrics. 2013;131(3):e843-9.

Disorders of the Esophagus

SK Mittal

GASTROESOPHAGEAL REFLUX DISEASE (GERD)

Definition of GER and GERD

Gastroesophageal reflux (GER) is defined as the passage of gastric contents into the esophagus with or without regurgitation and vomiting. GER is a normal physiological phenomenon and it occurs several times a day in healthy infants, children and adults. Most episodes of GER in healthy individuals last less than 3 minutes, occur in the postprandial period and cause few or no symptoms.[1] Post-prandial spitting of food is quite common in neonates and infants. This physiological reflux tends to reach its peak at 3 months of age and usually subsides by 6 months of age. As only less than 3% of infants continue to regurgitate or vomit feeds after 6 months, pathological GER should be suspected whenever vomiting or regurgitation persists beyond 6 months of age. In contrast, gastroesophageal reflux disease (GERD) is present when GER leads to troublesome symptoms and/or complications.

Pathophysiology

Contrary to the past when it was believed that GER during infancy and childhood was a consequence of poor or absent lower esophageal sphincter (LES) tone, now it is well known that baseline LES pressures are normal in pediatric patients, even in preterm infants. Currently, the primary mechanism of reflux has been demonstrated to involve increase in transient LES relaxation (TLESR). TLESR decreases the LES pressure by 0–2 mm Hg and may last up to 10 seconds, allowing gastric contents to reflux into the esophagus, thus causing the symptoms of GERD. Factors that may promote GER during TLESR includes increased intragastric liquid volumes (specially those associated with reduced viscosity) and certain body positions such as supine and slumped seated positions. Other factors that play a role in increasing reflux during TLESR includes straining, increased movements and coughing.

The self-limiting nature of GER in young infants may be attributable to other factors such as increasing angulation of the esophagus at the cardia and the assumption of upright posture besides introduction of semi-solid and solid food in the diet.

Clinical Manifestations

Recurrent vomiting and regurgitation of variable force and quantity are present in majority of infants with reflux, usually in the postprandial period. Features such as irritability, arching, choking, feed aversion and failure to thrive may be observed in severe cases as a result of the ensuing esophagitis. Older children may present with heartburn, chest pain, hematemesis, anemia, etc. Reflux esophagitis and its manifestations may occur even without any overt vomiting or regurgitation of feeds and may pose a diagnostic challenge.

The other manifestations include neonatal apnea, ALTE (acute life-threatening events), recurrent respiratory infections, recurrent wheezing, stridor, hoarseness, cough, chronic sinusitis, recurrent laryngitis, otitis media, dental erosions and arching (Table 3.1).

Above mentioned symptoms and signs (Table 3.1) are nonspecific for reflux. Not all children with GER have heartburn or irritability. Conversely, heartburn and irritability can be caused by conditions other than GER. Regurgitation, irritability and vomiting are common in infants with physiologic GER or GERD[2] but are indistinguishable from regurgitation, irritability, and vomiting caused by food allergy, colic, and other disorders. Individual symptoms in children generally are not highly predictive of findings of GERD. In a study of irritable infants younger than 9 months of age, regurgitation more than 5 times per day had a sensitivity of 54% and specificity of 71% for a reflux index (RI) >10%

Table 3.1: Symptoms and signs that may be associated with gastroesophageal reflux
Typical
• Recurrent regurgitation with/without vomiting especially continuing after 6 months of age
• Weight loss or poor weight gain/failure to thrive
• Irritability in infants
• Ruminative behavior
• Heartburn or chest pain
• Hematemesis/GI bleed/anemia
• Dysphagia, odynophagia
Atypical
• Nonregurgitating reflux
• Neonatal apnea
• Acute life-threatening event (ALTE) SIDS
• Recurrent respiratory infections
• Reactive airway disease/wheezing
• Stridor
• Cough
• Hoarseness
• Recurrent laryngitis/tracheitis especially in post-TOF cases
• Chronic sinusitis
• Dental erosions
• Dystonic neck posturing (Sandifer's syndrome)

Table 3.2: Warning signs requiring investigation in infants with regurgitation or vomiting suggesting complicated GER
• Epigastric distension/palpable mass in right hypochondrium
• Consistently forceful vomiting
• Onset or persistence of vomiting after 6 months of life
• Diarrhea
• Lethargy
• Fever
• Seizures
• Bulging fontanelle
• Constipation
• Abdominal tenderness or distension
• Bilious vomiting
• Gastrointestinal bleeding
• Hematemesis
• Hematochezia
• Failure to thrive
• Hepatosplenomegaly
• Macro/microcephaly
• Documented or suspected genetic/metabolic syndrome

by esophageal pH testing, whereas feeding difficulty, which is more difficult to define as an entity, had a sensitivity of 75% and specificity of 46%.[3]

GERD should be suspected in infants and children with symptoms mentioned earlier; but none of the symptoms are specific to GERD alone; so the major role of history and physical examination in the evaluation of GERD is to rule out other more worrisome disorders that present with vomiting and to identify complications of GERD listed in Table 3.2.

Parent- or patient-reported questionnaires based on clusters of symptoms have been developed, as individual symptoms do not consistently correlate with objective findings or response to medical treatment. Orenstein et al[4] developed a diagnostic questionnaire for GERD in infants, in which score of >7 (of 25 possible) on the initial instrument demonstrated a sensitivity of 0.74 and specificity of 0.94 during primary validation. However, when applied to a population in India, it had a sensitivity and specificity of only 43% and 79%, respectively, compared with pH-monitoring results.[5]

A 5-item questionnaire developed for children 7 to 16 years of age had a sensitivity of 75% and a specificity of 96% compared with pH monitoring during primary validation.[6]

Diagnostic Tests for GERD

Diagnosis of GER/GERD is largely clinical and usually does not require investigations. However, diagnostic tests may be required in some situations (Table 3.3).

Generally, in children younger than 2 years, the indications for work up/ investigations for GER include situations where complications of GERD are suspected clinically. These may include a generally unhappy baby, irritability during and after feeds, persistent vomiting, recurrent pneumonias, choking spells or near ALTEs, chronic cough, or a child who is failing to thrive.

Similarly in children older than 2 years, there are certain features that may warrant investigations for GER. These include persistence of vomiting since the child was less than 2 years, onset of vomiting recently, heartburn not responsive to 4 weeks of medical therapy. Investigations are also indicated in cases where there is a suspicion of complications of GER such as undiagnosed anemia, dysphagia, odynophagia, recurrent pneumonias and non-seasonal asthma.

Table 3.3: Indications to perform diagnostic tests for GER/GERD
• Uncertain diagnosis
• Atypical symptoms
• Symptoms associated with complications
• Inadequate response to therapy
• Recurrent symptoms
• Prior to anti-reflux surgery

GERD is confirmed, when tests shows excessive frequency or duration of reflux events, esophagitis, or a clear association of symptoms and signs with reflux events, in the absence of alternative diagnoses. Tests are useful to document the presence of pathologic reflux or its complications, to establish a causal relation between reflux and symptoms, to evaluate therapy, and to exclude other conditions. Although many tests have been used to diagnose GERD, no single test can address all these questions. Therefore, the tests must be carefully selected according to the information sought and the limitations of each test must be recognized. Importantly, a test cannot predict an individual patient's response to therapy.

Diagnostic Tests Available

- Upper GI barium studies
- Esophageal and gastric ultrasonography
- Nuclear scintigraphy
- Esophagoduodenoscopy and biopsy
- Esophageal 24 hr pH monitoring
- Motility studies
- Esophageal impedance
- Therapeutic trial

Barium Contrast Radiography

Although simple and easily available, the upper GI series is neither sensitive nor specific for diagnosing GERD. The sensitivity, specificity and positive predictive values range from 29% to 86%, 21% to 83%, and 80% to 82% respectively when compared with esophageal pH monitoring.[7,8] The brief duration of the upper GI series produces false-negative results whereas the frequent occurrence of non-pathological reflux during the test may cause false-positive results.

However, the upper GI series is useful in ruling out anatomical abnormalities like strictures, hiatus hernia, achalasia, tracheoesophageal fistula, intestinal malrotation or pyloric stenosis which are included in the differential diagnosis of infants and children with symptoms suggesting GERD.

Esophageal and Gastric Ultrasonography

Ultrasonography has been tried but generally not recommended as a test for GERD. The sensitivity of color Doppler ultrasound performed for 15 minutes postprandially is about 95% with a specificity of only 11%, when compared to 24-hour esophageal pH monitoring and there is no correlation between reflux frequency detected by ultrasound and reflux index detected by pH monitoring.[9]

Nuclear Scintigraphy

In gastroesophageal scintigraphy, food or formula labeled with [99]technetium is introduced into the stomach and region of interest—stomach, esophagus, and lungs are scanned for evidence of reflux and aspiration. The nuclear scan evaluates only postprandial reflux and demonstrates reflux independent of the gastric pH. It does not demonstrate presence or absence of esophagitis. Its primary utility is in infants less than 2 years of age. The advantages of this technique are that it demonstrates both acidic and nonacidic reflux, can evaluate gastric emptying (which may be delayed in children with GERD), and may even demonstrate aspirations. It is noninvasive.

Technique: Prokinetics are stopped for at least 24 hours before carrying out the test. The amount of milk/formula to be given must equal the normal feed volume for that infant. Scintigraphy is done for up to an hour after the feed. Occasionally it may be performed for 24 hours after feed which may help in detecting microaspiration and delayed gastric emptying.

Sensitivity and specificity of a 1-hour scintigraphy for the diagnosis of GERD are 15% to 59% and 83% to 100%, respectively, when compared with 24-hour esophageal pH monitoring.[10,11]

Endoscopy and Biopsy

The role of endoscopy and biopsy in the evaluation of GERD is primarily to demonstrate the effects of GERD on the esophagus in the form of esophagitis or stricture and not to demonstrate or document reflux directly. It therefore has limited application in the diagnosis of GERD but more helpful in establishing severity of reflux esophagitis. It is less useful in infants less than one year of age. The main indications for endoscopy and biopsy are situations where the complication of esophagitis is suspected, such as older children with recurrent abdominal pain, heartburn and chest pain; infants and younger children with symptoms like irritability, crying excessively during feeds, unexplained anemia and failure to thrive. It is also useful in evaluating empiric therapy failure, for preoperative evaluation and to rule out other conditions in the differential diagnosis such as eosinophilic or infective esophagitis, Crohn's disease, Barret's esophagus, etc.[12] Esophagoscopy combined with histological evaluation has more than 80% reliability in the diagnosis of GERD.

Reflux esophagitis is defined as the presence of visible breaks in the esophageal mucosa at or immediately above the gastroesophageal junction on endoscopic examination.[12] Mucosal erythema or an irregular Z-line is not a reliable sign of reflux esophagitis. Endoscopic classification system, is useful for evaluation of the severity of esophagitis and response to treatment.[13] The presence of endoscopically normal esophageal mucosa does not exclude a diagnosis of nonerosive reflux disease (NERD) or esophagitis of other etiology.[14] Multiple biopsies must be obtained as GERD may be patchy. Histologic observations include eosinophilia, elongation of papillae (rete pegs), basal hyperplasia, and dilated intercellular spaces (spongiosis) but may occur in other conditions also. When biopsies from lower esophagus show columnar epithelium, the term Barret's esophagus (BE) should be applied and the presence or absence of intestinal metaplasia be specified.[14,15] BE occurs with greatest frequency in children with underlying conditions putting them at high risk for GERD. The primary role for esophageal histology is to rule out other conditions in the differential diagnosis, such as eosinophilic esophagitis (EoE), Crohn disease, BE, and infection.

Esophageal pH Monitoring

Intraluminal esophageal pH monitoring measures the frequency and duration of acid esophageal reflux episodes. Most commercially available systems include a catheter for nasal insertion with 1 or more pH electrodes (antimony, glass, or ion-sensitive field effect) arrayed along its length and a system for data capture, analysis, and reporting. The recording device is a small box with high portability and allows maximum normal activity. Prokinetic agents should be discontinued at least 48 hours before, H-2 antagonist or PPI at least 3 to 4 days and antacids at least 24 hours before the investigation. Calibration is done before the procedure. For standard recording, the pH electrode is placed 2–3 cm above the lower esophageal sphincter under fluoroscopy. Patients are allowed normal diet and unrestricted activity for a 24-hour recording period. Patients or their mothers are instructed to record activities and events like eating, drinking, change of position and occurrence of symptoms and a symptom/activity diary is maintained. Data is collected in the recorder for 24 hours, then downloaded into a computer and finally graphic and numerical displays can be presented. It must be noted here that it is important to actually see the record to ensure absence of artifacts and to correlate with symptom diary. Only those episodes are relevant which are associated with occurrence of symptoms.

Interpretation of 24-hour esophageal pH monitoring
❏ A pH of 4 is regarded as the cut off level for acid GER.

The standard parameters calculated are:
❏ Total number of episodes with a pH <4
❏ No. of episodes lasting >5 min with a pH <4.0
❏ Percentage of time related to the total duration of the investigation with a pH <4 (reflux index).

In pH studies conducted with antimony electrodes, a RI >7% is considered abnormal, a RI <3% is considered normal, and a RI between 3% and 7% is indeterminate.[1,16]

The sensitivity and specificity is quoted as 87–93% and 93–97% respectively. In adult group of patients, the reproducibility of the test varies from 77–85%.[17,18]

The advantages of esophageal pH monitoring are that it detects episodes of acid reflux, determines association of acidic GER with symptoms, can assess the adequacy of antisecretory treatment and helps to select those children with wheezing or respiratory symptoms in which acid reflux may be an aggravating factor. However, its disadvantages include nondetection of nonacidic or weakly acidic reflux episodes.

In children with documented esophagitis, normal esophageal pH monitoring suggests a diagnosis other than GERD or alkaline reflux. Double lumen pH monitoring where another probe of pH monitor is kept at the upper end of the esophagus, is helpful in detecting high GER which is responsible for upper respiratory symptoms. Wireless capsule pH monitoring is a relatively new modification of the conventional pH probe. It offers the advantage of being more patient friendly with greater comfort in carrying out daily activities. Moreover, it allows for a longer, 48-hour period recording.[19] However, its limitations include an endoscopic placement, greater cost and variability in the records obtained on day 1 and day 2.

Motility Studies

Esophageal manometry measures esophageal peristalsis, upper and lower esophageal sphincter pressures, and the coordinated function of these structures during swallowing. Esophageal manometry may be abnormal in patients with GERD, but the observations are not sufficiently sensitive or specific to confirm a diagnosis of GERD, nor to predict response to medical or surgical therapy. It may be useful in patients who have failed acid suppression and who have negative endoscopy to search for a possible motility disorder, or to determine the position of the LES to place a pH probe. Manometric studies were critical in identifying TLESR as a causative mechanism for GERD. Recent studies indicate that there is no role for manometry in predicting outcome of fundoplication. Manometric studies are also important in confirming a diagnosis of achalasia or other motor disorders of the esophagus that may mimic GERD.

Combined Multiple Intraluminal Impedance (MII) and pH Monitoring

Multiple intraluminal impedance is a relatively new procedure in which changes in the esophageal impedance tracings caused by the passage of liquid, solid, gas, or mixed boluses are analyzed. If the impedance changes of a liquid bolus appear first in the distal channels and proceed sequentially to the proximal channels, they indicate retrograde bolus movement, which is GER. The upward extent of the bolus and the physical length of the bolus can also be evaluated.[20] MII can detect extremely small bolus volumes.

Combined measurement of pH and impedance (pH/MII) provides additional information as to whether refluxed material is acidic, weakly acidic, or nonacidic. The technology is especially useful in the postprandial period or at other times when gastric contents are nonacidic. The combination of pH/MII with simultaneous monitoring of symptoms using video-polysomnography or manometry has proven useful for the evaluation of symptom correlations between reflux episodes and apnea, cough, other respiratory symptoms, and behavioral symptoms.[21] Evaluation of MII recordings is aided by automated analysis tools. Normal values for all of the age groups have not yet been established.

Tests on Ear, Lung and Esophageal Fluids

Recent studies have suggested that finding pepsin, a gastric enzyme, in middle ear effusions of children with chronic otitis media, indicates that reflux is playing an etiologic role.[22] However, this relation has not been validated in controlled clinical trials.

Empiric Trial of Acid Suppression as a Diagnostic Test

In adults, empiric treatment with acid suppression, has been used for symptoms of heartburn, chronic cough, noncardiac chest pain, and dyspepsia. But, empiric therapy has only modest sensitivity and specificity as a diagnostic test for GERD, as compared to reference standard used (endoscopy, pH monitoring, symptom questionnaires),[23] and the appropriate duration of a "diagnostic trial" of acid suppression has not been determined. The 2-week "PPI test" lacks adequate specificity and sensitivity for use in clinical practice. In an older child or adolescent with symptoms suggesting GERD, an empiric PPI trial is justified for up to 4 weeks. However, in these cases also improvement following treatment does not confirm a diagnosis of GERD because symptoms may improve spontaneously or respond by a placebo effect.

Summary of the Diagnostic Techniques

It is advisable in such a scenario, to allow clinical presentation to dictate the diagnostic approach. For instance, in case of persistent vomiting or dysphagia, anatomical causes or severe esophagitis are to be investigated, preferably through barium studies and EGD. Alternatively, if the clinical presentation is wheezing,

apnea, or recurrent pneumonia, investigation is advisable with pH monitoring and nuclear scans. If seizure like activities are observed, especially with normal EEG's, it may be advisable to investigate the presence of reflux with pH monitoring and videographic recording. Lastly, if the presentation is of a feeding problem with a persistent failure of the baby to thrive, reflux esophagitis is to be investigated through an EGD along with biopsy.

Simplified Approach to Diagnosis and Management of GERD Based on Symptoms and Signs (Flow charts 3.1 and 3.2)

While investigating possible causes of recurrent pneumonia and suspected GER, it is advisable to exclude other potential causes, such as anatomical abnormality, aspiration during swallowing, foreign body, cystic fibrosis, immunodeficiency and neurological impairment. Tests useful in differentiating cases of recurrent pneumonia and suspected GER from these other conditions include flexible bronchoscopy with BAL for lipid laden

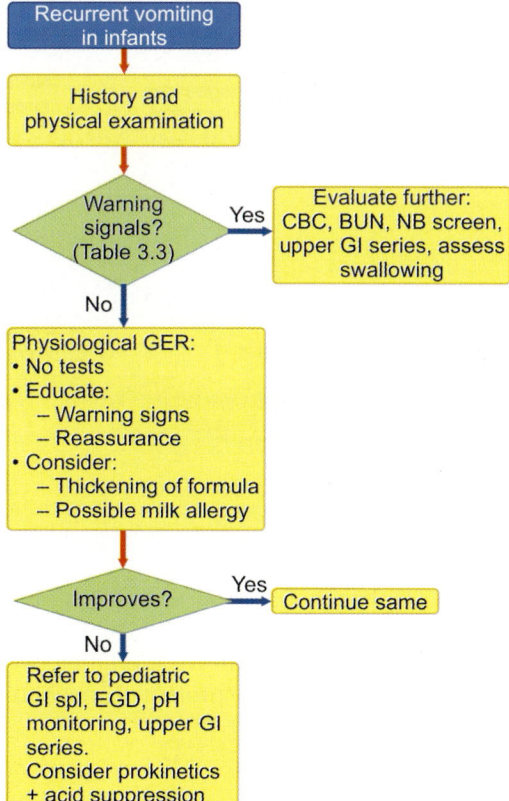

Flow chart 3.1: Recurrent vomiting in infants

[Modified and adapted from Joint Recommendations of the North American Society for Pediatric Gastroenterology, Hepatology and Nutrition (NASPGHAN) and the European Society for Pediatric Gastroenterology, Hepatology, and Nutrition (ESPGHAN), 2009]

Flow chart 3.2: Approach to older child with chronic heartburn

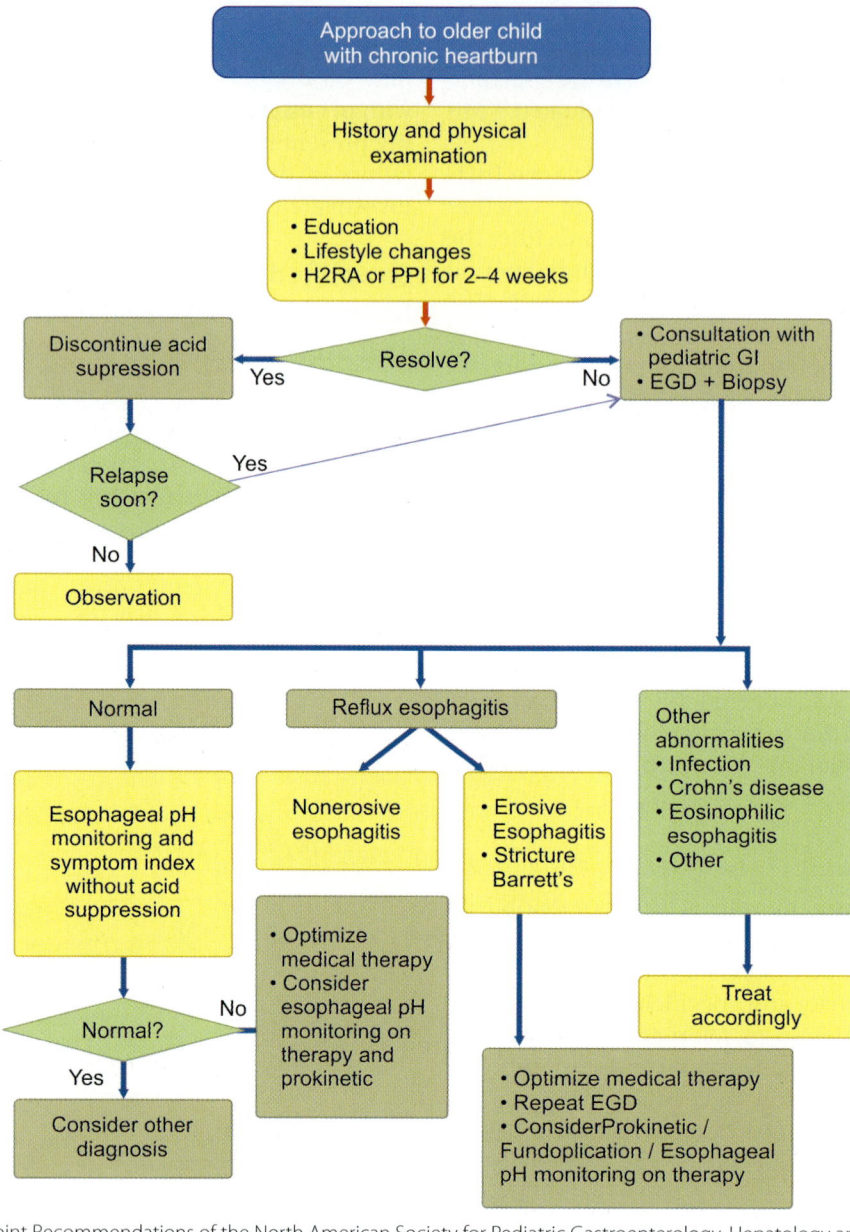

[*Modified and adapted from* Joint Recommendations of the North American Society for Pediatric Gastroenterology, Hepatology and Nutrition (NASPGHAM) and the European Society for Pediatric Gastroenterology, Hepatology and Nutrition (ESPGHAN), 2009.]

alveolar macrophages, nuclear scintigraphy, VSS (video fluoroscopic swallowing study), or FEEST (fiber-endoscopic swallowing evaluation), the latter two being for effectively evaluating airway protective mechanisms.

■ MANAGEMENT OF GERD

Physiological GER

Before initiating the management of GER in infants with recurrent vomiting, allergy to cow's milk protein (CMPI)

should be considered in the differential diagnosis. Response to stoppage of cow's milk feed within 2–3 weeks and relapse of symptoms after reintroduction of cow's milk is the only way to diagnose CMPI as laboratory investigations are hardly reliable.

For physiological GER, when the baby continues to gain weight adequately, only reassurance is required. If vomiting is very troublesome, then thickening of feeds may be advised. Adding feed thickeners such as rice cereal—the most commonly used thickening agent for formula, decreases the frequency of overt regurgitation, but it does not decrease the time with pH <4 (reflux index) measured by esophageal pH studies.[24,25] Thickening with 1 tablespoon per 2 oz of formula increases the energy density to ~27 kcal/oz (~0.95 kcal/mL).

Positioning Therapy for Infants

Several studies in infants have demonstrated significantly decreased acid reflux in the flat prone position compared with flat supine position.[26,27] However, there are significant concerns regarding the association of SIDS with the prone position and therefore prone position is recommended only in the awake infant who can easily be observed and specially in the postprandial period. During sleep, only the supine position is recommended.

Also, to be noted is the fact that the amount of reflux in supine infants with head elevated is equal to or greater than in infants supine and flat. The semisupine positioning in an infant exacerbates GER, and the full upright position appears to decrease measured reflux due to the effect of gravity, one study suggested that using formula thickened with rice cereal is more effective in decreasing the frequency of regurgitation than upright positioning after feeds.[26-28]

In older children, the left lateral position with head high is considered effective and better than the supine position for the management of reflux.

Lifestyle Changes in Children and Adolescents

Expert opinion suggests that children and adolescents with GERD should avoid caffeine, chocolate, alcohol, and spicy foods if they provoke symptoms. However, available literature does not support (or refute) the use of specific dietary changes to treat reflux beyond infancy. In an overweight individual, weight loss does decrease reflux, and is therefore recommended. Smoking should be avoided in those with GERD because it has been linked to adenocarcinoma of the esophagus in adults. Some studies have shown that chewing sugarless gum after a meal decreases reflux.[29]

■ PHARMACOLOGIC THERAPIES

Histamine-2 Receptor Antagonists (H2RA)

Histamine-2 receptor antagonists (H2RAs) decrease acid secretion by inhibiting histamine-2 receptors on gastric parietal cells. Gastric pH begins to increase within 30 minutes of administration and the effect lasts for 6 hours. Tachyphylaxis or dimunition of the response has been observed after 6 weeks of administration of H2RA drugs. Also, the efficacy of H2RA in achieving mucosal healing

and symptom relief is lesser than that of PPI.[30] H2RA are generally recommended only in older children and adolescent and that too for those with mild to moderate symptoms.

Side effects of H2RA in infants include irritability, head banging, headache, and somnolence.

The commonly used H2RA include ranitidine, famotidine, cimetidine and nizatidine. The usual dose of ranitidine is 2 mg/kg/day in 2 divided doses.

Proton Pump Inhibitors

Proton pump inhibitors (PPIs) act by inhibiting acid secretion by blocking the Na^+–K^+- ATPase, the final common pathway of parietal cell acid secretion. PPIs are more efficacious because of their ability to maintain intragastric pH at or above 4 for longer periods and to inhibit meal-induced acid secretion, this results in decrease in 24-hour intragastric acid volumes, thereby facilitating gastric emptying and decreasing the volume of reflux.[30,31] The effect of PPIs does not diminish with chronic use and their long-term use has also been found to be safe and effective on comparison with H2RAs. Side effects of PPIs include constipation, diarrhea, dizziness, headache and their long-term use may be associated with side effects of acid suppression like malabsorption of nutrients and drugs, and microbial overgrowth.

Proton pump inhibitors currently approved for use in children are omeprazole, lansoprazole, and esomeprazole. No PPI has been approved for use in infants younger than 1 year of age. The dose of omeprazole 1–3.3 mg/kg/day OD or divided BI and that of lansaprazole is 1.4 mg/kg/day OD.

Prokinetics

Available prokinetic agents include dopamine receptor blockers (metoclopropamide, domperidone), serotonin receptor (5HT3,4) agonists (cisapride, mosapride), and drugs with both effects (itopride).

Domperidone and ***metoclopramide*** are antidopaminergic agents that facilitate gastric emptying and also increase the LES tone. However, no RCT is available to demonstrate their clinical efficacy in children with GERD. They are poorly active and are associated with side effects like lethargy, irritability, gynecomastia, galacctorrhea, and extrapyramidal reactions. Their long-term use is, therefore, not recommended.

Cisapride is a mixed serotonergic agent, it acts by facilitating the release of acetylcholine at synapses in the myenteric plexus, leading to increased gastric emptying and improving esophageal and intestinal peristalsis. Clinical studies of cisapride in children with GERD showed significant reduction in the RI but with less consistent reduction in symptoms.[32] Cisapride's use has become restricted, it was found to produce prolongation of the QTc interval on electrocardiogram, increasing the risk of sudden death. Moreover it is not recommended to be used along with some other drugs like macrolide antibiotics, antifungal agents and antiviral agents that are also metabolized through cytochrome P450. **Mosapride,** on the other hand, has a better safety profile (than cisapride) vis a vis cardiac arrhythmias and does not interact with other cytochrome P450 inhibitors like macrolides, antifungals, antivirals, etc. Although used commonly in adults, its dose and use in children is not yet clearly defined.

Other prokinetic drugs like **bethanechol** (a direct cholinergic agonist), **erythromycin** (acts on motilin receptors) have uncertain efficacy and a high incidence of side effects limiting their use in clinical practice.[33]

Baclofen is a γ-amino-butyric-acid receptor agonist reduces both acidic and nonacidic reflux and also increases gastric emptying in children. However, it has unacceptable side effects like drowsiness, dizziness, fatigue and lowers seizure threshold that preclude its routine use.[1]

Other Agents

Antacids directly buffer gastric contents, thereby reducing heartburn and healing esophagitis. On-demand use of antacids may provide rapid symptom relief in some children and adolescents with NERD. Although, this approach appears to carry little risk, long-term use of antacids containing aluminum hydroxide is associated with side effects like increased plasma aluminum levels and those containing calcium carbonate with milk alkali syndrome (a triad of hypercalcemia, alkalosis and renal failure). Moreover, these agents have a short duration of action and need to be given 3–4 times a day. These agents, therefore, have limited use and are beneficial only for immediate relief in older children and adolescents on a need basis. Their routine or long-term use in the management of GERD is not recommended.[1]

Surface protective agents mostly comprise of alginate or sucralfate. Alginates are insoluble salts of alginic acid, a component of algal cell walls. Sucralfate is a compound of sucrose, sulfate, and aluminum which, in an acid environment forms a gel that binds to the exposed mucosa of peptic erosions. Although these agents have shown to be effective in decreasing symptoms and healing of nonerosive esophagitis in adults, the available data of their safety and efficacy in children is inadequate to warrant their routine use in the management of GERD in children.

Surgical Therapy

Fundoplication decreases reflux, including physiologic reflux by increasing the LES baseline pressure, decreasing TLESR and the nadir pressure during swallow-induced relaxation, increasing the length of the esophagus that is intra-abdominal, accentuating the angle of His, and reducing an HH if present.[34] Esophageal clearance, gastric emptying, or other GI dysmotility disorders are not corrected by fundoplication.[1]

Indications for surgical management of gastroesophageal reflux:
- ❑ Failure of medical therapy for gastroesophageal reflux (typically over 12 weeks) and infants and children who cannot be weaned off of acid-reducing medications.
- ❑ Those with an atypical presentation, especially respiratory, whose symptoms are clearly associated with gastroesophageal reflux (e.g. obstructive apnea temporally associated with reflux during pH monitoring. However, a period of medical therapy (including acid blockade) under close monitoring conditions should be attempted in many cases prior to recommending a surgical approach.
- ❑ Patients with complications of gastroesophageal reflux, such as aspiration, stricture of the esophagus, or Barrett esophagus should be considered for surgical treatment.
- ❑ Patients with neurologic impairment that requires feeding gastrostomy who are found to have pathologic reflux and remain medication dependent should also be considered for surgery.
- ❑ Patients with chronic reflux and recurrence of anastomotic stricture after repair of esophageal atresia should be considered for surgical treatment.

In a RCT comparing the efficacy and safety of laparoscopic fundoplication versus esomeprazole (20 mg qid) for treatment of adults with GERD, good to excellent symptom control was achieved in more than 90% of the treated adults in both groups. Dysphagia was present in 10% cases in the surgical group whereas, it was uncommon in the medically treated group. Quality of life measures were similar in both groups.[35] More recent long-term follow-up studies have demonstrated that relapse rates following fundoplication may also be considerable.

Corrosive Ingestion and Injury

Caustic Ingestion

Corrosive ingestion is a common pediatric problem. It is most common in children less than 3 years of age and more frequently observed in males.

Three types of chemicals can produce these injuries—alkalies (ph > 7), acids (ph < 7) and bleaches (ph = 7).

Alkalies cause the most severe injury and work through liquefaction necrosis. Once they form soap after coming in contact with fat, they become soluble and can diffuse deeper into the tissues thereby causing significant injury. The average household contains about half a dozen different cleaning products. Common sources of alkalies are various household cleaning solutions (containing 25% and 36.5% sodium or potassium hydroxide), drain cleaners (containing 25% and 36.5% of lye), etc. Acids work through coagulation necrosis, with formation of an eschar by the reaction. This coagulum serves to protect the tissues by limiting deeper penetration. Examples of strong acid sources include toilet bowl cleaners and metal cleaners (hydrochloric acid), car battery fluids (Sulfuric acid), anti-rust compounds (phosphoric acid), etc. The impression that acid burns are less serious than alkali burns is also a result of the infrequency with which these compounds are accidently consumed since they are mostly colored compounds with strong odors as against the alkali cleaners that are mostly colorless and odorless. Bleaches on the other hand are less harmful, can cause significant gastritis but rarely lead to esophageal burns or stricture formation.[36]

The amount, concentration and time of contact of the agent all factor into the severity of the burn. The initial contact of the agent will produce immediate changes in the mucosa which progresses over the next 3 days. Up to the transmural tissue, destruction leading to esophageal perforation and involvement of the mediastinum may occur acutely. Following the acute phase of the injury, a latent period begins, during which time stricture formation may occur. This process may proceed as rapidly as one month or over a period of years.[37]

Acute Corrosive Ingestion

A careful history with details of the brand name, type and amount of ingestion should be elicited. History of any ensuing vomiting after the ingestion should also be recorded since vomiting leads to an increased duration of contact with the caustic. Symptoms of hoarseness, stridor and dyspnea are noted. Odynophagia, drooling and refusal of food suggest a more severe injury. Substernal pain, abdominal pain, and rigidity suggest more grave injury and probably perforation of the stomach or esophagus.

Physical examination can reveal evidence of burns on the lips, chin, hands, oral cavity, pharynx, etc. The presence or absence of oral injuries is not predictive of esophageal injury and further evaluation should continue even if no findings are obvious.

Investigations

Blood investigations: Hemogram, serum electrolytes, liver and kidney fuction tests, coagulation profile and arterial blood gases are indicated in most cases. A WBC count of greater than $20,000/mm^3$ is an independent predictor of mortality in corrosive poisoing. Hypocalcemia may be observed with hydrogen fluoride poisoning. Arterial bood pH and base deficits also correlate with severity and adverse outcomes.

Radiology

Plain chest and abdominal X-rays may reveal features of perforation in the thorax or abdomen with findings of pneumothorax, pneumomediastinum or air under the diaphragm. Contrast studies are better avoided due to the high risk of aspiration and inflammation and a low sensitivity in detecting perforation.

CT scan of the neck/chest/abdomen is indicated where there is high suspicion of perforation but normal plain X-rays. Contrast enhanced CT is also useful in determining the esophageal thickness and predicting response to future stricture dilatation.

Endoscopy: The best time to do an esophagoscopy is within 24 to 48 hours of ingestion since by this time the injury would have demarcated itself well so that the degree of injury could be assessed. Endoscopy done after 48–72 hours increases the risk of perforation and also visualization is poor due to the presence of inflammatory exudate, tissue swelling and tissue necrosis.

Indications for upper GI endoscopy include corrosive ingestion by small children, symptomatic older children, children with altered mental status, intentional ingestion, patients with ingestions of large volumes and more concentrated products. The contraindications to endoscopy are any hemodynamic compromise, suspicion of GI perforation or peritonitis or mediastinitis and ingestion of very small amounts, asymptomatic patients with normal oral/upper airway.

Esophagoscopy is carried out to the upper limit of a severe burn beyond which the chances of perforation are high. On endoscopy, grade I is a superficial injury, grade II is transmucosal and grade III is transmural (Figs 3.1A and B). It is also important to note whether the injury is circumferential, which is most likely to lead to stricture formation.

Laryngoscopy may be required in patients with stridor and cough and extensive mouth burns. Chest and plain abdominal X-rays may be necessary in cases where aspiration and perforation is suspected.[38,39]

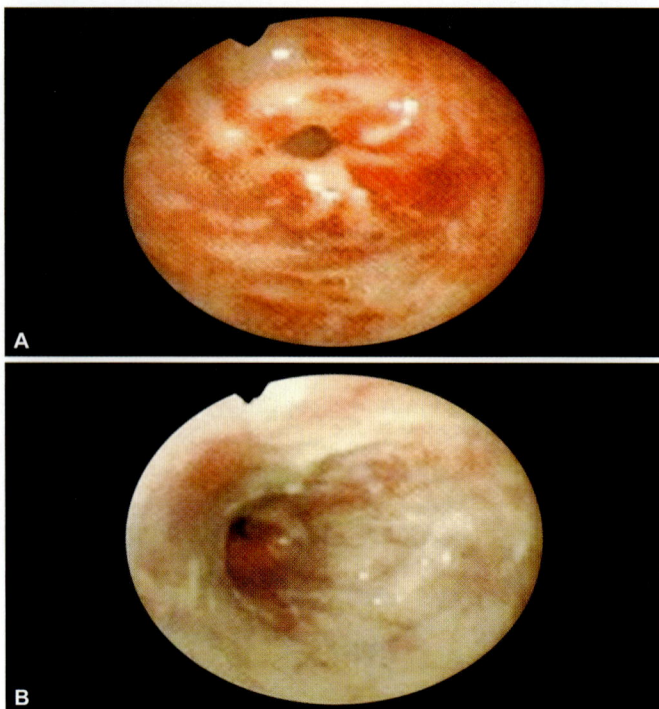

Figs 3.1A and B: Endoscopic view of the esophagus after ingestion of a household cleaning solution (alkali) showing marked erythema, ulcerations and sloughing of the esophageal mucosa

Management

In cases of minimal corrosive ingestion and no oropharyngeal burns on examination, the patient only needs to kept for observation.

In patients with history of large volume ingestions or in any symptomatic patient with signs like stridor, hoarseness of voice and respiratory distress, the patient requires admission to intensive care, airway management and hemodynamic stabilization.

The aim of treatment is to prevent permanent injury or stricture in the esophagus.

Initial treatment should begin with rinsing the mouth with water or milk. Drinking water or milk an lead to dilution and neutralization of the chemical but should not exceed 15–20 mL/kg since it can cause vomiting leading to further exposure of the esophagus.

Induced emesis and gastric lavage are contraindicated for the same reason. Nasogastric tube insertion should also not be attempted due to the risk of aspiration and perforation. Efforts to neutralize acids with alkali or vice versa should not be undertaken as heat generated by the neutralization reaction can seriously extend the damage that has already occurred.

Intravenous fluids and analgesics should be initiated for patient comfort.

Antibiotic use is controversial but may be useful in prevention of secondary infection.

Use of steroids in acute severe corrosive injury in an attempt to prevent stricture formation is debatable. Mild injury does not lead to stricture formation and therefore steroids have no role.

Prevention of secondary injury from gastric acid reflux is prevented by use of H_2 receptor antagonists or antacids.

Patients with more severe lesions may also require gastrostomy for enteral feeding or rarely even total parenteral nutrition (TPN).[40]

Subsequent Management

Despite all measures, stricture formation still develops in 10–15% of all esophageal burns. Management of strictures is primarily by dilatation. Barium esophagogram must be obtained to define the number and extent of strictures before embarking on program of dilatation (Fig. 3.2). Corrosive strictures tend to be most resistant to dilatation and usually require repeated dilatation.

Acid poisoning can often result in pyloric narrowing which can present as gastric outlet obstruction. This may need surgical management. Esophageal replacement surgery is reserved for cases where stricture dilatation fails.

The final consideration is the 1,000 times higher risk of development of esophageal carcinoma in some cases.

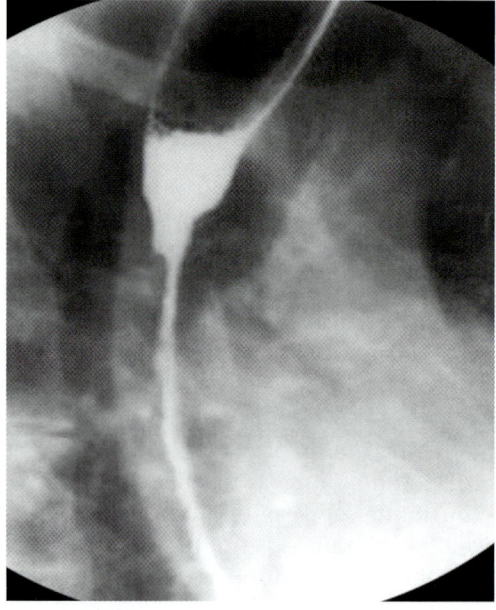

Fig. 3.2: Flouroscopic findings of esophageal stricture extending from the carina to the distal esophageal end in a case of corrosive poisoning

immunocompetent patients are treated with oral acyclovir along with use of antacids, sucralfate, etc.

Cytomegalovirus (CMV) esophagitis is best diagnosed by biopsy. Specific therapy for CMV esophagitis using ganciclovir may be helpful in immunocompromised hosts. CMV infection seems particularly common after liver and bone marrow transplant and is probably related to the use of the potent immunosuppressant cyclosporine A.

Bacterial esophagitis usually occurs as a superinfection of the viral or fungal esophagitis or secondary to trauma to the esophagus.

Eosinophilic Esophagitis

Eosinophilic esophagitis (EE) is a rare allergic inflammatory condition of the esophagus and is characterized by the infiltration of the esophageal mucosa with eosinophils. Symptoms of this condition include vomitings, regurgitation, dysphagia, epigastric pain and food refusal in small children. Sometimes, it is indistinguishable from GERD. Eosinophilic esophagitis can be associated with esophageal strictures and present with food impaction, dysphagia, heartburn, etc. It is more common in males and is usually not diagnosed by 7 years of age. Atopy in other forms and associated other food allergies are present in most patients. Patients have an elevated peripheral absolute eosinophil count and levels of IgE are also raised. Biopsy of the esophagus reveals more than 15–20 eosinophils/hpf (Fig. 3.11B). Grossly the esophageal mucosa may be normal or appear furrowed, granular or ringed (Fig. 3.11A). As against GER, erosive esophagitis is absent. There is poor response to anti-reflux agents clinically. Treatment strategies include dietary modifications to exclude food allergens, anti-allergic therapy and dilatation of strictures. An attempt to find out the offending allergen is made through allergy testing and if identified, it is eliminated from the diet. In case, this is not possible, the six common dietary allergens (milk, wheat, soy, egg, peanuts, tree nuts, seafood) are eliminated and response is looked for. If the patient is still symptomatic, he/she is put on an elemental amino-acid diet. Topical and systemic corticosteroids are used in patients whom do not respond to dietary modifications or in who the primary cause is not allergy. Other anti-inflammatory agents including leukotriene antagonists, anti-interleukins and antihistamines, have also be tried but with limited success.[49]

Esophageal Atresia and Tracheoesophageal Fistula

Esophageal atresia with or without tracheoesophageal fistula is a fairly common congenital malformation seen in newborns.

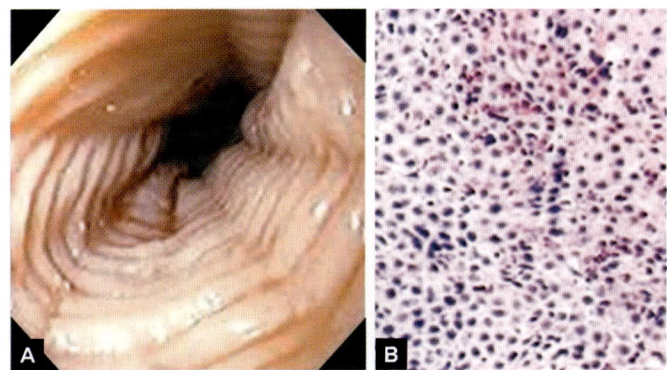

Figs 3.11A and B: Gross and microscopic appearance of eosinophilic esophagitis on upper GI endoscopy and biopsy

The incidence ranges from 1 in 3,000 to 1 in 5,000 live births. Prompt recognition, appropriate clinical management and early referral to a tertiary care center can result in significant reduction in the morbidity and mortality associated with this condition.[50]

Embryology

The esophagus and the trachea are derived from the primitive foregut. The trachea forms as a ventral diverticulum during 4th and 5th week of gestation, from the primitive pharynx (caudal part of the foregut). A tracheoesophageal septum develops at the site where the longitudinal tracheoesophageal folds fuse together. (Figs 3.12A and B). The septum divides the foregut into a ventral portion, the laryngotracheal tube and the dorsal portion (the esophagus). Esophageal atresia results if the tracheoesophageal septum is deviated posteriorly. This deviation causes incomplete separation of the esophagus from the trachea and results in a concomitant tracheoesophageal fistula.

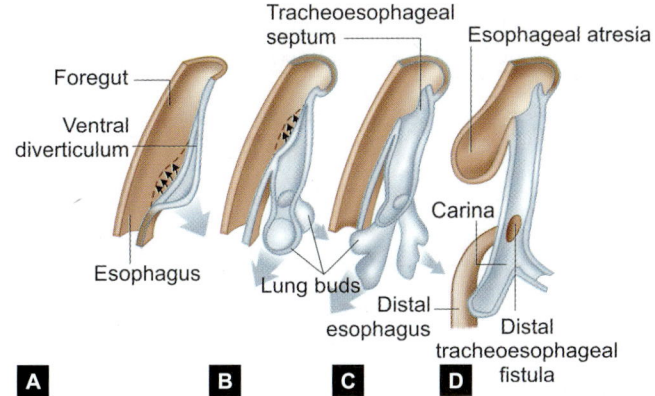

Figs 3.12A to D: Successive stages in the development of the tracheoesophageal septum during embryologic development [*Source:* Dwayne et al, Am Fam Physician. 1999;59(4):910-6.]

In case of isolated esophageal atresia without a tracheoesophageal fistula, the atresia is attributable to failure of the recanalization of the esophagus during the 8th week of gestation.

Pathology

Several anatomic variations of tracheoesophageal fistula (TEF) may occur. The classification system described by Gross of Boston is most often cited (Figs 3.13A to E).

According to this system, the types of esophageal atresia and the approximate incidence in all infants born with esophageal anomalies is as follows:

❑ Type A: Esophageal atresia (EA) without fistula or so called pure esophageal atresia (10%)
❑ Type B: Esophageal atresia with proximal TEF (1%)
❑ Type C: Esophageal atresia with distal TEF (85%)
❑ Type D: Esophageal atresia with proximal and distal TEFs (1%)
❑ Type E: TEF without esophageal atresia or so called H type fistula (4%).

In the most common variety, the fistula often enters the trachea close to the carina.

The proximal esophageal pouch is often hypertrophied and dilated secondary to the fetus efforts to swallow amniotic fluid. This muscular pouch pressing on the trachea can also be the cause of associated tracheomalacia at times.

Associated Defects

Additional congenital anomalies are present in approximately 50% of infants presenting with esophageal atresia with or without TEF. Among these, 25% of infants have cardiac defects, the most common ones being ventricular septal defect, patent ductus arteriosus and tetralogy of Fallot. GI malformations may occur in up to 16% infants with esophageal atresia, most common are imperforate anus, duodenal atresia, and malrotation. Renal and urological defects such as hypospadias, renal agenesis, ureteral malformations and horseshoe kidneys are commonly associated with esophageal atresia and TEF

and occur in up to 10% of cases. Musculoskeletal defects of the ribs and vertebra are common.

Trisomies 13, 18, 21 may be associated with esophageal atresia/TEF. 10% of the infants with CHARGE syndrome (coloboma of the iris, heart anomaly, choanal atresia, mental retardation, genital hypoplasia and ear abnormalities) have concurrent EA/TEF.

Opitz syndrome and VACTERAL syndrome (vertebral anomalies, renal atresia, cardiac anomalies, TEF, renal anomalies, limb anomalies) are X-linked syndromes associated with TEF. Up to 10% of infants with esophageal atresia/TEF have the VACTERAL syndrome. Fenigold syndrome, Pallister Hall syndrome, and anophthalmia-esophageal genital syndrome are other autosomal dominant syndromes that may be associated with EA/TEF.

Isolated esophageal atresia is associated with a higher incidence of other malformations than esophageal atresia with TEF.[51]

Clinical Presentation

Esophageal atresia may be suspected antenatally with ultrasound finding of polyhydramnios and absence of fetal stomach bubble.

At birth, inability to pass an appropriate size infant feeding tube up to the stomach in the newborn should make one highly suspicious of an underlying esophageal atresia. In the absence of atresia, a size 10 tube in the term infant and a size 8 tube in the preterm infant should reach the stomach after 17 cm of the tube has been inserted. In the presence of atresia, no more than 10–12 cm will be passed before resistance is encountered. Smaller size or softer tubes might coil in the upper pouch and this can be confirmed later on radiographs.

Classically, the newborn with esophageal atresia presents with copious, white, frothy bubbles of mucus in the mouth and sometimes the nose. The newborn may have respiratory distress, noisy breathing, choking, gagging, coughing and cyanosis.

If there is pure esophageal atresia without fistula, the abdomen will be scaphoid and if a TEF is present along

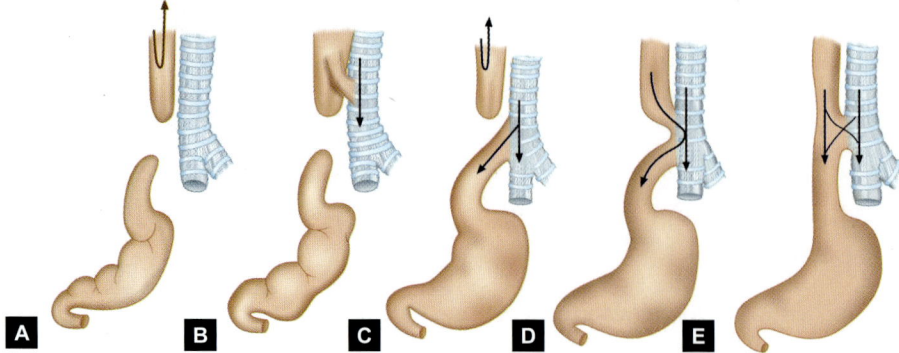

Figs 3.13A to E: Types of tracheoesophageal fistula

with esophageal atresia, abdominal distension may develop as air accumulates in the stomach.

Other associated anomalies as mentioned above should be looked for.

In all cases of esophageal atresia, chest radiographs (anteroposterior and lateral) should be obtained to confirm the position of the tube. The X-ray should include the entire abdomen. In cases of esophageal atresia, air in the stomach confirms the presence of distal fistula. In most other types (excluding the H type), the abdomen contains no gas. The chest X-ray also provides information about the cardiac silhouette, the location of the aortic arch, the presence of any associated vertebral or rib anomalies and pulmonary infiltrates if any. Contrast studies are seldom required and may increase the risk of aspiration pneumonitis.

Management

Once a diagnosis of esophageal atresia is made, preparation must be initiated for corrective surgery but immediately rushing the patient into the operating room is not required. Initial treatment of EA/TEF should involve stabilization of the newborn prior to transfer to a tertiary care center with pediatric surgery and intensive care services.

Measures should be taken to reduce the risk of aspiration. The infant should be nursed in a head high position at an angle of 30–45 degrees. The oral pharynx should be cleared and an 8 French sump tube placed for continuous suction of the upper pouch. Intravenous fluids should be started and oxygen initiated if required. In infants with severe respiratory distress, endotracheal intubation and ventilation may be required. Bag-mask ventilation is not appropriate since it may cause acute gastric distension in some cases. Empiric antibiotic therapy for pulmonary prophylaxis is recommened by many experts due to high risk of aspiration. The use of H_2 blockers like ranitidine may be helpful to prevent further reflux related complications in cases of tracheoesophageal fistulae with the distal esophagus.

Before surgical correction, the newborn should be thoroughly evaluated for the presence of other associated anomalies. Investigations such as chest X-ray, abdominal X-ray, echocardiogram and renal ultrasound should be obtained to rule out any underlying skeletal or cardiac anomalies, intestinal obstruction, malrotation and renal anomalies.

Healthy infants without pulmonary complications or other major anomalies can undergo primary repair in the first few days of life with very good survival.

Surgical repair may, however, be delayed in infants with low birth weight, pneumonia or other major anomalies. Such infants are usually treated with parenteral nutrition, gastrostomy and upper pouch suction until they are appropriate surgical candidates. The survival rate in this group is lower but in the range of 80–95%. Cardiac anomalies are usually the cause of death in these more complicated cases.

Surgery

Surgical ligation of the TEF and primary end-to-end anastomosis of the esophagus are performed wherever feasible. In very preterm babies or otherwise complicated baby, a primary closure may be delayed and initial surgery may just involve fistula ligation and a gastrostomy tube placement. If the gap between the two atretic segments is long (>3–4 cm), primary repair cannot be performed and in such cases a neoesophagus may be created by interposing either gastric, jejunal or colonic segments.

Postoperative Care

The intubated patient is transported to the neonatal intensive care unit (NICU). Antibiotics are continued till the chest drain is removed and the endotracheal tube is suctioned as necessary. Oral suctioning to a depth of no more than 7 cm from the lips is performed every half an hour for the first days, then every hour or as required from the second day onwards. Morphine is infused as necessary for management of postoperative pain and TPN commenced. Premature extubation and subsequent intubation in the setting of a freshly closed fistula invites reopening of the fistula. The chest drain should be observed for passage of any saliva since this may signal an anastomotic leak and this is often associated with respiratory distress.

Provided the baby is stable, a water-soluble contrast-enhanced study is done on day 6 or 7 to assess for leaks and to view the caliber of the repair. If the esophagus is patent and of adequate size, the baby can be fed orally. Next, the chest tube is removed and intravenous fluids disconnected as soon as the baby is feeding well. Oral ranitidine is prescribed for 6 months owing to the high incidence of gastroesophageal reflux in this group of patients and the risk of development of esophageal strictures.

Long-term follow-up: During follow-up, these children have a high probability of developing GER, recurrent aspiration pneumonia, tracheolaryngomalacia and recurrent laryngitis. Stricture at the anastomotic site is a frequent occurrence and may require repeated endoscopic dilatation.

REFERENCES

1. Joint Recommendations of the North American Society for Pediatric Gastroenterology, Hepatology, and Nutrition (NASPGHAN) and the European Society for Pediatric Gastroenterology, Hepatology, and Nutrition (ESPGHAN). J Pediatr Gastroenterol Nutr. 2009;49:4.

2. Iacono G, Merolla R, D'Amico D, et al. Gastrointestinal symptoms in infancy: a population-based prospective study. Dig Liver Dis. 2005;37:432-8.

3. Heine RG, Jordan B, Lubitz L, et al. Clinical predictors of pathological gastro-oesophageal reflux in infants with persistent distress. J Paediatr Child Health. 2006;42:134-9.

4. Orenstein SR, Shalaby TM, Cohn JF. Reflux symptoms in 100 normal infants: diagnostic validity of the infant gastroesophageal reflux questionnaire. Clin Pediatr (Phila). 1996;35:607-14.

5. Aggarwal S, Mittal SK, Kalra KK, et al. Infant gastroesophageal reflux disease score: reproducibility and validity in a developing country. Trop Gastroenterol. 2004;25:96-8.

6. Stordal K, Johannesdottir GB, Bentsen BS, et al. Gastroesophageal reflux disease in children: association between symptoms and pH monitoring. Scand J Gastroenterol. 2005;40:636-40.

7. Meyers WF, Roberts CC, Johnson DG, et al. Value of tests for evaluation of gastroesophageal reflux in children. J Pediatr Surg. 1985;20:515-20.

8. Gupta JP, Kumar A, Jain AK, et al. Gastro-esophageal reflux disease (GERD): an appraisal of different tests for diagnosis. J Assoc Physicians India. 1990;38(Suppl 1):S699-702.

9. Jang HS, Lee JS, Lim GY, et al. Correlation of color Doppler sonographic findings with pH measurements in gastroesophageal reflux in children. J Clin Ultrasound. 2001;29:212-7.

10. Seibert JJ, Byrne WJ, Euler AR, et al. Gastroesophageal refluxthe acid test: scintigraphy or the pH probe? AJR Am J Roentgenol. 1983;140:1087-90.

11. Arasu TS, Wyllie R, Fitzgerald JF, et al. Gastroesophageal reflux in infants and children comparative accuracy of diagnostic methods. J Pediatr. 1980;96:798-803.

12. Sherman P, Hassall E, Fagundes-Neto U, et al. A global evidence-based consensus on the definition of gastroesophageal reflux disease in children. Am J Gastroenterol. 2009;104:1278-95.

13. Lundell LR, Dent J, Bennett JR, et al. Endoscopic assessment of oesophagitis: clinical and functional correlates and further validation of the Los Angeles classification. Gut. 1999;45:172-80.

14. Vakil N, van Zanten SV, Kahrilas P, et al. The Montreal definition and classification of gastroesophageal reflux disease: a global evidence-based consensus. Am J Gastroenterol 2006;101:1900-20.

15. Dent J. Microscopic esophageal mucosal injury in nonerosive reflux disease. Clin Gastroenterol Hepatol. 2007;5:4-16.

16. TF TONG, DKK NG. A Review of Esophageal pH Monitoring for the Diagnosis of Gastroesophageal Reflux in Children. HK J Paediatr (new series). 2002;7:112-7A.

17. Mahajan L, Wyllie R, Oliva L, et al. Reproducibility of 24-hour intraesophageal pH monitoring in pediatric patients. Pediatrics. 1998;101:260-3.

18. Vandenplas Y, Helven R, Goyvaerts H, et al. Reproducibility of continuous 24 hour oesophageal pH monitoring in infants and children (see comments). Gut. 1990;31:374-7.

19. Hochman JA, Favaloro-Sabatier J. Tolerance and reliability of wireless pH monitoring in children. J Pediatr Gastroenterol Nutr. 2005;41:411-5.

20. Wenzl TG. Invited review: investigating esophageal reflux with the intraluminal impedance technique. J Pediatr Gastroenterol Nutr. 2002;34:261-8.

21. Wenzl TG. Evaluation of gastroesophageal reflux events in children using multichannel intraluminal electrical impedance. Am J Med. 2003;115(Suppl 3A):161S-5S.

22. Tack J. Review article: the role of bile and pepsin in the pathophysiology and treatment of gastro-oesophageal reflux disease. Aliment Pharmacol Ther. 2006;24(Suppl 2):S10-6.

23. Numans ME, Lau J, de Wit NJ, et al. Short-term treatment with proton-pump inhibitors as a test for gastroesophageal reflux disease: a meta-analysis of diagnostic test characteristics. Ann Intern Med. 2004;140:518-27.

24. Khoshoo V, Ross G, Brown S, et al. Smaller volume, thickened formulas in the management of gastroesophageal reflux in thriving infants. J Pediatr Gastroenterol Nutr. 2000;31:554-6.

25. Craig WR, Hanlon-Dearman A, Sinclair C, Taback S, Moffatt M. Metoclopramide, thickened feedings, and positioning for gastro-oesophageal reflux in children under two years. Cochrane Database Syst Rev. 2004:CD003502.

26. Meyers WF, Herbst JJ. Effectiveness of positioning therapy for gastroesophageal reflux. Pediatr. 1982;69:768-72.

27. Tobin JM, McCloud P, Cameron DJ. Posture and gastro-oesophageal reflux: a case for left lateral positioning. Arch Dis Child. 1997;76:254-8.

28. Chao HC, Vandenplas Y. Effect of cereal-thickened formula and upright positioning on regurgitation, gastric emptying, and weight gain in infants with regurgitation. Nutrition. 2007;23:23-8.

29. Avidan B, Sonnenberg A, Schnell TG, et al.Walking and chewing reduce postprandial acid reflux. Aliment Pharmacol Ther. 2001;15:151-5.

30. Van Pinxteren B, Numans ME, Bonis PA, Lau J. Short-term treatment with proton-pump inhibitors, H_2-receptor antagonists and prokinetics for gastro-oesophageal reflux disease-like symptoms and endoscopy negative reflux disease. Cochrane Database Syst Rev. 2006:CD002095.

31. Khan M, Santana J, Donnellan C, Preston C, Moayyedi P. Medical treatments in the short-term management of reflux oesophagitis. Cochrane Database Syst Rev. 2007:CD003244.

32. Dalby-Payne JR, Morris AM, Craig JC. Meta-analysis of randomized controlled trials on the benefits and risks of using cisapride for the treatment of gastroesophageal reflux in children. J Gastroenterol Hepatol. 2003;18:196-202.

33. Euler AR. Use of bethanechol for the treatment of gastroesophageal reflux. J Pediatr. 1980;96:321-4.

34. Vandenplas Y, Hassall E. Mechanisms of gastroesophageal reflux and gastroesophageal reflux disease. J Pediatr Gastroenterol Nutr. 2002;35:119-36.

35. Lundell L, Attwood S, Ell C, et al. Comparing laparoscopic antireflux surgery with esomeprazole in the management of patients with chronic gastro-oesophageal reflux disease: a 3-year interim analysis of the LOTUS trial. Gut. 2008;57:1207-13.

36. Lupa M, Magne J, Amendee R. Update on the diagnosis and treatment of caustic ingestion. Oschner J. 2009;9(2):54-9.

37. Kay M, Wyllie R. Caustic ingestions in children. Current Opinion in Pediatrics; 2009.

38. Lahoti D, Broor SL. Corrosive injury to the upper gastrointestinal tract. Ind J Gastroenter. 1993;12:135-41.

39. Lakshmi CP, Vijayahari R, Kante V. A hospital based epidemiological study of corrosive alimentary injuries with particular reference

to the Indian experience. The National Medical Journal of India. 2013;26:1.

40. Ramulu Naik RR, Vadivelan M. Corrosive Poisoning. Indian Journal of Clinical Pediatrics. 2012;23:3.

41. Richter JE. Peptic strictures of the esophagus. Gastroenterol Clin North Am. 1999;28(4):875-91.

42. Bansal A, Peter JK, Marquardt GH. Treatment of GERD complications, Barrett's, peptic stricture and extraesophageal syndromes. Clinical Gastroenterolgy. 2010;24(6):961-8.

43. Mittal SK, Kalra KK, Khanijo CM, Rajeshwari K. Benign oesophageal strictures in children of north India. Trop Gastroenterol. 2000;21(1):37-40.

44. Uyemura MC. Foreign body ingestion in children. Am fam Physician. 2005;72(2):287-91.

45. Kay M, Wyllie R. Pediatric foreign bodies and their management. Current gastroenterology reports. 2005;7(3):212-18.

46. Gilger M, Jain A, McOmber M. Foreign bodies of the esophagus and the gastrointestinal tract in children. UpToDate, 2009.

47. Park W, Vaezi M. Etiology and pathogenesis of achalasia: the current understanding. Am J Gastroenterol. 2005;100(6):1404-14.

48. Francis, DL; Katzka, DA . Achalasia : Update on the disease and its treatment. Gastroenterology. 2010;139(2):369-74.

49. Noel Richard J, Putnam Philip E, Rothenberg Marc E. Eosinophilic esophagitis. New England Journal of Medicine. 2004;351(9):940-1.

50. Clark DC. Esophageal atresia and tracheoesophageal fistula. Am Fam Physician. 1999;59:910.

51. Goyal A, Jones MO, Couriel JM, Losty PD. Esophageal atresia and tracheoesophageal fistula. Arch Dis Child Fetal Neonatal Ed. 2006;91: F381.

Chapter

4

Neurogastroenterology and Motility Disorders

Paolo Quitadamo, Efstratios Saliakellis, Osvaldo Borrelli, Nikhil Thapar

▌ INTRODUCTION

Gut motility disorders comprise a heterogeneous group of disorders that result from disruption of the functional integrity of the intrinsic neuromusculature of the gastrointestinal (GI) tract. This intrinsic neuromusculature includes the smooth muscle layers, the intrinsic nervous system of the GI tract (enteric nervous system or ENS) and the interstitial cells of Cajal. The contribution of each of these components to function can be compromised by alterations in structure (ranging from absence to derangement in numbers and/or anatomy) or of function (complete or partial failure in physiological function). This pathology can be primary or secondary to a number of insults, e.g. infections, inflammation, toxins etc. In children disorders may be congenital being present from birth or acquired later in life. Finally involvement of the enteric neuromusculature can be patchy/segmental or affect the gastrointestinal tract diffusely.

Neurogastroenterology is the study of the interface of all aspects of the gastrointestinal tract or digestive system with the different branches of the body's nervous system including the enteric, central and autonomic nervous systems. The combined terms 'Neurogastroenterology and motility' are designed to encompass the study of all the components of the enteric neuromusculature and their modulating influences and represents one of the fastest growing areas in gastroenterology clinical practice and research. This chapter aims to address some of the most common neurogastroenterology and motility conditions seen in clinical practice ranging from those with defined pathology to those which fall under the umbrella of functional gastrointestinal disorders. The latter comprise some of the commonest but challenging disorders and the term 'functional' reflects the fact that in the majority of such conditions no organic cause can be found. It should also be noted that at the present time many functional disorders, e.g. abdominal pain-related functional GI disorders, represent symptom complexes that can further be subdivided into more discrete entities, e.g. irritable bowel syndrome, functional abdominal pain, etc. depending on the nature, location and associations of the symptoms. Clinicians will often rely on the presence or absence of 'red flags', e.g. associated weight loss, severe or significant symptoms, etc. to decide whether patients are likely to have organic or functional disorders. Exhaustive investigations in the latter are likely to prove fruitless, expensive and perpetuate 'illness behaviors' in the patients.

▌ ABDOMINAL PAIN-RELATED FUNCTIONAL GASTROINTESTINAL DISORDERS

Introduction

Abdominal pain-related functional gastrointestinal disorders (FGID) constitute a spectrum of conditions characterized by the presence of recurrent abdominal pain in the absence of any defined pathology.[1] In the past these disorders fell under the single term 'Recurrent abdominal pain' (RAP) but have since been re-categorized under an international initiative (Rome Foundation) to improve the diagnosis and classification of such conditions. The Rome III criteria[2,3] are currently being utilized (summarized in Tables 4.1 to 4.5).

RAP is frequently encountered as a presenting complaint in pediatrics.[4,5] In the majority of patients no organic disease is identified.[6] Despite its benign nature the persistence of symptoms can result in significant stress to children and their families as well as clinicians concerned at the possibility of missing an underlying pathology. With the implementation of the Rome III criteria, abdominal pain-related FGID, have been framed as a positive diagnosis rather than one of exclusion,[3] which will hopefully facilitate the reduction of unnecessary diagnostic procedures and expedite the initiation of appropriate treatment.[7]

Epidemiology

The prevalence of childhood abdominal pain-related FGID in western countries has been estimated to be between 0.3 to 19%.[8] Various definitions and diagnostic criteria used for such disorders prior to the development of the ROME III criteria are likely to have accounted for the wide range of the reported prevalence.

Pathophysiology

The pathophysiological model for abdominal pain-related FGIDs is undoubtedly multifactorial.[9] It has been proposed that various mechanisms such as genetics, early life events, environmental, gastrointestinal and psychosocial factors act together in a complex interplay ultimately resulting in an alteration to the gut-brain axis.[10-16] Afferent signals from the gastrointestinal tract transmitted via the pain pathways are subsequently amplified and the patient's perception of painful stimuli is in turn enhanced.[17] These phenomena have been defined as visceral hypersensitivity and central hypervigilance respectively.[14]

Clinical Presentation

According to the Rome III criteria, the diagnosis of abdominal pain-related FGIDs relies on the absence of any evidence of possible organic disease that could account for patient's symptomatology and a distinct clinical picture. The latter proposes to allow abdominal pain-related FGIDs to be divided into five disorders; (i) Functional abdomen pain (FAP)—when abdominal pain (intermittent or continuous) is present at least once a week for a period of ≥2 months prior to the diagnosis along with criteria insufficient for the diagnosis of other abdominal pain-related FGIDs; (ii) Functional abdomen pain syndrome (FAPS)—when the criteria of FAP are present for at least 25% of the time along with some loss of functioning on a daily basis and/or the presence of somatic symptoms, such as headache, sleeping difficulties and limb pain; (iii) Functional dyspepsia (FD)—when there is pain (persistent or recurrent) or discomfort localized in the upper abdomen (above the level of umbilicus) at least once a week for a period of ≥2 months prior to diagnosis along with criteria insufficient for the diagnosis of irritable bowel syndrome (IBS); (iv) Abdominal migraine—when there are paroxysms of intense and acute periumbilical pain (duration ≥ 1 hour) that affects child's normal activities and is associated with ≥ 2 of the following symptoms—anorexia,

Table 4.1: 'Red flag' or alarm features that may suggest the presence of an underlying organic pathology for recurrent abdominal pain in children

From history
- Onset of symptoms <5 years of age
- Presence of constitutional symptoms (e.g. fever, weight loss)
- Presence of nocturnal symptoms (e.g. pain that awakens the child, diarrhea)
- Gastrointestinal bleeding
- Vomiting
- Dysphagia
- Persistent right upper or lower abdominal quadrant pain
- Presence of referred pain (back, shoulders and extremities)
- Dysuric symptoms
- Family history of inflammatory bowel disease, celiac or peptic ulcer disease

From physical examination
- Faltering growth, delayed puberty
- Hepatosplenomegaly
- Jaundice
- Signs of perianal disease (tags, fissures and fistulas)
- From first-line blood test
- Anemia, neutropenia or thrombocytopenia
- Hypoalbuminemia
- Elevated inflammatory markers (white blood cell count, erythrocyte sedimentation rate, C-reactive protein)

nausea, vomiting, headache, photophobia and pallor. The episodes of pain are followed by intervals of usual health (duration—weeks to months). The aforementioned criteria must be present at least once a week for a period of ≥2 months prior to diagnosis; (v) IBS when there is abdominal discomfort or pain associated with ≥2 of the following at least 25% of the time—improvement with defecation, onset of pain associated with a change in the frequency of bowel motions, onset of pain associated with a change in the consistency of stools and duration of the abovementioned criteria at least once a week for a period of ≥2 months prior to the diagnosis.[3]

During history taking, physical examination and interpretation of first-line blood tests, there are certain features that may suggest the presence of an underlying organic pathology. Physicians need to be aware of these "red-flag" signs/symptoms, which are summarized in Table 4.1.[1]

The identification of alarm features should guide the diagnostic procedure toward excluding an organic disease. Amongst the myriad of pathologies that could potentially present with abdominal pain (Table 4.2) below lists those most frequently encountered in pediatrics.

Diagnostic Investigations

Laboratory tests, imaging studies and endoscopic procedures should be performed wisely and guided by

Table 4.2: Potential organic disorders as differential diagnoses of recurrent abdominal pain

Gastrointestinal system
- Gastroesophageal reflux
- Peptic ulcer disease
- Celiac disease
- Eosinophilic gastrointestinal disease
- Food allergy
- Inflammatory bowel disease
- Chronic constipation
- Malrotation
- Hernias
- Intussusception
- Tumors (e.g. lymphoma)

Pancreatic and hepatobiliary
- Cholelithiasis
- Cholecystitis
- Chronic hepatitis
- Chronic pancreatitis

Respiratory system
- Pneumonia

Genitourinary system
- Nephrolithiasis
- Pyelonephritis/Cystitis
- Ureteropelvic junction obstruction
- Hematocolpos

Musculoskeletal system
- Trauma
- Tumors

Other systems
- Sickle cell disease
- Leukemia
- Diabetes mellitus
- Porphyria
- Familial mediterranean fever
- Lead poisoning

the information obtained from the history and physical examination. Although there is lack of evidence to evaluate the usefulness of blood tests as a discriminatory tool between functional and organic disease, a limited number of first line tests may be warranted. It has been proposed that these should include a full blood count with differential, erythrocyte sedimentation rate, C-reactive protein, celiac serology, urinalysis, urine culture, and fecal examination for ova and parasites.[18,19] Extensive diagnostic investigations should be avoided as they are usually not clinically indicated, are of significant financial cost and ultimately impair the physician-patient relationship as they increase patient's uncertainty regarding the diagnosis and the overall treatment plan.[1]

Treatment

The management plan of the childhood FAP should be based on the biopsychosocial model for FGID and needs to incorporate a multidisciplinary approach specifically developed to each child's symptomatology and identifiable triggers.[17]

Dietary interventions (such as food elimination diets) and use of probiotics have shown favorable results in certain groups of patients with FAP, however more data are needed in order to fully evaluate their therapeutic efficacy.[20,21]

Psychosocial interventions (e.g. parental education, family therapy, relaxation, distraction, hypnotherapy, biofeedback) are also very effective in reducing the severity and maintenance of somatic symptoms in children with abdominal pain-related FGID.[22] Indeed it has been shown that hypnotherapy in particular is a highly beneficial therapeutic modality even when compared to conventional medical care resulting in long-term remission in children with either FAP or IBS.[23,24] More work needs to address the modalities and resources needed to deliver hypnotherapy in the broader clinical arena.

Certain groups of drugs, such as antidepressants (e.g. tricyclic antidepressants, serotonin reuptake inhibitors), antispasmodics (e.g. peppermint oil, hyoscyamine), cyproheptadine and prokinetics (e.g. domperidone, erythromycin) have been reported to be successful in the treatment of childhood FAP and are used widely, albeit variably.[25-29] There is, however, a clear lack of well-controlled trials to precisely support the efficacy of long-term of the aforementioned medications in the pediatric population. Thus the benefit of their use in clinical practice is yet to be elucidated.[30] With regard to complementary and alternative medicine (herbal preparations, acupuncture) there are currently no sufficient data to support their potential therapeutic role in childhood FAP.[18,31]

Overall, robust randomised placebo-controlled trials are needed to assess these agents especially given reports of substantial placebo effects of up to 50%.[32]

Prognosis

Long-term follow-up of children with RAP reveals that 35–50% of them will eventually progress to complete resolution of their symptoms, whereas at least 25% will continue to experience abdominal pain in adulthood. Amongst children with RAP those who had been given a clear and simple explanation of their condition along with the physician's reassurance were less likely to express extra-abdominal complaints or relapse later in life.[33–35] Male gender, onset of symptoms at an age younger than 6 years, duration of symptoms >6 months, low educational and socioeconomic status, presence of a so-called 'painful family' and an increased number of surgical procedures (eg tonsillectomy, appendectomy) have been established as poor prognostic indicators for the long-term outcome of children with RAP.[33,35]

Conclusion

Abdominal pain-related FGIDs may result in a significant impairment of the well being of children and their families as well. The role of the physician is crucial in advising the family to adopt appropriate parenting styles, which create a supportive and loving environment that subsequently reduces the anxiety caused in children by minor injuries/illnesses and other stressful situations that they may encounter.

The diagnostic approach and therapeutic management of a child presenting with RAP may be challenging. A detailed history combined with a thorough clinical examination as suggested by the Rome III criteria remains the cornerstone for diagnosis. Baseline laboratory investigations may aid the establishment of a positive diagnosis of FGID, thereby leading to prompt appropriate management and better long-term outcomes.

FUNCTIONAL CONSTIPATION

Introduction

Chronic constipation is a common problem in children with a reported prevalence of between 0.7% and 29.6% (median 12%).[36] Most often it is defined as a delay or difficulty in defecation present for at least 2 weeks sufficient to cause significant distress to the patient.[37] A normal pattern of stool evacuation is commonly thought to be a sign of health in children of all ages. Especially during the first months of life, parents pay close attention to the frequency and the characteristics of their babies' defecation. Any deviation from what they think is normal may trigger a call to the nurse or a visit to the pediatrician. Thus, it is not surprising that approximately 3% of general pediatric outpatient visits and 25% of pediatric gastroenterology consultations are related to a perceived defecation disorder.[38] Chronic constipation is an important source of anxiety for parents who often worry that a serious disease is causing the symptom, accepting that beyond the neonatal period, the most common cause of constipation in children is functional with only a small minority of children thought to have an organic cause.

Pathophysiology

Functional constipation is defined as constipation without objective evidence of a pathological condition and is thought to result from painful bowel movements with consequent voluntary withholding of feces, by a child who wants to avoid unpleasant defecation. Several events can lead to painful defecation, such as toilet training, changes in routine or diet, stressful events, intercurrent illness, deliberate avoidance or unavailability or of toilets, e.g. at school, or the child's postponing defecation because he or she is too busy. Withholding feces can lead to protracted fecal stasis in the colon with resorption of fluids leading to both a change in stool consistency and an increase in their overall size. The passage of large, hard stools that painfully stretch the anus may frighten the child and result in a fearful determination to avoid all defecation. Such children respond to the urge to defecate by contracting their anal sphincter and gluteal muscles, attempting to withhold stool.[39,40] Eventually, the rectum habituates to the stimulus of the enlarging fecal mass, and the urge to defecate slackens. After a while, such retentive behavior becomes an automatic reaction. As the rectal wall stretches, fecal soiling may occur, angering the parents and frightening the child.[41] After several days without a bowel movement, irritability, abdominal distension, cramps, and decreased oral intake may appear.

Diagnosis

Currently, the most widely accepted criteria to diagnose childhood functional constipation are the Rome III criteria.[2,3] There are two sets of criteria based on the age of the patient (i.e. below and above the age of 4 years) and the diagnosis is based on careful clinical history and examination. The history should include both a personal (e.g. age at first passage of meconium and onset of symptoms, acquisition of developmental milestones and growth parameters, associated symptoms including bilious vomiting or rectal bleeding, etc.) as well as family history (e.g. gastrointestinal disease, allergy, other non-gastrointestinal disorders etc.). Examination should focus on general well-being, growth parameters, the abdomen for organomegaly, distention and masses, inspection of the anus, as well as examination of the lumbosacral spine and neurology. Table 4.3 lists a number of 'red flags' that should alert the clinician to the possibility of organic

Table 4.3: Red flags
Main red flags which may suggest organic constipation
• Delayed passage of meconium after birth (> 48 hours)
• Early onset (first months of life)
• Family history of Hirschsprung disease
• Growth failure
• Abnormal examination of lumbosacral spine (sacral dimple, patch of hair, gluteal cleft deviation)
• Abnormal neurological examination of anal reflexes and/or lower limbs
• Abnormal anus (position, scars, fistulae)
• Other significant signs or symptoms (blood in stools in the absence of visible anal fissures, massive abdominal distention, bilious vomiting, fever)
• Unusual history and examination findings (consistent empty rectal ampulla on rectal examination, absence of withholding or fecal incontinence, extreme anal phobia)

disease underlying the constipation. The presence of one or more of these should raise the suspicion for organic cause of constipation and need for further workup. It should be noted that this list is not exhaustive.

According to the Rome III criteria the diagnosis of functional constipation in a child below the age of 4 years is considered secure when there are present (31 month prior to diagnosis) at least two of the following criteria: (i) two or fewer defecations per week (ii) at least one episode/week of incontinence after the acquisition of toileting skills; (iii) history of excessive stool retention; (iv) history of painful or hard bowel movements; (v) presence of a large fecal mass in the rectum; (vi) history of large diameter stools which may obstruct the toilet.[2] The same criteria (accepting retentive posturing as a sign of stool retention) can be applied to children with a developmental age greater than 4 years of age where the diagnosis of functional constipation is based on the presence of two or more of the criteria being fulfilled at least once per week for at least 2 months before diagnosis and there should also be insufficient criteria for the diagnosis of IBS.[3]

Investigations

A thorough history and physical examination is usually sufficient to allow the practitioner to establish whether the child requires further investigation or has functional constipation. The presence of 'red flags should alert the clinician to the possible need for further testing to exclude organic pathology. Metabolic tests, such as serum calcium level and thyroid function tests, X-ray abdomen, barium enema, anorectal manometry, suction rectal biopsy, colonic manometry, magnetic resonance imaging of the lumbosacral spine, and psychological evaluation may be helpful in order to rule out a possible organic cause of constipation. These should be performed in liaison with a pediatric gastroenterologist.

Treatment

The general approach to the child with functional constipation includes four sequential phases—parental education, elimination of the fecal mass if present, maintenance therapy to prevent fecal reaccumulation, and close follow-up for a sufficient time-period to adjust medications as necessary.[1,42] The education of the family should include the demystification of constipation and an explanation of its pathogenesis. Moreover, parents are encouraged to maintain a consistent, positive, and supportive attitude in all aspects of treatment. If a fecal mass is present, disimpaction must be carried out before initiation of maintenance therapy and may be accomplished by either the oral or rectal route. The

oral approach is less invasive and gives a sense of power to the child, but adherence to the treatment regimen may be a problem, particularly given the increased fecal incontinence seen with the use of polyethylene glycol.[43] The rectal approach is faster but is invasive and may become more challenging with repeated use. Oral (with polyethylene glycol) and rectal disimpaction have been shown to equally effective[43] and the choice of treatment is best determined after discussing the options with the family and child. Disimpaction with oral medication has been successfully reported with high doses of mineral oil, polyethylene glycol electrolyte solutions, or both.[44-48] Rectal disimpaction may be performed with phosphate, saline, or mineral oil enemas alone or in combination.[49,50] Once the impaction has been removed, the treatment focuses on maintenance therapy to prevent recurrence. This treatment consists of dietary interventions, behavioral modification, and laxatives to assure that bowel movements occur at normal intervals with good evacuation. Multiple laxatives have been routinely used in the treatment of childhood constipation with a number of new agents currently being trialed, mostly in adults.[51] At the present time published evidence suggests that polyethylene glycol 3350 should be the laxative of first choice in pediatrics for functional constipation.[42,51-54] Enemas do not appear to carry any added benefit and should not be used routinely for maintenance therapy.[55] Increased intake of fluids and the use of absorbable and nonabsorbable carbohydrate, and more recently pro- and pre-biotics, are commonly advised as methods to soften stools and improve defecation frequency. Current evidence, however, does not support their routine use as supplementation over and above a normal intake, for the treatment of functional constipation.[51] Finally, an important component of treatment includes behavior modification and regular toilet habits, including unhurried time on the toilet after meals, although on their own these are unlikely to result in long-term sustained benefit.[56] Surgical interventions have little role in the management of functional constipation although there have been reports of success with the use of antegrade continence enemas in children with an intractable course.[57] Data on transcutaneous and sacral nerve stimulation is emerging and does not yet have a routine place in treatment.[58]

Prognosis and Long-term Outcomes

A systematic review of functional constipation follow-up studies suggested that almost two-thirds of children are found to be free from symptoms after 6 to 12 months of laxative treatment. Recovery rates appear to be better with early and sustained intervention with laxative treatment. Outcomes showed no relation with defecation frequency or positive family history and studies have been unable to identify a group of children at most risk of poor prognosis.[59-61] Long-term treatment and follow-up, with early therapeutic interventions of relapses remains an integral part of successful management of functional constipation.[42,62]

CHRONIC INTESTINAL PSEUDO-OBSTRUCTION

Introduction

Chronic intestinal pseudo-obstruction (CIPO) comprises a rare and heterogeneous group of conditions that variably affect one or more of the intrinsic gut components that govern intestinal motility namely the enteric nerves, muscles and interstitial cells of Cajal (ICCs) or affect their modulating influences. This impairs the ability of the intestine to propel its contents and CIPO is defined and characterized by repetitive episodes or continuous symptoms and signs of intestinal obstruction in the absence of a fixed, lumen-occluding lesion, which may be associated with radiological evidence of dilated bowel with fluid levels.[62,63] Although the true incidence and prevalence of CIPO conditions across the world are unclear, scanty epidemiological data suggest they are rare with an estimated incidence of approximately 1 in 40,000 live births.[64]

Pathophysiology

Conditions can be classified by whether they primarily affect intestinal smooth muscle (myopathies), nerves (neuropathies) or ICCs (mesenchymopathies) and can further be subdivided into primary or secondary, congenital or acquired, inheritance and what area of the gut they primarily involve.[63] CIPO in children most commonly occurs sporadically, is congenital and primary, and affects the intestine diffusely. At the present time, although mesenchymopathies have been implicated in a few reports, the majority of conditions are classified as neuropathies and myopathies.[65-69] For the majority this is adequately achieved through appropriate, often specialized, functional assessment and histopathology.

CIPO may also occur in association with other conditions affecting other systems of the body. Most commonly affected, more so in myopathies than neuropathies, is the urinary tract.[67] Specific conditions include hollow visceral myopathy and Megacystis—microcolon intestinal hypoperistalsis syndrome.[70] Other associations include connective tissue disorders, muscular dystrophies and autonomic disorders. CIPO may also occur secondary to intestinal surgery and a range of toxins, endocrine and metabolic defects. More recently, neuropathic viruses have been implicated in adult patients with CIPO.[71]

The genetics of CIPO is poorly characterized. In those that have been reported there appears to be a heterogeneous pattern of inheritance consisting of autosomal recessive (AR), autosomal dominant (AD) and X-linked (XL).[72] Genes implicated include those for the transcription factor Sox10 (AD), filamin A (XL), and the L1 cell adhesion molecule (XL). CIPO is also seen in the context of mitochondrial disorders caused by mutations in the thymidine phosphorylase [mitochondrial neurogastrointestinal encephalomyopathy (MNGIE) syndrome] or in the polymerase-gamma genes (MNGIE without leukoencephalopathy).[73]

Clinical Presentation

Patients with CIPO typically present with recurrent or continuous sub-occlusive episodes, which resemble intestinal mechanical obstruction. Patients with congenital CIPO typically present early in life with the majority being diagnosed within the first few weeks and months of life. Some of these will present in utero with a dilated urinary tract or abdominal distention. Approximately, a third of children with congenital CIPO have intestinal malrotation.[67]

Symptoms vary according to age at presentation and the part of the gastrointestinal tract primarily affected. They commonly include vomiting (which is often bilious) and abdominal distension. Other symptoms variably include abdominal pain, anorexia, poor weight gain, constipation and diarrhea. Other symptoms may result from involvement of other organ systems, e.g. urinary tract (megacystis with increased bladder compliance and capacity and poor detrusor contractility, ureterohydronephrosis, recurrent UTIs). A most severe condition involving both the intestine and urinary system is megacystis-microcolon intestinal hypoperistalsis syndrome.[71] Symptoms may also be secondary to complications, e.g. diarrhea from bacterial overgrowth. Exacerbation of symptoms may be precipitated by various causes including intercurrent infections and stress.

The clinical course is generally characterized by relapses and remissions leading, in a small proportion, to gradual decompensation of intestinal function and ultimately to intestinal failure. This is more likely in severe cases, and those presenting late and/or that have been inadequately treated.

Diagnosis

Although this may be suspected from the clinical history (including family history) and course of the disease, it is often difficult because of the varied clinical presentation and limitations in the availability of specific or specialized diagnostic testing. Plain abdominal radiographs classically show a dilated gastrointestinal tract, which may contain air-fluid levels. Contrast studies often show marked delays in intestinal transit and may reveal other abnormalities, such as malrotation and microcolon. Water-soluble contrast should be used instead of barium to prevent insipissation of contrast. Unfortunately, children with CIPO often undergo repeated and complex gastrointestinal surgery (including resection of dilated loops of bowel), which is neither diagnostic nor curative, before a diagnosis is finally made. A diagnosis of pseudo-obstruction should be suspected if there are symptoms of a generalized dysmotility (vomiting, abdominal distension and constipation) especially when they occur recurrently or chronically with no symptom free intervals. Associated urinary symptoms and autonomic nervous system dysfunction may also be suggestive. Review of previous radiological studies and histopathology may be helpful.

A more definitive diagnosis relies on following a number of specific steps:

❑ *Exclusion of any mechanical obstructive lesion* of the gastrointestinal tract (X-rays, contrast studies or by previous exploratory surgery).
❑ *Confirmation of abnormal motility* (functional motility testing, e.g. esophageal manometry, electrogastrography, gastric emptying studies, bowel transit studies, small and large bowel manometry). An abnormal small intestinal (antroduodenal) manometry study, with disruption of the phasic fasting motor activity, is classically associated with CIPO.[73]
❑ *Search for an underlying cause* for the pseudo-obstruction, including potentially treatable ones. This may include, for example, assessment of hematological parameters, blood chemistry, metabolic screening, toxicology, infections, connective tissue diseases, etc. Histopathological assessment is often valuable in the diagnosis and classification of CIPO. Limitations and variability in expertise and availability of specialized histopathological tools are a significant problem. International initiatives are underway to improve the diagnostic yield and ultimate classification of CIPO disorders.[74-76]

Pediatric condition falcification has been recognized in children presenting with potential CIPO.[77] Small intestinal manometry in such children is often normal in direct contrast to those suffering from CIPO.

Treatment

Unfortunately, the management of CIPO has seen little real progress and essentially remains supportive to:
❑ Maintain nutrition
❑ Preserve growth and development
❑ Limit symptoms and improve quality of life
❑ Limit complications such as bacterial overgrowth and life-threatening sepsis.

Nutrition aims to maintain maximally tolerated enteral feeds with use of parenteral nutrition (PN) as required. In our experience although most of the CIPO children had ileostomy formation to decompress the bowel and reduce afterload, three quarters of the myopathic CIPO remained dependent on PN as a main source of nutrition and fluid long-term as opposed to just over a third of the neuropathic CIPO patients *(N Thapar, unpublished)*. Maintaining patients on maximally tolerated enteral nutrition preserves intestinal viability, enhances adaptation and limits associated complications e.g. hepatic cholestasis. Regimes to achieve this include specialized feeds and diets that transit the intestine most effectively and contain minimal residue. Continuous rather than bolus feeds via a gastrostomy or jejunostomy may be required.[78-80]

Drug use is largely limited to control of inflammation and immunomodulation, and of bacterial overgrowth, with variable success reported with prokinetics.[80,81] The best studied and apparently most effective motility agents such as cisapride and tegaserod are no longer available, given safety concerns. Newer agents are being developed but not routinely available at present. Many current regimes to enhance intestinal motility are anecdotal or based case reports and include the use of, for example, the somatostatin analog octreotide in combination with erythromycin.[81] Sepsis by bacterial translocation or infection of central venous lines is a major consideration and antibiotic use is a valuable part of treatment.

Surgery remains the most common intervention in patients with pseudo-obstruction with roles in diagnosis, feeding, symptom relief, bowel decompression, bypassing of diseased segments, etc.[82] In our practise the majority of children with CIPO will have formation of an ostomy early in the course of the disease. Maintaining bowel decompression (nasogastric tubes, venting gastrostomies or jejunostomies, surgical stomas) is valuable not only for symptomatic relief but also helps limit further deterioration in effective motility secondary to chronic distension. It often reduces pseudo-obstructive episodes and enhaces the tolerance of enteral feeding.[80,81,83] Electrical pacing of the gastrointestinal wall using implantable pacemakers provides a potential therapy but remains experimental at present.

Small bowel transplantation remains the only definitive cure with a number of centres reporting improved outcomes and survival.[83.]

Prognosis

Intestinal pseudo-obstruction remains a serious life-threatening disease with devastating effects for patients and their families, including significantly impaired quality of life.[84] The mortality is not clear but is thought to be in the order of 20–30% long-term.[66,67] Increasing expertise in both the surgical and medical management has contributed to an improved prognosis especially to prevent complication such as sepsis and PN related liver disease. Outcomes from intestinal transplantation appear to be showing some improvement.[83,84]

Summary and Future Perspectives

CIPO presents a relatively rare but challenging group of conditions. Despite prolonged experience diagnosis remains difficult and management largely supportive. Initiatives to improve diagnosis and classification of disorders should help the identification and development of appropriate treatments. Recent advances raise possibilities for the use of novel pharmacologic agents and perhaps others such as cellular therapies to restore function.

GASTROINTESTINAL AND NUTRITIONAL PROBLEMS IN NEUROLOGICALLY IMPAIRED CHILDREN

Introduction

The current increasing survival of children with severe central nervous system damage has created a major challenge for medical care. Although, the primary problems for individuals with neurodevelopmental disabilities are physical and mental incapacities, several clinical papers have reported that brain injuries may often result in significant gastrointestinal (GI) dysfunction.[85-88] The enteric nervous system includes as many of not more nerve cells than the spinal cord and thus it is not surprising that any insult to the central nervous system may affect the complex integrated capacities underlying feeding and nutrition.[89] Gastrointestinal and nutritional problems in neurologically impaired children have been recently recognized as an integral part of their disease, often leading to growth failure and worsened quality of life for both children and caregivers. The increased awareness of such conditions, together with a better understanding of their etiology and interplay, is essential to achieve an optimal global management of this group of children.

Feeding and Nutritional Aspects

Historically, severe malnutrition has been accepted as an unavoidable and irremediable consequence of neurological impairment. Poor nutritional status was often marked by linear growth failure, decreased lean body mass, and diminished fat stores.[90,91] Over the past two to three decades, the development of multidisciplinary feeding programs providing comprehensive evaluation and management of feeding disorders in children with developmental disabilities have been proven to improve nutritional status and impact upon quality of life and a reduction in hospitalization rates.[92] Studies on small numbers of children with developmental disabilities have demonstrated that adequate nutritional support, provided by less invasive enteral access methods and better tolerated enteral formulae, may improve weight, muscle mass, subcutaneous energy stores, peripheral circulation, the healing of decubitus ulcers and general well-being, whilst at the same time decreasing irritability and spasticity.[93,94]

The true prevalence of undernutrition in neurologically impaired children is unknown. It has been estimated that approximately one-third are undernourished and many exhibit the consequences of malnutrition.[7] Yet, the prevalence and severity of malnutrition increases in parallel with the duration and severity of neurological impairment.[95-97] The predominant nutritional deficit is in energy intake, given that only 20% of these children regularly ingest 100% of their estimated average requirement. Moreover, half of the children with severe disabilities consumed less than 81% of the reference nutrient intake for copper, iron, magnesium, and zinc, influenced largely by their large consumption of milk.[98]

Nutritional support is essential for the care of neurologically impaired children. An individualized management plan accounting for the child's nutritional status, feeding ability, and medical condition should be determined. Energy requirements must be individualized considering muscle tone, mobility, activity level, altered metabolism and growth. In order to increase energy intake, the easiest and least invasive approach is to improve oral intake. Food caloric density may be increased by adding modular nutrients, modifying recipes or using high-calorie formulae. Children who cannot chew effectively may be able to receive the same foods blended into a puree of acceptable consistency. Those who can tolerate solids but not liquids can have commercial thickeners added to their fluids. Oral feeding skills may be improved with rehabilitation therapy, even if the results are often disappointing.[99-101] Adequate positioning of the child during meals and appropriate food temperature are also important. However, oral intake can be maintained as long as the child is growing well, there is no risk of aspiration, and the feeding time remains within acceptable limits. When oral intake is insufficient, unsafe, or too time-consuming enteral nutrition should be initiated.

The type of enteral access will depend on the anticipated duration of enteral nutrition support as well as the clinical status of the child. Nasogastric tubes are minimally invasive but are easily dislodged and may be associated with local complications such as otitis, sinusitis, congestion, and skin irritation. Therefore, nasogastric feeds should only be used for short-term nutritional support (usually less than three months). When long-term enteral nutrition support is required, a gastrostomy should be considered. Although more invasive, gastrostomies are more convenient and esthetically acceptable. Gastrostomy placement has been shown to reduce feeding time, food-related choking episodes, frequency of chest infections, family stress, and to improve weight and nutritional status significantly in children with severe neurologic impairment.[95,102] Percutaneous gastrostomy (PEG), however, is not without complications or concerns. Minor catheter infections, perforation and an overall reduced length of survival have being described in both adult and pediatric populations.[103-107]

The anatomy and function of the stomach should be carefully evaluated before the placement of the feeding tube. The coexistence of gastroesophageal reflux may require a simultaneous fundoplication, and delayed gastric emptying may necessitate consideration of pyloroplasty or duodenal placement of the distal portion of the tube. Physiologically designed formulas of increased caloric and protein density can be used for gastric and nasogastric infusion, as palatability is no longer an issue. The choice between bolus and drip may depend on esophagogastric function, the volume to be delivered, or the home care needs of the child and his or her caregivers. Often patients may benefit from a combination of daytime bolus and nocturnal continuous feeds, with the latter providing 30-50% of the child's nutrient needs thus allowing more freedom for daily activities. When safety of oral feeding is not an issue, these enteral techniques can merely supplement the child's own nutrition, with caregivers continuing to feed the child actively. This dual feeding method often provides great satisfaction to parents and caregivers given the mealtime interaction is improved when there is no longer need for force-feeding of medication or nourishment.

Gastrointestinal Problems

Chronic gastrointestinal disorders are very common in neurologically impaired children, with a reported prevalence of up to 92% 108. Dysphagia, rumination,

gastro-oesophageal reflux (GOR), delayed gastric emptying, abdominal pain and constipation have all been described in this group of children, potentially contributing to feeding difficulties and carrying challenging long-term management issues.

Dysphagia

Oro-motor dysfunction is a frequent concomitant issue and often one of the first signs of neuromuscular impairment. Related swallowing problems have been shown to affect up to 90% of neurologically impaired children, and is a major contributor to malnutrition.[86] This is not surprising since the development of oral-motor skills mirrors general neurological maturation and requires coordination of the movement of several striated muscles in the mouth, pharynx and esophagus, which are under the control of six cranial nerves, the brain stem and the cerebral cortex. In addition, anatomic abnormalities such as cleft palate, laryngeal clefts, and tracheoesophageal fistula may accompany neurologic deficits as part of congenital or genetic syndromes. Dysphagia may manifest as distress during meals (including coughing, choking, and refusal of feeding), chronic or episodic aspiration-related respiratory disorders, and failure to thrive. Barium swallow, cine-swallow, radionuclide esophageal clearance scan, and oesophageal manometry may all be of some help in the clinical assessment. Successful management of dysphagia is central to the child's well-being and ability to achieve his or her potential. Neurologically impaired children often show greater problems with liquid foods, thus requiring the use of thickener products. Oral motor exercise approaches using sensory modalities may help improving muscle strength and oral coordination. Nevertheless, in most cases, the presence of unsafe swallows and/or prolonged distressing mealtimes finally leads to the use of enteral rather than oral nutrition.

Gastroesophageal Reflux

Several reports have demonstrated a high incidence of Gastroesophageal reflux (GOR) in children with neurological impairment. Increased intra-abdominal pressure secondary to spasticity and scoliosis, prolonged supine position,, and coexisting hiatal hernia have been attributed as contributing factors to the increased frequency of GOR. Central nervous system dysfunction, however, is likely to be the primary cause, with GOR being part of the generalized dysmotility of the foregut or indeed the entire intestine. Decreased resting pressure and increased frequency of transient relaxations of the lower esophageal sphincter, together with esophageal motility abnormalities, are probably a consequence of neuromuscular incoordination.

Currently the most accurate way of diagnosing GOR is 24-hour oesophageal pH impedance recording, which allows not only the quantification of reflux episodes but also helps in establishing the temporal relationship between GOR and the symptom complex in question. The diagnostic work-up should then include upper GI endoscopy with multiple esophageal biopsies and upper GI barium study, in order to evaluate the mucosa and to look for the possible presence of strictures, diverticuli, or hiatal herniae. Radionuclide studies such as gastric scintigraphy should also be performed, given the higher incidence of delayed gastric emptying which may contribute to GOR.[109,110] An esophageal manometry evaluating visceral motility may be helpful to detect the underlying pathophysiological mechanisms, especially when surgery is being considered.

Although children with neurologic impairment are more likely to have intractable reflux and eventually require some surgical procedures, medical therapy should be tried first. When surgery is required, the Nissen fundoplication is currently the most widely used technique to strengthen the anti-reflux barrier and relieve symptoms.

Constipation

Infrequent stool passage and hard bowel movements are very common in neurologically impaired children. Total and segmental colonic transit times have been reported to be prolonged and delayed mainly at the level of the left colon and rectum in this group of children, implying a probable defect in gut innervation.[88] The problem is usually exacerbated by prolonged immobility, inadequate fiber intake, and concurrent medications. Unfortunately, recognition and effective management of constipation are often postponed because other disabilities overshadow those related to defecation. The therapeutic approach needs to be tailored to the individual patient. Oral or rectal disimpaction should be followed by promotion of regular bowel habit, through dietary modification, positioning, and use of laxative medications. A significant number of children with neurological impairment needs to be on chronic doses of laxatives. This medical management is usually effective in enabling regular defecation, but where it fails, consideration should be given to a surgically placed appendicostomy.

▌CYCLICAL VOMITING SYNDROME

Introduction

Cyclic vomiting syndrome (CVS) is a disorder characterized by recurrent, stereotypical episodes of intense nausea and vomiting lasting few hours to days interspersed with symptom-free periods of varying length.[111] In the majority of cases the underlying mechanisms remain unknown and patients are labeled as having idiopathic CVS. In children, the incidence of new cases has been reported to be 3.15/100,000 children per year, suggesting that CVS is more common than previously thought.[112] Although CVS may occur in all age groups the average age at initial diagnosis is 5 years with often a delay in diagnosis of several years. In children with CVS, there is a recognized association with a personal history of headache or migraine (in up to 45%) and family history of migraine. CVS has a substantially negative impact on children's quality of life, given that hospital admissions during the acute phase are rather common and that the condition significantly affects children' activities of daily living and academic time.[113]

Pathophysiology

The pathogenesis of CVS remains poorly understood and different mechanisms have been suggested including mitochondrial DNA (mtDNA) mutations responsible for deficits in cellular energy production, heightened hypothalamic-pituitary-adrenal (HPA) axis activation and autonomic nervous system (ANS) dysfunction.[114-116] A unifying theory has recently been hypothesized suggesting that psychological and physical stress conditions initiate the cascade of HPA axis activation by releasing corticotrophin-releasing factor (CRF), which in turn inhibits the foregut motility by activating the inhibitory motor neurons in the dorsal motor nucleus of the vagus, and increases the adrenergic tone by activating the locus ceruleus in the lateral floor of the fourth ventricle. In concert, during stress conditions when needs are increased the impaired cellular energy production due to mtDNA mutations is unable to meet the heightened demand and predisposes individuals to the onset of vomiting cycle, and perpetuates the dysfunction of the autonomic neurons because of their high energy requirement.

Clinical presentation

CVS has a typical on-off temporal pattern and is usually characterized by 4 different phases: 1. *The interepisodic or well phase*, which occurs between the vomiting episodes when the child is relatively symptom-free, and lasts weeks to months. 2. *The prodromal phase*, which is usually characterized by intense nausea, anorexia, pallor, lethargy and headache, and lasts minutes to hours. Usually, during this phase the child is still able to take and retain oral medication. 3. *The emetic phase*, during which the most common symptoms are intense nausea, vomiting, retching, listlessness, pallor, hypothermia or low grade fever, prostration, abdominal pain, diarrhea, photophobia, phonophobia and hypertension in the Sato variant. The episodes may last from hours to days (up to 10 days), with a median duration of 24–27 hours. The frequency of the emetic phases ranges from 1 to 70 per year with an average of 12 episodes a year, and the number of emeses during each attack is at least 4 times/hour for at least 1 hour. It usually occurs early morning (2–4 AM) or upon awakening (6–8 AM), and each episode tends to be stereotypical for each patient regarding the time of onset, the duration, intensity and symptomatology. Many patients show unusual specific behavior features during the attacks aimed at lessening the intense nausea, such as being irritable, verbally abusive, and demanding, taking long hot showers or baths, drinking compulsively, and remaining in the fetal position in a dark and quite room. Finally, various complications may occur as consequence of intense and repetitive episodes of vomiting including dehydration and electrolytes imbalance, peptic esophagitis, gastritis and hematemesis due to Mallory-Weiss tears, weight loss and dental caries. Specific triggering factors are identified in almost two third of patients including psychological stressors (holiday, birthday, vacation, parental or interpersonal conflict), physical stressors (lack of sleep, excess physical exhaustion, menses), infections (upper respiratory infections, sinusitis) and dietary factors (glutamate, chocolate, cheese, allergy). 4. *The recovery phase*, which begin when vomiting and nausea terminate and end when the child return to the normal activity.

Diagnosis

The diagnosis of CVS is primarily based on history and clinical presentation fulfilling the diagnostic criteria developed by North American Society for Pediatric Gastroenterology, Hepatology and Nutrition, in the absence of other possible causes with similar presentation.[117] These include the presence of all of the following: (i) at least 5 attacks in any interval, or a minimum of 3 attacks during a 6 month period (ii) episodic attacks of intense nausea and vomiting lasting 1 hour to 10 days and occurring at least 1 week apart (iii) stereotypical pattern and symptoms in the individual patient (iv) vomiting during attacks occurs at least 4 times/hour for at least 1 hour (v) return to baseline health between episodes and (vi) no evidence of organic disorder that could possibly account for the patient's symptomatology.[117]

There are no specific tests to diagnose CVS, and currently the basic assessment includes FBC, amylase, lipase, liver function test, basic metabolic profile (glucose, BUN and electrolytes), and upper gastrointestinal contrast study to rule out anatomical abnormalities. In the presence of warning signals, such as bilious vomiting, severe abdominal pain, abdominal tenderness,

episodes triggered by either fasting or high-protein meals, and abnormal neurological findings, further specific investigations should be promptly considered and tailored to the individual patient presentation. For instance, if there is a suspicion of metabolic and endocrine disorders additional laboratory tests, such as lactate, pyruvate, organic acid and amino acid analysis, plasma carnitine and acylcarnitine, plasma cortisol levels, and urinary prophyrins should be performed. Abdominal ultrasound, abdominal CT scan and upper gastrointestinal endoscopy should be considered in the presence of gastrointestinal alarm symptoms and signs. Finally, brain magnetic resonance imaging should be performed if a patient has neurologic manifestations. The differential diagnosis of disorders mimicking CVS is extensive and partially summarised in Table 4.4.

Management

The treatment of CVS is aimed at avoiding the trigger factors, terminating the acute phase, and preventing or reducing

---

Table 4.4: Differential diagnosis of cyclical vomiting in children and adolescents

Gastrointestinal disorders
- Bowel obstruction (malrotation with volvulus, duplication cyst, and intermittent intestinal intussusception)
- Inflammatory diseases (gastritis, duodenitis, peptic ulcer disease IBD)
- Pancreatic diseases (pancreatitis and pancreatic pseudocyst)
- Hepatobiliary disease (hepatitis)

Infections
- Enteritis
- Otitis media, chronic sinusitis, and hepatitis

Neurologic disorders
- Migraine
- Epilepsy
- Space occupying central nervous system lesions (hydrocephalus, posterior fossa tumors, subdural hematoma, and subdural effusion)
- Familial dysautonomia

Metabolic and endocrine disorders
- Diabetes mellitus, Addison disease, and pheochromocytoma
- Aminoaciduria, organic aciduria, fatty acid oxidation disorders, mitochondrial disorders, and urea cycle defects

Medications and toxins
- Antibiotics, NSAID, laxatives, hormones, etc.

Urologic/gynecological disorders
- Pelviureteric junction obstruction
- Nephrolithiasis

Miscellaneous disorders
- Abdominal migraines
- Asthma
- Benign paroxysmal positional vertigo

the frequency and intensity of acute episodes. Supportive and abortive measures during the acute episode include a dark and quiet environment, intravenous fluid, rescue agents as Ondansetron, Lorazepam and Chlorpromazine, and in older children Sumatriptan as an abortive agent.[118] Prophylactic therapies are usually provided for those children with high recurrence and severity of episodes, and include as first-line agents Cyproheptadine, Pizotifen, and Amitriptiline, and Propanolol as a second line approach.[118] In the last few years, the use of mitochondrial supplements, such as Riboflavin, L-carnitine and CoQ10, have been gradually increased based upon evidence of their efficacy in migraine.

Prognosis

Although the above treatments are effective in more than two third of cases, the management remains unsatisfactory in a significant number of the children who are referred to tertiary and quaternary centers.

REFERENCES

1. Chiou E, Nurko S. Functional abdominal pain and irritable bowel syndrome in children and adolescents. Therapy. 2011;8:315-31.
2. Hyman PE, Milla PJ, Benninga MA, Davidson GP, Fleisher DF, et al. Childhood functional gastrointestinal disorders: neonate/toddler. Gastroenterology. 2006;130:1519-26.
3. Rasquin A, Di Lorenzo C, Forbes D, Guiraldes E, Hyams JS, Staiano A, et al. Childhood functional gastrointestinal disorders: child/adolescent. Gastroenterology. 2006;130:1527-37.
4. Starfield B, Hoekelman RA, McCormick M, Benson P, Mendenhall RC, Moynihan C, et al. Who provides health care to children and adolescents in the United States? Pediatrics. 1984;74:991-7.
5. Crushell E, Rowland M, Doherty M, Gormally S, Harty S, Bourke B, et al. Importance of parental conceptual model of illness in severe recurrent abdominal pain. Pediatrics. 2003;112:1368-72.
6. Chiou E, Nurko S. Management of functional abdominal pain and irritable bowel syndrome in children and adolescents. Expert Rev Gastroenterol Hepatol. 2010;4:293-304.
7. Tam YH, Chan KW, To KF, Cheung ST, Mou JW, Pang KK, et al. Impact of pediatric Rome III criteria of functional dyspepsia on the diagnostic yield of upper endoscopy and predictors for a positive endoscopic finding. J Pediatr Gastroenterol Nutr. 2011;52:387-91.
8. Chitkara DK, Rawat DJ, Talley NJ. The epidemiology of childhood recurrent abdominal pain in Western countries: a systematic review. Am J Gastroenterol. 2005;100:1868-75.
9. Hyams JS, Hyman PE. Recurrent abdominal pain and the biopsychosocial model of medical practice. J Pediatr. 1998;133:473-8.
10. Buonavolonta R, Coccorullo P, Turco R, Boccia G, Greco L, Staiano A. Familial aggregation in children affected by functional gastrointestinal disorders. J Pediatr Gastroenterol Nutr. 2010;50:500-5.
11. Drossman DA, Li Z, Leserman J, Toomey TC, Hu YJ. Health status by gastrointestinal diagnosis and abuse history. Gastroenterology. 1996;110:999-1007.
12. Saps M, Lu P, Bonilla S. Cow's-milk allergy is a risk factor for the development of FGIDs in children. J Pediatr Gastroenterol Nutr. 2011;52:166-9.
13. Campo JV, Bridge J, Lucas A, Savorelli S, Walker L, Di Lorenzo C, et al. Physical and emotional health of mothers of youth with functional abdominal pain. Arch Pediatr Adolesc Med. 2007;161:131-7.
14. Yacob D, Di Lorenzo C, Bridge JA, Rosenstein PF, Onorato M, Bravender T, et al. Prevalence of pain-predominant functional gastrointestinal disorders and somatic symptoms in patients with anxiety or depressive disorders. J Pediatr. 2013;163:767-70.
15. Bonilla S, Saps M. Early life events predispose the onset of childhood functional gastrointestinal disorders. Rev Gastroenterol Mex. 2013;78:82-91.
16. Saps M, Bonilla S. Early life events: Infants with pyloric stenosis have a higher risk of developing chronic abdominal pain in childhood. J Pediatr. 2011;159:551-4 e551.
17. Tanaka Y, Kanazawa M, Fukudo S, Drossman DA. Biopsychosocial model of irritable bowel syndrome. J Neurogastroenterol Motil. 2011;17:131-9.
18. Di Lorenzo C, Colletti RB, Lehmann HP, Boyle JT, Gerson WT, Hyams JS, et al. Chronic Abdominal Pain In Children: a Technical Report of the American Academy of Pediatrics and the North American Society for Pediatric Gastroenterology, Hepatology and Nutrition. J Pediatr Gastroenterol Nutr. 2005;40:249-61.
19. Dodge JA. Recurrent abdominal pain in children. Br Med J. 1976;1:385-7.
20. Gomara RE, Halata MS, Newman LJ, Bostwick HE, Berezin SH, Cukaj L, et al. Fructose intolerance in children presenting with abdominal pain. J Pediatr Gastroenterol Nutr. 2008;47:303-8.
21. Guandalini S, Magazzu G, Chiaro A, La Balestra V, Di Nardo G, Gopalan S, et al. VSL#3 improves symptoms in children with irritable bowel syndrome: a multicenter, randomized, placebo-controlled, double-blind, crossover study. J Pediatr Gastroenterol Nutr. 2010;51:24-30.
22. Huertas-Ceballos A, Logan S, Bennett C, Macarthur C. Psychosocial interventions for recurrent abdominal pain (RAP) and irritable bowel syndrome (IBS) in childhood. Cochrane Database Syst Rev. 2008:CD003014.
23. Rutten JM, Reitsma JB, Vlieger AM, Benninga MA. Gut-directed hypnotherapy for functional abdominal pain or irritable bowel syndrome in children: a systematic review. Arch Dis Child. 2013;98:252-7.
24. Vlieger AM, Rutten JM, Govers AM, Frankenhuis C, Benninga MA. Long-term follow-up of gut-directed hypnotherapy vs standard care in children with functional abdominal pain or irritable bowel syndrome. Am J Gastroenterol. 2012;107:627-31.
25. Saps M, Youssef N, Miranda A, Nurko S, Hyman P, Cocjin J, et al. Multicenter, randomized, placebo-controlled trial of amitriptyline in children with functional gastrointestinal disorders. Gastroenterology. 2009;137:1261-9.
26. Campo JV, Perel J, Lucas A, Bridge J, Ehmann M, Kalas C, et al. Citalopram treatment of pediatric recurrent abdominal pain and

comorbid internalizing disorders: an exploratory study. J Am Acad Child Adolesc Psychiatry. 2004;43:1234-42.

27. Ford AC, Talley NJ, Spiegel BM, Foxx-Orenstein AE, Schiller L, Quigley EM, et al. Effect of fibre, antispasmodics, and peppermint oil in the treatment of irritable bowel syndrome: systematic review and meta-analysis. BMJ. 2008;337:a2313.

28. Sadeghian M, Farahmand F, Fallahi GH, Abbasi A. Cyproheptadine for the treatment of functional abdominal pain in childhood: a double-blinded randomized placebo-controlled trial. Minerva Pediatr. 2008;60:1367-74.

29. Tack J. Prokinetics and fundic relaxants in upper functional GI disorders. Curr Opin Pharmacol. 2008;8:690-6.

30. Huertas-Ceballos A, Logan S, Bennett C, Macarthur C. Pharmacological interventions for recurrent abdominal pain (RAP) and irritable bowel syndrome (IBS) in childhood. Cochrane Database Syst Rev. 2008:CD003017.

31. Lembo AJ, Conboy L, Kelley JM, Schnyer RS, McManus CA, Quilty MT, et al. A treatment trial of acupuncture in IBS patients. Am J Gastroenterol. 2009;104:1489-97.

32. Benninga MA, Mayer EA. The power of placebo in pediatric functional gastrointestinal disease. Gastroenterology. 2009;137(4):1207-10.

33. Apley J, Hale B. Children with recurrent abdominal pain: how do they grow up? Br Med J. 1973;3:7-9.

34. Christensen MF, Mortensen O. Long-term prognosis in children with recurrent abdominal pain. Arch Dis Child. 1975;50:110-4.

35. Magni G, Pierri M, Donzelli F. Recurrent abdominal pain in children: a long term follow-up. Eur J Pediatr. 1987;146:72-4.

36. Mugie SM, Benninga MA, Di Lorenzo C. Epidemiology of constipation in children and adults: a systematic review. Best Pract Res Clin Gastroenterol. 2011;25(1):3-18.

37. Baker S, Liptak G, Colletti R, et al. Evaluation and treatment of constipation in infants and children: recommendations of the North American Society for Pediatric Gastroenterology, Hepatology and Nutrition. Constipation Guideline Committee of the North American Society for Pediatric Gastroenterology, Hepatology and Nutrition. J Pediatr Gastroenterol Nutr. 2006;43(3):e1-13.

38. Molnar D, Taitz LS, Urwin OM, Wales JK. Anorectal manometry results in defecation disorders. Arch Dis Child. 1983;58:257-61.

39. Partin JC, Hamill SK, Fischel JE, Partin JS. Painful defecation and fecal soiling in children. Pediatr. 1992;89:1007-9.

40. Borowitz SM, Cox DJ, Tam A, et al. Precipitants of constipation during early childhood. J Amer Board Fam Pract. 2003;16:213-8.

41. Hyman PE, Fleisher D. Functional fecal retention. Pract Gastroenterol. 1992;31:29-37.

42. Mugie SM, Di Lorenzo C, Benninga MA. Constipation in childhood. Nat Rev Gastroenterol Hepatol. 2011;8(9):502-11.

43. Bekkali NL, van den Berg MM, Dijkgraaf MG, van Wijk MP, Bongers ME, Liem O, et al. Rectal fecal impaction treatment in childhood constipation: enemas versus high doses oral PEG. Pediatrics. 2009;124(6):e1108-15.

44. Tolia V, Lin CH, Elitsur Y. A prospective randomized study with mineral oil and oral lavage solution for treatment of faecal impaction in children. Aliment Pharmacol Ther. 1993;7:523Y9.

45. Gleghorn EE, Heyman MB, Rudolph CD. No-enema therapy for idiopathic constipation and encopresis. Clin Pediatr. 1991;30:667-72.

46. Ingebo KB, Heyman MB. Polyethylene glycol-electrolyte solution for intestinal clearance in children with refractory encopresis: a safe and effective therapeutic program. Am J Dis Child. 1988;142:340-2.

47. Youssef NN, Peters JM, Henderson W, et al. Dose response of PEG 3350 for the treatment of childhood fecal impaction. J Pediatr. 2002;141:410-4.

48. Ferguson A, Culbert P, Gillett H, Barras N. New polyethylene glycol electrolyte solution for the treatment of constipation and faecal impaction. Ital J Gastroenterol Hepatol. 1999;31(Suppl 3):S249Y52.

49. Nurko SS, Garcia Y, Aranda JA, et al. Treatment of intractable constipation in children: experience with Cisapride. J Pediatr Gastroenterol Nutr. 1996;22:38-44.

50. Cox DJ, Sutphen J, Borowitz S, et al.. Simple electromyographic biofeedback treatment for chronic pediatric constipation/encopresis: Preliminary report. Biofeedback Self Regul. 1994;19:41-50.

51. Hoekman DR, Benninga MA. Functional constipation in childhood: current pharmacotherapy and future perspectives. Expert Opin Pharmacother. 2013;14(1):41-51.

52. Baker S, Liptak G, Colletti R, et al. Evaluation and treatment of constipation in children: summary of updated recommendations of the North American Society for Pediatric Gastroenterology, Hepatology and Nutrition. J Pediatr Gastroenterol Nutr. 2000;30(1):109.

53. Staiano A. Use of polyethylene glycol solution in functional and organic constipation in children. Ital J Gastroenterol Hepatol. 1999;31(Suppl 3):S260-3.

54. Pashankar DS, Bishop WP, Loening-Baucke V. Long-term efficacy of polyethylene glycol 3350 for the treatment of chronic constipation in children with and without encopresis. Clin Pediatr. 2003;42:815-9.

55. Bongers ME, van den Berg MM, Reitsma JB, Voskuijl WP, Benninga MA. A randomized controlled trial of enemas in combination with oral laxative therapy for children with chronic constipation. Clin Gastroenterol Hepatol. 2009;7(10):1069-74.

56. Lowery SP, Srour JW, Whitehead WE, Schuster NM. Habit training as treatment of encopresis secondary to chronic constipation. J Pediatr Gastroenterol Nutr. 1985;4:397-401.

57. Mugie SM, Machado RS, Mousa HM, et al. Ten-Year Experience Using Antegrade Enemas in Children. J Pediatr. 2012;161:700-4.

58. Van Wunnik BP, Baeten CG, Southwell BR. Neuromodulation for constipation: sacral and transcutaneous stimulation. Best Pract Res Clin Gastroenterol. 2011;25:181-91.

59. Pijpers MA, Bongers ME, Benninga MA, Berger MY. Functional constipation inchildren: a systematic review on prognosis and predictive factors. J Pediatr Gastroenterol Nutr. 2010;50(3):256-68.

60. Bongers MEJ, van Wijk MP, et al. Long-term prognosis for childhood constipation: clinical outcomes in adulthood. Pediatrics. 2010;126:e156-62.

61. van den Berg MM, van Rossum CH, de Lorijn F, et al. Functional constipation in infants: a follow-up study. J Pediatr. 2005;147:700-4.

62. Rudolph CD, Hyman PE, Altschuler SM, Christensen J, Colletti RB, Cucchiara S, et al. Diagnosis and treatment of chronic intestinal pseudo-obstruction in children: report of consensus workshop. J Pediatr Gastroenterol Nutr. 1997;24:102-12.

63. Hyman P, Thapar N. Pediatric neurogastroenterology: gastrointestinal motility and functional disorders in children, clinical gastroenterology. Faure, Di Lorenzo Thapar (Eds). Springer Inc. 2013;257-70.

64. Vargas JH, Sachs P, Ament ME. Chronic intestinal pseudo-obstruction syndrome in pediatrics. Results of a national survey by members of the North American Society of Pediatric Gastroenterology and Nutrition. J Pediatr Gastroenterol Nutr. 1989;7:323-32.

65. Mousa H, Hyman PE, Cocjin J, Flores AF, Di Lorenzo C. Long-term outcome of congenital intestinal pseudoobstruction. Dig Dis Sci. 2002 Oct;47(10):298-305

66. Heneyke S, Smith VV, Spitz L, Milla PJ. Chronic intestinal pseudo-obstruction: treatment and long term follow up of 44 patients. Arch Dis Child. 1999 Jul;81(1):21-27.

67. Streutker CJ, Huizinga JD, Campbell F, Ho J, Riddell RH. Loss of CD117 (c-kit)- and CD34-positive ICC and associated CD34-positive fibroblasts defines a subpopulation of chronic intestinal pseudo-obstruction. Am J Surg Pathol. 2003;27:228-35.

68. Jain D, Moussa K, Tandon M, Culpepper-Morgan J, Proctor DD. Role of interstitial cells of Cajal in motility disorders of the bowel. Am J Gastroenterol. 2003;98:618-24.

69. Struijs MC, Diamond IR, Pencharz PB, Chang KT, Viero S, Langer JC, et al. Absence of the interstitial cells of Cajal in a child with chronic pseudo-obstruction. J Pediatr Surg. 2008 Dec;43(12):e25-9.

70. Gosemann JH, Puri P. Megacystis microcolon intestinal hypoperistalsis syndrome: systematic review of outcome. Pediatr Surg Int. 2011 Oct;27(10):1041-6.

71. De Giorgio R, Ricciardiello L, Naponelli V, Selgrad M, Piazzi G, Felicani C, et al. Chronic intestinal pseudo-obstruction related to viral infections. Transplant Proc. 2010 Jan-Feb;42(1):9-14.

72. Panza E, Knowles CH, Graziano C, Thapar N, Burns AJ, Seri M, et al. Genetics of human enteric neuropathies. Prog Neurobiol. 2012 Feb;96(2):176-89.

73. Borrelli O, Giorgio V, Thapar N. Antroduodenal Manometry. Pediatric Neurogastroenterology: Gastrointestinal Motility and Functional Disorders in Children, Clinical Gastroenterology. Faure, Di Lorenzo Thapar (Eds). Springer Inc. 2013;91-105.

74. Knowles et al. Acta Neuropathol. 2009;118:271-301.

75. Knowles et al. Gut. 2010;59:882-7.

76. Knowles et al. Neurogastroenterol Motil. 2011;23:115-24.

77. Hyman PE, Bursch B, Beck D, DiLorenzo C, Zeltzer LK. Discriminating pediatric condition falsification from chronic intestinal pseudo-obstruction in toddlers. Child Maltreat. 2002 May;7(2):132-7.

78. Di Lorenzo C, Flores AF, Buie T, Hyman PE. Intestinal motility and jejunal feeding in children with chronic intestinal pseudo-obstruction. Gastroenterology.1995 May;108(5):1379-85.

79. Gariepy CE, Mousa H. Clinical management of motility disorders in children. Semin Pediatr Surg. 2009 Nov;18(4):224-38.

80. Di Lorenzo C, Youssef NN. Diagnosis and management of intestinal motility disorders. Semin Pediatr Surg. 2010 Feb;19(1):50-8.

81. Di Lorenzo C, Lucanto C, Flores AF, Idries S, Hyman PE. Effect of sequential erythromycin and octreotide on antroduodenal manometry. J Pediatr Gastroenterol Nutr. 1999 Sep;29(3):293-6.

82. Mugie SM, Di Lorenzo C. From ACE to replace: role of surgery and transplantation in motility disorders. J Pediatr Gastroenterol Nutr. 2011 Dec;53(Suppl 2):S59-61.

83. Millar AJ, Gupte G, Sharif K. Intestinal transplantation for motility disorders. Semin Pediatr Surg. 2009 Nov;18(4):258-62.

84. Schwankovsky L, Mousa H, Rowhani A, DI Lorenzo C, Hyman PE. Quality of life outcomes in congenital chronic intestinal pseudo-obstruction. Dig Dis Sci. 2002 Sep;47(9):1965-8.

85. Reilly S, Skuse D, Poblete X. Prevalence of feeding problems and oral motor dysfunction in children with cerebral palsy: a community survey. J Pediatr. 1996;129:877-82.

86. Sondheimer JM, Morris BA. Gastroesophageal reflux among severely retarded children. J Pediatr. 1979;94:710-4.

87. Staiano A, Del Giudice E. Colonic transit and anorectal manometry in children with severe brain damage. Pediatrics. 1994;94:169-73.

88. Ravelli AM, Milla PJ. Vomiting and gastroesophageal motor activity in children with disorders of the central nervous system. J Pediatr Gastroenterol Nut. 1998;26:56-63.

89. Menkes JH, Ament ME. Neurologic disorders of gastroesophageal function. Advances in Neurology. 188;49:409-16.

90. Patrick J, Boland M, Stoski D, Murray GE. Rapid correction of wasting in children with cerebral palsy. Dev Med Child Neurol. 1986;28:734-9.

91. Stallings VA, Cronk CE, Zemel BS, Charney EB. Body composition in children with spastic quadriplegic cerebral palsy. J Pediatr. 1995;126:833-9.

92. Schwartz SM, Corredor J, Fisher-Medina J, et al. Diagnosis and treatment of feeding disorders in children with developmental disabilities. Pediatrics. 2001;108:671-6.

93. Rempel GR, Colwell S, Nelson RP. Growth in children with cerebral palsy fed via gastrostomy. Pediatrics. 1988;857-62.

94. Sanders KD, Cox K, Cannon R, et al. Growth response to enteral feeding by children with cerebral palsy. J Parenter Enteral Nutr. 1990;14:23-6.

95. Stallings VA, Charney EB, Davies JC, Cronk CE. Nutritional status and growth of children with diplegic or hemiplegic cerebral palsy. Dev Med Child Neurol. 1993;35:997-1006.

96. Stevenson RD, Hayes RP, Cater LV, Blackman JA. Clinical correlates of linear growth in children with cerebral palsy. Dev Med Child Neurol. 1994;36:135-42.

97. Sánchez-Lastres J, Eirís-Puñal J, Otero-Cepeda JL, Pavón-Belinchón P, Castro-Gago M. Nutritional status of mentally retarded children in north-west Spain. I. Anthropometric indicators. Acta Paediatr. 2003;92:747-53.

98. Sullivan PB, Juszczak E, Lambert BR, et al. Impact of feeding problems on nutritional intake and growth: Oxford feeding study II. Dev Med Child Neurol. 2002;44:461-7.

99. Gisel EG. Effect of oral sensorimotor treatment on measures of growth and efficiency of eating in the moderately eating-impaired child with cerebral palsy. Dysphagia. 1996;11:48-58.

100. Pinnington L, Hegarty J. Effects of consistent food presentation on oral-motor skill acquisition in children with severe neurological impairment. Dysphagia. 2000;15:213-23.

101. Rogers B. Feeding method and health outcomes of children with cerebral palsy. J Pediatr. 2004;145:S28-32.

102. Brant CQ, Stanich P, Ferrari Jr. AP. Improvement in children's nutritional status after enteral feeding by PEG: an iterim report. Gastrointest Endosc. 1990;50:183-8.

103. Arvedson JC, Rogers BT. Pediatric swallowing and feeding disorders. J Med Speech-Lang Pathol. 1993;1:203-21.

104. Gauderer MW. Percutaneous endoscopic gastrostomy: a 10-year experience with 220 children. J Pediatr Surg. 1991;26:288-92.

105. Eyman RK, Grossman HJ, Chaney RH, Call TL. Survival of profoundly disabled people with severe mental retardation. Am J Dis Child. 1993;147:329-36.

106. Ashwal S, Eyman RK, Call TL. Life expectancy of children in a persistent vegetative state. Pediatr Neurol. 1994;10:27-33.

107. Strauss D, Kastner T, Ashwal S, White J. Tubefeeding and mortality in children with severe disabilities and mental retardation. Pediatrics. 1997; 99:358-62.

108. Del Giudice E, Staiano A, Capano G, et al. Gastrointestinal manifestations in children with cerebral palsy. Brain Dev. 1999;21:307-11.

109. Fonkalsrud EW, Foglia RP, Ament ME, et al. Operative treatment for the gastroesophageal reflux syndrome in children. J Pediatr Surg. 1989;24(6):525-9.

110. Okada T, Sasaki F, Asaka M, et al. Delay of gastric emptying measured by 13C-acetate breath test in neurologically impaired children with gastroesophageal reflux. Eur J Pediatr Surg. 2005 Apr;15(2):77-81.

111. Li BU, Balint JP. Cyclic vomiting syndrome: evolution in our understanding of a brain-gut disorder. Adv Pediatr. 2000;47: 117-60.

112. Fitzpatrick E, Bourke B, Drumm B, et al. The incidence of cyclic vomiting syndrome in children: population-based study. Am J Gastroenterol. 2008;103:991-5.

113. Drumm BR, Bourke B, Drummond J, McNicholas et al. Cyclical vomiting syndrome in children: a prospective study. Neurogastroenterol Motil. 2012;24:922-7.

114. Li BU, Misiewicz L. Cyclic vomiting syndrome: a brain-gut disorder. Gastroenterol Clin North Am. 2003;32:997-1019.

115. Boles RG, Adams K, Li BU. Maternal inheritance in cyclic vomiting syndrome. Am J Med Genet A. 2005 Feb 15;133A:71-7.

116. Wang Q, Ito M, Adams K, et al Mitochondrial DNA control region sequence variation in migraine headache and cyclic vomiting syndrome. Am J Med Genet A. 2004;131:50-8.

117. Li BU, Lefevre F, Chelimsky GG, et al. North American Society for Pediatric Gastroenterology, Hepatology, and Nutrition consensus statement on the diagnosis and management of cyclic vomiting syndrome. J Pediatr Gastroenterol Nutr. 2008;47:379-93.

118. Sudel B, Li BU. Treatment options for cyclic vomiting syndrome. Curr Treat Options Gastroenterol. 2005;8:387-95.

Chapter 5

Disorders of the Stomach and Small Intestine

Ravinder Goyal, BR Thapa, Rimjhim Shrivastava, Srikanth KP

CONGENITAL ANOMALIES OF THE STOMACH

The primary function of the stomach is to act as a reservoir for large quantities of recently ingested food and release its contents intermittently in the duodenum, which is of much smaller capacity. The volume of stomach ranges from about 30 mL in a neonate to 1.5 to 2 L in adulthood.[1]

The stomach is recognizable by the 4 weeks of gestation as a dilation of the distal foregut which becomes well defined by 6 weeks of gestation. The muscular layers become visible by 9 weeks and various types of epithelium of the gastric mucosa get differentiated by 12 weeks of gestation which by 16 weeks start secreting their respective cellular products. Several trophic factors as transforming growth factor-β1, basement membrane proteins called laminins, fibroblast growth factors 10 and 2, and proteins in the hedgehog pathway have been shown to be involved in gastric epithelial differentiation.[2]

As the stomach undergoes enlargement, there is a differential growth in the form of the dorsal aspect growing more rapidly than the ventral aspect forming the greater curvature. During 7–8 weeks of gestation stomach rotates 90 degrees around its craniocaudal axis orienting the greater curvature to the left (the dorsal aspect) and the lesser curvature (ventral aspect) to the right. Due to the combined effects of rotation and the ongoing differential growth, the stomach lies transversely in the mid and left upper abdomen with the greater curvature being more elongated than the lesser curvature.[1] Further, in the course the continued differential expansion of the superior part of the greater curvature gives rise to the fundus and cardiac incisure by the end of the seventh week. The stomach can be visualized in fetal ultrasonography at around 11–12 weeks of gestation as a cystic structure in the left hypochondrium.[3]

Congenital anomalies of the stomach are among the least frequently encountered malformations of the gastrointestinal tract, with very few case reports in the literature. Hypertrophic pyloric stenosis is the only serious gastric disorder seen frequently in infancy but is not of embryonic origin.[4] Most gastric defects are sporadic, isolated, and idiopathic and may have some syndromic associations. Patients present with variable features, during the neonatal period or later in life depending upon the anomaly and degree of gastric outlet obstruction. Various congenital anamolies of the stomach are given in Table 5.1.

Table 5.1: Congenital anomalies of the stomach[1]				
Anomaly	Incidence	Age at onset	Presentation	Management
Atresia	3:100,000	Infancy	Nonbilious vomiting	Gastroduodenostomy, gastrojejunostomy
Diaphragm	As above	Any age	Failure to thrive, vomiting	Incision or excision, pyloroplasty
Pyloric stenosis	1–8:1000	Infancy	Nonbilious vomiting, pyloric mass, visible peristalsis	Pyloromyotomy, endoscopic dilation
Volvulus	Rare	Any age	Vomiting, refusal to feed	Reduction, gastropexy
Microgastria	Rare	Infancy	Vomiting, malnutrition	Continuous drip feeding, jejunal reservoir pouch
Duplication	Rare	Any age	Abdominal mass, vomiting	Excision or partial gastrectomy
Diverticulum	Rare	Any age	Mostly asymptomatic	Usually not required

Gastric Atresia or Stenosis

These anomalies are uncommon, with a reported incidence of 1 to 3 per 100,000 newborns.[5,6] Most common part to be affected is pylorus or antrum. Though, most cases are sporadic, some may be inherited as autosomal recessive. Many genetic defects can be associated with this anomaly as junctional epidermolysis bullosa, multiple intestinal atresias, Down syndrome, or aplasia cutis congenit.[7]

Clinical Features

Neonates with complete obstruction present with forceful, persistent nonbilious vomiting following the first feed, leading to metabolic derangements, dehydration or shock. The abdomen is generally scaphoid unless gastric distention is present. In partial obstructions symptoms may not appear until childhood or even adulthood or may have failure to thrive and recurrent abdominal discomfort.

Diagnosis

Diagnosis can be made by abdominal radiographs showing gaseous distention of the stomach (*single bubble appearence*) and a gasless intestine. Contrast study may demonstrate complete obstruction of the stomach or thin, linear filling defect due to an incomplete prepyloric membrane. Ultrasonography may demonstrate the diaphragm as an echogenic band. Upper gastrointestinal endoscopy may aid the diagnosis by direct visualization.

Management

❏ This includes patient stabilization and gastric decompression. If the symptoms are mild in the form of only delayed gastric emptying low-residue feeds and gastric emptying drugs may be successful.

❏ Surgical: It provides the definitive therapy and may range from simple excision for complete or incomplete antral membranes and pyloroplasty for pyloric membranes to gastroduodenostomy/gastrojejunostomy for atretic gap.

❏ Endoscopic therapy: Newer modalities using a snare, papillotome, laser, or dilation via balloon have been described especially in case of diaphragm, pre-pyloric webs and pyloric stenosis.

Gastric Duplication

Of all the gastrointestinal duplications 20% are gastric. It is generally contiguous with the stomach, along the greater curvature or posterior wall, contains all layers of the gastric wall and share a common blood supply and outer smooth muscle coat with the stomach. Gastric duplication cysts if lined by gastric and pancreatic mucosa, may lead to peptic ulcer disease and pancreatitis. It may have connection with other abdominal organs as colon or pancreas or rarely stomach. The embryological defects proposed for this are errors in separation of notochord (split notochord theory) and endoderm, persistence of embryonic diverticula, and persistence of vacuoles within the epithelium of the primitive foregut.[8]

Clinical Features

The child presents classically in infancy, although can present at any age. Common observed symptoms are nonbilious vomiting, weight loss, failure to thrive, abdominal pain and distension. There may be a palpable abdominal mass on examination. It may complicate as the cyst enlarges and present with obstruction of gastric emptying or compression of adjacent structures. Also, it may have ulceration, bleeding, or inflammation of the mucosa within the cyst, hemorrhage, or perforation with peritonitis or fistula formation. Ectopic pancreatic tissue is commonly seen. Communicating duplication cyst may present with recurrent bouts of hematemesis.

Diagnosis

Abdominal radiograph shows displacement and extrinsic compression of gastric lumen. Contrast radiography may demonstrate the duplication via a mass effect on the stomach. Other imaging modalities as ultrasonography, computed tomography (CT) scan, magnetic resonance cholangiopancreatography (MRCP), Tc-99m pertechnetate, and endoscopy with endoscopic ultrasonography (EUS) may also demonstrate the lesion. Peristalsis identified by EUS in a juxtaenteric cyst is specific for a duplication cyst and may be considered as a diagnostic feature.

Management

The treatment of choice is surgical excision of the duplication cyst. When the cyst and stomach have a common muscle layer, excision is not possible. In such cases, debulking, cyst-gastrostomy, or partial gastrectomy may be done. Resection of aberrant or ectopic pancreatic tissue should also be done.

Gastric Volvulus

Gastric volvulus constitutes a surgical emergency and was first described by Berti in 1866. Generally the stomach is resistant to abnormal rotation, owing to the fixations at the gastroesophageal junction and pylorus, in addition to four gastric ligaments. Volvulus constitutes abnormal rotation of one part of the stomach around another, with resulting obstruction at the pylorus or cardia and/or ischemia. The majority of congenital gastric volvuli are a result of gastric malfixation, especially at the gastroesophageal junction, diaphragmatic complications (e.g. congenital diaphragmatic hernia), and absence or laxity of gastric ligaments.

Clinical Features

The incidence of gastric volvulus are unknown. According to a study there have been 581 cases of gastric volvulus in children reported between 1929 and 2007.[9] The time of presentation is within the first few months of life. Acute volvulus presents with classic symptoms as unproductive retching, localized epigastric distension and inability to pass a nasogastric tube (Borchardt triad). Chronic gastric volvulus is associated with mild and nonspecific symptoms such as dysphagia, epigastric discomfort or fullness, bloating, and heartburn, particularly after meals for months to years.

Diagnosis

On plain X-ray mesenteroaxial volvulus shows spherical distended stomach. Air-fluid levels in fundus and antrum can be seen. Beaking can be seen at esophagogastric junction. Organoaxial volvulus is difficult to diagnose on plain images.[9] A barium meal will confirm the diagnosis. Upper endoscopy in absence of ischemia may show twisting of the gastric folds.

Management

- *Conservative:* Improvement over time has been reported with conservative treatment like positioning infants in the prone or upright position after meals in less affected children and chronic cases.
- *Surgery:* Reduction of volvulus by open or laparoscopic surgery can be done to prevent gastric ischemia, necrosis, and perforation in acute volvulus. If the stomach is viable, gastropexy or gastrostomy is performed.
- *Endotherapy:* Endoscopic detorsion can be done under fluoroscopy.[10]

Inantile Hypertrophic Pyloric Stenosis

Inantile hypertrophic pyloric stenosis (IHPS) is form of gastric outlet obstruction caused by hypertrophy of circular muscle surrounding the pyloric channel. The incidence of IHPS ranges from 1 to 8 in 1000 live births. The etiology remains unknown but some autosomal dominant forms have been reported.[11] The first-born

male infants are more at risk. Association has been found with Turner's syndrome, trisomy 18, Cornelia de Lange syndrome, esophageal atresia, Hirschsprung's disease, phenylketonuria, and congenital rubella syndrome.[12]

Clinical Features

The presentation is generally after 3–4 weeks of age, but can present in the first week also. The infant has mild spitting, which progresses to projectile, forceful non-bilious vomiting following feeds. Subsequently, infant may become wasted and severely dehydrated with decreased urine and stool output. Due to chloride loss in the vomitus marked metabolic alkalosis develops. On examination there is classically presence of a palpable pyloric mass and visible peristaltic waves (Fig. 5.1). The mass may be seen from the level of the umbilicus to near the epigastrium and is palpable in 70% to 90% of affected infants. Peristaltic waves are best observed during feeding of the naked and noncrying infant.

Diagnosis

In an infant with typical presentation, with a palpable mass and visible peristalsis usually no further studies are required. If in doubt, a definitive diagnosis can be made on radiologic studies. X-ray abdomen shows a distended stomach with paucity of gas beyond the stomach. Abdominal ultrasonography confirms the diagnosis and is the diagnostic study of choice. It demonstrates the range of length of the hypertrophied canal from 14 mm to more than 20 mm. A negative ultrasonographic study shows a normal pyloric ring and a distensible antropyloric portion of the stomach. Barium contrast study can be the

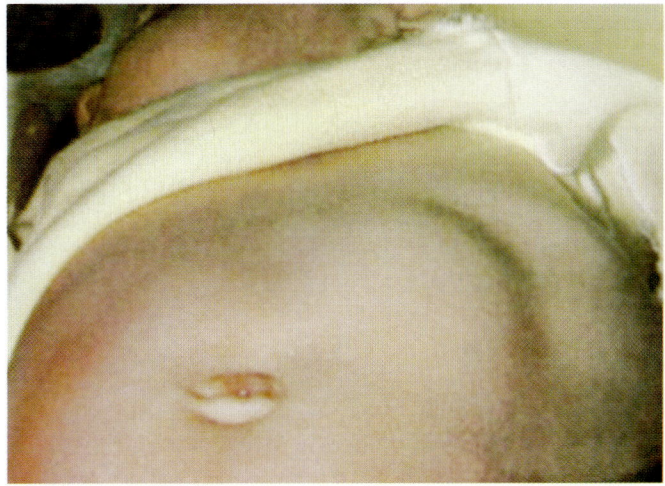

Fig. 5.1: Visible peristalsis in IHPS [*Courtesy:* Dr Shashank Shrotriya, MCh (Ped Surg), Pune, Maharashtra, India]

first choice if other conditions as gastroesophageal reflux, or other upper gastrointestinal disorders are to be ruled out. It shows characteristically elongated narrow pylorus (*double channel*) with indentation of the adjacent antrum and duodenum by the pyloric mass (*shoulders*).

Management

❑ *Medical:* Fluid and electrolyte replacement should be done to correct dehydration and hypochloremic metabolic alkalosis. Anticholinergic medications can improve the symptoms transiently but have got high failure rate.
❑ *Surgical:* Ramstedt pyloromyotomy (Figs 5.2 and 5.3) is the definitive therapy in which a longitudinal incision is

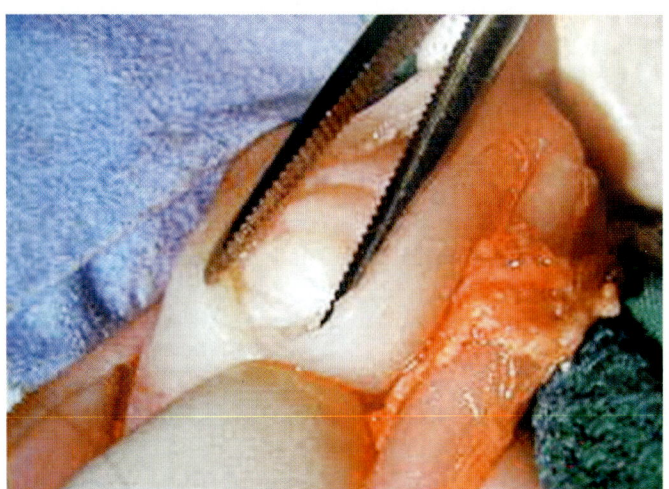

Fig. 5.2: Intraoperative hypertrophic pylorus [*Courtesy:* Dr Shashank Shrotriya, MCh (Ped Surg), Pune, Maharashtra, India]

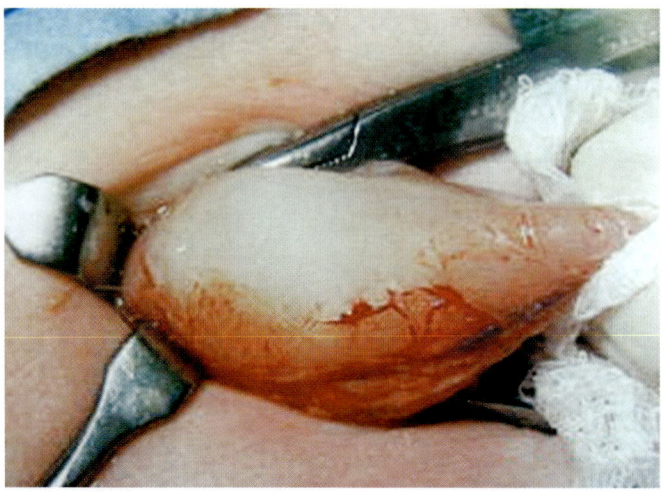

Fig. 5.3: Pyloromyotomy in IHPS [*Courtesy:* Dr Shashank Shrotriya, MCh (Ped Surg), Pune, Maharashtra, India]

taken through the hypertrophied pyloric muscle down to the submucosa on the anterior surface of the pylorus. Alternatively pyloric traumamyoplasty can be done where the hypertrophic pylorus muscle is disrupted at two places. Laparoscopic pyloromyotomy can also be done. Endoscopic treatment is possible in experienced hands. The prognosis following surgery is excellent.

Microgastria

Microgastria is small, tubular or saccular, stomach of reduced capacity which is incompletely rotated and is associated with a megaesophagus, resulting from a failure of gastric enlargement during embryogenesis. It is extremely rare condition. The etiology is unknown. It is almost always associated with other congenital anomalies like duodenal atresia, nonrotation of the midgut, ileal duplication, hiatal hernia, asplenia, partial situs inversus, or renal, upper limb, cardiac, pulmonary, skeletal, or spinal anomalies, though isolated forms have also been described. Microgastria should be excluded in patients presenting with VACTERL (vertebral, anal, cardiac, tracheal, esophageal, renal, and limb) association and midline defects.

Clinical Features

The patient presents with postprandial vomiting and gastroesophageal reflux and recurrent chest infections due to aspirations. Malnutrition, failure to thrive, and growth retardation commonly associated.

Diagnosis

Upper gastrointestinal contrast study confirms the diagnosis which shows a small, tubular stomach in an abnormal position.

Management

❑ *Conservative:* This includes frequent small-volume feedings or continuous-drip feedings in stomach or via jejunostomy.
❑ *Surgical:* To increase the capacity of the stomach double-lumen Roux-en-Y pouch anastomosed to the greater curvature of the stomach (*Hunt-Lawrence jejunal pouch*).

GASTRITIS: *H. PYLORI* AND PEPTIC ULCER DISEASE, AND NON-*H. PYLORI* ULCERS

Gastric secretion is composed of mucus, hydrochloric acid, proteases and gastrin hormone. It has a pH of 1.5 to 3.5. The acid plays a key role in digestion of proteins, calcium, iron, vitamin B_{12} and suppression of growth of bacteria thus preventing enteric infections. The surface of the gastric mucosa is lined by a simple mucus- secreting columnar epithelium.[13] Gastritis is defined as microscopic evidence of inflammation affecting the gastric mucosa. It can be acute or chronic. Peptic ulcers, by definition, are deep mucosal lesions that disrupt the muscularis mucosa coat of the gastric or duodenal wall.[14] Gastritis and peptic ulcer disease can be divided into two major categories, primary and secondary, on the basis of the underlying etiology owing to the difference in the natural history.[15] Most cases of primary or unexplained gastritis are now known to be caused by Helicobacter pylori (H. pylori). Primary duodenal ulcer disease is very rare in children under 10 years of age and primary gastric ulcers rarely occur in children.[16]

Helicobacter pylori

Helicobacter pylori is a gram negative, flagellate, spiral and highly motile organism with special affinity for gastric mucosa, antrum being the most commonly affected part. It produces abundant urease which aids in colonization and is the basis of rapid urease test (RUT) during endoscopy, the urea breath test as well as an antigen for serological test.[17] In vitro, it thrives well in neutral or close to neutral pH (i.e. pH 5.5– 7.5) and may die at more acidic or alkaline pH levels. H. pylori is difficult and tedious to culture as they grow slowly and require specialized culture media as well as a controlled microaerophilic environment.[18] H. pylori infection is almost always acquired in early childhood and persists throughout life unless a specific treatment is given.

Gastritis and Peptic Ulcer

H. pylori causes chronic gastritis which is usually asymptomatic but leads to several diseases as peptic ulcer disease and gastric malignancies typically occurring in adulthood.[19] A meta-analysis including 24 randomized controlled trials and randomized comparative trials including 2,102 patients with peptic ulcer disease (PUD) revealed that the 12-month ulcer remission rate was 97% for gastric ulcer, and 98% for duodenal ulcer in patients successfully eradicated of H. pylori infection.[20]

Epidemiology

Helicobacter pylori infection is one of the most widely spread chronic bacterial infections in the world. It infects at least 50% of the world's human population. Low socio-economic condition and crowding are regarded as the most important risk factors for its acquisition. Children are typically infected by 10 years of age and spontaneous elimination of bacteria and subsequent reinfection is quite common.[18]

Transmission

Due to passively transferred immunity from the mother, infants are rarely infected in the developed world. However, H. pylori is commonly seen in infants of developing countries. H. pylori is mainly acquired in children through feco-oral route. Gastro-oral route of transmission has also been recognized via regurgitation and vomiting. Other modes of transmission like contaminated water and oral-oral route by kissing and feeding of pre masticated food is also known.[21]

Pathogenesis

The mechanisms of H. pylori infection and the spectrum of disease is not clearly understood. One theory suggest its mechanism as immune-mediated toxicity and direct toxicity mediated by toxin secretion. Another theory suggest that it acts also acts by altering the regulation of acid secretion.[14,18]

Clinical Features

Many clinical pictures have been attributed to H. pylori infection as acute gastritis, chronic gastritis, duodenal ulcer, gastric ulcer, etc. The age group affected is commonly older than 8–10 years and mostly are males. Symptoms are age dependent. Infants and young children present with vomiting or upper gastrointestinal bleeding whereas older children with ulcer may have abdominal pain and/or vomiting. They have epigastric localization of pain which is often nocturnal and is relieved by meal or antacids. Severe cases may have hematemesis and weight loss. Children with H. pylori-associated gastritis without ulcer are asymptomatic in the majority of cases. H pylori has been suspected to be one of the causes of recurrent abdominal pain but population-based studies failed to show any association in children.[22-24] Anemia and growth failure has also been reported with H. pylori infection. MALT lymphoma and carcinoma have been well correlated with H. pylori infection in adult population.

The most frequent complication of peptic ulcer disease is gastrointestinal bleeding with hematemesis and/or melena and perforation with or without peritonitis.[25]

Diagnosis

There is no single test which can be considered the gold standard for the diagnosis of H. pylori.[26]

Endoscopic Diagnostic Tests

❑ **Rapid urease test**: This is also called 2 minute endoscopic test and detects active *H. pylori* infection. Gastric biopsies are obtained and placed into an agar gel or on a reaction strip containing urea, a buffer, and a pH-sensitive indicator. A change in color of the pH sensitive indicator signifies a positive result. It has a sensitivity of >90% and specificity of >95%. The patient should not have been on a proton pump inhibitors (PPI) within 1–2 weeks or any antibiotic or bismuth within 4 weeks of endoscopy.[27]

❑ **Histology (Figs 5.4 and 5.5)**: If the patient has not been on PPI, antibiotics or bismuth, gastric biopsies can be taken. It has been considered the gold standard for detection of *H. pylori*. It is recommended that a minimum of three biopsies should be obtained, one from the incisura angularis, one from the greater curvature of the corpus, and one from the greater curvature of the antrum, to maximize the diagnostic yield. It has a sensitivity and specificity of >95% but the high cost and need for trained personnel limits its use.[28]

❑ **Culture**: It is highly specific test for the detection of active *H. pylori* infection but it is less sensitive than RUT and histology. Moreover, it is very costly and requires special media for culture. The culture positivity is also very low.

❑ **Polymerase chain reaction**: It is highly specific and sensitive than other tissue based tests but presently it is restricted to research area.

Nonendoscopic Diagnostic Tests

❑ **Antibody detection**: It detects IgG antibodies specific to *H. pylori* in serum, whole blood, or urine. It is typically detected 21 days after *H. pylori* infection and remains positive for a long duration. It is of low cost, widely available and gives rapid result but has a low sensitivity and specificity of around 75–85%. It cannot differentiate between old and new infection, so having epidemiological importance.

❑ **Urea breath test (UBT)**: It measures the production of labelled CO_2 in the expired breath. It has a sensitivity and specificity of more than 95%. It is currently recommended that bismuth and antibiotics should be withheld for at least 28 days and a PPI for 7–14 days prior to the UBT.

❑ **Fecal antigen testing**: It identifies *H. pylori* antigen in the stool by enzyme immunoassay. It has a very high sensitivity and specificity of 95% before antibiotic treatment but it declines after antibiotic treatment.

Treatment of H. pylori-related Gastritis and PUD

The greatest possibility of *H. pylori* eradication lies with the first course of therapy.

Children infected with *H. pylori* and having peptic ulcer disease should receive treatment to eradicate the infection.[29] Various drugs and their dosage are mentioned in Table 5.2. Following are the various regimens for *H. pylori* infection:

❑ **Triple drug regimen:** This is the first line of treatment comprising one proton pump inhibitor (PPI) and two antibiotics twice in a day (amoxicillin plus clarithromycin or metronidazole) for 10 to 14 days, for example:
  • Amoxicillin + clarithromycin + PPI
  • Amoxicillin + metronidazole + PPI
  • Bismuth salts + amoxicillin + metronidazole

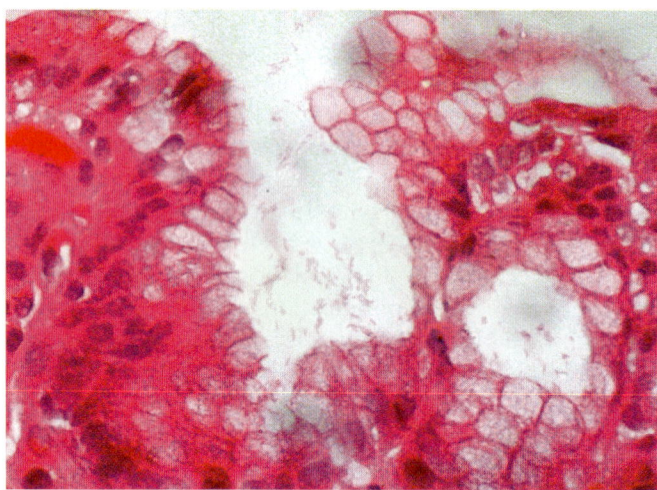

Fig. 5.4: *Helicobacter pylori* gastritis. The spirally shaped organisms demonstrated by the routine H&E stain (*Courtesy*: Dr KK Prasad, PGI, Chandigarh, India)

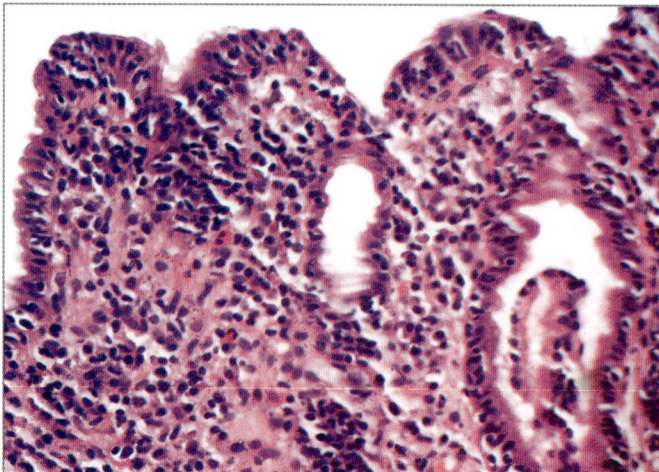

Fig. 5.5: Lymphocytic gastritis. The gastric foveolar and pit epithelium shows distinct intraepithelial lymphocytosis. (*Courtesy*: Dr KK Prasad, PGI, Chandigarh, India)

❑ **Sequential therapy**: It involves dual therapy with a PPI and amoxicillin for 5 days followed sequentially by 5 days of triple therapy (a PPI with clarithromycin and metronidazole).

❑ **Second line or salvage therapy** (up to 14 days)

The first line therapy fails to eradicate the organism in 5–30% patients. In such patients quadruple therapy is given. This includes PPI, bismuth, metronidazole, and amoxicillin. After 4–8 weeks of completion of the regimens the eradication of the organism should be confirmed with reliable noninvasive tests like 13C-urea breath test or fecal antigen test.

Table 5.2: Various drugs and dosage for *H. pylori* eradication	
Amoxicillin	50 mg/kg/day (Max 1 g bid)
Clarithromycin	20 mg/kg/day (Max 500 mg bid)
Omeprazole	1–2 mg/kg/day (Max 20 mg bid)
Metronidazole	20 mg/kg/day (Max 500 mg bid)
Bismuth subsalicylate	8 mg/kg/day (Max 262 mg qid)
Ranitidine bismuth citrate	1 tablet qid

Prognosis

After completion of the drug therapy, successful eradication is generally seen which is followed by clinical improvement and ulcer healing. Relapse of peptic ulcer disease is rarely seen after 5 years of age. However, children with chronic gastritis have a more unpredictable clinical outcome, even if *H. pylori* is eradicated.[30,31]

Helicobacter pylori -Negative Gastritis

Usually the medications available for *H. pylori* eradicates the organism and prevents recurrence, but 20% of them have recurrences and may develop ulcers.[32]

The exact prevalence and pathogenesis of *H. pylori*-negative gastritis is not clearly understood. Recent studies have suggested *Helicobacter pylori*-negative gastritis may be quite common and there is high prevalence (over 90%) and severity of chronic gastritis in this group of population.[33] Apart from being chronic, the gastritis can also be active. In a recent study comprising 491 adults who underwent elective upper gastrointestinal endoscopy, forty-one (20.5%) had *H. pylori*-negative gastritis; thirty (73.2%) had chronic gastritis, five (12.2%) had active gastritis, and six (14.6%) had both. It was equally distributed in the antrum, corpus, and both antrum and corpus.[34]

Four criteria have been proposed for *H. pylori*-negative gastritis:

1. The triple staining at seven gastric sites should be negative (two antrum, four corpus, and one cardia).
2. Culture for *H. pylori* should be negative.
3. IgG serology for *H. pylori* should be negative.
4. Patient should not have received any treatment for *H. pylori*.[34]

Etiology

There are two possibilities for the histological diagnosis of *H. pylori*-negative gastritis. One is false-negative cases where the organism is absent in spite of it being true *H. pylori* gastritis, and the other, true positive cases that may mimic *H. pylori* infection.[35]

False-negative conditions can be seen in previously treated *H. pylori* infection. If the patient does not remember being treated for *H. pylori* infection, false-negative results may be seen. In such cases, IgG serology can be done, which remains positive for a long duration, even 3–4 years.[36]

Also, if there is previous use of PPI false negative reporting may be done. In a study about 68% of *H. pylori*-negative gastritis patients either had a history of PPI use or were currently on PPI. Also, it has been observed that long-term lansoprazole treatment was associated with reduction in acute and chronic inflammation in the stomach.[37,38]

True positive cases include reactive gastropathy with focal activity, focally active gastritis and carditis, autoimmune gastritis, granulomatous gastritis, lymphocytic gastritis, and other infections. Some organisms can also mimic features of gastritis as *Mycobacterium avium*-intracellulare, herpes simplex and cytomegalovirus.[34]

The prognosis of *H. pylori*-negative gastritis is not known. In two different randomised control trials the proportion of non-*H. pylori* ulcer has been estimated as 52% in United States and 42% in Australia.[39] According to a theory some idiopathic ulcers may occur due to the colonization of *H. pylori* in the duodenum. The conventional RUT is negative in these patients as only gastric biopsies are taken.[40] Such patients present with longer duration of ulceration, frequent recurrences with more severe dyspepsia and higher degree of morbidity as compared to patients with *H. pylori* positive ulcers. They are generally older, sicker and have frequent upper gastrointestinal bleeding episodes.[41]

H. pylori-negative gastritis does not warrant any treatment.[34] However, it has been reported that *H. pylori* negative ulcer patients respond well to proton pump inhibitors.[42]

Gastric Neoplasms

Gastric neoplasms are uncommon in the pediatric age group (Table 5.3). Overall incidence in pediatric age group is less than 0.1%. In a large study spanning over more than 40 years, only 3 cases of primary gastric neoplasms were detected.[43] Unlike adult population, primary gastric adenocarcinoma is very rare in pediatric population whereas lymphoma and sarcoma are the most common neoplasms followed by some benign tumors.[44]

Table 5.3: Various gastric neoplasms in children		
Benign	Malignant	Miscellaneous
Gastric polyps	Lymphoma	Hemangioma
• Sporadic	Adenocarcinoma	Lipoma
• Familial polyposis coli	Gastrointestinal stromal tumor	Inflammatory myofibroblastic tumor
• Peutz-Jeghers syndrome	Leiomyosarcoma	Hamartoma
• Juvenile polyposis		Langerhans cell histiocytosis
Gastric teratoma		
Leiomyoma		

Gastric Lymphoma

In children, small bowel is the most frequent site for gastrointestinal lymphoma followed by stomach which constitutes about 2.5 to 17% of total gastrointestinal lymphoma cases,[45,46] whereas in adult population stomach is the most frequent site followed by small bowel.

Various underlying conditions predispose a child to lymphomatous transformation and lymphoma.[47,48] These are:
❑ Primary immunodeficiency disorders
  • Severe combined immunodeficiency
  • Common variable immunodeficiency disease
  • X-linked agammaglobulinemia
  • Ataxia telangiectasia
  • Wiskott-Aldrich syndrome
❑ Acquired immunodeficiency disorder like HIV positive patients
❑ H. pylori infection related lymphoma.

Gastric lymphomas usually present with pain abdomen, lump abdomen, gastrointestinal bleeding or occasionally as gastric outlet obstruction. Most of these tumors are high grade neoplasms and carry a poorer prognosis, mostly being lymbhoblastic or large cell anaplastic types. Surgical

resection followed by chemotherapy and radiotherapy is the main mode of treatment.[46,49]

Adenocarcinoma

Gastric adenocarcinoma is extremely rare in pediatric population, but whenever they occur in younger population, these tumors carry poorer clinical and histological markers as compared to older population. In a large study spanning over 10 years no pediatric case of gastric adenocarcinoma was found.[50]

Exact risk factors involved in causation of gastric adenocarcinoma in children are not well known. Genetics probably plays an important part because around 10 to 25% young patients have a positive family history.[51] Various risk factors which are commonly associated with gastric adenocarcinoma in adult population like H. pylori infection, pernicious anemia and hypertrophic gastropathy are not found in pediatric population. Certain diseases in children like immunoglobulin A deficiency, common variable immunodeficiency syndrome, ataxia telangiectasia, familial polyposis coli, Peutz-Jeghers syndrome and prior exposure to radiotherapy and chemotherapy have been reported to be associated with it.[52,53]

The most common presentation is with abdominal pain, vomiting, anorexia and weight loss. Abdominal lump can be palpated in more than two third of the cases.[54] Histology is usually similar to that of adult onset disease but probably mucinous and signet ring cell type histological pattern is slightly more common in children.

Various treatment protocols based on experience in adult population have been tried in pediatric patients, but overall prognosis remains to be poor.[51]

Gastrointestinal Stromal Tumor

This mesenchymal tumor is again a rare entity in childhood. These tumors occur sporadically or as a part of carney triad which comprise of functional extra-adrenal paraganglioma, pulmonary chondroma and gastric epitheloid stromal sarcoma.[55]

Interstitial cells of Cajal, also known as pacemakers cells, are the cells implicated in the origin of this tumor. These tumors express both KIT and CD34 on their surface.

60–70% cases are found in the stomach. Majority of them measure between 3–15 cm in size. Most common presentation in childhood is in the form of gastrointestinal bleeding or obstruction. Other less common presentations like pain abdomen, fever, weight loss and lump abdomen have also been reported.[56] All gastrointestinal stromal tumors should be treated as potentially malignant tumors which is based on the size of the tumor and histological details of the tumor.

Gastric Teratoma

Although this is a rare tumor, but this definitely needs a mention because it exclusively occurs in pediatric population mainly in male children younger than 2 years of age. It arises from pluripotent cells and is composed of elements from ectoderm, endoderm as well as mesoderm. Usual presentation is with large abdominal mass with or without obstruction and sometimes upper gastrointestinal bleeding due to ulceration of the mucosa. Preoperative imaging sometimes show tumoral calcifications which are due to presence of teeth or bone within the tumor. Histology typically show elements from all the three germ layers. It is a benign tumor and surgical excision alone is usually curative.[57,58]

Gastric Polyps

Although colon is the most common site for polyps, but less frequently stomach is also the site for various types of polyps. They can be sporadic or a part of a polyposis syndrome. They can be adenomatous, juvenile, hamartomatous or fundic gland type depending on the histology.

Familial adenomatous polyposis (FAP) is the most common polyposis syndrome of childhood. Both adenomatous as well as fundic gland type of polyps are seen with a tendency for malignant transformation, but mostly occurring beyond pediatric age group.[59] Endoscopic polypectomy is the treatment of choice but regular endoscopic surveillance is needed to find out new adenomas as well as to pick up malignancy at an early stage.

Around 40% of Peutz-Jeghers patients present with gastric polyps. These are mostly asymptomatic, but antral obstruction as well as upper gastrointestinal bleeding can also occur. These hamartomatous polyps have a typical histology similar to colonic polyps found in this syndrome. Malignancy can occur in these polyps but at a much lower rate.[59,60]

Polyps in the stomach are also commonly found in the juvenile polyposis syndrome especially in generalized juvenile polyposis syndrome as well as in fatal infantile variety of juvenile polyposis.[60,61] These hamartomatous polyps have a typical histology with presence of large cystic spaces inside the polyp. Periodic upper GI endoscopy is indicated because of underlying malignant potential.

Conclusion

Gastric tumor are uncommon in pediatric age group. But these tumors should always be kept in the differential diagnosis in any child presenting with mass in the upper abdomen, pain, vomiting and hemorrhage.

CONGENITAL ANOMALIES OF SMALL INTESTINE

The ultimate digestive function is carried out by the small intestine and is the primary site of absorption of the nutrients. Duodenum originates from the terminal portion of the foregut and cephalic part of the midgut while the rest of the small intestine develops from the midgut. As the stomach rotates during the 7–8 weeks of gestation, the duodenum becomes C-shaped and rotates to the right while the fourth portion becomes fixed in the left upper abdominal cavity. Due to the proliferation of cells in the 8 weeks of gestation, the lumen of the duodenum is obliterated. The midgut rapidly lengthens with formation of the primary intestinal loop. Due to rapid differential growth of abdominal organs, loops of small intestine herniate into umbilical region during 6 weeks of gestation (*physiologic umbilical herniation*). At around 8 weeks of gestation, it rotates 270 degrees around the axis of superior mesenteric artery and continues to elongate with jejunum and ileum forming a number of coiled loops within the peritoneal cavity. As the body grows and relative size of solid organs decrease, midgut returns into abdominal cavity by 10 weeks of gestation and rotates another 180 degrees around superior mesenteric artery. The cranial limb emerges first and settles on the left side of the body. The lumen of small intestine becomes patent at 12 weeks of gestation and the gradual development of digestive function becomes complete by 34 weeks of gestation.[62,63]

Duodenal Atresia and Stenosis

Duodenal obstruction (atresia/stenosis) is the most common cause of proximal (high) intestinal obstruction in newborns occurring 1 per 5,000 to 10,000 live births, affecting boys more commonly than girls.[64] Atresia is caused by failure of canalization during the 7 weeks of gestation whereas stenosis may be a result of failure to re-canalize due to malrotation with or without volvulus, duodenal web, annular pancreas or duplication cysts.

Types

❏ *Type 1:* Mucosal membrane or diaphragm (complete/perforated) without discontinuity of the muscle coats, most commonly seen.

❑ *Type 2:* Blind-ending proximal and distal segments of duodenum connected by a fibrous band.
❑ *Type 3:* Same as type 2 but separated by a gap, least common.
❑ *Double duodenal atresia:* Two defects or a combination of above defects in the same patient.[63,65]

Clinical Features

In atresia there is persistent, bilious vomiting from the first hours of life, usually following the first feed. The infant has flat, minimally distended or scaphoid abdomen

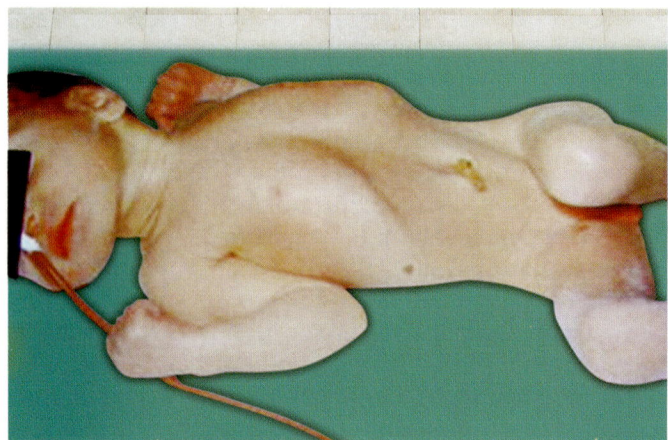

Fig. 5.6: Scaphoid abdomen in duodenal atresia [*Courtesy*: Dr Shashank Shrotriya, MCh (Ped Surg), Pune, Maharashtra, India]

(Fig. 5.6). Presentation may be delayed in duodenal stenosis where recurrent vomiting and failure to thrive are the main symptoms. About 50% of affected patients have associated congenital anomalies associated with pancreas, gastrointestinal tract, cardiovascular, central nervous or renal system rarely, biliary tract anomalies. Down syndrome is associated with about 30% of patients of duodenal atresia.[66]

Diagnosis

In duodenal atresia plain X-ray abdomen classically shows presence of air in the stomach and in the first portion of the duodenum (*double bubble sign*) (Fig. 5.7). No gas is visible throughout the distal intestine. Direct visualization by endoscopy may be useful in duodenal stenosis. Contrast study confirms the diagnosis (Fig. 5.8) and protrusion of the duodenal membrane if present, into the third or fourth part of the duodenum (*Windsock sign*).

Management

❑ *Medical:* It involves decompression, and correction of dehydration and electrolyte imbalance.
❑ *Surgical:* It is the definitive therapy. This includes resection of the membrane or side-to-side or end-to-side duodenoduodenostomy or duodenojejunostomy depending upon the defect. Prognosis is usually good (early postoperative survival rate up to 90%) in absence of genetic abnormalities.[67]

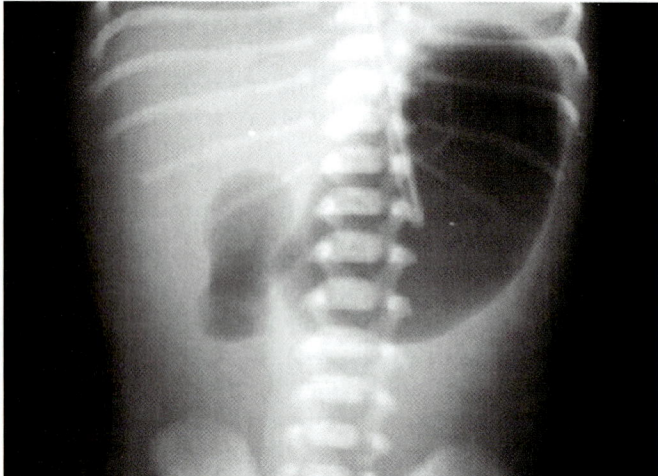

Fig. 5.7: Plain X-ray abdomen showing double bubble sign in duodenal atresia [*Courtesy*: Dr Shashank Shrotriya, MCh (Ped Surg), Pune, Maharashtra, India]

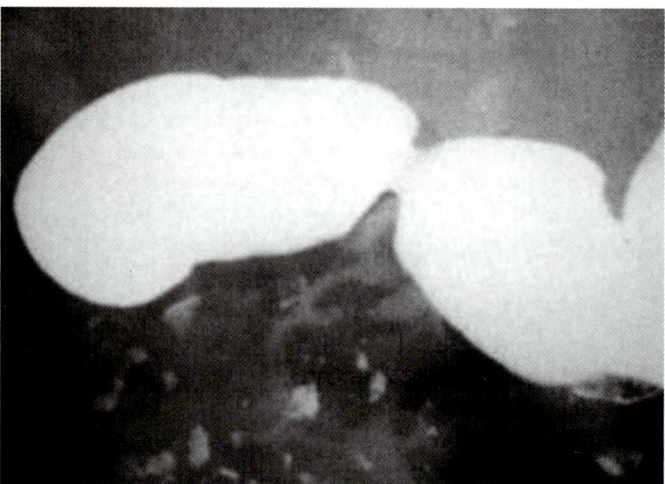

Fig. 5.8: Contrast study showing duodenal atresia [*Courtesy*: Dr Shashank Shrotriya, MCh (Ped Surg), Pune, Maharashtra, India]

□ Endotherapy: Type 1 duodenal atresia can be managed by endoscopic balloon dilation.

Small Intestinal Duplication

Duplication cysts are congenital tubular or spherical cysts attached to the alimentary canal anywhere between the mouth and the anus. This can be communicating or non-communicating types. The term duplication was suggested by Gross and the first case of duodenal duplication was reported by Sanger in 1880 in a still born female.[67,68]

It is most commonly seen in the ileocecal region (44%) while duplication cyst of duodenum is very rare entity constituting around 2–12% of gastrointestinal duplication cysts.[69] They usually lie on the mesenteric side of the small intestine. Tubular type of duplications may communicate with the adjacent intestinal lumen.

Histologic Criteria for Duplication Cysts[62]

□ Presence of gastrointestinal mucosa: It is typically that of the adjacent part of the gastrointestinal tract, but in 15% gastric mucosa and very rarely pancreatic mucosa can be seen.
□ Presence of smooth muscle layer in the wall.
□ Associated with the duodenal wall.

Types[70]

□ *Type 1:* Parallel type—the duplication is on the border of one leaf of mesentery and the straight artery to the duplication is separated from the straight artery to the bowel, more commonly seen.

□ *Type 2:* Intramesenteric type—the duplication is located in between the both leaves of the mesentery and the straight arteries passes over the both surfaces of the duplication to reach the bowel.

Clinical Features

The child may remain asymptomatic for years. They may present with an abdominal mass or obstruction of the adjacent intestinal lumen, vomiting, decreased oral intake, abdominal distension and periumbilical tenderness. An abdominal mass may be palpable. Ulceration, hemorrhage within the cyst, pancreatitis, and biliary obstruction can also be seen. The communicating duplication cyst manifest with massive GI bleeding.

Diagnosis

Abdominal ultrasonography may show unilocular cystic structure with echogenic mucosa surrounded by thin hypoechoic halo of muscle layer and peristaltic waves. Radiology may demonstrate obstruction or compression effect. Computed tomography or magnetic resonance (Fig. 5.9) may demonstrate an encapsulated cyst.[71] ERCP may demonstrate a compressible periampullary mass. Diagnosis of communicating duplication cyst is very difficult. At times barium studies may show doubling of the loop.

Management

Surgery is the treatment of choice where complete or partial excision can be done (Fig. 5.10). Endoscopic drainage and removal has also been tried.

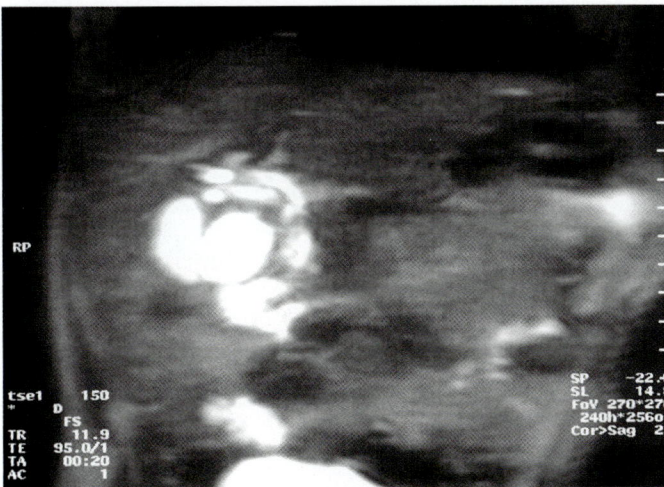

Fig. 5.9: Magnetic resonance of a child with duplication of gallbladder with double gallbladder, a rarest of rare condition

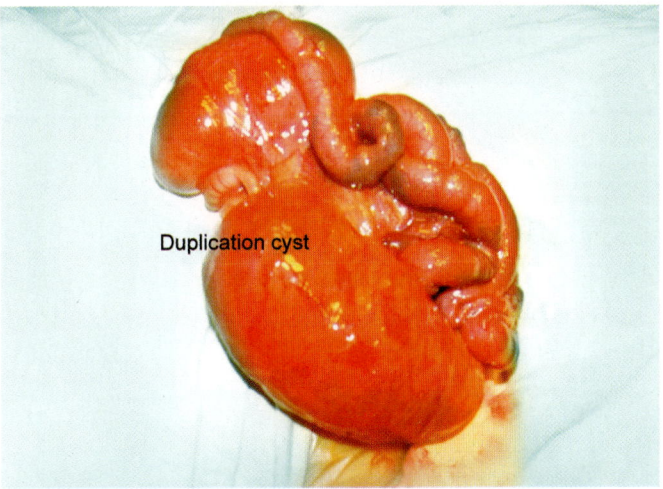

Fig. 5.10: Duplication cyst of ileum [*Courtesy:* Dr Shashank Shrotriya, MCh (Ped Surg), Pune, Maharashtra, India]

Malrotation and Midgut Volvulus

This is a consequence of errors in the normal embryonic development of the midgut. The child may present in the newborn, neonatal period or even later in childhood and adulthood. The true incidence of malroation is unknown, however, a prevalence of 1 in 500 live births has been reported. A classification has been proposed depending on the the stage of rotation at which normal embryonic development of the midgut was interrupted. Most anomalies of midgut rotation occur during the second stage of rotation.

Defects in the first and third stages of rotation are uncommon and generally involves the cecum. Second stage rotational defects are:

❑ *Nonrotation:* This is most commonly seen where there is complete failure of the second stage of rotation, positioning the small intestine to the right of the midline and the colon to the left.

❑ *Reverse rotation:* This is rare and most commonly seen in adults. In this the midgut rotates 180 degrees clockwise, resulting in a net 90 degrees of clockwise rotation positioning colon behind the superior mesenteric artery.

❑ *Malrotation:* Here the proximal midgut fails to rotate around the mesenteric vessels, positioning jejunum and ileum to the right of the superior mesenteric artery and the cecum in the subpyloric region.[62]

Clinical Features

Intestinal malrotation may present acutely as bowel obstruction and intestinal ischemia associated with midgut volulus in newborns, or chronically in older children as vague abdominal discomfort and malnutrition. It may be associated with other congenital anomalies as intestinal atresia, omphalocele or gastroschisis or congenital diaphragmatic hernia. Commonly seen features are bilious emesis, abdominal distention, abdominal pain, vomiting, diarrhea, abdominal tenderness or even melena. Intestinal ischemia may result in peritonitis and hypovolemic shock.[72]

Diagnosis

Upper gastrointestinal contrast study may delineate the site of the duodenojejunal junction (Fig. 5.11). Ultrasonography may demonstrate superior mesenteric vein located to the left of the superior mesenteric artery, suggesting malrotation. If a child is having acute onset of bilious vomiting and peritoneal signs, no diagnostic studies should be performed if they delay surgical intervention.

Management

Surgery offers the definitive treatment (Figs 5.12 and 5.13). Ladd's procedure is the operation of choice which constitutes Ladd's bands, if present, widening of the mesentery, appendectomy, and fixation of the small intestine on the right and the colon on the left side of the abdomen.

Jejunal and Ileal Atresia

Atresia of the jejunum and ileum is twice as common as duodenal atresia and occurs in 1 out of 500 live births. Jejunal atresias (Fig. 5.14) are more common than ileal atresias. Isolated jejunal atresia are more likely to be associated with other congenital abnormalities.

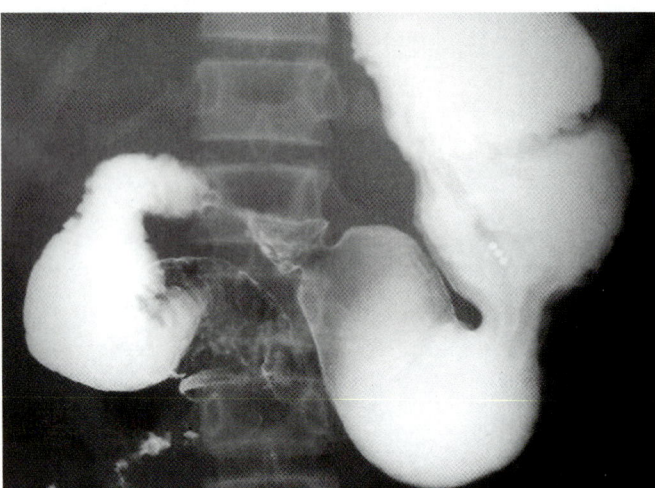

Fig. 5.11: Contrast study in malrotation showing duodenal-jejunal flexure to the left [*Courtesy:* Dr Shashank Shrotriya, MCh (Ped Surg), Pune, Maharashtra, India]

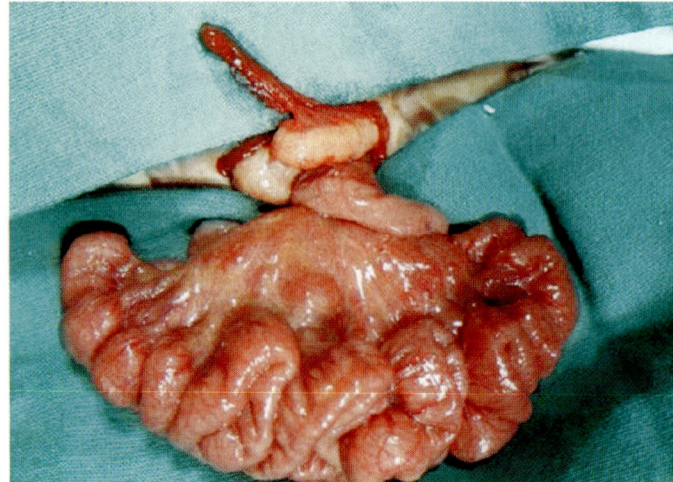

Fig. 5.12: Midgut volvulus [*Courtesy:* Dr Shashank Shrotriya, MCh (Ped Surg), Pune, Maharashtra, India]

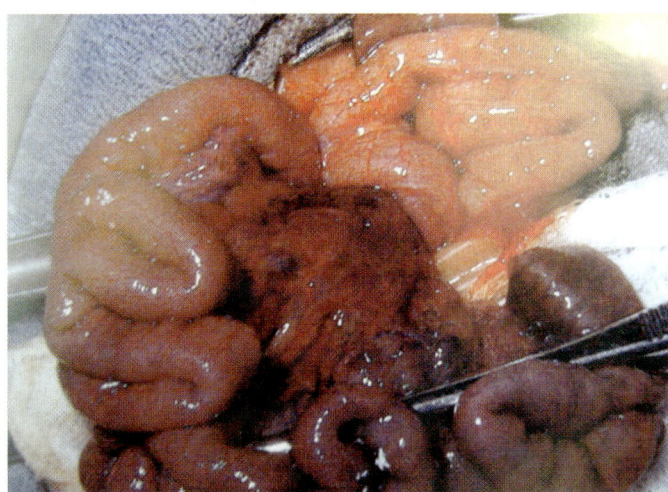

Fig. 5.13: Gangrenous midgut due to malrotation [*Courtesy*: Dr Shashank Shrotriya, MCh (Ped Surg), Pune, Maharashtra, India]

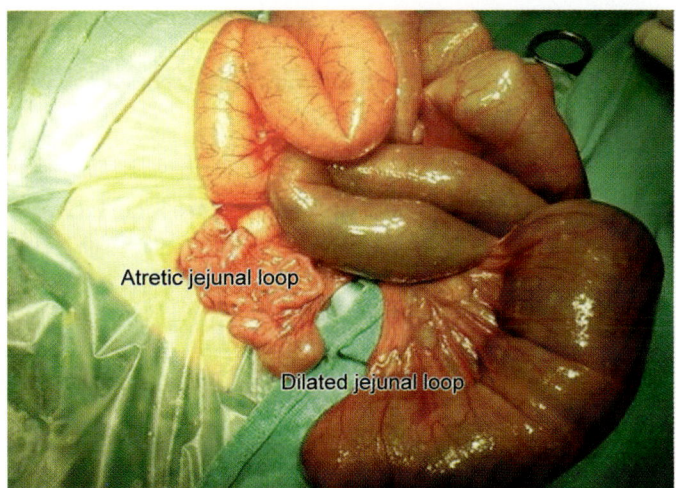

Atretic jejunal loop

Dilated jejunal loop

Fig. 5.14: Intraoperative photograph of jejunal atresia (Type III) [*Courtesy*: Dr Shashank Shrotriya, MCh (Ped Surg), Pune, Maharashtra, India]

Types

❑ *Type I:* Mucosal obstruction caused by an intraluminal epithelial membrane with intact bowel wall.
❑ *Type II:* The blind ends are connected by a fibrous cord, constitutes 35% of intestinal atresias.
❑ *Type III:* The two blind ends are completely separated by a V-shaped mesenteric defect (IIIa) or are associated with a significant mesentric defect with loss of the normal blood supply to the distal bowel (IIIb). Type IIIb is also known as *Apple peel* or *Christmas tree* deformity.
❑ *Type IV:* Presence of multiple atresias resembling a string of sausages and comprises 5% of all intestinal atresias.[63]

Clinical Features

Neonates with jejunal or ileal obstruction present with bilious vomiting depending on the level of obstruction and a distended abdomen. The child fails to pass meconium. The symptom is usually less severe than in duodenal obstruction. The etiology considered are vascular accidents, such a thromboembolic occlusion, hypoxia or volvulus. The ischemic event may also lead to the perforation and meconium peritonitis.

Diagnosis

Plain X-ray abdomen show dilatation of pre-atretic loops. In jejunal atresia only a few loops of distended jejunum are present in the left upper abdomen, while in ileal atresia (Fig. 5.15) many dilated loops can be seen. A barium enema or ultrasonography may be required in complicated cases with an abnormally distended and painful abdomen to exclude meconium ileus or meconium peritonitis.

Management

Definitive treatment is surgical resection of the atretic portion of the bowel with an end-to-end anastomosis. Postoperatively, parentral nutritional may be required until bowel function is restored. Prognosis is determined by the length and function of the remaining bowel.[73]

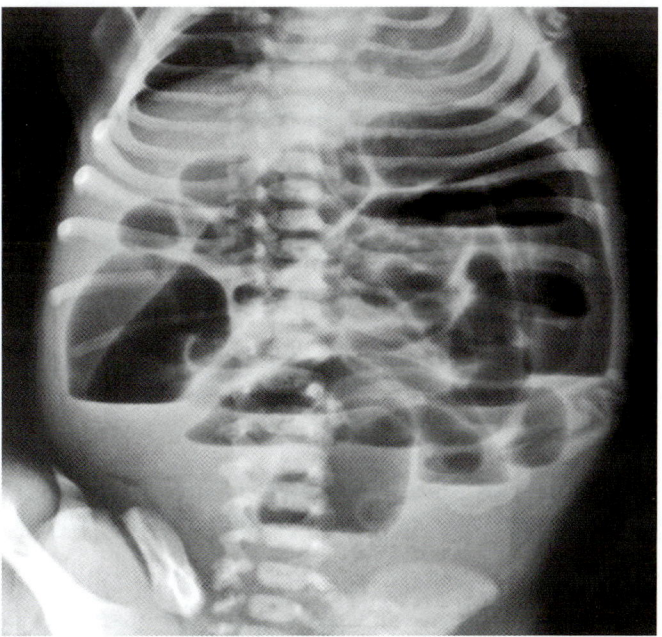

Fig. 5.15: Plain X-ray of ileal atresia showing multiple air-fluid levels [*Courtesy:* Dr Shashank Shrotriya, MCh (Ped Surg), Pune, Maharashtra, India]

Megacystis-Microcolon-Malrotation-Intestinal-Hypoperistalsis Syndrome (MMMIHS)

MMMIHS is a rare autosomal recessive disorder first described in 1976 by Berdon in five newborn girls. The main features are abdominal distension, distended nonobstructive urinary bladder, microcolon, intestinal hypoperistalsis and malrotation of the small intestine. It is three to four times more prevalent in females. It is usually lethal within the first year of life.[74]

Clinical Features

Patient presents with vomiting, failure to pass meconium, absent spontaneous micturition along with distension of abdomen.

Diagnosis

Plain X-ray abdomen shows a highly distended abdomen caused by a distended urinary bladder.

Barium study may demonstrate dilated small bowel without peristaltic activity and microcolon. Ultrasonography demonstrate large urinary bladder with dilated ureters and pyelocaliceal systems.

Management

Nutritional support is the mainstay of treatment. Palliative surgery such as jejunostomy or cystostomy can be done.[75] Bowel transplantation has also been tried. The overall prognosis is considered to be poor and treatment has been shown to be generally ineffective.

Small Intestinal Bacterial Overgrowth

Normally, human colon contains bacteria at a concentration of 100 billion organisms/mL, whereas stomach and upper small bowel contain very insignificant amount of bacteria.[76] In certain conditions these colonic bacteria proliferate in the small intestine and cause their ill effects like steatorrhea and anemia, leading to syndrome known as small intestinal bacterial overgrowth syndrome (SIBO). SIBO is also known by various other names like stagnant loop,[77] small bowel stasis,[78] contaminated small bowel[79] or blind loop syndrome.[80]

At birth gut is sterile, but very soon after birth bacteria start colonizing the intestine. Normally small intestine has mainly aerobic gram-positive population of bacteria which shifts to predominant anaerobic gram-negative type in the colon. Similarly bacterial counts also go on increasing as one travels from proximal parts of the small intestine to the colon (Table 5.4).[76]

Table 5.4: Normal distribution of bacteria within the gastrointestinal tract	
Proximal small intestine	Distal small intestine and colon
<10 million organisms/mL	>100000 million organisms/mL
Aerobic, mainly gram-positive flora predominates	Anaerobic, facultative anaerobic and mainly gram-negative flora predominates
Streptococcus	Bacteroides, E. coli
Lactobacillus, Neisseria	Bifidobacterium, Clostridium

There are some protective forces inside the human body normally which do not allow the bacterial overgrowth to occur. On the other side, any defect in these protective forces makes one prone to develop bacterial overgrowth and its ill effects subsequently.

Factors preventing bacterial overgrowth in the small intestine:
- Gastric acidity[81]
- Normal peristaltic movements and migratory motor complexes of the small intestine[82]
- Antibacterial properties of pancreatic enzymes, bile acids and other digestive secretions[83]
- Mucus[84]
- Ileocecal valve[85]
- Antibodies secreted by normal mucosa like IgG and IgA, activated T cells and macrophages—less important role[76]

Factors predisposing to the development of small intestinal bacterial overgrowth:
- Anatomic abnormalities of the GI tract like strictures, stenosis, duplications, webs, diverticula and blind loops leading to stasis and hence bacterial overgrowth[86]
- Motility problems like in premature neonates, scleroderma, diabetes mellitus and pseudo-obstruction
- Increased bacterial load in colo-enteric fistulas, achlorhydria due to chronic PPI use or pernicious anemia, loss of ileocecal valve function[76]
- Decreased host immune response especially in severe protein-energy malnutrition and primary or secondary immune deficiencient states.[87]

Pathophysiology

Increased number of bacteria in small intestinal bacterial overgrowth change the intraluminal secretions and also produce various toxins, enzymes and other metabolic products which are responsible for producing various local as well as systemic side effects of it.[76]

Most important is the deconjugation of bile salts by anaerobic bacteria leading to impaired absorption of triglycerides, fat soluble vitamins and other lipid molecules, clinically manifesting as steatorrhea.[88] Intraluminal bacteria also consume vitamin B_{12} and also produce ceramides which inhibit vitamin B_{12} absorption in ileum leading to vitamin B_{12} deficiency and result in magaloblastic anemia not correctable by intrinsic factor.[89]

Mucosa also suffer damage due to the toxins and enzymes produced by bacteria. It causes patchy lesions of subtotal villous atrophy as well as subepithelial inflammation. Brush border disaccharidases as well as monosaccharide transport across the mucosa is impaired[76] Absorption of some of these toxins lead to systemic manifestations of small intestinal bacterial overgrowth in the form of arthritis, dermatitis, vasculitis as well as hepatobiliary injury.[90]

Clinical Features

Clinical symptoms does not occur in all patients, being manifested only in one-third of cases, varying from mild complaints to severe disabling symptoms.[91] Younger patients are more severely affected because of immaturity of mucosal defence mechanisms.[76]

Diarrhea is most common symptom which brings a child into notice of a physician. Stools may be greasy or watery and explosive due to underlying fat and carbohydrate malabsorption. Diarrhea is usually associated with abnormal growth parameters like wasting and stunting. Loose stools are commonly associated with abdominal distension, nausea and vomiting.[76]

Deficiency signs due to vitamin D and B complex group are very commonly found in severly affected patients. Vitamin B_{12} deficiency anemia is uncommon during pediatric age group due to adequate body stores,[76] but iron deficiency is more common due to mucosal losses of iron. Serum folic acid levels are elevated due to bacterial production of folic acid.[92]

Small intestinal bacterial overgrowth is an important cause of pain abdomen in some children.[93] It may also manifest as arthralgias, tenosynovitis and vasculitic episodes.[90] It is also involved in the causation of SBP as well as in causation of NASH related liver injury.[94] It also alters the metabolism of oral digoxin as well as antipyrine.[76]

Diagnosis of SIBO

A detailed history and examination is the first and most important step in making a diagnosis of SIBO. Initial tests performed should be a complete hemogram, red blood cell indices, peripheral blood picture, serum iron studies, blood vitamin B_{12} and folic acid levels, stool fat estimation and barium meal follow through. In some cases a duodenal biopsy with serological markers is required to rule out celiac disease.[76]

Specific tests for diagnosing SIBO are breath tests and duodenal fluid aspirate for culture of the bacteria. Culture of coliforms or anaerobic bacteria with a count of >10^5 colony forming units/mL confirms the diagnosis of SIBO. Although duodenal aspirate is considered the gold standard test for diagnosing SIBO, it is an invasive procedure which requires sedation, passing of a catheter per orally with requirement of fluoroscopy with associated radiation hazards or an endoscope, making it a less preferred test in day-to-day clinical practice.[95]

Breath Tests

Breath tests are the preferred noninvasive tests available for diagnosing SIBO. These tests depend on the ability of intestinal bacteria to deconjugate C14 or 13 labeled bile acids to produce CO_2 gas labeled with C14 or 13, which can be detected in expired air or production of H_2 gas by bacteria when they come in contact with substrates like lactulose, glucose or lactose, leading to detection of H_2 gas in the expired air.[96]

Tests based on radiolabeled isotopes like C14 or 13 are not preferred in pediatric age group due to deleterious effects of radiation on young children. Usually lactulose or glucose based H_2 breath tests are preferred in children. Glucose-based tests are more specific but less sensitive than lactulose based test, as well as glucose is less palatable than lactulose, making lactulose-based test as the preferred choice in children.[96]

Breath tests also have certain limitations like difficulty in collecting breath samples in young children, false-positive or negative results with certain food products or use of antibiotics or due to altered gastric emptying or intestinal transit time, apart from some technical difficulties encountered during conduction of these tests.[76,96]

Treatment

Most important is correction of the underlying predisposing condition if possible. But most patients require antibiotics because predisposing condition is either inapparent or is not easily correctable by surgical or medical management.

Antibiotics like metronidazole, tetracycline, chloramphenicol, lincomycin which are active against bacteroides are the preferred drugs. Metronidazole is the drug of choice in children and usually prescribed for 2–4 weeks. In case of relapse a repeat course of same drug for a longer period or an alternative drug can be used. Other drugs which can be used are trimethoprim-sulphamethoxazole and amoxicillin-clavulanic acid.[1] In a recent study in IBS children with SIBO, rifaximin at a dose of 600 mg/day for one week was effective in treating SIBO and improvement in gastrointestinal symptoms of IBS was also noted.[97] Probiotics like lactobacillus GG and lactobacillus plantarum have been found useful in SIBO in children with short bowel syndrome. Octreotide has been found useful in scleroderma associated SIBO.[98]

Apart from drug therapy and correction of underlying predisposing condition, improving the nutritional status of the patient is of utmost importance. A low fat diet rich in medium chain triglycerides is most preferred diet. Fat-soluble vitamins should be supplemented especially.[76]

REFERENCES

1. Semrin MG, Russo MA. Anatomy, Histology, Embryology, and Developmental Anomalies of the Stomach and Duodenum. Sleisenger and Fordtran's Gastrointestinal and Liver Disease. 9th ed. 2010;1:773-85.
2. Christine AG, Sherin UD. Avery's diseases of the newborn. 9th ed. 2013.pp.973-8.
3. Baert AL, Knauth LM, Sartor GK. Radiological Imaging of the digestive tract in infants and children. p.109.
4. Teresa B, Isabel T, Julia G, Consuelo P, Maria L, Manuel L. Congenital Anomalies of the Upper Gastrointestinal Tract. Radiographics. 1999;19:855-72.
5. Al-Salem AH. Pyloric atresia associated with duodenal and jejunal atresia and duplication. Pediatr Surg Int. 1999;15:512-4.
6. Okoye BO, Parikh DH, Buick RG, Lander AD. Pyloric atresia: five new cases, a new association, and a review of the literature with guidelines. J Pediatr Surg. 2000;35:1242-5.
7. Al-Salem A, Nawaz A, Matta H, Jacobsz A. Congenital pyloric atresia: the spectrum. Int Surg. 2002;87:147-51.
8. Kedinger M, Simon-Assmann PM, Lacroix B, et al. Fetal gut mesenchyme induces differentiation of cultured intestinal endodermal and crypt cells. Dev Biol. 1986;113:474-83.
9. Randolph KC, Kenneth WG, Mark LW. Gastric Volvulus in Infants and Children. Pediatrics. 2008;122:e752-62.
10. Michaud L, Gottrand F, Ategbo S, et al. Pitfalls of endoscopy for diagnosis of pyloric stenosis. J Pediatr Gastroenterol Nutr. 1995; 21:483.
11. Holder-Espinasse M, Ahmad Z, Hamill J, et al. Familial syndromic duodenal atresia: Feingold syndrome. Eur J Pediatr Surg. 2004; 14:112-6.
12. MacMahon B. The continuing enigma of pyloric stenosis of infancy: a review. Epidemiology. 2000;17:195-201.
13. Schubert ML, Peura DA. Control of gastric acid secretion in health and disease. Gastroenterology. 2008;134:1842.
14. Marion R, Billy B, Brendan D. Helicobacter pylori and Peptic Ulcer Disease. In: Pediatric Gastrointestinal Disease by W Allan Walker. 4th ed. p.491-512.
15. Drumm B, Rhoads JM, Stringer DA, et al. Peptic ulcer disease in children: etiology, clinical findings, and clinical course. Pediatrics. 1988;82:410-4.
16. Drumm B. Helicobacter pylori in the pediatric patient. Gastroenterol Clin North Am. 1993;22:169-82.
17. Hassall E, Dimmick JE. Unique features of Helicobacter pylori disease in children. Dig Dis Sci. 1991;36:417-23.
18. Suerbaum S, Michetti P. Helicobacter pylori infection. N Engl J Med. 2002;347:1175-86.
19. Gormally SM, Kierce BM, Daly LE, et al. Gastric metaplasia and duodenal ulcer disease in children infected by Helicobacter pylori. Gut. 1996;38:513-7.
20. Leodolter A, Kulig M, Brasch H, et al. A meta-analysis comparing eradication, healing and relapse rates in patients with Helicobacter pylori-associated gastric or duodenal ulcer. Aliment Pharmacol Ther. 2001;15:1949-58.
21. Brown LM. Helicobacter pylori: Epidemiology and routes of transmission. Epidemiol Rev. 2000;22:283-97.
22. Murphy MS, Eastham EJ, Jimenez M, et al. Duodenal ulceration: review of 110 cases. Arch Dis Child. 1987;62:554-8.
23. De Giacomo C, Valdambrini V, Lizzoli F. et al. A population-based survey on gastrointestinal tract symptoms and Helicobacter pylori infection in children and adolescents. Helicobacter: 2002; 7:356-63.
24. O'Donohoe JM, Sullivan PB, Scott R. et al. Recurrent abdominal pain and Helicobacter pylori in a community-based sample of London children. Acta Paediatr. 1996;85:961-4.
25. Helicobacter and Cancer Collaborative Group. Gastric cancer and Helicobacter pylori: a combined analysis of 12 case control studies nested within prospective cohorts. Gut 2001; 49: 347–353.
26. BenjaminCY, Wong CY. American College of Gastroenterology Guideline on the Management of Helicobacter pylori Infection. Am J Gastroenterol. 2007;102:1808-25.
27. Midolo P, Marshall BJ. Accurate diagnosis of Helicobacter pylori. Urease tests. Gastroenterol Clin N Am. 2000;29:871-8.
28. El-Zimaity HM. Accurate diagnosis of Helicobacter pylori with biopsy. Gastroenterol Clin N Am. 2000;29:863-9.
29. Koletzko S, Jones NL, Goodman KJ, Gold B, Rowland M, Cadranel S, et al. Evidence-based guidelines from ESPGHAN and NASPGHAN for Helicobacter pylori infection in children. J Pediatr Gastroenterol Nutr. 2011;53:230-43.
30. Oderda G, Forni M, Dell'Olio D, Ansaldi N. Cure of peptic ulcer associated with eradication of Helicobacter pylori. Lancet .1990; 335:1599.
31. Drumm B, Koletzko S, Oderda S. On behalf of the European Pediatric Task force on Helicobacter pylori. Helicobacter pylori infection in children: a consensus statement. J Pediatr Gastroenterol Nutr. 2000;30:207-13.
32. Laine L, Hopkins RJ, Girardi LS. Has the impact of Helicobactor pylori therapy on ulcer recurrence in the United States been overstated? A meta analysis of rigorously designed trials. Am J Gastroenterol. 1998;93:1409-15.
33. Peura DA, Haber MM, Hunt B, Atkinson S. Helicobacter pylori-negative gastritis in erosive esophagitis, nonerosive reflux disease or functional dyspepsia patients. J Clin Gastroenterol. 2010 Mar;44:180-5.
34. Nordenstedt H, Graham DY, Kramer JR, Rugge M, Verstovsek G, et al. Helicobacter pylori-negative gastritis: prevalence and risk factors. Am J Gastroenterol. 2013;108:65-71.

35. Genta RM, Lash RH. *Helicobacter pylori*-negative gastritis: seek, yet ye shall not always find. Am J Surg Pathol. 2010;34:e25-34.

36. Cutler AF, Prasad VM, Santogade P. Four-year trends in *Helicobacter pylori* IgG serology following successful eradication. Am J Med. 1998;105:18-20.

37. Haber MM, Hunt B, Freston JW. et al. Changes of gastric histology in patients with erosive oesophagitis receiving long-term lansoprazole maintenance therapy. Aliment Pharmacol Ther. 2010;32:83-96.

38. Zavros Y, Rieder G, Ferguson A. et al. Genetic or chemical hypochlorhydria is associated with inflammation that modulates parietal and G-cell populations in mice. Gastroenterol. 2002;122:119-33.

39. Freston JW. Review article:role of proton pump inhibitors in non-*H. pylori* related ulcer. Aliment Pharmacol Therapy. 2001;15:2-5.

40. Pietroiusti A, Forlini A, Magrini A, et al. Isolated *H. pylori* duodenal colonization and idiopathic duodenal ulcers. Am J Gastroenterol. 2008;103:55-61.

41. Chow DK, Sung JJ. Non-NSAID non-*H. pylori* ulcer disease. Best Pract Res Clin Gastroenterol. 2009;23:3-9.

42. Bytzer P, Teglbjaerg PS. Danish Ulcer Study Group. *Helicobactor pylori*-negative duodenal ulcers: prevalence, clinical characteristics, and prognosis-results from a randomised trial with 2-year follow-up. Am J Gastroenterol. 2001;96:1409-16.

43. Bethel CA, Bhattacharyya N, Hutchinson C. et al. Alimentary tract malignancies in children. J Pediatr Surg. 1997;32:1004-8.

44. Goldthorn JF, Canizaro PC. Gastrointestinal malignancies in infancy, childhood and adolescence. Surg Clin North Am. 1986;66:845-61.

45. Gurney KA, Cartwright RA, Gilman EA. Descriptive epidemiology of gastrointestinal non-Hodgkin's lymphoma in a population based registry. Br J Cancer. 1999;79:1929-34.

46. Takahashi H, Hansmann ML. Primary gastrointestinal lymphoma in childhood (up to 18 years of age). A morphological, immunohistochemical and clinical study. J Cancer Res Clin Oncol. 1990;116:190.

47. Filipovich AH, Mathur A, Kamat D, et al. Lymphoproliferative disorders and other tumors complicating immunodeficiencies. Immunodeficiency. 1994;5:91-112.

48. Kahn E. Gastrointestinal manifestations in pediatric AIDS. Pediatr Pathol Lab Med. 1997;17:171-208.

49. Ciftci AO, Tanyel FC, Kotiloglu E, Hicsonmez A. Gastric lymphoma causing gastric outlet obstruction. J Pediatr Surg. 1996;31:1424-6.

50. Grabiec J, Owen DA. Carcinoma of the stomach in younger persons. Cancer. 1985;56:388-96.

51. Michalek J, Kopecna L, Tuma J, et al. Gastric carcinoma in a 9-year-old boy. Pediatr Hematol Oncol. 2000;17:511-5.

52. Haerer AF, Jackson JF, Evers CG. Ataxia-telangiectasia with gastric adenocarcinoma. JAMA. 1969;210:1884-7.

53. Fraser KJ, Rankin JG. Selective deficiency of IgA immunoglobulins associated with carcinoma of the stomach. Australas Ann Med. 1970;19:165-7.

54. Mcneer G. Cancer of the stomach in the young. Am J Roentgenol Rad Ther Nucl Med. 1941;45:537.

55. Carney JA. Gastric stromal sarcomas, pulmonary chondroma and extra-adrenal paraganglioma (carney triad):natural history, adrenocortical component and possible familial occurrence. Mayo Clin Proc. 1999;74:543-52.

56. Berman J. O'Leary TJ. Gastrointestinal stromal tumor workshop. Hum Pathol. 2001;32:78-82.

57. Matsukuma S, Wada R, Daibou M, et al. Adenocarcinoma arising from gastric immature teratoma. Report of a case in an adult and a review of the literature. Cancer. 1995;75:2663-8.

58. Cairo MS, Grosfeld JL, Weetman RM. Gastric teratoma: unusual cause for bleeding of the upper gastrointestinal tract in the newborn. Pediatrics. 1981;67:721-4.

59. Erdman SH, Barnard JA. Gastrointestinal polyps and polyposis syndrome in children. Curr Opin Pediatr. 2002;14:576-82.

60. Coffin M, Pappin AL. Polyps and neoplasms of the gastrointestinal tract in childhood and adolescence. Gastrointest Dis. 1997;20:127-71.

61. Rustgi AK. Hereditary gastrointestinal polyposis and nonpolyposis syndromes. N Engl J Med. 1994;331:1694-702.

62. Ellen Kahn,Fredric Daum. Anatomy, Histology, Embryology, and Developmental Anomalies of the Small and Large Intestine . In: Sleisenger and Fordtran's Gastrointestinal and Liver Disease. 9th ed. 1623-41.

63. David AL, Simon EK. Congenital Anomalies. In: Pediatric Gastrointestinal Disease by W. Allan Walker. 4th ed. p:561-72.

64. Escobar MA, Ladd AP, Grosfeld JL, West KW, et al. Duodenal atresia and stenosis: long-term follow-up over 30 years. J Pediatr Surg. 2004;39:867-71.

65. Stringer MD, Brereton RJ, Drake DP, et al. Double duodenal atresia/stenosis: a report of four cases. J Pediatr Surg. 1992;27:576-80.

66. Dalla Vecchia LK, Grosfeld JL, West KW, et al: Intestinal atresia and stenosis: A 25-year experience with 277 cases. Arch Surg. 1998;133: 490-7.

67. Gross RE, GW Holocomb, Farner S. Duplication of the Alimentary Tract. Pediatrics.1952;9:449.

68. William YI, Corinne F, William TF,Theodore A. Duodenal Duplication: Case Report and Literature Review. Ann Surg. 1965;162:910-16.

69. Chen JJ, Lee HC, Yeung CY, et al. Meta-analysis: the clinical features of the duodenal duplication cyst. J Pediatr Surg. 2010;45:1598-606.

70. Long Li, Zhang Jin-Zhe, Wang Yan-Xia. Vascular classification for small intestinal duplications: Experience with 80 cases. JPediatr Surg. 1998; 33;1243-5.

71. Menon P, Rao KLN,Thapa BR, Goyal R, et al. Duplicated gall bladder with duodenal duplication cyst. J Pediatr Surg. 2013;48(4):E25-8.

72. Powell DM, Othersen HB, Smith CD. Malrotation of the intestine in children: the effect of age on presentation and therapy. J Pediatr Surg. 1989;14:777-80.

73. Rescorla FJ, Grosfeld JL. Intestinal atresia and stenosis: Analysis of survival in 120 cases. Surgery.1985; 98:668-76.

74. Berdon WE, Baker DH, Blanc WA, Gay B, Santulli TV, Do-novan C. Megacystis–microcolon–intestinal hypoperistalsis syndrome: a new cause of intestinal obstruction in the newborn: report of radiologic findings in five newborn girls. Am J Roentgen. 1976; 126:957-64.

75. Manop J, Chamnanvanakij S, Wattanasarn C. Megacystis Microcolon Intestinal Hypoperistalsis Syndrome (MMIHS): A Case Report in Thailand. J Med Assoc Thai. 2004;87:1385-8.

76. Lichtman SN. Bacterial overgrowth. In: Walker WA, Durie PT, Hamilton JR, et al (Eds). Pediatric Gastrointestinal Disease, 3rd edn. Ontario BC Decker. 2000:569-81.

77. Gorbach SL, Tabaqchali S. Bacteria, bile and small bowel. Gut 1969;10:963-72.

78. Ament MF, Shimoda SS, Sanders DP. Pathogenesis of steatorrhea in three cases of small intestinal stasis syndrome. Gastroenterology. 1972;63:728.

79. Gracey M. The contaminated small bowel syndrome: pathogenesis, diagnosis and treatment. Am J Clin Nutr. 1979;32:234-43.

80. Ellis H, Smith ADM. The blind loop syndrome. Monogr Surg Sci. 1977;4:193-7.

81. Giannella RA, Broitman SA, Zamcheck N. Influence of gastric acidity on bacterial and parasitic enteric infections: a prospective. Ann Intern Med. 1973;78:271-6.

82. Scott LD, Cahall DL. Influence of interdigestive myoelectric complex on enteric flora in the rat. Gastroenterology. 1982;82:737-45.

83. Rubinstein E, Mark Z, Haspel J, et al. Antibacterial activity of the pancreatic fluid. Gastroenterology. 1985;88:927-32.

84. Sherman P, Fleming N, Forstner J, et al. Bacteria and the mucus blanket in experimental small bowel bacterial overgrowth. Am J Pathol. 1987;126:527-34.

85. Griffen WO, Richardson JD, Medley ES. Prevention of small bowel contamination by the ileocecal valve. South Med J. 1971;64:1056-9.

86. Bishop RF, Anderson CM. The bacterial flora of the stomach and small intestine in children with intestinal obstruction. Arch Dis Child. 1960;35:487-91.

87. Mata LJ, Jiminez F, Cordon M, et al. Gastrointestinal flora of children with protein-calorie malnutrition. Am J Clin Nutr. 1972;25:1118-26.

88. Hill mj, Drassar BS. Degradation of bile salts by human intestinal bacteria. Gut. 1986;9:22-7

89. Brandt LJ, Bernstein LH, Wagle A. Production of vitamin B12 analogues in patients with small bowel bacterial overgrowth. Ann Intern Med. 1977;87:546-51.

90. Klinkhoff AV, Stein HB, Schlapper OL, Boyka WB. Postgastrectomy blind loop syndrome and the arthritis-dermatitis syndrome. Arthritis Rheum. 1985;28:214.

91. King CE, Toskes PP. Small intestinal bacterial overgrowth. Gastroenterology. 1979;76:1035-55.

92. Hoffbrand AV, Tabaqchali S, Mollin DL. High serum folate levels in intestinal blind-loop syndrome. Lancet. 1966;i:1339-42.

93. De Boissieu D, Chaussain M, Badoual J, et al. Small-bowel bacterial overgrowth in children with diarrhea, abdominal pain or both. Pediatr. 1996;128:203-7.

94. Runyon BA, Sugano S, Kanel G, Mellencamp MA. A rodent model of cirrhosis, ascites and bacterial peritonitis. Gastroenterology. 1991;100:489-93.

95. Gasbarrini A, Lauritano EC, Gabrielli M, Scarpellini E, Lupascu A, Ojetti V, et al. Small intestinal bacterial overgrowth: diagnosis and treatment. Dig Dis. 2007;25:237-40.

96. Khoshini R, Dai SC, Lezcano S, Pimentel M. A systematic review of diagnostic tests for small intestinal bacterial overgrowth. Dig Dis Sci. 2008;53:1443-54.

97. Scarpellini E, Giorgio V, Gabrielli M, Filoni S, Vitale G, Tortora A, et al. Rifaximin treatment for small intestinal bacterial overgrowth in children with irritable bowel syndrome. Eur Rev Med Pharmacol. Sci. 2013;17:1314-20.

98. Goan D, Garmendia C, Murrielo NO, et al. Effect of Lactobacillus strains on bacterial overgrowth related chronic diarrhea. Medicina. 2002;62:159-63.

Acute Diarrhea

AK Patwari

INTRODUCTION

Diarrhea is usually defined as passage of 3 or more loose or watery stools in a 24 hour period, a loose stool being one that would take the shape of a container. However, from a practical standpoint, it is the recent change in consistency and character of stool and water content rather than the number of stools that is important. Infants who are exclusively breastfed normally pass several soft or semi-liquid stools each day; for them, it is practical to define diarrhea as an increase in stool frequency or liquidity that is considered abnormal by the mother.

EPIDEMIOLOGY

Diarrhea continues to be one of the major causes of mortality in children under five years of age and is responsible for 11% of deaths in this age group, globally. In India, 13% of children under five years of age die due to diarrhea in 2010, according to data from the Child Health Reference Group (CHERG).[1] A child below five years of age suffers from an average of 2-3 episodes of diarrhea per year. Most of the diarrheal episodes occur during the first 2 years of life (highest incidence at 6-12 months of age) and about 10% of diarrheal episodes are dysentery (stools contain blood).[2] Low socioeconomic status, bottle-feeding, measles, severe malnutrition and immunodeficiency are known risk factors.

ETIOLOGY

In developing countries, the organisms most frequently associated with acute watery diarrhea include Enterotoxigenic *Escherichia coli* (ETEC), Enteropathogenic *Escherichia coli* (EPEC), *Shigella* and *Campylobacter jejuni*. *Vibrio cholerae* O1 and O139 is an important organism in endemic areas and during epidemics of cholera. Non-typhoidal *Salmonella* is a common organism in areas where commercially processed foods are widely used

and is also implicated in hospital outbreaks. Most of these organisms produce watery diarrhea. Rotavirus is a common cause of severe diarrhea, vomiting and fever leading to rapid dehydration. In 2005, 113,000 rotavirus deaths were reported in India, according to data from the million deaths study.[3]

The main pathogens causing acute dysentery are *Shigella*, *Campylobacter jejuni* and less frequently Enteroinvasive *Escherichia coli* (EIEC) or non-typhoidal salmonella. Epidemics of dysentery are usually caused by *S. dysenteriae type 1*. *Entamoeba histolytica* can cause dysentery in adults but is a less common cause in young children.

Diarrhea may also be caused by a number of antibacterial agents like ampicillin, cotrimoxazole, chloramphenicol, amoxicillin, clindamycin etc. Pseudomembranous colitis is the most severe form of antibiotic-associated diarrhea.

A study on acute diarrhea , conducted from 2007–2009 reported infection with a single organism in 39% and mixed infection in 48% of under-five children suffering from acute diarrhea. Common causative organisms were rotavirus (48.1%), *Vibrio cholera* O1 (16.4%), *Giardia* (14.2%), EAEC (12%), adenovirus (11.6%), *Cryptosporidium* (11%), *C. jejuni* (9.3%), *Shigella* (7.9%) and *E. histolytica* (4%). An increase in *Vibrio cholerae* O1 infection and polymicrobial etiology were the two important observations in this study.[4]

PATHOGENESIS

Most enteropathogens can cause diarrhea by more than one mechanism. Therefore, the clinical presentation depends upon the underlying pathophysiological changes taking place in the gastrointestinal tract. Three clinical types of diarrhea have been defined, each one occurring due to a different pathogenetic mechanism and necessitating a different approach to treatment.

Secretory Diarrhea: It is characterized by acute watery diarrhea with profound loss of water and electrolytes due to sodium pump failure as a result of the action of identified toxins. This group is at risk for rapid development of dehydration and electrolyte imbalance. Common causes are ETEC and *V. cholerae*.

Invasive Diarrhea (Dysentery): Intestinal mucosal cells are actually invaded by the microorganisms, which set up an inflammatory reaction clinically presenting with blood and mucus in the stools. This group is prone to develop complications like intestinal perforation, toxic megacolon, rectal prolapse, convulsions, septicemia and hemolytic uremic syndrome.

Osmotic Diarrhea: Injury to enterocytes may result in damage to the mucosal brush border and epithelial destruction leading to decreased mucosal disaccharidase activity. Clinical presentation is characterized by passage of large, frothy, explosive and acidic stools. High osmolar solutions given orally such as carbonated soft drinks and oral rehydration solutions (ORS) with high sugar content can also result in osmotic diarrhea. In this type of diarrhea, in addition to the possibility of the child developing dehydration, hypernatremia is a serious concern.

CLINICAL FEATURES

Diarrhea in children can present as acute watery diarrhea, dysentery or persistent diarrhea.

Acute watery diarrhea: It refers to diarrhea that begins acutely, lasts for less than 14 days, with passage of frequent loose or watery stools and without visible blood. Vomiting may occur and fever may be present. Loss of large volume of water and electrolytes can result in dehydration and dyselectrolytemia.

Dysentery: It is the term used for diarrhea with visible blood and mucus. Dysentery is often associated with fever and tenesmus (painful spasmodic contractions of the rectal and anal musculature). Common clinical features of dysentery include anorexia, rapid weight loss and complications like renal failure and encephalopathy.

Persistent diarrhea: An episode of diarrhea, presumed to be caused by infectious agents that begins acutely but is of longer duration (>14 days), as compared to acute diarrhea. The episode may begin either as acute watery diarrhea or as dysentery.

Approach to a Patient with Acute Diarrhea

Diagnosis of acute diarrhea is based on clinical history of passing frequent, loose or watery stools, with or without vomiting, fever, abdominal pain or blood in the stools. Many children may have symptoms and signs of other associated illnesses like cough, skin rashes/measles or urinary symptoms.

PRINCIPLES OF TREATMENT

Apart from general assessment of the child, the following principles are followed in management of a child with acute diarrhea:

- ❏ Assessment of hydration status
- ❏ Appropriate feeding to provide optimal energy and nutrient requirements
- ❏ Zinc supplementation
- ❏ Treatment of associated problems
- ❏ Identification of risk factors for diarrheal morbidity and mortality
- ❏ Correction of electrolyte and acid-base imbalance
- ❏ Prevention.

Assessment of Dehydration

Dehydration, the immediate consequence of diarrheal diseases, remains the primary focus in patient management. Dehydration is a frequent and serious consequence of acute watery diarrhea including cholera, but some cases of dysentery may also present with dehydration. Prolonged and recurrent episodes of diarrhea adversely affect the nutritional status of a child and thereby significantly contribute to the vicious cycle of malnutrition and infection.

Young children are more susceptible to develop dehydration due to a limited urinary concentrating capacity of the kidneys, more insensible loss of water through skin and lungs owing to a large surface area and rapid breathing, and their dependence on adults to replace their fluid losses. Loss of water and electrolytes in the diarrheal stool results in depletion of the extra cellular fluid volume (ECFV), electrolyte imbalance and the clinical manifestation of dehydration. Even though intracellular and extracellular fluid compartments are equally depleted in diarrhea, the measurement of ECFV show mostly a depletion of the extracellular compartment.[5] The explanation for this is that ECFV contracts in "two directions"—out in the stools and into the cell, so that the net measured loss of volume is largely contributed by the ECFV. Continued ECFV contraction is the root cause of all the physiological changes taking place in dehydration and reversion to normal is more readily accomplished by rehydrating solutions which more closely approximate the composition of the extracellular fluid.[6]

In the past, higher mortality which was reported soon after admission, was mostly due to uncorrected volume depletion or electrolyte imbalance.[7] These observations highlight the importance of the "first day" in fluid therapy of severe dehydration and the need for prompt replacement of losses, particularly in severe secretory diarrhea like cholera, which results in rapidly progressing dehydration, metabolic acidosis and other electrolyte imbalance. The first symptom of dehydration appears after fluid loss of about 5% of body weight. When fluid loss reaches 10%, shock often sets in and the cascade of events that follows can culminate in death, unless there is immediate intervention. Without treatment, severe episodes literally wring out body fluids from the victim faster than they can be replaced. Rehydration, orally or intravenously, is the only effective therapy.

Compensatory Mechanisms

Contraction of the ECFV consequent to loss of water and electrolytes in diarrheal stools, leads to increase in renin, angiotensin, aldosterone and antidiuretic hormone (ADH) secretion and decrease in the glomerular filtration rate (GFR). All these changes lead to compensatory retention of salt and water but proportionately more of the latter. The first palpable response to ECFV contraction is thirst and if water is administered, it will be mostly retained due to the effect of ADH. In addition, water may also be generated internally by steroids and catecholamines. Therefore, retention of water by these mechanisms results in isotonic or hypotonic dehydration. Pre-existing or uncorrected potassium deficiency can also perpetuate hypotonicity.[8-10] Comparison of various intravenous regimens containing high or low sodium have shown that rational treatment should reverse all the compensatory events by restoring volume quickly, correcting acidosis and reducing potassium deficit with solutions approximating the composition of the extracellular fluid. The more hypotonic the fluid is with respect to sodium, less efficient and slower will be correction of the ECFV contraction.

Prevention and Treatment of Dehydration

A number of clinical signs and symptoms can help in detecting dehydration. However, a simple assessment chart can be referred to for a rapid assessment of dehydration and administration of appropriate fluids for prevention and treatment of dehydration (Table 6.1).

Management of 'No Dehydration': The objective of treatment is prevention of dehydration and malnutrition (Plan A). The management can be successfully carried out at home, by the mother/caretaker who is advised to (Table 6.2): (i) give more fluids than normal (Table 6.2), ORS or homemade food-based solutions, (ii) continue feeding, and (iii) bring the child back after 2 days, or earlier if he has any of the danger signs (thirsty, irritable/restless, fever, high purge rate, repeated vomiting, blood in the stool, eating or drinking poorly, lethargic).

Management of 'Some Dehydration': The objective of treatment is to treat dehydration and electrolyte imbalance, and to continue feeding. These children should be rehydrated with ORS (Table 6.3) under supervision in a health facility (Plan B).

Correction of dehydration

- For correction of fluid and electrolyte deficit on account of dehydration, administer 50–100 mL/kg body weight (75 mL/kg) of ORS, over a period of 4 hours. If the child demands more, administer more ORS. Breastfeeding should be continued.
- Older children should have free access to plain water.

Table 6.1: Assessment of hydration status in a patient with diarrhea

Clinical Signs			
General condition	Well, alert	Restless, irritable	Lethargic or unconscious
Eyes	Normal	Sunken	Sunken
Thirst*	Drinks normally, not thirsty	Drinks eagerly, thirsty	Drinks poorly, not able to drink
Skin pinch	Goes back quickly	Goes back 'slowly'	Goes back 'very slowly'
Decide hydration Status			
	The patient has no signs of dehydration	If the patient has two or more signs, there is 'some dehydration'	If the patient has two or more signs, there is 'severe dehydration'
Treatment Plan	Plan A	Plan B	Plan C

* In a young infant less than 2 months of age, thirst is not assessed and decision regarding 'some' or 'severe dehydration' is made if 'two' of the three signs are present

Table 6.2: Guidelines for replacement of fluid and electrolytes in children with 'No Dehydration' (Plan A)

Age	After each loose stool, offer*:
< 6 months	Quarter glass or cup (50 mL)
7 months to 2 years	Quarter to half glass or cup (50 mL–100 mL)
2–5 years	Half to one glass or cup (100–200 mL)
Older children	As much as the child can take

* Fluids which can be offered include ORS, lemon water, butter milk, rice kanji, lentil soup, light tea, etc.

❏ Acceptance of ORS, purge rate and vomiting should be closely monitored.

Reassess after 4 hours
❏ If still dehydrated, repeat deficit therapy (Plan B) and also offer milk/food.
❏ If rehydrated, treat as 'no dehydration' with maintenance therapy with ORS as in Plan A.
❏ If oral rehydration therapy (ORT) is not successful, treat as 'severe dehydration' with intravenous fluids as in Plan C.

Management of 'Severe Dehydration': The primary objective is to quickly rehydrate the child in a hospital with facilities for intravenous (IV) fluid therapy. Ringer's lactate is the preferred solution for rehydration and is given as 100 mL/kg over 6 hours in infants < 1 year and over 3 hours in older children (Table 6.4). If Ringer's lactate is not available, other alternatives like normal saline may be used .

Rehydration of Severely Malnourished Children: Rehydration of severely malnourished children deserves special

Table 6.3: Low osmolarity ORS formulation recommended by WHO/UNICEF

Reduced osmolarity ORS	grams/ liter	Reduced osmolarity ORS	mmol/ liter
Sodium chloride	2.6	Sodium	75
Glucose, anhydrous	13.5	Chloride	65
Potassium chloride	1.5	Glucose, anhydrous	75
Trisodium citrate, dihydrate	2.9	Potassium	20
		Citrate	10
		Total osmolarity	**245**

Table 6.4: Deficit fluid therapy for 'severe dehydration' (Plan C)

	Infants (< 1 year)	Older Child (> 1 year)
Volume of Ringer's lactate	30 mL/kg body weight within first 1 hour, followed by 70 mL/kg body weight over next 5 hours	30 mL/kg body weight within ½ hour, followed by 70 mL/ kg body weight over next 2½ hours
Monitoring	Assess for improvement every 1-2 hours: • If not improving, give IV infusion more rapidly • Encourage oral feeding by giving ORS 5 mL/ kg/hour, along with IV fluids, as soon as the child is able to drink *Reassess hydration status:* • After 6 hours (infants) and 3 hours (Older children) assess hydration status and choose appropriate plan for hydration (Plan A, B or C)	

attention owing to certain pathophysiological changes in water and electrolyte status peculiar to protein-energy malnutrition (PEM). Dehydration may be over or under estimated in the clinical setting of marasmus or edema, respectively. These children are at risk to develop hypoglycemia and electrolyte imbalance. Rehydration with ORS solution should be preferred because IV fluid administration may inadvertently result in overhydration and, in some cases, even congestive cardiac failure. Therefore, it is recommended that severely malnourished children are slowly rehydrated, carefully monitored and feeding is initiated early.

Oral rehydration therapy: The concept of oral rehydration therapy (ORT) has revolutionized the management of diarrhea with the discovery of coupled active transport of glucose and sodium in the small bowel, resulting in the passive absorption of water and other electrolytes, even during episodes of copious diarrhea. Oral rehydration therapy (ORT) includes: (a) ORS solution of recommended composition, (b) solution made from sugar and salt (if prepared correctly), (c) food-based solutions with appropriate concentration of salt, like lentil soup, rice, kanji, butter milk etc., and (d) plain water administered along with continued feeding.

Low Osmolarity Oral Rehydration Salts (ORS) Solution: The standard WHO-ORS, used for over three decades, has saved millions of lives but did not decrease diarrheal duration or stool output. More effective low osmolarity ORS (Table 6.3) is now recommended as the universal solution for treatment and prevention of dehydration for all causes of diarrhea and at all ages.

Nutritional Management During and After a Diarrheal Episode

Diarrhea is a major cause of malnutrition owing to low food intake during the illness, reduced nutrient absorption in the intestine, and increased nutrient requirement as a result of infection. Poor appetite, vomiting, oral thrush/ stomatitis and the common practice of withholding or diluting food are some of the reasons for poor intake during an episode of diarrhea. Reduced nutrient absorption in the intestines, and increased requirements as a result of infection contributes to energy and nutrient depletion. Repeated and prolonged episodes of diarrhea have even more deleterious effects and may eventually result in growth failure, intercurrent infections, severe malnutrition and even death. Therefore, food intake should never be restricted during or following diarrhea. Instead, the goal should be to maintain the intake of energy and other nutrients at as high a level as possible. When this is achieved even with only 80–95 percent carbohydrates,

70 percent fat. and 75 percent nitrogen being actually absorbed during acute diarrhea, sufficient nutrients can be absorbed to support continued growth and weight gain.[11] Continued feeding also speeds the recovery of normal intestinal function, including the ability to digest and absorb various nutrients. In contrast, children whose food is restricted or diluted usually lose weight, have prolonged diarrhea and recover intestinal function more slowly.[12]

Nutritional management in acute diarrhea and dysentery optimally utilizes intestinal absorptive capacity, which is achieved effectively in the child with diarrhea, by feeding small, frequent, energy-dense food taking into consideration the age, preillness feeding pattern and state of hydration of the child (Table 6.5). Feeding is continued in infants and children with no dehydration and resumed as early as possible in those with some dehydration. If the child is dehydrated, *during the phase of dehydration,* breastfeeding should be continued and normal feeding resumed after dehydration is corrected. However, in severely malnourished children some food should also be offered as soon as possible during the phase of rehydration.[13] *After the phase of dehydration,* the dietary management during a diarrheal includes: (i) Continued breastfeeding on demand; (ii) Young infants who consume animal milk should continue to take undiluted milk as before their illness; (iii) Children 6 months of age and older should receive energy rich mixture of soft weaning foods in addition to breast milk or animal milk; (iv) Energy rich food (thick preparations of staple food with extra vegetable oil or animal fats), potassium rich foods (legumes, banana) and carotene containing foods (dark green leafy vegetables, red palm oil, carrots, pumpkins) should be given to the child in sufficient quantity. In young children, these foods should be well cooked and mashed to facilitate easy digestion. Owing to loss of appetite or vomiting, children may need to be frequently encouraged to eat. It is helpful to give food frequently in small amounts (six times a day or more).

Prolonged and recurrent episodes of diarrhea adversely affect the nutritional status of a child and thereby significantly contribute to the vicious cycle of malnutrition and infection.[14] After an episode of diarrhea, a child should receive more food than usual for at least two weeks after diarrhea stops. During this period, the child may consume up to 150 cal/kg of body weight per day. A practical approach is to give the child at least one extra meal each day with energy rich foods.[13]

Zinc Supplementation for Treatment of Diarrhea

Zinc deficiency is common in children in developing countries because of intake of predominantly vegetarian diets and the high content of dietary phytates. Increased fecal losses during many episodes of diarrhea aggravate pre-existing zinc deficiency. WHO and Indian Academy of Pediatrics recommend zinc supplementation as an adjunct to ORS in the treatment of diarrhea. The National IAP Task Force and Government of India recommend that all children older than 6 months suffering from diarrhea should receive a uniform dose of 20 mg of elemental zinc as soon as diarrhea starts and continue for a total period of 14 days. Children aged 2 to 6 months should be advised 10 mg per day of elemental zinc for a total period of 14 days.[15,16]

Treatment of Associated Problems

Antibiotics for Dysentery and Cholera: Diarrhea in young children is often infective in origin. However, it is important to remember that most of these infections are self limiting and antibiotic therapy does not significantly alter the clinical course. Antibiotic therapy in most of these cases, therefore, is not only unnecessary but may lead to undesired side effects and consequences. Antibiotic therapy should be reserved only for cases of dysentery and suspected cholera (Table 6.6). Therefore, every infant or child with diarrhea

Table 6.5: Feeding during diarrhea	
Stage of hydration	*Recommended schedule of feeding*
During rehydration phase	
• Breastfed infants	• Continue breastfeeding
• Nonbreastfed infants	• Should be preferable given only ORS till they are rehydrated
	• Animal milk/ food should be offered, if rehydration takes longer than 4 hours
• Severely malnourished children	• Offer some food as soon as possible
After rehydration phase	
• Breastfed infants	• Breastfeed more frequently
• Non-breastfed infants	• Offer undiluted milk as before
• Infants 6–12 months	• Give easily digestible energy rich complementary foods in addition to breast/animal milk • Encourage to eat at least 3 times a day in breastfed infants and 5 times in non breastfed infants
For Older children	• Give thick preparation of staple food with extra vegetable oil or animal fats, rich in potassium (legumes, banana), carotene (dark green leafy vegetables, red palm oil, carrot, pumpkin) • Encourage to eat at least 6 times a day

needs to be carefully evaluated for the presence of blood in the stools (which indicates dysentery) and to identify cases of suspected cholera (high purge rate with severe dehydration in a child above 2 years of age in an area where cholera is known to be present). For the management of dysentery, it is assumed that the cause is shigellosis and therefore an oral antibiotic to which *Shigella* are sensitive should be prescribed. Owing to widespread resistance to trimethoprim-sulfamethoxazole (TMP-SMX) and reported resistance to nalidixic acid, the Indian Academy of Pediatrics Task Force recommends ciprofloxacin (15 mg/kg two times daily × 3 days) as a first line drug in areas where resistance to cotrimoxazole exceeds 30%. The child should be examined again after 2 days and if the mother still observes blood in stool, an alternative antibiotic needs to be prescribed for the next 2–5 days. For proven as well as suspected cases of cholera, single dose doxycycline (6 mg/kg) has been recommended in children > 2 years.[16]

Antibiotics in Severely Malnourished Children: In severe acute malnutrition (SAM), the usual signs of infection such as fever are often absent, yet multiple infections are common. Hypoglycemia and hypothermia are often signs of severe infection.[17] Therefore, it is assumed that all malnourished children have an infection on their arrival in the health facility and should be treated with broad spectrum parenteral antibiotics like ampicillin or crystalline penicillin with gentamicin.[16,17]

Associated non-gastrointestinal infections: Associated infections like pneumonia, meningitis and urinary tract infection should also be carefully looked for and appropriately treated.

Table 6.6: Antimicrobials used to treat specific causes of diarrhea in children

Causes	Drugs of choice	Doses
Cholera	First line: Doxycycline	Single dose of 6 mg/kg orally (Maximum 200 mg)
	Second line: Ciprofloxacin	Single dose of 15 mg/kg
Dysentery	First line: Ciprofloxacin	15 mg/kg two times a day orally x 3 days
	Second line: Pivmecillinam	20 mg/kg four times a day orally x 5 days
	Ceftriaxone	50–100 mg/kg once a day intramuscularly x 2–5 days
Amebic dysentery	Metronidazole	30 mg/kg/day in 3 divided doses orally x 5–10 days
Acute giardiasis	Metronidazole or Tinidazole	15 mg/kg/day in 3 divided doses orally x 5 days

Risk Factors for Diarrheal Morbidity and Mortality

Early home therapy with ORT at the onset of a diarrheal episode remains the treatment of choice in almost all cases of diarrhea. However, it may be necessary to identify on the first day of an episode of diarrhea, signs and symptoms which indicate an increased likelihood of developing dehydration. Alteration in thirst (increased in a normal child and decreased in a severely dehydrated child), 6 or more loose stools, presence of fever, vomiting and a reduction in appetite[18] are some of the clinical features, which help to recognize potentially severe cases who should be kept under close surveillance. Associated major infections (pneumonia, septicemia or meningitis), severe wasting and severe stunting have been reported as risk factors for fatal diarrhea and therefore such children must be identified and targeted for intensive intervention.[19]

Correction of Electrolyte and Acid-base Imbalance

Most cases with acute watery diarrhea can be managed appropriately with oral rehydration therapy and zinc supplementation and children with dysentery respond very well to antibiotics. However, the following complications may be encountered:

Electrolyte Imbalance

With appropriate use of oral rehydration therapy, access to plain water and continued feeding, the risk of electrolyte disturbances is minimized. However, following electrolyte disturbance may be encountered in some cases:

Hypernatremia: Some children with diarrhea, especially young infants, develop hypernatremic dehydration which usually follows use of hypertonic drinks (canned fruit juices, carbonated cold drinks, incorrectly prepared salt and sugar solutions, ORS with high glucose content). Children with hypernatremic dehydration (serum sodium >150 mEq/L, osmolality >295 mOsm/kg) are extremely thirsty, out of proportion to their other signs of dehydration and sometimes have convulsions. These children can be successfully treated with low osmolarity ORS. However, if the child is unable to drink orally, Ringer's lactate can be initially given to treat shock and later switch over to ORT with low osmolarity ORS.

Hyponatremia: Patients who ingest only large amount of water or watery drinks that contain very little salt, may present with hyponatremia (serum sodium 130 mEq/L, osmolality <275 mOsm/kg), which may be clinically associated with lethargy and seizures. ORS is a safe and effective therapy for hyponatremia as well. For children who are unable to drink orally, intravenous infusion of Ringer's lactate can effectively treat hyponatremia.

Hypokalemia: Inadequate replacement of potassium losses during diarrhea can lead to potassium depletion and hypokalemia (serum potassium <3 mEq/L), which may result in muscle weakness, paralytic ileus, renal impairment and cardiac arrhythmias. Severe potassium depletion, particularly in malnourished children, may lead to acute onset flaccid paralysis ranging from neck flop to quadriparesis and even respiratory paralysis.[20] The potassium deficit can be corrected by using ORS solution for rehydration therapy and by feeding potassium rich foods (e.g. banana, fresh fruit juices) during and after diarrhea. Oral potassium supplementation (2 mEq/kg/day) is indicated in malnourished children. In transient flaccid paralysis due to hypokalemia, potassium can be administered parenterally by using 15 percent solution of potassium chloride (1 mL=2 mEq of potassium) but not exceeding 40 mEq/L of IV fluids adequate dehydration.[21]

Hypoglycemia

Continued feeding during an episode of diarrhea minimizes the risk of getting hypoglycemia. However some children, particularly those severely malnourished, are at a risk of becoming hypoglycemic. Early feeding can prevent hypoglycemia in these cases. If a child develops symptoms of hypoglycemia (lethargy, cold and clammy skin), he/she should be immediately given glucose/milk and kept warm.

Metabolic Acidosis

During acute diarrhea, large amounts of bicarbonate may be lost in the stool. If the kidneys continue to function normally, most of the lost bicarbonate is replaced and a serious base deficit does not develop. Metabolic acidosis tends to correct spontaneously in most of the cases as the child is properly rehydrated. ORS solution contains adequate bicarbonate/citrate to counter acidosis in less severe cases. However, in severe dehydration, compromised renal function leads to rapid development of base deficit and metabolic acidosis. Hypovolemic shock as a consequence of rapid loss of water and electrolytes in severe diarrhea results in excessive production of lactic acid, which may further contribute to metabolic acidosis. Rapid intravenous infusion of Ringer's lactate, which contains 28 mEq/L of lactate (metabolized to bicarbonate), is recommended in severe dehydration. However, in the presence of circulatory failure, bicarbonate precursors (e.g., citrate, lactate) may not be readily metabolized in

the body. If the patient presents with severe metabolic acidosis (pH < 7.20, serum $HCO_3^- < 8$ mEq/L), sodium bicarbonate in a bolus dose of 2-3 mEq/kg is administered to correct acidosis. The serum potassium concentration must be very carefully monitored as correction of acidosis in a patient with low potassium can lead to life-threatening hypokalemia.

Acute Renal Failure

Severe dehydration and shock lead to decreased renal blood flow resulting in pre-renal type of acute renal failure. Immediate replacement of fluids and a fluid challenge is usually sufficient to restore kidney function unless the renal failure is irreversible. In that case, the child requires hospitalization and managed as per acute renal failure protocol.

Hemolytic Uremic Syndrome (HUS)

Some children with invasive diarrhea due to *Shigella dysenteriae* or *Enteroinvasive E. coli* may have HUS due to nephrotoxins liberated by these organisms. These children develop intravascular hemolysis with acute renal failure. This is a serious condition and needs to be managed in a hospital setting.

Prevention: Diarrheal diseases can be prevented to a great extent by improving infant feeding practices and personal and domestic hygiene. Some of the interventions which are feasible and cost-effective include: (i) promotion of exclusive breastfeeding up to 6 months of age; (ii) improved complementary feeding practices; (iii) use of clean drinking water and sufficient water for personal hygiene; (iv) hand washing; (v) use of sanitary toilets; (vi) safe disposal of the stool of young children and (vii) measles vaccination.

Rotavirus vaccines: Recent studies have demonstrated safety and efficacy of two new live, oral, attenuated rotavirus vaccines (RVV) in middle and high income countries thereby suggesting a combined preventive and treatment strategy (vaccine, low osmolarity ORS and zinc supplementation) to significantly reduce child mortality. However, the diversity of rotavirus strains and high prevalence of mixed infections are unique features of rotavirus epidemiology in India. Vaccine manufacturers in India have started working on indigenous rotavirus vaccine development. Three such vaccines have been developed and phase II studies have shown about 90% protection in Indian children. With the development of the Indian vaccines, the cost is expected to decrease significantly, making them affordable for a larger Indian population and feasible to introduce in the public health system of the country.

REFERENCES

1. Liu L, Johnson HL, Cousens S, Perin J, Scott S, et al. Global, regional, and national causes of child mortality: an updated systematic analysis for 2010 with time trends since 2000. Lancet. 2012;379:2151-61.

2. Shah D, Choudhury P, Gupta P, Mathew JL, et al. Promoting appropriate management of diarrhea: A systematic review of literature for advocacy and action: UNICEF-PHFI Series on Newborn. Indian Pediatr. 2012;49:627-49.

3. Morris SK, Awasthi S, Khera A, Bassani DG, Kang G, Parashar UD, et al. Million Death Study Collaborators. Rotavirus mortality in India: estimates based on a nationally representative survey of diarrhoeal deaths. Bull World Health Organ. 2012;90:720-7.

4. Nair GB, Ramamurthy T, Bhattacharya MK, et al. Emerging trends in the etiology of enteric pathogens as evidenced from an active surveillance of hospitalized diarrhoeal patients in Kolkata, India. Gut Pathogens. 2010;2(1):4.

5. Mahalanabis D, Wallace CK, Kallen RJ, Mondal A. Pierce NE. Water and electrolyte losses due to cholera in infants and small children: a recovery balance study. Pediatrics. 1970;45:374-85.

6. Hirschhorn N. The treatment of acute diarrhea in children. A historical and physiological perspective. Am J Clin Nutr. 1980;33:637-63.

7. Nalin DR. Mortality from cholera and other diarrheal diseases at a cholera hospital. Trop Geog Med. 1972;24:101-6.

8. Hirschhorn N. The management of acute diarrhea in children: An overview. In: Progress in Drug Resistant Tropical Disease II, Vol. 19. Basel Birkhauser Verlag. 1975;527.

9. Fleming BJ, Genuth SM, Goul AB. Laxative-induced hypokalemia, sodium depletion and hyper-reninemia. Effects of potassium and sodium replacement on the renin-angiotensin-aldosterone system. Ann Intern Med. 1975;83:60-2.

10. Knochel JP. Role of glycoregulatory hormones in potassium homeostasis. Kidney Int. 1977;11:443-52.

11. Arora NK, Bhan MK. Nutritional management of acute diarrhea. Indian J Pediatr. 1991;58:763-7.

12. Brown KH, Gastanaduy AS, Saavedra JM. Effect of continued oral feeding on clinical and nutritional outcome of acute diarrhea in children. J Pediatr. 1988;112:191-200.

13. Jelliffe DB, Jelliffe EFP. Dietary management of Young Children with Acute Diarrhea, 2nd edn. Geneva, WHO/UNICEF, 1991.

14. Patwari AK.. Diarrhoea and malnutrition interaction. Indian J Pediatr. 1999; 66:S124-34.

15. Bhatnagar S, Bhandari N, Mouli UC, Bhan MK. Consensus statement of IAP National Task Force: Status Report on Management of Acute Diarrhea. Indian Pediatr. 2004;41:335-48.

16. Government of India. Integrated Management of Neonatal and Childhood Illness. Training Modules for Physicians. Ministry of Health and Family Welfare. 2009.

17. World Health Organization. Management of the Child with a Serious Infection or Severe Malnutrition. WHO/FCH/CAH/00.1, WHO, Geneva, 2000;1-146.

18. Victora CG, Kirkwood BR, Fuchs SC, Lombardi C, Barros FC. Is it possible to predict which diarrhea episodes will lead to life-threatening dehydration. Int J Epidemiol. 1990;19:736-41.

19. Sachdev HPS, Kumar S, Singh KK, Satyanarayana, Puri KK. Risk factors for fatal diarrhea in hospitalized children in India. J Pediatr Gastroenterol Nutr. 1991;12:76-81.

20. Chhabra A, Patwari AK, Aneja S, et al. Neuromuscular manifestations of diarrhoea related hypokalemia. Indian Pediatrics. 1995;32:409-15.

21. Kallen RJ. The management of diarrheal dehydration in infants using parenteral fluids. Pediatr Clin North Amer. 1990;37:265-86.

Chapter

7

Chronic and Persistent Diarrhea

Sarah Paul, John Matthai

INTRODUCTION

Diarrhea is a common childhood illness and a major cause for death among children below 5 years of age. Rational use of antibiotics, oral rehydration solution, promotion of breastfeeding and decline in malnutrition have made a major difference in the outcome of children with acute diarrhea. However, chronic and persistent diarrhea continue to remain a challenge to pediatricians.

Definitions

The word diarrhea is derived from Greek and signifies an increase in the fluidity and frequency of stools. It is classified as acute, chronic and persistent diarrhea. Most acute diarrheal episodes resolve in 7 days, a few may last up to 14 days. If it lasts more than 14 days, it is either chronic or persistent diarrhea. The term protracted diarrhea is not in use now.

Persistent Diarrhea

This is an episode of diarrhea of presumed infectious etiology, which starts acutely but lasts for more than 14 days.

Chronic Diarrhea

This has an insidious onset and lasts for more than 14 days. It is usually noninfectious and associated with malabsorption.

Malabsorption

Any condition in which there is a persistent disturbance of the digestive-absorptive process across the intestinal mucosa.

Protracted Diarrhea

This is a clinical entity characterized by diarrhea lasting for more than 2 weeks, starting before 3 months of age with severe nutritional disturbances and negative stool culture for enteropathogens. With better investigative facilities such babies are now known to have one of the congenital causes of diarrhea.

CHRONIC DIARRHEA

The etiology of chronic diarrhea varies according to the age of the child and usually involves a persistent disturbance in the digestive process. The normal process of digestion involves a series of sequential steps—solubilization (fats and fat soluble vitamins by miscelle formation), digestion (by specific digestive enzymes), intestinal transit (by peristalsis), mucosal absorption (by diffusion or carrier mediated transport) and postmucosal transport of absorbed substrates.[1]

Chronic diarrhea is a consequence of a disturbance in one of the above processes.[2] It can, therefore, be broadly classified depending on the basic defect involved:
- *Abnormal digestion:* Pancreatic disease, cholestasis
- *Defective absorption:* Celiac disease
- *Altered gut transit:* Motility disorders, short gut
- *Secretory tumors:* VIPoma
- *Metabolic diseases:* Acrodermatitis
- *Drugs and chemicals:* Antibiotics.

The list of causes of chronic diarrhea is exhaustive and the common causes are listed in Table 7.1.

Epidemiology

The true incidence of chronic diarrhea in developing countries is not known as diagnostic facilities are often

Table 7.1: Causes of chronic diarrhea

Common causes		Uncommon causes at all ages
Below 1 year	Over 1 year	
Cow's milk protein allergy	Celiac disease	Congenital enzyme defects
Urinary tract infection	Giardiasis, amebiasis	Acrodermatitis enteropathica
Celiac disease	Irritable bowel syndrome	Lymphangiectasia
Toddler's diarrhea	Cow's milk protein allergy	Pancreatic insufficiency
Immunodeficiency states	Drug induced	Bacterial overgrowth
Intractable diarrhea of infancy	Inflammatory bowel disease	Pseudomembranous colitis
Short bowel syndrome	Immunodeficiency	VIPoma
		Hyperthyroidism
		Zollinger-Ellison syndrome

limited. Celiac disease and parasitic infections are the more commonly recognized etiologies in the developing countries.[3] Allergy and immune-mediated causes are more common in the western countries.[4]

Evaluation of a Child with Chronic Diarrhea

A careful history and physical examination are invaluable in diagnosis and adequate time should be spent on them before investigations are done. The history should confirm the presence of a diarrhea. It is important to differentiate over flow incontinence secondary to constipation. History of blood/mucus is suggestive of dysentery and possible large bowel diarrhea, while visible oil in stools would point to pancreatic disease. A careful weaning and dietary history should be obtained in relation to the age of the child. A history of abdominal pain may suggest obstruction or pancreatic insufficiency. A previous history of abdominal surgery may suggest a blind loop bacterial overgrowth or short gut. Ask for a family history of celiac disease, Crohn's disease, cystic fibrosis or allergic disorders.

Growth should be plotted in a growth chart and a detailed examination must be done. Look carefully for dehydration, anemia, oral thrush, edema (hypoalbuminemia), signs of vitamin and mineral deficiencies, clubbing (Celiac disease, Crohn's disease and cystic fibrosis) and abdominal distension (obstruction, paralytic ileus, hypokalemia)

It may be possible to differentiate small bowel from large bowel diarrhea. In the former children are dehydrated with vitamin and mineral deficiency. Stools are pale, large volume and explosive with fat or carbohydrate malabsorption. Large bowel diarrhea is associated with abdominal pain and tenesmus and systemic symptoms. The stools are of smaller volume with blood and copious mucus and no malabsorption or steatorrhea.

Investigations

General

❑ **Stool examination:** Microscopy may detect ova and cysts, the presence of blood and also fat globules and fatty acid crystals. Culture for enteric pathogens and assay for C difficile toxin are helpful in specific settings. polymerase chain reaction (PCR) and enzyme-linked immunosorbent assay (ELISA) for antigen detection are used in opportunistic infections like *Cryptosporidium*.

❑ **Stool osmotic gap:** The stool osmotic gap is helpful in differentiating secretory from osmotic diarrhea. It can be calculated by subtracting twice the Na and potassium from 290. Values over 100 are seen in osmotic diarrhea, while in secretory diarrhea it is below 50.

❑ **Biochemical tests:** In addition to detecting electrolyte imbalance, hypoalbuminemia, and hyperglobulinemia are helpful in diagnosis. Tests for confirmation of malabsorption of fat, protein and carbohydrate are of value in specific situations. Prolonged prothrombin time may be secondary to prolonged antibiotic use and altered gut flora or a concomitant liver disease.

❑ **Hematology:** Peripheral smear is useful in determining the type of anemia and detecting acanthocytes in abetalipoproteinemia. Lymphopenia can be seen in immunodeficiency and intestinal lyphangiectasia, while thrombocytosis and raised ESR suggests chronic inflammatory diarrhea.

Specific Tests

❑ *Tests of malabsorption:* Fecal fat estimation in 72-hour sample by Van de Kramer method is the gold standard and values above 4.5 g/day are considered abnormal. Chymotrypsin and elastase levels in stool are reduced in pancreatic insufficiency. D-xylose test is abnormal (serum levels <20 mg/dL) in proximal small bowel disease. Folate malabsorption can be detected by serum or RBC levels. In situations where the serum vitamin B_{12} levels are low, a schilling test can be used to distinguish between gastric and ileal disease.

❑ *Endoscopy:* Histopathology is an important investigation in chronic diarrhea. Celiac disease, Crohn's disease and intestinal lymphangiectasia are confirmed by histology. Duodenal aspirate can be tested for parasites and also sent for culture to detect bacterial overgrowth.

- *Imaging studies:* These are useful in pancreatic disease, intestinal tuberculosis and tumors.
- *Specific tests:* Antiendomyseal Abs and TTGA in celiac disease, RAST for cow's milk protein allergy, anti-enterocyte Abs in autoimmune enteropathy, HIV and immunoglobulin levels in immunodeficiency and sweat chloride test in cystic fibrosis.

Specific Etiology

Celiac disease and food allergies are dealt with separately and hence omitted from this discussion.

- **Chronic nonspecific diarrhea (CNSD):** This is a common cause of diarrhea between 6 months and 4 years.[5] The child is well thriving with no vitamin or mineral deficiency and passes 4–5 loose stools containing undigested vegetable matter during the day time. Stool examination is normal. Parental reassurance and diet modification (high fat, low carbohydrate, low fruit juice, high fiber diet) suffice in most instances. A positive diagnosis will prevent unnecessary medications.
- **Giardiasis and amoebiasis:** Giardiasis is the most common chronic parasitic infection and is acquired by ingesting infective cysts in food and water.[6] The parasite inhabits the upper small intestine and chronic infection can result in malabsorption, lactose intolerance and failure to thrive. Microscopic examination of a freshly passed stool or duodenal aspirate will reveal the trophozoites or cysts. Duodenal biopsy may show flattened villi and the organism. Metronidazole is the drug of choice, while nitazoxanide, tinidazole and furazolidone are alternatives. Amoebiasis is caused by *Entamoeba histolytica* and infection occurs by ingestion of contaminated food or water. The trophozoites of the organism have characteristic diagnostic features on microscopy but the cyst forms are indistinguishable from E Dispar which is a nonpathogenic amoeba.[7] The trophozoites most commonly establish in the cecum and ascending colon, but the rectosigmoid can also be affected in severe infection. Diagnosis is made on microscopy of a fresh stool for the presence of trophozoites with erythrocytes within the cytoplasm (erythrophgocytic trophozoites). Proctosigmoidoscopy may reveal chronic ulcers with normal intervening mucosa. Serology is usually negative if infection is limited to the gut. Metronidazole, tinidazole or ornidazole are the drugs of choice. Diloxanide furoate or iodoquinol is used as a cysticidal drug to eradicate intestinal carrier state. The stool should be re examined after a full course of therapy.
- **Congenital immunodeficiency:** Congenital immuno-deficiency syndromes most commonly associated with chronic diarrhea are X-linked agammaglobulinemia, selective IgA deficiency and common variable immunodeficiency. Gastrointestinal manifestations include recurrent giardiasis, bacterial overgrowth, chronic viral enteritis and nonspecific enteropathy or enterocolitis. Those with IgA deficiency have an increased risk of celiac disease and Crohn's disease. In addition to treatment of the specific etiology, parenteral immunoglobulin may be beneficial in some cases.[8]
- **Acquired immunodeficiency:** Patients with CD 4 counts below 200 cells/mL are at an increased risk of opportunistic infection. Impaired mucosal immunity and altered function of enterocytes predisposes to opportunistic infections and bacterial overgrowth. Common infections include *Salmonella*, *Shigella*, *Campylobacter*, cytomegalovirus, *Candida*, *Cryptococcus*, *Cryptosporidium*, *Isospora* and *Giardia*. Patients with severe chronic diarrhea without an identifiable pathogen and mucosal biopsy shows partial villus atrophy with increased intraepithelial are deemed to have HIV enteropathy.[9] It is important to remember that antiretroviral drugs of the protease inhibitor class like lopinavir and nelfinavir can also cause diarrhea.
- **Abetalipoproteinemia:** In these patients, mutation in the MTP (microsomal transport protein) gene leads to impaired chylomicron formation and transport from the intestine and liver.[10] Children have failure to thrive from early infancy and chronic diarrhea which is worse with intake of fat. Neurological involvement appears by around five years. Chylomicrons, LDL and VLDL are very low or absent in plasma and duodenal biopsy shows lipid droplet filled enterocytes. Restriction of fat intake, with supplementation of MCT, fat soluble vitamins and vitamin E in very high doses (1000–2000 mg in infants, 5000–10,000 mg in older children) may show some benefit.
- **Acrodermatitis enteropathica:** These children are unable to absorb zinc in the intestine and present with perianal eczematous rash, alopecia and chronic diarrhea soon after weaning. Serum zinc and alkaline phosphatase levels are low. Infants respond to high dose zinc supplementation (1–2 mg daily in infants, 30–40 mg daily in older children).
- **Intestinal lymphangiectasia:** These patients have dilated lacteals in the small intestine causing leakage of lymph and protein losing enteropathy resulting in lymphopenia, hypocalcemia, hypoalbuminemia and hypogammaglobulinemia. Increased fecal alpha

1 antitrypsin levels confirms enteric protein loss.[11] Barium study shows thickening of jejunal folds with patchy nodular hyperlucencies in the mucosa. Dilated lymphatics can be demonstrated on lymphangiography. Upper GI endoscopy done after a fatty meal will enable better visualization of the prominent lymphatics with the leaking lymph seen as white spots on the mucosa. Histopathology reveals the characteristic dilated lacteals. High protein, low fat diet with only medium chain triglycerides as well as supplementation with calcium and fat soluble vitamins helps reduce the diarrhea. Exclusion of long chain triglycerides reduces lymph flow and prevents rupture of lymphatics. MCTs are directly absorbed into the portal circulation and so can be safely used. Localized lymphangiectasia can be excised.

❑ **Short gut syndrome:** This refers to symptoms and signs that occur after intestinal resection or a congenitally short gut. Symptoms are likely if the small intestine is less than 70 cm with an intact colon or less than 150 cm without any colon. Presence of the colon is crucial, since it can reabsorb substantial amounts of water, sodium and short chain fatty acids and thus limit the consequences of a short intestine. The remaining small intestine always adapts over time, and so most patients will improve in a few years.[12] Total parenteral nutrition initially, followed by gradually increasing oral feeding is beneficial.

❑ **Bacterial overgrowth:** The normal proximal small intestine is predominantly colonized by aerobic flora ($<10^2$–10^3 organisms/mL). The presence of $>10^5$ colony forming units/mL of colonic type bacteria (gram negative bacteria, strict anaerobes and enterococci) are diagnostic of bacterial overgrowth. Children with anatomic structural abnormalities, abnormal motility, abnormal communication between proximal and distal gut, immunodeficiency and achlorhydria are prone for small intestinal bacterial overgrowth. Diagnosis is based on culture of direct aspirate of small bowel contents and hydrogen breath testing. Barium meal with follow through demonstrates the underlying anatomic abnormality. Cyclical courses of antibiotics (metronidazole, gentamicin, cotrimoxazole, rifaximin, ciprofloxacin and tetracycline) are the treatment of choice.[13] Role of probiotics is still unproven.

❑ **Drug induced diarrhea:** Drugs can cause diarrhea by increased GI motility, mucosal injury and by altering the intestinal flora. Antibiotics can cause diarrhea by altering the flora or damaging the mucosa. *Clostridium difficile* colitis can result from prolonged antibiotic use. Chemotherapeutic drugs can cause mucositis and lead to diarrhea. Sorbitol which is the base in many liquid preparations can cause osmotic diarrhea. Laxative abuse is not uncommon in adolescent children. Metoclopramide can cause diarrhea by increasing the gut motility. Withdrawal of the offending drug suffices in most cases. *Clostridium difficile* diarrhea needs specific treatment with vancomycin or metronidazole. Probiotics have been reported to reduce the incidence of antibiotic associated diarrhea, but the effects are strain specific.[14]

❑ **Intractable diarrhea of infancy:** These are a difficult group to manage with a poor outcome and prognosis.[15] They are divided into two broad groups.

• **Without villous atrophy:** This includes the congenital transport defects, ileal bile acid receptor defect, congenital glucose galactose malabsorption, etc. Stool electrolytes estimation can be done in specialized centers. Diagnosis is based on a clinical picture with the serum electrolytes. Elimination diets are available to assess response.

• **With villous atrophy:** This includes defects due to congenital epithelial structure and function like microvillous inclusion disease, tufting enteropathy and the autoimmune enteropathies. Diagnosis is based on intestinal biopsy with antienterocyte, anticolonic antibodies and genetic studies. Steroids and immunosupression may have a role in autoimmune enteropathies.

❑ **Hormone-mediated diarrhea:** Neuroendocrine tumors though rare are a diagnostic challenge. They may present with profuse secretory diarrhea. Diagnosis requires estimation of serum gastrin, VIP, somatostatin and calcitonin. Tumor-III octreotide scintigraphic scan or an endoscopic ultrasound is useful. Surgical excision, if possible is curative.

Prognosis and Outcome

Prognosis depends on the underlying cause of chronic diarrhea. Nutritional support and correction of micronutrient deficiencies is essential in all children. Special formulas and parenteral nutrition has helped to decrease morbidity and mortality. Outcome largely depends on the primary diagnosis, early recognition and adequate therapy.

▌PERSISTENT DIARRHEA

Persistent diarrhea is now essentially a disease of the developing countries where malnutrition and infection co-exist.[16] According to the WHO, persistent diarrhea accounts for one third of all deaths from diarrhea in children below 5 years in the developing countries. Mortality from persistent diarrhea is 13.9% compared to only 0.7% in acute diarrhea.[17] The risk of a diarrheal episode becoming persistent is related to the age and nutritional status of the child, and the burden of diarrheal episodes. Other risk factors include previous infections, recent introduction of animal milk, irrational usage of antibiotics, and lack of breast milk.[18] The pathogenesis is multifactorial-ongoing mucosal injury from prolonged or sequential infections in a host with malnutrition, vitamin/mineral deficiency and compromised immune status. It is believed that persisting inflammation and defective mucosal repair leads to poor nutrient absorption as well as increased permeability to bacterial and dietary antigens.[19]

Since defective nutrient absorption is the fundamental problem, nutritional therapy is the cornerstone of treatment.[20] Treatment should be started early to ensure better results. Milk cereal mixes are as good as milk free diet in the early stages. Milk-free diet with simple carbohydrates is better for those with severe disease. Monosaccharide-based diet is required only for those who do not respond. The energy density of the feeds should not be more than 1 kcal/g and a daily intake of 100 cal/kg should be targeted. Most children have dehydration and electrolyte imbalance at admission, which will need correction. Sepsis is present in more than 50% of hospitalized infants with persistent diarrhea.[21] Parenteral third generation cephalosporin is recommended. Oral vitamin A (<6 months 50,000 IU, 6–12 months 100,000 IU) and a dose of parenteral vitamin K should be given at admission. Infants with severe disease also need supplementation with the following—multivitamins (twice the RDA), folic acid (5 mg day 1, then 1 mg/day), zinc (2 mg/kg/day) and copper (0.3 mg/kg/day) for two weeks and 50% magnesium sulphate 0.2 mL/kg/dose twice daily for 2–3 days.[22] Available data does not justify use of probiotics in treatment. Severe malnutrition, unusual enteropathogens and severe systemic infection are reasons for poor outcome.[23] Special formulae like extensively hydrolyzed 100% bovine casein infant formulas and elemental amino acid formulae are therapeutic options, but are too expensive for routine use in developing countries. Parenteral nutrition is life saving in those who do not tolerate any oral feeds. Re-feeding syndrome can occur due to aggressive and rapid nutritional therapy in chronically undernourished children.[24] It is characterized by hypophosphatemia, hypokalemia, hypomagnesemia and thiamine deficiency. It may present with muscle weakness, seizures, congestive heart failure, arrhythmia, altered sensorium and even sudden death. Carbohydrate and protein rich food cause increased secretion of insulin which causes anabolism and intracellular movement of phosphate, potassium and magnesium. It can be prevented by slower increase in calorie intake and lower supplementation of electrolytes and vitamins.

REFERENCES

1. Schmitz J. Maldigestion and Malabsorption. In Walker AW, goulet O, et al (Eds). Pediatric Gastroenterol disease. New York. BC Dekker Inc. 2004;8-20.
2. Srivasatava A. Chronic diarrhea and malabsorption. In Bavdekar A, Matthai J, et al (Eds). Pediatric Gastroenterology. New Delhi Jaypee Brothers. 2013;54-73.
3. Rastogi A, Malhotra V, Uppal B, et al. Etiology of chronic diarrhea in tropical children. Tropical Gastroenterology. 1998;19:45-9.
4. Lee WS, Boey CCM. Chronic diarrhea in infants and young children: causes, clinical features and outcome. J Pediatr Child Health. 1999;35:260-3.
5. Kneepkens CM, Hoekstra JH. Chronic nonspecific diarrhea of childhood: pathophysiology and management. Pediatr Clin North Am. 1996;43:375-90.
6. Ortega YR, Adam RD. Giardia: Overview and update. Clin Infect Dis. 1997;25:545-9.
7. Haque R, Huston CD, Hughes M, Houtp E, Petri WA. Amebiasis. N Engl J Med. 2003;348:1565-73.
8. Khodadad A, Aghamohammadi A, Parvaneh N, Rezaei N, Mahjoob F, Bashashati M, et al. Gastrointestinal Manifestations in Patients with Common Variable Immunodeficiency. Dig Dis Sci. 2007;52:2977-83.
9. Wilcox CM, Saag MS. Gastrointestinal complications of HIV infection: changing priorities in the HAART era Gut. 2008;57:861-70.
10. Peretti N, Sassolas A, Roy CC, Deslandres C, Charcosset M, Castagnetti J, et al. Guidelines for the diagnosis and management of chylomicron retention disease based on a review of the literature and the experience of two centers. Orphanet J Rare Dis. 2010;5:24.
11. Marjet JA, Braamskamp M, Dolman DM, Tabbers MM. Clinical practice Protein-losing enteropathy in children. Eur J Pediatr. 2010;169:1179-85.
12. Scolopio JS. Short bowel syndrome. J Parenteral and Enteral Nutrition. 2002;26:S11-6.
13. Quigley Eamonn MM, Abu-Shanab A. Small Intestinal Bacterial Overgrowth. Infect Dis Clin N Am. 2010;24:943-59.
14. Hempel S, Newberry SJ, Maher AR, Wang Z, Miles JN, Shanman R, et al. Probiotics for the prevention and treatment of antibiotic-associated diarrhea: a systematic review and meta-analysis. JAMA. 2012;307:1959-69.
15. Sherman PM, Mitchell DJ, Cutz E. Neonatal enteropathies: defining the causes of protracted diarrhea of infancy. J Pediatr Gastroenterol Nutr. 2004;38:16-26.
16. Matthai J. for Pediatric Gastroenterology chapter of IAP. Chronic and persistent diarrhea in infants and young children. Status statement. Ind Pediatr. 2011;48:37-42.
17. Bhan MK, Bhandari N, Sazawal S, Clemens J, Raj P, Levine MM, et al. Descriptive epidemiology of persistent diarrhoea among young children in rural northern India. Bull World Health Organ. 1989;67(3):281-8.
18. Bhutta ZA, Ghishan F, Lindley K, Memon IA, Mittal S, Rhoads JM. Persistent and chronic diarrhea and malabsorption. J Pediatr Gastroenterol Nutr. 2004;39(2):S711-6.

19. Sullivan PB. Studies of the small intestine in persistent diarrhea and malnutrition: the Gambian experience. J Pediatr Gastroenterol Nutr. 2002;34(1):S11-3.

20. Bhan MK, Bhandari N, Bhatnagar S, Bahl R. Epidemiology and management of persistent diarrhoea in children of developing countries. Ind J Med Res. 1996;104:103-14.

21. Bhutta ZA, Nizami SQ, Thobani S. Factors determining recovery during nutritional therapy of persistent diarrhoea: the impact of diarrhea severity and intercurrent infections. Acta Paediatr. 1997;86:796-802.

22. Khatun UH, Malek MA, Black RE, Sarkar NR, Wahed MA, Fuchs G, et al. A randomized controlled clinical trial of zinc, vitamin A or both in undernourished children with persistent diarrhea in Bangladesh. Acta Paediatr. 2001;90:376-80.

23. Bhatanagar S, Bhan MK, Singh KD, Srivastav R. Prognostic Factors in Hospitalized Children with Persistent Diarrhea: Implications for Diet Therapy. J Pediatr Gastroenterol Nutr. 1996;23(2):151-8.

24. Afzal NA, Addai S, Fagbemi A, et al. Refeeding syndrome with enteral nutrition in children: a case report, literature review and clinical guidelines. Clin Nutr. 2002;21:515-20.

Chapter

8

Celiac Disease

Bhupinder Sandhu, Nkem Onyeador

DEFINITION

Celiac disease (CD) is defined as an immune-mediated systemic disorder elicited by the ingestion of gluten and related prolamines in genetically susceptible individuals. It is characterized by the presence of a variable combination of gluten-dependent clinical manifestations, CD-specific autoantibodies and HLA-DQ2 or HLA-DQ8 haplotypes, and small bowel enteropathy.[1]

HISTORICAL BACKGROUND

In 250 AD, a Greek physician named Aretaeus of Cappadocia described in his writings some of the clinical features of as yet an unrecognized disease state. When depicting his patients he referred to them as having "koiliakos," which meant "suffering in the bowels." Francis Adams translated these observations from Greek to English for the Sydenham Society of England in 1856.[2]

"If the stomach be irretentive of the food and if it pass through undigested and crude, and nothing ascends into the body, we call such persons celiacs".

The clinical features of what is now known as celiac disease (CD) were first accurately described as the 'celiac affection' by the English physician and pediatrician Samuel Gee in a lecture to medical students at Great Ormond Street Hospital in London in 1887. He theorized about the importance of diet in its treatment. He stated[3]:

"To regulate the food is the main part of treatment. The allowance of farinaceous foods must be small, but if the patient can be cured at all, it must be by means of diet."

It was not until 1950 that the Dutch pediatrician, Willem Dicke linked and established the role of wheat and rye flour in the pathogenesis of the disease. In the late 1940s he astutely observed that the variations in the weight, stool frequency and overall well-being of his celiac patients on his ward were dependent on the type of food (a porridge called 'gruel') being served. Depending on availability of supply, during some months the gruel served would be wheat flour based whilst at other times it would be rice or potato flour based.[4] Collaborating with his Dutch colleagues including biochemist van de Kamer, they discovered increases in fecal fat output in CD patients consuming wheat and rye flour compared to those consuming rice, oats, potato, or corn flour.[5] Similar work was then carried out by Charlotte Anderson and colleagues in the United Kingdom[6] which confirmed the findings. Subsequently, a protein called gluten in wheat, barley and rye was identified as the causative agent.

The next major contribution to our understanding of the disease came with the advent of peroral biopsy of the small intestinal mucosa. In 1957, an English physician, Margot Shiner performed the first jejunal biopsy in a child using an adult biopsy tube that she had described in 1956.[7,8] This was of great diagnostic importance in CD. The histological changes of enteropathy visualized in the small bowel biopsies at diagnosis and their normalization on a gluten free diet formed the basis for the diagnostic criteria published in 1969 by ESPGAN (European Society of Pediatric Gastroenterology and Nutrition).[9] The diagnosis of CD was to be based on histological features, thus requiring small bowel biopsy in all suspected cases.

Research over the past 30 years has dramatically changed the initial perception of CD as a rare enteropathy to a relatively common multiorgan systemic disease with a strong genetic predisposition. The advent and availability of highly sensitive CD-specific autoantibody tests and CD-specific human leukocyte antigen (HLA) testing has led to the modification of the diagnostic criteria so that in a small selected number of children with symptoms, the diagnosis can be reliably made based on very high autoantibody levels (greater than ten times the upper limit of the normal range) and positive HLA testing without mandatory small bowel biopsy.

EPIDEMIOLOGY

Until the 1970s the global prevalence of CD in the general population was estimated at being around 0.03%.[10] It was perceived to be more common in the Caucasian population in Europe, Australasia and North America where wheat is a staple food. With the advent of endoscopic biopsy techniques (in the 1970s), identification of HLA-DQ2 and HLA-DQ8 (in the late 1980s and early 1990s), and development of sensitive and specific serological tests (since the 1990s), the diagnostic pick up rate increased greatly. Over time, cases were reported in other parts of the world, including North India, Sudan, Saudi Arabia, Lebanon and Iraq. CD was thought to be very uncommon in China but CD cases have recently been reported in children with chronic diarrhoea.[11] Whilst CD is said to remain relatively uncommon in sub-Saharan Africa and in African-American populations it is unclear whether this is due to genetic factors or under diagnosis.

Finnish, Italian and British studies based on population screening reveal the prevalence of CD in children to be around 1%.[12-14] Studies on prevalence of CD in various countries worldwide are listed in Table 8.1.[15-28] There appears to be an increasing prevalence of diagnosed CD[29] and since the 1990s a trend towards earlier diagnosis of CD has also been observed.[30] However, recent studies in the United Kingdom suggest despite free access to the National Health Service around 90% of cases may be remaining undiagnosed and hence clinical CD represents only the 'tip of the iceberg'.[31]

CD may present at any age after gluten has been introduced into the diet but peaks in early childhood and later adulthood. CD affects more females than males with a ratio of 2:1 in line with many autoimmune diseases. Whilst the incidence and prevalence of CD may be increasing, heightened awareness of the condition together with the availability of highly specific and sensitive screening tests is uncovering a larger number of previously undiagnosed patients who may have 'silent' or 'subclinical' symptoms. This has important health consequences as patients without overt clinical signs remain at risk from the long term detrimental effects of the disease.

The prevalence of CD may be set to increase in many developing countries due to the progressive 'Westernisation' of the diet.[32] This is particularly true in many Asian countries where industrialization and increased income has resulted in a decreased intake of rice per capita and an associated increased intake of wheat-based products.[33]

GENETICS

Celiac disease is one of the most common genetic diseases. It is strongly linked to an underlying genetic susceptibility, which was suggested by early observations that CD tends to affect several members of the same family.

The prevalence of CD amongst first degree relatives is estimated between 2.8%[34] and 17.2%.[35] This rises to 30–40% in HLA matched siblings and 80% in monozygotic twins.[36,37]

The strongest genetic association of CD is with the HLA class II DQ locus. There are seven HLA-DQ variants (DQ2 and DQ4-9). The most important HLA-DQ molecules in CD are DQ2 and DQ8. These genes code for receptors that bind to gliadin peptides that subsequently activate the T cell response. The vast majority of people with CD have one of these two types of the HLA-DQ protein. DQ2 is most commonly found as the subtype DQ2.5 (alleles DQA1*0501 and DQB1*0201) but can also be found as DQ2.2 (DQA1*0201 and DQB1*0202). DQ8 is usually subtype DQ8.1 (DQA1*0301 and DQB1*0302). Nearly all individuals with CD are DQ2 (95%) and/or DQ8 (~5%) positive[1] (compared with 25–40% in the general population in USA and Europe).[38] Only 4% of DQ2 positive individuals go on to develop CD.[39] The presence of CD associated HLA haplotypes DQ2 and DQ8 are necessary but not sufficient to develop CD.

Specific HLA genotypes are associated with greater risk of developing CD. For instance, family studies have shown that individuals who are DQ2.5 homozygous or DQ2.5/DQ2.2 heterozygous are 5 times more likely to develop CD compared to DQ2/DQX heterozygous individuals.[40] There is also some evidence that CD develops earlier and in a more severe form in children that are homozygous for DQ2.5.[41,42] The frequency of these genes varies geographically. For instance, DQ2.5 has an increased frequency in peoples of Northern and Western Europe descent, particularly in

Table 8.1: Prevalence of celiac disease in children in different countries world-wide	
Country	*Prevalence*
Europe and North America	
• Finland	1%[12]
• Germany	0.2%[15]
• Italy	0.54–0.9%[14,16,17]
• Netherlands	0.5%[18]
• Sweden	1.3%[19]
• United Kingdom	1.0%[13]
• USA	0.9–0.31%[20]
Asia and The Middle East	
• India (North)	1%[21]
• Iran	0.6%[22]
• Saudi Arabia	2.2%[23]
• Turkey	0.47%[24,25]
• Jordan	0.8%[26]
North Africa	
• Algeria	5.6%[27]
• Tunisia	0.64%[28]

Ireland and the Basque region, and in portions of North Africa and North India.[43]

The increased prevalence of these CD genotypes in the present population is also not fully explained. It would be expected that given the characteristics of the disease and its strong genetic predisposition that over time the genotype would undergo evolutionary negative selection, particularly in countries where agricultural farming has long been practised. This evolutionary model principle was first proposed by Simoons in 1978[44] when it was applied to explain the drop in prevalence of lactose intolerance from nearly 100% in ancestral populations to less that 5% in some current European populations. This appears not to be the case with CD. Rather there is evidence of positive selection in CD genotypes. It is thus proposed that, similar to diseases such as sickle cell, where the heterozygous trait conferred some protection against malaria, that somehow the genotype may be beneficial by providing protection against bacterial infections and hence has been favored by a process of natural selection.[45]

Other genetic factors have been reported in CD. In recent years, two genome-wide association studies (GWAS) and one fine-mapping project have identified up to 57 non-HLA single-nucleotide polymorphisms (SNP) that contribute to CD susceptibility.[46-49] At present about 54% of the genetics of CD can be explained by HLA plus the 57 non-HLA SNP compared to 40% by HLA alone.[50]

PATHOGENESIS

Celiac disease is induced by the ingestion of gluten, which is derived from wheat, barley and rye. Gluten refers to the entire protein component of wheat; gliadin is the alcohol-soluble fraction of gluten that contains the toxic constituents.[51] The gliadin when in α-gliadin fraction form passes through the epithelial barrier of the small intestine during periods of increased intestinal permeability and interacts with the antigen presenting cells (APC) in the lamina propria. This leads to an inflammatory reaction mediated by the innate and adaptive immune systems. The adaptive immune response is mediated by CD4+ T cells that recognise gliadin peptides, which are bound to HLA class II molecules on DQ2 or DQ8 APC. The pro-inflammatory cascade produces cytokines, particularly interferon-γ.[52]

CLINICAL FEATURES AND PATTERNS OF DISEASE

Clinical Features

"*The single most important step in diagnosing celiac disease is to first consider the disorder by recognizing its myriad of clinical features*" (*National Institute of Health consensus statement, 2004*).[53]

Celiac disease is a multiorgan systemic disorder and therefore by its very nature its presentation in individuals can vary widely from gastrointestinal (GI) symptoms (such as chronic diarrhea, abdominal pain/bloating and failure to thrive) to nongastrointestinal symptoms (such as anemia, short stature and delayed puberty) (Table 8.2) to no symptoms at all. CD should be an early consideration in the differential diagnosis in a child presenting with any combination of persistent diarrhea, steatorrhea, abdominal pain and bloating and failure to thrive.

Iron deficiency anemia that does not respond to iron supplementation is the most common biochemical abnormality seen in children and adults. Arthritis and arthralgia can also be part of the spectrum of clinical features at diagnosis. Children from poor socioeconomic backgrounds and in children with darker skin who do not have adequate exposure to sunlight, rickets may be one of the presenting features of CD.[54,55] Short stature is a well-recognized extraintestinal manifestation. Previous studies have shown that in some populations, 10% of patients with isolated short stature were found to have CD.[56]

As the severity of symptoms at presentation does not normally correlate with the severity of the underlying pathology, it is important to diagnose all patients with CD. Failure to appreciate the variable clinical manifestations of CD can lead to delay in diagnosis.

Patterns of Disease

Celiac disease can be recognized as being symptomatic (classical or non-classical presentation) or asymptomatic (detected by screening) (see Screening for Celiac Disease on page 89).

Classical Celiac Disease

The classical form is characterized by intestinal villous atrophy and typical symptoms of malabsorption including diarrhea, steatorrhea, abdominal distension, poor growth

Table 8.2: Clinical and biochemical features of celiac disease
Gastrointestinal manifestations: Recurrent abdominal pain, abdominal bloating/distension, flatulence, chronic or recurrent diarrhea, steatorrhea, failure to thrive, weight loss, anorexia, nausea, vomiting, constipation, aphthous stomatitis.
Extraintestinal manifestations: Anemia (usually iron deficiency), short stature/growth failure, pubertal delay, dermatitis herpetiformis, irritability, muscle wasting, chronic fatigue, arthralgia/arthritis, transaminitis, cryptogenic hepatitis, rickets, dental hypoplasia, infertility.

and failure to thrive. Muscle wasting of the buttocks is also often described. Parents may also report behavioral changes, including irritability, clinginess, withdrawal and low mood.[57] These symptoms characteristically begin after the introduction of gluten into the diet, between 6 months and 24 months of age, but can occur at any age.

Ironically, the so called 'classical' presentation is a misnomer as this presentation of CD is becoming less common in the pediatric population, particularly in the developed world.

At the end of the spectrum of the classical presentation is the 'celiac crisis'. This is characterized by marked abdominal distension, explosive watery diarrhea, with ensuing dehydration, electrolyte imbalances, lethargy and hypotension. Although rarely seen, this can cause significant morbidity and mortality if left untreated.

Nonclassical Celiac Disease

The nonclassical form is seen in a significant proportion of patients with CD. It is characterized by enteropathy of the small intestinal mucosa but only minor intestinal symptoms rather than the florid malabsorptive presentation described above. Patients can also present with extraintestinal signs and symptoms, such as anemia, rickets, hepatitis, dermatitis herpetiformis as well as developmental and behavioral problems. Older children may present with constipation and abdominal pain but no malabsorption. Patients with mono-symptomatic disease (other than diarrhea or steatorrhea) usually have nonclassical CD.[58]

▌ INVESTIGATIONS (FLOW CHART 8.1)

Children presenting with symptoms suggestive of CD should have serological testing. In addition other differential diagnoses and co-existing pathology should be excluded.

Any patient presenting with chronic diarrhea should have stool sent for microscopy and culture, ova, cysts and parasites to look for evidence of gastroenteritis, which can co-exist with CD, particularly in developing countries.

Flow chart 8.1: Diagnostic approach to celiac disease

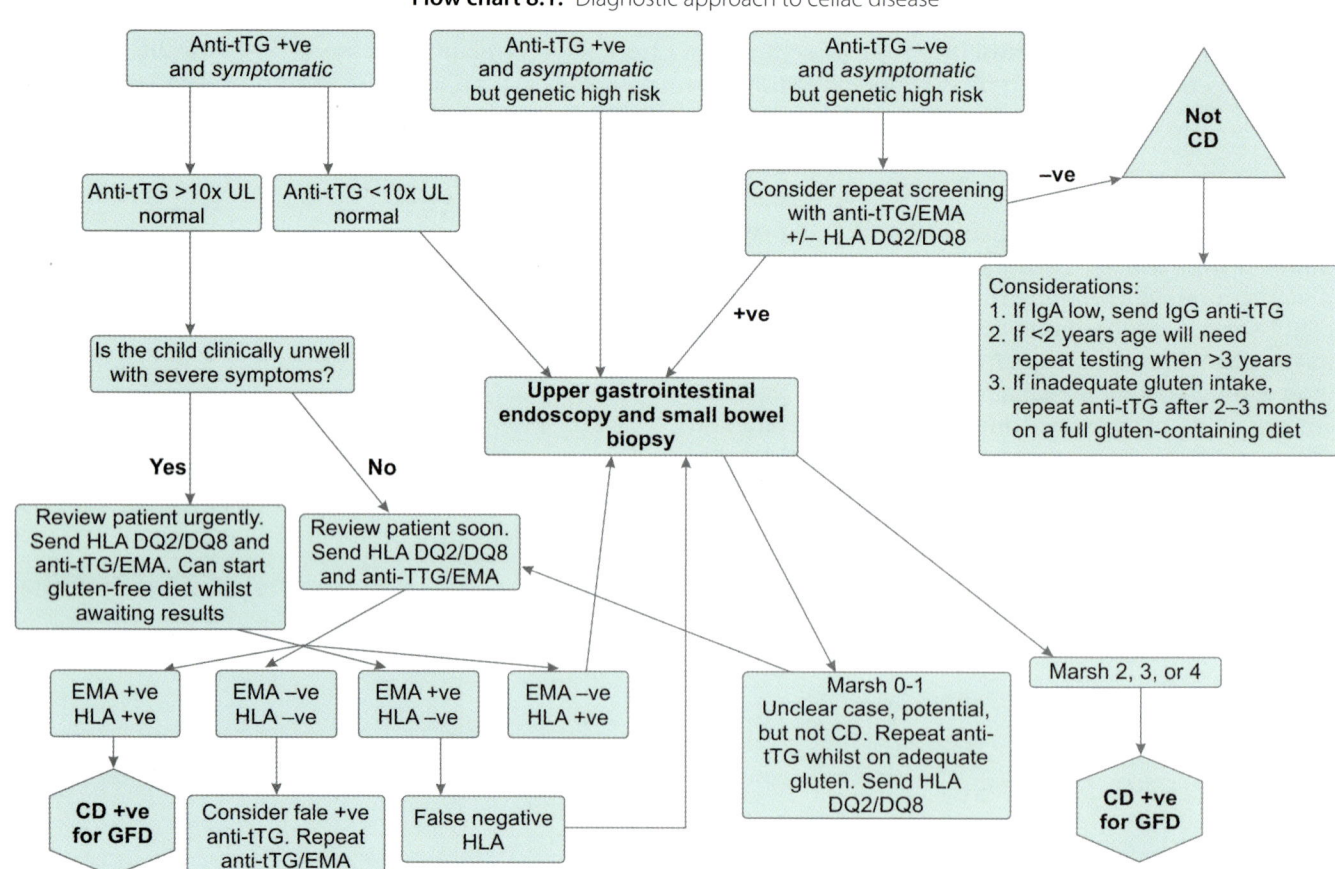

Abbreviations: Anti-tTG—anti-tissue transglutaminase antibody; Anti-EMA—anti-endomysial antibodies; CD +ve—celiac disease positive; FH—family history; UL normal—upper limit of normal range; GFD—gluten-free diet.

Other causes of chronic diarrhea, abdominal pain and poor weight gain should be considered.

First line blood investigations should in addition to CD serology include a full blood count, ferritin and liver function tests. Due to malabsorption, iron deficiency anemia is common in CD. Occasionally, deficiencies in vitamin D and even vitamin E can occur. Vitamin D deficiency may present with clinical or biochemical rickets and vitamin D or E deficiency may present with muscle weakness and motor developmental delay. In patients presenting with suspected rickets a wrist X-ray should be performed.

Serological Tests

Serologic screening for CD has evolved markedly over the past two and a half decades, and tests with high sensitivity and specificity are now readily available. Antibodies used for screening for CD include both IgA and IgG anti-tissue transglutaminase antibodies (tTG), IgA anti-endomysial antibodies (IgA-EMA), and conventional antigliadin antibodies (AGA). Of the aforementioned, IgA tTG and IgA EMA appear highly accurate to diagnose CD and are the cornerstones of laboratory diagnosis.[1]

Every child with positive antibodies for CD should be reviewed by a Pediatrician or Pediatric Gastroenterologist.

Antigliadin Antibodies (AGA)

Initially AGA-IgA and IgG were used for screening but they have poor sensitivity and specificity for CD screening and therefore have essentially been replaced by newer serologic screening tests. Elevated levels of AGA-IgA and IgG have been found in many other conditions associated with increased permeability of the GI tract such as food allergies, cow's milk protein allergy, gastrointestinal infections, irritable bowel syndrome, and inflammatory bowel disease.

Whilst some studies have suggested that AGA has a particularly increased sensitivity specifically in children under the age of 2, current guidelines recommend against using AGA in the diagnosis of CD, even in young children.[1] Instead of adding AGA serology, children with a high clinical suspicion for CD who are otherwise seronegative ought to proceed to having endoscopy and small bowel biopsy.

Anti-tissue Transglutaminase (tTG) and Anti-endomysial Antibodies (EMA)

Initial CD screening for children typically begins with either tTG-IgA or EMA-IgA; both tests have superior accuracy compared to AGA, and both are highly sensitive and specific in the pediatric population. Although EMA has been considered the 'gold standard' of screening for CD due to its high specificity, because it uses direct immunofluorescence, it is more expensive and labor intensive than tTG-IgA. Since the discovery of tTG-IgA, the autoantigen in CD and the antigen to which EMA binds, antibodies to tTG have become useful as one of the most sensitive and specific screening tests for CD. It is performed either using enzyme-linked immunosorbent assay (ELISA) or radio-immunoassay (RIA) techniques which make it cheaper, and therefore more accessible than EMA.

Initial testing for CD requires that the child is on an adequate gluten-containing diet prior to and at the time of serological testing. An estimation of total IgA and quantitative IgA anti-tTG antibody levels is taken from the individual at this time. CD cannot be diagnosed solely on the basis of IgA anti-tTG antibody level test. Findings of a raised anti-tTG level or positive EMA require further diagnostic investigation (see Flow chart 8.1).

In symptomatic children, if the IgA anti-tTG level is less than 10-fold the upper limit of normal (ULN) then a small bowel biopsy is recommended for a histological diagnosis.[1] If the IgA anti-tTG level is greater than 10-fold ULN, then a second blood test for EMA or anti-tTG and HLA-DQ typing is required. A positive EMA (or repeat high level anti-tTG if EMA not available) and the presence of HLA-DQ2 or HLA-DQ8 typing confirms the diagnosis of CD in symptomatic patients without the need for small bowel biopsy.[38]

HLA Typing

CD is an immune-mediated disease which is strongly dependent on the HLA-DQ2 and DQ8 haplotype. It has a high negative predictive value; if a child does not have DQ2 or DQ8 haplotypes then CD is highly unlikely. Therefore, typing for HLA can be used to exclude a diagnosis of CD, which can be particularly useful in screening at risk groups (see Screening for Celiac Disease on page 130). HLA typing for DQ2 and DQ8 is also recommended in children in whom there is a strong suspicion of CD (symptomatic and anti-tTG greater than 10-fold ULN) in order to add strength to the diagnosis, particularly when small bowel biopsies will not be performed (see Flow chart 8.1).

Endoscopy and Histology

In the majority of suspected cases of CD, biopsies of the duodenum are required to confirm a diagnosis of CD. Prior to the modification of ESPGHAN guidelines for the diagnosis of CD in 2012, diagnostic criteria were based on histological features typical of CD identified in small bowel and therefore endoscopic evaluation was an essential requirement in diagnosing CD. Indeed previously those diagnosed with CD under the age of two would have required a gluten challenge at a later stage and repeat biopsy to confirm the diagnosis.

Small bowel biopsy remains the current best practice for diagnosing most cases of CD. A lifelong gluten-free diet has considerable psychological, social and economic consequences and hence it is important that CD is correctly diagnosed.

There is consensus within the ESPGHAN guidelines on CD that a minimum of five biopsies should be taken from the second or third part of duodenum (minimum of four biopsies), and also from the duodenal bulb (minimum of one biopsy),[1] which can increase diagnostic yield.[59 60]

The histological features of the small bowel in CD have a variable severity, not necessarily related to clinical severity, may be patchy and in some cases be isolated to the duodenal bulb only.[1] Typically, the histological findings will include an increased number of intraepithelial lymphocytes (IEL) of >25/100 cells and progress to mucosal villous atrophy of variable grade. There are several histological classifications.[61-63] The Marsh-Oberhuber classification[62] is widely used and is summarized in Table 8.3.

In order to obtain an accurate diagnosis, adequate tissue sampling must be combined with correct orientation and interpretation by experienced histopathologists. Finding enteropathy in isolation should not be considered pathognomonic for pediatric CD. Whilst CD is the commonest cause of these histological changes, other differential diagnoses should still be considered and correlated with the clinical presentation. Other causes of villous atrophy including cow's milk protein allergy, tropical sprue, giardiasis, protein-energy malnutrition, microvillous atrophy, autoimmune enteropathy, gastroenteritis and post-gastroenteritis syndromes and immunodeficiencies (e.g. HIV/AIDS)[64] should be considered. This is particularly important in developing countries where malnutrition and gut infections are more likely to co-exist.

SCREENING FOR CELIAC DISEASE

Whilst mass population screening for CD remains a controversial topic and has currently not been recommended or adopted,[65] there should be a very low threshold for screening in 'subclinical' or 'at risk' groups. Current recommendations for CD screening in the pediatric population suggest a systematic process of case-finding, targeting at risk groups, particularly those with diseases associated with CD and those with a positive family history in first degree relative.[1,66] CD is associated with a number of genetic and autoimmune conditions[1,67-77] (Table 8.4) and children with these conditions should be screened for CD.

Pre-test counseling is advised when screening for CD. Where appropriate, the parent and child should be informed about the impact of a positive result, including the potential requirement of small bowel biopsy to confirm diagnosis.

Immunoglobulin A (IgA) Deficiency

Selective IgA deficiency is a common primary immune deficiency characterized by low levels of IgA. It can be asymptomatic or present with recurrent respiratory and gastrointestinal infections. IgA deficiency is associated with an increased prevalence of CD. This is of particular

Table 8.3: Marsh-Oberhuber classification[62]	
Classification	Morphology of duodenal mucosal biopsy of extraintestinal manifestations
Type 0	Normal architecture with or without increase IEL ≤40/100 enterocytes
Type 1	Normal architecture and increased IEL ≥40/100 enterocytes
Type 2	Normal architecture and increased IEL ≥40/100 enterocytes with crypt hyperplasia
Type 3a	Partial villous atrophy; villi blunt and shortened with an increase in crypt height. IEL ≥40/100 enterocytes
Type 3b	Subtotal villous atrophy; villi atrophic. IEL ≥40/100 enterocytes
Type 3c	Total villous atrophy; absence of rudimentary villi. IEL ≥40/100 enterocytes
Type 4	Atrophic hypoplastic lesion with flat mucosa. Normal crypt height, no inflammation, normal IEL count

Table 8.4: Conditions associated with celiac disease and their prevalence	
Condition	Prevalence of CD
Type 1 diabetes	2–10%[1,67]
Juvenile chronic arthritis	1.5–2.5%[68,69]
Down syndrome	6.3%[70]
Turner syndrome	6.4%[71]
Williams syndrome	9.5%[72]
IgA nephropathy	4%[73]
IgA deficiency	3%[74,75]
Autoimmune thyroid disease	3.3%[76]
Autoimmune liver disease	13.5%[77]

importance in screening and diagnosis as screening tests are usually IgA based. As IgA deficiency is associated with CD, total IgA should be measured in all children at initial diagnostic screening. Children who have total serum IgA levels less than 0.2 g/L should have additional testing done with IgG specific antibodies (anti-tTG IgG, or anti-EMA IgG). However, it should be noted than neither of the IgG specific antibodies are as specific as the IgA antibodies and therefore biopsy is recommended in symptomatic patients with IgA deficiency even if there are IgG anti-tTG serology negative.

Dermatitis Herpetiformis

Dermatitis herpetiformis (DH) is a cutaneous manifestation strongly associated with CD and CD-related HLA haplotypes. It is characterized by symmetrical, herpetiform clusters of pruritic vesicles and papules visible on the skin, especially on the elbows, buttocks and knees. This presentation is less common in children than adults, however, the vast majority of children presenting with DH will have CD. Skin biopsy reveals IgA deposits in the dermal papillae whilst concomitant small bowel biopsy will usually show villous atrophy at diagnosis, even if otherwise asymptomatic.

Parents should be reassured that after one to three months of treatment on a gluten free diet, 82% of DH skin lesions will have cleared, although occasionally treatment with dapsone will be required.[78]

When to Screen Asymptomatic but at Risk Groups

Most screening should start after the age of three years when there is adequate gluten in the diet for at least one year. It is important that adequate gluten content be maintained in the diet of the child before and during CD screening. It is recommended that children with parents or siblings who have CD and children with conditions associated with CD (Table 8.4) undergo CD autoantibody serological testing.

In asymptomatic children with associated conditions and negative anti-tTG antibodies, consider HLA typing. If HLA DQ2/DQ8 is positive, continued surveillance is recommended with repeat anti-tTG serological testing every two to three years or sooner if they become symptomatic. Small bowel biopsy should be performed if the anti-tTG becomes positive. If HLA DQ2/DQ8 testing is negative then development of CD is very unlikely and hence CD antibody serological surveillance can stop to be re-evaluated only if the child becomes symptomatic in later life.

Categories of Celiac Disease Identified on Screening

Asymptomatic Celiac Disease

Asymptomatic CD is characterized by patients with positive CD autoantibody serology but no gastrointestinal or extra-intestinal symptoms and similarly no clinical response to a gluten-free diet. All these patients should have a small bowel biopsy to confirm the diagnosis.

Subclinical Celiac Disease

Subclinical CD is usually picked up during screening of high genetic risk groups (see Table 8.4). These patients will have a positive CD autoantibody screen. On retrospection the patient with subclinical CD may report some mild gastrointestinal symptoms and a subtle decrease in wellbeing, which had not previously been recognized. The patient will usually see some positive improvement whilst on the gluten-free diet. Some studies have shown that children with subclinical CD have decreased height z-scores which correlate with the degree of mucosal damage.[79] All these patients should have a small bowel biopsy to confirm the diagnosis.

Potential Celiac Disease

The presence of CD-associated autoantibodies with normal jejunal mucosa indicates potential CD. This presentation is becoming more common due to increased awareness of CD and more active case finding, particular in at risk groups. These patients may or may not have symptoms and signs to suggest CD at the time of diagnosis. These children may or may not develop a gluten-dependent enteropathy. Some data suggests that approximately a third of these patients will develop a histological gluten enteropathy.[80] One of the challenges in the definition of this group is the variability in the adequacy of the biopsies that are deemed to exclude the diagnosis of active CD. CD is patchy in nature and at least four biopsies should be taken from the duodenum and at least one from the duodenal bulb as this may be the only location of histological changes.[60] Inadequate biopsies can change a diagnosis of CD to potential CD.

MANAGEMENT OF CELIAC DISEASE

Acute Management

Currently a life-long gluten-free diet (GFD) is the only accepted treatment for children and adults with CD. This should be commenced as soon as the diagnosis is confirmed.

Children may occasionally present acutely unwell in a 'celiac crisis' condition. In such cases where there is a high index of suspicion demonstrating a fulminant malabsorpative state with severe dehydration and electrolyte abnormalities, the management should involve fluid resuscitation and correction of electrolyte imbalances whilst commencing a gluten-free diet.

In developing countries, severely malnourished patients presenting with CD are at significant risk of life-threatening refeeding syndrome which may mimic a celiac crisis state. Typically these patients may present with worsening of their clinical state and electrolyte imbalance (particularly hypophosphatemia) after the introduction of a gluten-free diet. Early recognition and appropriate management of refeeding syndrome in such cases is crucial and can save lives.[81,82]

Long-term Management

Pediatric dietetic support is essential in the early weeks and months of establishing a strict gluten-free diet. Children and their parents should be followed up at 3–6 monthly intervals for the first year (or longer if ongoing dietary compliancy issues). After the first year, most children can be reviewed annually.

Children who were previously symptomatic often notice improvement after a few weeks on a GFD and parents will often comment on improved appetite, energy levels and behavior in younger children. Some children may become very sensitive to gluten in the diet if it is inadvertently ingested whilst some will not notice. It is important that the child and parent appreciate that even small amounts of gluten ingested regularly can cause mucosal damage and long-term complications although the child may remain clinically asymptomatic.

Historically oats were also excluded in GFD mainly because of they were ground in the same mills that ground the wheat thus resulting in cross-contamination. However, only 5% of individuals with CD will be sensitive to oats. Oats can, therefore, be eaten as long as they are uncontaminated 'gluten-free' oats. It is advisable that oats only be introduced to the diet at a later stage when the child is well established on the GFD and completely symptom free, preferably with normalization of anti-tTG level. Oats can then be introduced into the diet with careful monitoring of clinical and serological response.

Monitoring

Children with CD and their families require ongoing long-term support preferably by a Pediatric Gastroenterologist or a Pediatrician with a special interest in CD. This is essential to ensure long-term adherence to GFD. After the initial diagnosis and commencement of GFD, a repeat anti-tTG level should be performed after 6 months which should demonstrate a fall in anti-tTG level. At the same time the consultation should include a symptom review, physical examination with assessment of growth parameters and micronutrient status (particular iron and vitamin D status). If the child is well and anti-tTG antibodies have normalized, then anti-tTG can be repeated annually, particularly to help identify poor dietary compliance.

Gluten Challenge

Historically, gluten challenge formed part of the diagnostic criteria for CD in children. Nowadays, the gluten challenge is reserved for those patients where diagnostic doubt lingers. For instance a child may be very symptomatic on gluten but have negative biopsy results whilst being HLA-DQ2 or DQ8 positive. This child may have been started on a GFD with clinical improvement. In such a case, it would be prudent to repeat anti-tTG and if positive to perform a repeat biopsy after an optimum of at least 3 months on adequate gluten-containing diet. This could be expedited to 6-8 weeks should the child become very symptomatic. The challenge should be performed either before or after the pubertal period so as not to affect growth.

The gluten challenge requires an adequate amount of gluten in the diet (10–15 g/day). 2–3 g of gluten is contained in one medium slice of bread or four tablespoons of cooked pasta. It is, therefore, advised that gluten containing food should be incorporated into two or three meals per day during the gluten challenge. Whilst this may exacerbate symptoms temporarily parents should be counselled beforehand about the need for adequate gluten in the diet for histological changes to be seen to confirm the diagnosis.

PROGNOSIS

In individuals with CD that adhere to a lifelong strict gluten-free diet, the prognosis is excellent. They usually see full resolution of symptoms, appropriate catch-up growth and weight gain, reversed bone demineralization and resolution of micronutrient deficiencies. The previous increased risk of gut-related lymphoma decreases to the rate of the normal population.

A lifelong GFD is well-tolerated therapy and most children and the supporting parent(s) are motivated to continue to ensure strict adherence. However, the GFD is difficult to maintain for several reasons including gluten cross-contamination of food products, high cost of gluten-free products and perceived 'social burden' of a lifelong restricted diet[83] (Table 8.5).

Table 8.5: Barriers to dietary adherence in children with celiac disease

- High cost of gluten-free products
- Reduced palatability of gluten-free foods
- Poor labeling of food products clearly stating whether gluten-free
- Inadequate dietary counselling pre- and postcommencing diet
- Social burden of lifelong lifestyle modification
- Absence of symptoms when gluten re-introduced into the diet
- Social, cultural and peer pressures
- Child's limited developmental capacity to comprehend diagnosis
- Transitioning into adolescence
- Lack of social or family support system
- Limited access to resources and support groups
- Parental illiteracy (in developing world)
- Lack of availability of gluten-free products (in developing world)

COMPLICATIONS OF CELIAC DISEASE

Despite the challenges of adhering to GFD strict compliance remains of paramount importance to avoid morbidity and the complications associated with untreated CD. Childhood complications of CD include growth failure, delayed puberty, malnutrition and micronutrient deficiencies, which can lead to anemia and in a few cases, rickets and delayed motor development. In adulthood the complications can progress to osteoporosis, infertility, recurrent miscarriages, intestinal adenocarcinoma and enteropathy associated T-cell lymphoma.[84,85] Parents and children should be counselled accordingly.

Some patients may have persisting associated lactose intolerance secondary to CD. This is caused by damage to the brush border of the small intestine that produces lactase, the enzyme responsible for breaking down lactose to glucose and galactose. The lactose intolerance is usually temporary and reversible once GFD has been established and the enteropathy has resolved. In those with lactose intolerance, lactose should be introduced gradually into the diet after three months on a strict GFD, however, it can take up to 2 years for complete healing and functioning of the brush border. If symptoms do persist, this should prompt consideration of other differential diagnoses (such as cow's milk protein enteropathy). In older children/adults of non-Caucasian origin, there is an increased likelihood of lactose intolerance and hence lactose may also need to be reduced or permanently excluded from the diet to control symptoms.

REFRACTORY CELIAC DISEASE

Refractory CD is characterized by the persistence or recurrence of malabsorptive symptoms and signs with villous atrophy despite a strict gluten-free diet for more than 12 months in the absence of other causes of villous atrophy.[58] This is rare in childhood. Generally, these patients will be negative for CD autoantibodies at the time of diagnosis of refractory CD. However, the persisting presence of elevated levels of anti-tTG or EMA autoantibodies does not rule out refractory CD, although dietary compliancy issues should be considered in the first instance.[58] Treatment of refractory CD involves nutritional support, repletion of micronutrients and strict GFD.

FUTURE RESEARCH

In the past decade CD research interest has included therapeutic alternatives to GFD for patients with CD (Table 8.6).

These alternatives include use of genetically modified gluten,[86] gluten peptide vaccination[87,88] and use of a zonulin inhibitor.[89] A tissue transglutaminase inhibitor may also have a role in preventing the breakdown of gluten fragments.[90] The role of probiotics in modifying GI disease has received increasing attention. *Bifidobacterium lactis* bacteria have been shown to inhibit the toxic effects induced by wheat gliadin in epithelial cell culture.[91] Probiotics may have a role in refractory CD. Currently, none of these measures have been investigated in the pediatric population where the risk of harm compared to a safe current gold standard of the GFD may be unethical. Any immunomodulatory approach will need to have the same excellent safety profile of GFD with the added benefit of avoiding dietary restriction.

Table 8.6: New potential therapeutic agents and their mode of action

Therapeutic agent	Mode of action
Genetically modified gluten[86]	Transamidation of gliadin decreases gluten exposure
Gluten peptide vaccination[87,88]	Creates immune tolerance to gluten fragments. Causes desensitization to gluten
Zonulin inhibitor[89]	Increases intestinal permeability by decreasing zonulin signaling protein at tight junction
Tissue transglutaminase inhibitors[90]	Inhibit tissue transglutaminase from breaking down to gluten fragments, averting subsequent immune response
Probiotics[91]	Genetically modified bacteria that detoxify gliadin and promote intestinal healing

SOURCES OF PATIENT/PARENT INFORMATION

There are a number of national CD support groups worldwide that offer information, guidance and support for patients and their families. These include Celiac UK in the United Kingdom (www.coeliac.org.uk), Celiac Australia (www.coeliac.org.au) and the Celiac Disease Foundation in North America (www.celiac.org).

REFERENCES

1. Husby S, Koletzko S, Korponay-Szabo IR, Mearin ML, Phillips A, Shamir R, et al. European Society for Pediatric Gastroenterology, Hepatology, and Nutrition guidelines for the diagnosis of coeliac disease. J Pediatr Gastroenterol Nutr. 2012;54(1):136-60.
2. Adams F. The extant works of Aretæus, The Cappadocian. 1856.
3. Gee S. On the Coeliac Affection. St Bartholomews Hospital Reports. 1888;24:17-20.
4. Anderson CM. Chapter 1: Evolution of Successful Treatment in 'Coeliac Disease' Ed Marsh M.N. Oxford: Blackwell Scientific Publications, 1992.
5. Dicke WK, Weijers HA, Van De Kamer JH. Coeliac disease. II. The presence in wheat of a factor having a deleterious effect in cases of coeliac disease. Acta Paediatr. 1953;42(1):34-42.
6. Anderson CM, French JM, Sammons HG, Frazer AC, Gerrard JW, Smellie JM. Coeliac disease; gastrointestinal studies and the effect of dietary wheat flour. Lancet. 1952;1(6713):836-42.
7. Sakula J, Shiner M. Coeliac disease with atrophy of the small-intestine mucosa. Lancet. 1957;273(7001):876-7.
8. Shiner M. Duodenal biopsy. Lancet. 1956;270(6906):17-9.
9. Meeuwisse GW. Round table discussion. Diagnostic criteria in coeliac disease. Acta Paediatrica Scandinavica. 1970;59:461-3.
10. Green PH, Jabri B. Coeliac disease. Lancet. 2003;362(9381):383-91.
11. Wang XQ, Liu W, Xu CD, Mei H, Gao Y, Peng HM, et al. Celiac disease in children with diarrhea in 4 cities in China. J Pediatr Gastroenterol Nutr. 2011;53(4):368-70.
12. Maki M, Mustalahti K, Kokkonen J, Kulmala P, Haapalahti M, Karttunen T, et al. Prevalence of celiac disease among children in Finland. N Engl J Med. 2003;348(25):2517-24.
13. Bingley PJ, Williams AJ, Norcross AJ, Unsworth DJ, Lock RJ, Ness AR, et al. Undiagnosed coeliac disease at age seven: population based prospective birth cohort study. BMJ. 2004;328(7435):322-3.
14. Tommasini A, Not T, Kiren V, Baldas V, Santon D, Trevisiol C, et al. Mass screening for coeliac disease using antihuman transglutaminase antibody assay. Arch Dis Child. 2004;89(6):512-5.
15. Henker J, Losel A, Conrad K, Hirsch T, Leupold W. Prevalence of asymptomatic coeliac disease in children and adults in the Dresden region of Germany. Dtsch Med Wochenschr. 2002;127(28-29):1511-5.
16. Catassi C, Fabiani E, Ratsch IM, Coppa GV, Giorgi PL, Pierdomenico R, et al. The coeliac iceberg in Italy. A multicentre antigliadin antibodies screening for coeliac disease in school-age subjects. Acta Paediatr Suppl. 1996;412:29-35.
17. Castano L, Blarduni E, Ortiz L, Nunez J, Bilbao JR, Rica I, et al. Prospective population screening for celiac disease: high prevalence in the first 3 years of life. J Pediatr Gastroenterol Nutr. 2004;39(1):80-4.
18. Csizmadia CG, Mearin ML, von Blomberg BM, Brand R, Verloove-Vanhorick SP. An iceberg of childhood coeliac disease in the Netherlands. Lancet. 1999;353(9155):813-4.
19. Carlsson AK, Axelsson IE, Borulf SK, Bredberg AC, Ivarsson SA. Serological screening for celiac disease in healthy 2.5-year-old children in Sweden. Pediatrics. 2001;107(1):42-5.
20. Hoffenberg EJ, MacKenzie T, Barriga KJ, Eisenbarth GS, Bao F, Haas JE, et al. A prospective study of the incidence of childhood celiac disease. J Pediatr. 2003;143(3):308-14.
21. Sood A, Midha V, Sood N, Avasthi G, Sehgal A. Prevalence of celiac disease among school children in Punjab, North India. J Gastroenterol Hepatol. 2006;21(10):1622-5.
22. Dehghani SM, Haghighat M, Mobayen A, Rezaianzadeh A, Geramizadeh B. Prevalence of celiac disease in healthy Iranian school children. Ann Saudi Med. 2013;33(2):159-61.
23. Aljebreen AM, Almadi MA, Alhammad A, Al Faleh FZ. Seroprevalence of celiac disease among healthy adolescents in Saudi Arabia. World J Gastroenterol. 2013;19(15):2374-8.
24. Dalgic B, Sari S, Basturk B, Ensari A, Egritas O, Bukulmez A, et al. Prevalence of celiac disease in healthy Turkish school children. Am J Gastroenterol. 2011;106(8):1512-7.
25. Ertekin V, Selimoglu MA, Kardas F, Aktas E. Prevalence of celiac disease in Turkish children. J Clin Gastroenterol. 2005;39(8):689-91.
26. Nusier MK, Brodtkorb HK, Rein SE, Odeh A, Radaideh AM, Klungland H. Serological screening for celiac disease in schoolchildren in Jordan. Is height and weight affected when seropositive? Ital J Pediatr. 2010;36:16.
27. Catassi C, Ratsch IM, Gandolfi L, Pratesi R, Fabiani E, El Asmar R. et al. Why is coeliac disease endemic in the people of the Sahara? Lancet 1999;354(9179):647-8.
28. Ben Hariz M, Kallel-Sellami M, Kallel L, Lahmer A, Halioui S, Bouraoui S, et al. Prevalence of celiac disease in Tunisia: mass-screening study in school children. Eur J Gastroenterol Hepatol. 2007;19(8):687-94.
29. Lohi S, Mustalahti K, Kaukinen K, Laurila K, Collin P, Rissanen H, et al. Increasing prevalence of coeliac disease over time. Aliment Pharmacol Ther. 2007;26(9):1217-25.
30. Rampertab SD, Pooran N, Brar P, Singh P, Green PH. Trends in the presentation of celiac disease. Am J Med. 2006;119(4):355 e9-14.
31. Ravikumara M, Nootigattu VK, Sandhu BK. Ninety percent of celiac disease is being missed. J Pediatr Gastroenterol Nutr. 2007;45(4):497-9.
32. Fasano A, Catassi C. Clinical practice. Celiac disease. N Engl J Med. 2012;367(25):2419-26.
33. FAO (Food & Agriculture Organization of the United Nations); World agriculture: towards 2015/2030 : summary report. Rome: FAO, 2002.
34. Vitoria JC, Arrieta A, Astigarraga I, Garcia-Masdevall D, Rodriguez-Soriano J. Use of serological markers as a screening test in family members of patients with celiac disease. J Pediatr Gastroenterol Nutr. 1994;19(3):304-9.
35. Book L, Zone JJ, Neuhausen SL. Prevalence of celiac disease among relatives of sib pairs with celiac disease in US families. Am J Gastroenterol. 2003;98(2):377-81.

36. Nistico L, Fagnani C, Coto I, Percopo S, Cotichini R, Limongelli MG, et al. Concordance, disease progression, and heritability of coeliac disease in Italian twins. Gut. 2006;55(6):803-8.

37. Greco L, Romino R, Coto I, Di Cosmo N, Percopo S, Maglio M, et al. The first large population based twin study of coeliac disease. Gut. 2002;50(5):624-8.

38. Giersiepen K, Lelgemann M, Stuhldreher N, Ronfani L, Husby S, Koletzko S, et al. Accuracy of diagnostic antibody tests for coeliac disease in children: summary of an evidence report. J Pediatr Gastroenterol Nutr. 2012;54(2):229-41.

39. Wolters VM, Wijmenga C. Genetic background of celiac disease and its clinical implications. Am J Gastroenterol. 2008;103(1):190-5.

40. van Belzen MJ, Koeleman BP, Crusius JB, Meijer JW, Bardoel AF, Pearson PL, et al. Defining the contribution of the HLA region to cis DQ2-positive coeliac disease patients. Genes Immun. 2004;5(3):215-20.

41. Congia M, Cucca F, Frau F, Lampis R, Melis L, Clemente MG, et al. A gene dosage effect of the DQA1*0501/DQB1*0201 allelic combination influences the clinical heterogeneity of celiac disease. Hum Immunol. 1994;40(2):138-42.

42. Jores RD, Frau F, Cucca F, Grazia Clemente M, Orru S, Rais M, et al. HLA-DQB1*0201 homozygosis predisposes to severe intestinal damage in celiac disease. Scand J Gastroenterol. 2007;42(1):48-53.

43. Kaur G, Sarkar N, Bhatnagar S, Kumar S, Rapthap CC, Bhan MK, et al. Pediatric celiac disease in India is associated with multiple DR3-DQ2 haplotypes. Hum Immunol. 2002;63(8):677-82.

44. Simoons FJ. The geographic hypothesis and lactose malabsorption. A weighing of the evidence. Am J Dig Dis. 1978;23(11):963-80.

45. Zhernakova A, Elbers CC, Ferwerda B, Romanos J, Trynka G, Dubois PC, et al. Evolutionary and Functional Analysis of Celiac Risk Loci Reveals SH2B3 as a Protective Factor against Bacterial Infection. American Journal of Human Genetics. 2010;86(6):970-77.

46. Dubois PC, Trynka G, Franke L, Hunt KA, Romanos J, Curtotti A, et al. Multiple common variants for celiac disease influencing immune gene expression. Nat Genet. 2010;42(4):295-302.

47. Hunt KA, Zhernakova A, Turner G, Heap GA, Franke L, Bruinenberg M, et al. Newly identified genetic risk variants for celiac disease related to the immune response. Nat Genet. 2008;40(4):395-402.

48. Trynka G, Hunt KA, Bockett NA, Romanos J, Mistry V, Szperl A, et al. Dense genotyping identifies and localizes multiple common and rare variant association signals in celiac disease. Nat Genet. 2011;43(12):1193-201.

49. Trynka G, Zhernakova A, Romanos J, Franke L, Hunt KA, Turner G, et al. Coeliac disease-associated risk variants in TNFAIP3 and REL implicate altered NF-κB signalling. Gut 2009;58(8):1078-83.

50. Kumar V, Wijmenga C, Withoff S. From genome-wide association studies to disease mechanisms: celiac disease as a model for autoimmune diseases. Semin Immunopathol. 2012;34(4):567-80.

51. Green PH, Cellier C. Celiac disease. N Engl J Med. 2007; 357(17):1731-43.

52. Nilsen EM, Jahnsen FL, Lundin KE, Johansen FE, Fausa O, Sollid LM, et al. Gluten induces an intestinal cytokine response strongly dominated by interferon gamma in patients with celiac disease. Gastroenterology. 1998;115(3):551-63.

53. National Institute for Health (NIH) Consensus Development Conference on Celiac Disease. NIH Consens State Sci Statements 2004;21(1):1-23.

54. Assiri A, Saeed A, AlSarkhy A, El Mouzan MI, El Matary W. Celiac disease presenting as rickets in Saudi children. Ann Saudi Med. 2013;33(1):49-51.

55. Thalayasingam B. Coeliac disease as a cause of osteomalacia and rickets in the Asian immigrant population. Br Med J (Clin Res Ed) 1985;290(6475):1146-7.

56. Cacciari E, Salardi S, Volta U, Biasco G, Lazzari R, Corazza GR, et al. Can antigliadin antibody detect symptomless coeliac disease in children with short stature? Lancet. 1985;1(8444):1469-71.

57. Dewar DH, Ciclitira PJ. Clinical features and diagnosis of celiac disease. Gastroenterology. 2005;128(4 Suppl 1):S19-24.

58. Ludvigsson JF, Leffler DA, Bai JC, Biagi F, Fasano A, Green PH, et al. The Oslo definitions for coeliac disease and related terms. Gut. 2013;62(1):43-52.

59. Mangiavillano B, Masci E, Parma B, Barera G, Viaggi P, Albarello L, et al. Bulb biopsies for the diagnosis of celiac disease in pediatric patients. Gastrointestinal endoscopy 2010;72(3):564-68.

60. Gonzalez S, Gupta A, Cheng J, Tennyson C, Lewis SK, Bhagat G, et al. Prospective study of the role of duodenal bulb biopsies in the diagnosis of celiac disease. Gastrointest Endosc. 2010;72(4):758-65.

61. Corazza GR, Villanacci V, Zambelli C, Milione M, Luinetti O, Vindigni C, et al. Comparison of the interobserver reproducibility with different histologic criteria used in celiac disease. Clin Gastroenterol Hepatol. 2007;5(7):838-43.

62. Oberhuber G, Granditsch G, Vogelsang H. The histopathology of coeliac disease: time for a standardized report scheme for pathologists. Eur J Gastroenterol Hepatol. 1999;11(10):1185-94.

63. Marsh MN. Gluten, major histocompatibility complex, and the small intestine. A molecular and immunobiologic approach to the spectrum of gluten sensitivity ('celiac sprue'). Gastroenterology. 1992;102(1):330-54.

64. Katz AJ, Grand RJ. All that flattens is not "sprue". Gastroenterology 1979;76(2):375-7.

65. Collin P. Should adults be screened for celiac disease? What are the benefits and harms of screening? Gastroenterology. 2005;128(4 Suppl 1):S104-8.

66. Hill ID, Dirks MH, Liptak GS, Colletti RB, Fasano A, Guandalini S, et al. Guideline for the diagnosis and treatment of celiac disease in children: recommendations of the North American Society for Pediatric Gastroenterology, Hepatology and Nutrition. J Pediatr Gastroenterol Nutr. 2005;40(1):1-19.

67. National Institute for Health and Clinical Excellence (NICE): Coeliac Disease: Recognition and Assessment of Coeliac Disease. London: National Institute for Health and Clinical Excellence, 2009.

68. George EK, Hertzberger-ten Cate R, van Suijlekom-Smit LW, von Blomberg BM, Stapel SO, van Elburg RM, et al. Juvenile chronic arthritis and coeliac disease in The Netherlands. Clin Exp Rheumatol. 1996;14(5):571-5.

69. Lepore L, Martelossi S, Pennesi M, Falcini F, Ermini ML, Ferrari R, et al. Prevalence of celiac disease in patients with juvenile chronic arthritis. J Pediatr. 1996;129(2):311-3.

70. Carnicer J, Farre C, Varea V, Vilar P, Moreno J, Artigas J. Prevalence of coeliac disease in Down's syndrome. Eur J Gastroenterol Hepatol. 2001;13(3):263-7.

71. Bonamico M, Pasquino AM, Mariani P, Danesi HM, Culasso F, Mazzanti L, et al. Prevalence and clinical picture of celiac disease in Turner syndrome. J Clin Endocrinol Metab. 2002;87(12):5495-8.

72. Giannotti A, Tiberio G, Castro M, Virgilii F, Colistro F, Ferretti F, et al. Coeliac disease in Williams syndrome. J Med Genet 2001;38(11):767-8.

73. Collin P, Syrjanen J, Partanen J, Pasternack A, Kaukinen K, Mustonen J. Celiac disease and HLA DQ in patients with IgA nephropathy. Am J Gastroenterol. 2002;97(10):2572-6.

74. Cataldo F, Lio D, Marino V, Picarelli A, Ventura A, Corazza GR. IgG(1) antiendomysium and IgG antitissue transglutaminase (anti-tTG) antibodies in coeliac patients with selective IgA deficiency. Working Groups on Celiac Disease of SIGEP and Club del Tenue. Gut. 2000;47(3):366-9.

75. Bottaro G, Cataldo F, Rotolo N, Spina M, Corazza GR. The clinical pattern of subclinical/silent celiac disease: an analysis on 1026 consecutive cases. Am J Gastroenterol. 1999;94(3):691-6.

76. Valentino R, Savastano S, Tommaselli AP, Dorato M, Scarpitta MT, Gigante M, et al. Prevalence of coeliac disease in patients with thyroid autoimmunity. Horm Res. 1999;51(3):124-7.

77. Caprai S, Vajro P, Ventura A, Sciveres M, Maggiore G. Autoimmune liver disease associated with celiac disease in childhood: a multicenter study. Clin Gastroenterol Hepatol. 2008;6(7):803-6.

78. Ermacora E, Prampolini L, Tribbia G, Pezzoli G, Gelmetti C, Cucchi G, et al. Long-term follow-up of dermatitis herpetiformis in children. J Am Acad Dermatol. 1986;15(1):24-30.

79. Hoffenberg EJ, Emery LM, Barriga KJ, Bao F, Taylor J, Eisenbarth GS, et al. Clinical features of children with screening-identified evidence of celiac disease. Pediatrics. 2004;113(5):1254-9.

80. Tosco A, Salvati VM, Auricchio R, Maglio M, Borrelli M, Coruzzo A, et al. Natural history of potential celiac disease in children. Clin Gastroenterol Hepatol. 2011;9(4):320-5; quiz e36.

81. Agarwal J, Poddar U, Yachha SK, Srivastava A. Refeeding syndrome in children in developing countries who have celiac disease. J Pediatr Gastroenterol Nutr. 2012;54(4):521-4.

82. Catassi C. Celiac crisis/refeeding syndrome combination: new mechanism for an old complication. J Pediatr Gastroenterol Nutr. 2012;54(4):442-3.

83. Whitaker JK, West J, Holmes GK, Logan RF. Patient perceptions of the burden of coeliac disease and its treatment in the UK. Aliment Pharmacol Ther. 2009;29(10):1131-6.

84. Cellier C, Delabesse E, Helmer C, Patey N, Matuchansky C, Jabri B, et al. Refractory sprue, coeliac disease, and enteropathy-associated T-cell lymphoma. French Coeliac Disease Study Group. Lancet. 2000;356(9225):203-8.

85. Rampertab SD, Forde KA, Green PH. Small bowel neoplasia in coeliac disease. Gut. 2003;52(8):1211-4.

86. Gianfrani C, Siciliano RA, Facchiano AM, Camarca A, Mazzeo MF, Costantini S, et al. Transamidation of wheat flour inhibits the response to gliadin of intestinal T cells in celiac disease. Gastroenterology. 2007;133(3):780-9.

87. Keech CL, Dromey J, Chen Z, Anderson RP, McCluskey J. 355 Immune Tolerance Induced by Peptide Immunotherapy in An HLA Dq2-Dependent Mouse Model of Gluten Immunity. Gastroenterology. 2009;136(5):A-57.

88. Brown G DJ, Marjason JK, et al. A phase 1 study to determine safety, tolerability and bioactivity of Nexvax in HLADQ2+ volunteers with celiac disease following a long-term, strict gluten-free diet. Gastroenterology. 2011;140:S437-8.

89. Paterson BM, Lammers KM, Arrieta MC, Fasano A, Meddings JB. The safety, tolerance, pharmacokinetic and pharmacodynamic effects of single doses of AT-1001 in coeliac disease subjects: a proof of concept study. Aliment Pharmacol Ther. 2007;26(5):757-66.

90. Siegel M, Khosla C. Transglutaminase 2 inhibitors and their therapeutic role in disease states. Pharmacol Ther. 2007;115(2):232-45.

91. Lindfors K, Blomqvist T, Juuti-Uusitalo K, Stenman S, Venalainen J, Maki M, et al. Live probiotic Bifidobacterium lactis bacteria inhibit the toxic effects induced by wheat gliadin in epithelial cell culture. Clin Exp Immunol. 2008;152(3):552-8.

Chapter

9

Inflammatory Bowel Disease

Boosba Vivatvakin, Palittiya Sintusek

■ INTRODUCTION

Inflammatory bowel disease (IBD) is characterized by chronic and relapsing inflammation of the gastrointestinal tract. It is classified into Crohn's disease (CD) and ulcerative colitis (UC).

CD is characterized by skip and recurrent ulcers throughout the gastrointestinal tract. These inflammatory lesions are deep and involve transmural layers of bowel causing stenosis, stricture, microperforation and fistula.

UC is characterized by recurring inflammation of the mucosal layer of the large intestine extended continuously upwards from rectum.

The genetic predisposition of IBD in many patients can demonstrate the overactive immune response to gut microbiome.[1,2] The environmental factors (e.g. infection; smoking) trigger the interaction between luminal bacteria and gut immune cells in different pathways with different clinical manifestation of IBD.[3,4]

■ INFLAMMATORY BOWEL DISEASE

The etiology of IBD is not clearly understood. Many studies have hypothesized that the main causative factors of the diseases are genetic susceptibility triggered by environmental factors, microbial factors and also immune factors. Many advanced studies have been done over the last decade to find evidence to cope with these diseases. There are four main factors associated with IBD:[5]

Genetic Susceptibility

Both CD and UC have a genetic predisposition. This concept is supported by studies about the probability of IBD existence in families and twins. For example, initial family-based linkage studies of IBD implicated the NOD2 gene in CD and the MHC region in UC for increasing susceptibility. To date, many new genes have been widely identified as shown in Table 9.1, family and twin studies about IBD in Table 9.2.

Table 9.1: Demonstration of IBD susceptibility loci[6]		
CD	Both CD and UC	UC
Cellular innate immunity	Th17	Epithelial barrier
NOD2	IL23R*	ECM1
ATG16	IL12B*	HNF4A
IRGM	STAT3*J	CDH1
LRRK2	AK2*	LAMB1
	TYK2	GNA12
Immune-mediated	Immune-mediated	Immune-mediated
PTPN22	MST1*	IFNγ/ IL26
CCR6	IL10*	IL8RA/IL8RB
IL2RA	CARD9*	IL2/IL21
IL18RAP	REL*	IL7R
IL27	PRDM1*	TNFRSF9
ERAP2	TNFSF15*	TNFRSF14
ITLN1	ICOSLG*	FCGR2A
CCL2/CCL7	IL1R2*	IRF5
TNFSF11	YDJC	LSP1
BACH2	SMAD3	
TAGAP	PTPN2	
VAMP3		
Others	Others	Others
DENNDIB	NKX2-3*	OTUD3/PLA2G2E
DNMT3A	CREM*	DAP
GCKR	C11Orf30*	PIM3
THADA	ORMDL3*	CAPN10
SP140	RTEL1*	
PRDX5	PTGER4*	
ZPF36L1	KIF21B*	
ZMIZ1	CDKAL1	
MUC1/SCAMP3	ZNF365	
CPEB4		
FADS1		
5q31 (IBD5)		
	HLA : DRB*103	

Table 9.2: Demonstration of the occurrence of genetic impact in IBD[7]
The occurrence of affected first-degree relatives in a proband with CD and UC
• First-degree relatives with CD : 2.2–13.6%
• First-degree relatives with any forms of IBD : 5.2–15.6%
• First-degree relatives with UC : 7.1–11.3%
• First-degree relatives with any forms of IBD : 8.1–13.8%
Concordance rates for CD and UC
• Monozygotic twin: both have CD 20–50%
both have UC 20–50%
• Dizygotic twin: both have CD 0–7%
both have UC 0–7%

Table 9.3: Demonstration of proinflammatory cytokines in IBD		
Cytokine	CD	UC
Innate immune response		
• IL-1ß	↑	↑
• IL-6	↑	↑
• IL-8	↑	↑
• IL-12	↑	Normal
• IL-18	↑	Normal
• IL-23	↑	Normal
• IL-27	↑	Normal
• TNFα	↑	↑
• TL1A	↑	↑
Adaptive immune response		
• IL-5	Normal	↑
• IL-13	Normal	↑
• IL-17	↑	↑
• IL-21	↑	Normal
• IL-22	↑	↑
• IFN-γ	↑	↑
• LIGHT	↑	↑
• TL1A	↑	↑

Microbial Factors

Infectious organisms causing IBD are an accepted proposition even though the etiology remains unclear. There are two hypotheses:[8]

❑ Dysbiosis of the normal flora
  • Increased mucosa-associated bacteria
  • Decreased *Faecalibacterium prausnitzii* and *Bacteroides fragilis*
❑ Pathological organisms causing inflammation and abnormal immunoregulation
  • More recently an intracellular enteric pathogen as entero-adhesive *Escherichia coli* (EAEC) and *Mycobacterium avium* subspecies *paratuberculosis* (MAP) have been described as being associated with CD, but its potential etiological role remains unclear.

Due to these hypotheses, antibiotics or probiotics usage to balance intestinal microflora may be helpful in some patients.

Immune Factors[9]

Inflammation is the most common type of reaction from offending agents. The gut is very susceptible to inflammation. When the gut has excessive physical response, it will cause chronic injury leading to anatomical and functional defects. Both cellular and molecular mechanisms induce an abnormal immune mucosal response.

The main mechanisms believed to cause IBD as described below:

❑ Primary bacterial abnormality (normal flora or/and pathologic organism) induced inflammation.
❑ Primary deficiency in microbial clearance (innate or/and adaptive immunity).
❑ Primary defect in immunoregulation that cannot control process of ongoing inflammation, including abnormalities of defensin, dendritic cell, autophagy and NOD2/CARD15 genes.

Some studies have postulated about the abnormal cytokine response in IBD. CD has T-helper cell (Th1) specific response and Th17 CD4 T-cell differentiation while UC has a predominant Th2 specific response. Then in the second step, there are no difference in cytokine responses with INFα, IL-1ß, IL-6 triumphirate and TL1A (tumor necrosis factor-like ligand). As a result, we use anti-TNFα, anti-IL6 and anti-TL1A for treatment of both CD and UC. The cytokine response in IBD is shown in Table 9.3.

Environmental Factors[9]

An explanation for the higher frequency of IBD in western countries has been attributed to the "hygiene hypothesis" which postulates that the fundamental lifestyle change from high to low microbial exposure. Exposure to fewer microbial antigens early in life has prepared to tackle challenges later on, and mounting immune response causing inability to eliminate offending agents insulting chronic inflammation.

Other environmental factors are considered as risk factors for IBD, including smoking, diet, drugs, geography and social status, increased stress, the enteric flora, altered intestinal permeability, and appendectomy.

Clinical Manifestations

CD and UC have some similar clinical settings ,but many clinical symptoms differ as in Table 9.4.[10,11] The histopathological studies also are different as in Table 9.5.[12]

Table 9.4: Comparison of CD and UC

Feature	CD	UC
Rectal bleeding	Sometimes	Common
Diarrhea, mucus, pus	Variable	Common
Abdominal pain	Common	Variable
Abdominal mass	Common	Not present
Growth failure	Common	Variable
Perianal disease	Common	Rare
Rectal involvement	Occasional	Universal
Pyoderma gangrenosum	Rare	Present
Erythema nodosum	Common	Less common
Mouth ulceration	Common	Rare
Thrombosis	Less common	Present
Colonic disease	50-75%	100%
Ileal disease	Common	Rare
Stomach-esophageal disease	More common	Chronic gastritis can be seen
Strictures	Common	Rare
Fissures	Common	Rare
Fistulas	Common	Rare
Toxic megacolon	None	Present
Sclerosing cholangitis	Less common	Present
Risk for cancer	Increased	Greatly increased
Discontinuous (skip) lesions	Common	Not present
Transmural involvement	Common	Unusual
Crypt abscesses	Less common	Common
Granulomas	Common	None
Linear ulcerations	Uncommon	Common

The clinical manifestations of CD overlap with the presentations of UC, but the diagnostic investigation can distinguish both diseases.

Crohn's Disease

Investigation[10]

Complete blood counts show anemia due to deficiencies of iron, B_{12} or folic acid. Leukocytosis, thrombocytosis relate to the inflammation. Serum ferritin correlates well with iron storage in bone marrow and low serum albumin results from malnutrition and intestinal protein loss. There are leukocytes in stool and high level of fecal calprotectin and lactoferrin reflect the severity of CD.

The serological markers of anti-Saccharomyces cerevisiae antibody (ASCA) and antibody to the outer core membrane of *E. coli* (anti-Omp-C) have high specificity to CD. ASCA can be positive 55-60% in children with CD but can be positive in 5-10% of patient with celiac disease and NSAID gastropathy.[13,15,17] Anti-Omp-C; anti-I2 and anti-CBirl flagellin antibodies have been also frequent positive in CD with fistula and stricture.[14,18,19]

Imaging Studies

The evolution of imaging studies helps clinicians to make a better decision to diagnosis and evaluate the complications of CD.

Contrast studies either air contrast or double contrast is better than single contrast study to assess mucosal details, colonic distensibility and stricture.[16]

Table 9.5: Histological features that allow the physician to distinguish among acute self-limited colitis (ASLC), ulcerative colitis (UC), and Crohn's disease (CD)[12]

ASLC Feature	UC (n=44)	ASLC vs UC (n=56)	CD (Pa)	ASLC vs CD (n=26)	UC vs CD (Pa)	(Pa)
Distorted crypt architecture	0	32	<0.00001	7	<0.005	0.01
Mixed lamina propria inflammation	0	15	<0.001	7	<0.001	NS
Villous surface	0	22	<0.00001	3	<0.047	<0.11
Granuloma	1b	3...	NS	16	<0.0017	<0.00001
Crypt atrophy	0	16	<0.0001	3	<0.048	<0.047
Basal lymphoid aggregates	0	12	<0.0011	3	NS	NS
Surface erosions	4	21	<0.0011	2	NS	<0.007
Superficial isolated giant cell	7	3	NS	0	NS	NS
Basal isolated giant cell	1	6	NS	3	NS	NS
Polymorphonuclear cells in surface epithelium	9	19	NS	3	NS	<0.04

NS = not significant

MRI can be used to assesses wall thickening, fat inflammation, abscesses or mesenteric inflammation.

Endoscopy is used to differentiate between CD and UC by pattern and area of mucosal involvement. CD is characterizes by skip lesions (areas of inflammation inter-spread with normal mucosa), "cobblestone" appearance and transmural inflammation. Video capsule endoscopy (VCE) can demonstrate the lesions located in the jejunum and proximal ileum. The significant risk of capsule retention in the strictured intestine limits the use of this investigation.[15]

Ulcerative Colitis

The typical presentations of ulcerative colitis are chronic diarrhea with blood and mucus. Furthermore, tenesmus and recurrent abdominal pain especially in the night time are also common. However up to 30% of patient with proctitis complain of hard stools.

In case of fulminant colitis fever, severe anemia, hypoalbuminemia, leukocytosis and more than 5 bloody stools per day for 5 days are present (Table 9.6). Anorexia, weight loss and delayed puberty are less common than in Crohn's disease. About 2% of ulcerative colitis patients develop primary sclerosing cholangitis. Chronic active hepatitis is also found. Erythema nodosum characterized as raised tender, erythematous nodules on extremities and pyoderma gangrenosum are found in both CD and UC. Seronegative arthritis of large joints and ankylosing spondylitis can be found. Secondary amenorrhea is common during active disease.

The pattern of clinical remission and relapse occur differently in individual patients. After treatment, only 5% of children with UC have prolonged remission. But in area of the high incidence of enteric infection, the infection may mimic a disease flare. The use of nonsteroidal anti-inflammatory drugs and stress may exacerbate the symptoms.

The risk of colon cancer occurs after 8-10 years of disease thus the patients who have had UC for more than 10 years should be under colonoscopic surveillance every year to look for mucosal dysplasia.

Despite the burden of chronic illness; most of the patients can maintain normal school and work. The disease affects the quality of life during acute flare and some children are anxious for fear of relapse. The life expectancy of the UC patient is the same as for the normal population.

Investigations

Complete blood count, liver biochemistry and stool examination and culture to find the potential cause of colitis should be done. Fecal inflammatory markers, e.g. fecal calprotection and lactoferin are done to assess disease activity and distinguish from irritable bowel syndrome (IBS).[11]

Serologic markers of pANCA (peripheral anti-nuclear antibody) and ANCA have been developed to improve the diagnosis of UC. Patients with UC have 50-80% positivity for pANCA while CD patients have 30% positivity for pANCA.[13,17]

ASCA[18] is less specific for ulcerative colitis than Crohn's disease, because ASCA appears to be related with small bowel disease. The OMP-C and anti-I12 are also found more in CD.

These serological markers can be used in the patient with "indeterminate colitis." The pANCA+, ASCA- is more common in UC compared with pANCA-, ASCA+ in CD's patient.[19]

Endoscopy[16,20]

Sigmoidoscopy with biopsy is sufficient to confirm the diagnosis and useful to start treatment. Patient with increased disease activity should not undergo colonoscopy for the risk of perforation. Total colonoscopy can be done with caution after the active disease has been controlled. The aim of colonoscopy is to distinguish CD and establish the extent of disease. Histology of terminal ileal biopsies may help to exclude other diagnoses (e.g. TB, Behcet's syndrome, lymphoma, vasculitis) as well as assess the extension of IBD.

The characteristic of UC is continuous inflammation beginning in the rectum and extending upwards. The earliest sign is loss of normal reticular pattern of rectal mucosa, mucosal edema and erythema. As the disease progress, mucosa becomes granular, friable with contact bleeding. Linear, punctate, annular or serpiginous ulcerations occurs in the later stage. Finally the ulceration pattern may turn to diffuse colitis, pseudopolyp formation and "cobble stone" appearance.

Ulcerative proctitis is the most common presentation in the adolescent and adult. It is defined as inflammation limited to the distal 15-20 cm from anal verge. The symptoms typically are bloody stool, urgency and constipation.

Left-sided colitis is also commonly found with symptoms of urgency, tenesmus, rectal bleeding and left lower quadrant abdominal pain.

Pancolitis or extensive colitis is defined as the inflammation extending to the transverse or right colon. The symptoms comprise watery diarrhea, rectal bleeding, urgency, tenesmus and diffuse abdominal pain. Weight loss and other systemic symptoms are also noted. Unlike adults, over 90% of children with UC have a pancolitis making a full length colonoscopy advisable.

Toxic megacolon is the most severe form and manifests with fever; severe abdominal cramps, abdominal distension with rebound tenderness.

The clinical severity of UC has been established by Truelove and Witts and has been widely accepted and used since 1955 with some modifications as shown in Table 9.6.[21]

Imaging Study

Barium studies have been replaced with colonoscopic biopsy to demonstrate the histopathology. In severe colitis or toxic megacolon, plain abdominal radiography can give the bowel wall outline showing the presence or absence of haustration. The sacroiliac joint and lumbosacral spine can be evaluated for sacroilitis or ankylosing spondylitis.

Computed tomography (CT) of the abdomen can demonstrate the presence of an abscess or perforation.

Magnetic resonance imaging (MRI) is the tool to show intra-abdominal abscess or other complication.

Video capsule endoscopy (VCE) can be used in indeterminate colitis to differentiate small bowel lesions in CD.

Severity of Disease

Several criteria as in Table 9.6 have been set to assess the severity of the inflammatory bowel disease, both CD and UC in regard to consider proper treatment and follow up.

Activity Index

Crohn activity index (CDAI)[22-25] as in Table 9.7 and pediatric Crohn activity index (PCDAI)[23] and modified PCDAI can be used in children and adolescents as in Table 9.8 as well as pediatric ulcerative colitis activity index (PUCAI)[26] shown in Table 9.9 is also widely used to monitor the treatment plan.

Nutritional Management[27-30]

Malnutrition is predominantly found in CD than in UC. Factors leading to malnutrition in IBD include loss of appetite, anorexia, increased caloric requirement due to hypercatabolism from inflammation, malabsorption of nutrients, loss of protein, iron, electrolytes from intestinal ulcerations and from side effects of pharmacological treatment.

The aims of treatment are treating the deficiencies and reducing the inflammation. Specific supplementation for calcium, magnesium, fat soluble vitamin B_{12} and protein especially in the patients who have ileal resection or intestinal fistula.

Ileal resection promotes the loss of bile acid and malabsorption of B_{12}. Bile acid diarrhea occurs in the early phase of bowel resection. Later in the disease course low bile salt pool can cause fat malabsorption. Cholestyramine is worsens fat absorption. Unabsorbed fatty acids enter the colon and are hydroxylated by bacteria to be hydroxylated fatty acid which stimulates colonic water and salt secretion. The treatment of fat malabsorption is to reduce

Table 9.6: Severity of UC described by Truelove and Witts compared with Werlin and Qrand[21]		
Feature	*Truelove and Witts*	*Werlin and Grand*
Bloody stools	≥ 6 per day	≥ 5 per day
Fever	Mean evening temperature ≥ 37.5° C (100° F) or higher than 37.7° C on at least 2 of 4 days at any time of the day	≥ 37.8 ° C (100° F) during the first hospital temperature
Tachycardia	Mean pulse rate ≥ 90 /min	≥ 90 /min
Anemia	Hb ≤ 10.5 g/dL	Hct ≤ 30%
Sedimentation rate	≥ 30 mm/h	-
Hypoalbuminemia	-	Serum albumin < 3.0 g/dL

Table 9.7: Crohn's disease activity index (CDAI)* [24,25]	
Variable	*Scale*
Liquid or very soft stools	Stool count summed daily for 7 days
Abdominal pain	Sum of 7 days of daily ratings as : 0 = none, 1 = mild, 2 = moderate, 3 = severe
Features of extraintestinal disease	Any of the following present during the 7 days a. Arthritis or arthralgia b. Skin or mouth lesions, including pyoderma gangrenosum, erythema nodosum, aphthous stomatitis c. Iritis or uveitis d. Anal fissure, fistula, or perirectal abscess e. Other external fistula f. Fever > 37.8°C (100°F)
Opiates for diarrhea	0 = no, 1 = yes
Abdominal mass	0 = none, 2 = questionable, 5 = definite
Hematocrit value	Males : 47 % Females: 42 %
% Body weight below standard	100 x [1-(body weight/standard weight)]

* To calculate the CDAI, the scale is multiplied by the weighting factor for each variable and then all eight weighted variables are added.

TABLE 9.8: PCDAI and modified PCDAI parameters[26]

	Items	Score
History (Recall, 1 wk)— PCDAI only	None	0
Abdominal pain	Mild—brief, does not interfere with activities	5
	Mod/severe—daily, longer lasting, affects activities, nocturnal	10
	0–1 liquid stools, no blood	0
Stools per day	Up to 2 semiformed with small blood or 2–5 liquid	5
	Gross bleeding, or 6 liquid, or nocturnal diarrhea	10
Patient functioning	Well, no limitations of activities	0
General well-being	Below par occasional difficulty in maintaining age-appropriate activities	5
	Very poor, frequent limitation of activities	10
Examination—PCDAI only		
Weight	Weight gain or voluntary weight stable/loss	0
	Involuntary weight stable, weight loss 1%–9%	5
	Weight loss 10%	10
	<1 channel decrease	0
Height (at diagnosis)	1, <2 channel decrease	5
	>2 channel decrease	10
	Height velocity 1SD	0
Height (at follow-up)	Height velocity <1SD,> 2SD	10
	Height velocity 2SD	
	No tenderness, no mass	0
Abdomen	Tenderness, or mass without tenderness	5
	Tenderness, involuntary guarding, definite mass	10
	None, asymptomatic tags	0
Perirectal disease	1–2 indolent fistula, scant drainage, no tenderness	5
	Active fistula, drainage, tenderness, or abscess	10
	Fever 38.5°C for 3 days in past week, definite arthritis, uveitis	
Erythema nodosum, Pyoderma gangrenosum		
Extraintestinal manifestations	None	0
	1	5
	≥2	10

Contd...

Contd...

Laboratory—PCDAI and mod PCDAI

Hct, %	<10y (>33),11–19F (34), 11–14M (35),15–19 M (37)	0
	<10 y (28 – 32),11–19 F(29 – 33),11–14 M (30 – 34),15–19 M (32 – 36)	2.5
	10 y (<28), 11–19 F (<29), 11–14 M (<30), 15–19 M (<32)	5
	<20	0
ESR, mm/h	20–50	2.5
	>50	5
	<3.5	0
Alb, g/dL	3.1–3.4	5
	<3.0	10
Additional laboratory—mod PCDAI only		
CRP, mg/L	<5	0
	5–10	2.5
	>10	5

PCDAI score reproduced from (1). Alb ¼ albumin; CRP ¼ C-reactive protein; ESR ¼ erythrocyte sedimentation rate; Hct ¼ hematocrit; PCDAI ¼ Pediatric Crohn Disease Activity Index. (From Turner Gastroenterology 2007;133:423–32.)

the long chain fatty acids and substitute with medium chain fatty acids. To increase the caloric density, complex carbohydrate can be added to the diet together with high peptide or high protein content.

Nutrients are rich in n-3 fatty acids or fish oil may have anti-inflammatory activity due to inhibition of prostaglandin and leukotriene synthesis.

Also MCT oil may have direct anti-inflammatory effect by modulating the expression of cytokines.

Adding prebiotics to the diet with or without probiotics may promote butyrate formation. Colonic butyrates serve to activate anti-inflammatory nuclear transcription factor NF-Kapppa B.

Enteral feeding with modular semielemental or elemental diet via nasogastric or nasojejunal tube improves the nutritioinal deficiencies especially in the anorexic patient. Studies in adults show the beneficial effect on nutritioinal treatment in reducing disease activity and reduction of mesalamine and steroid dosage.

Pharmacological Treatment of IBD

5-Aminosalicylic Acid Compound (ASA)[31-34]

The approach of free 5-ASA to the site of inflammation depend on the dissolving of 5-ASA granules which are pH dependent. Asacol granules dissolve at pH > 7 and release 5-ASA primarily in the colon and terminal ileum. Pentasa,

5-ASA in cellulose coated released 5-ASA at pH > 6, so 35% of 5-ASA are released in the small intestine and may be useful in small intestinal CD. But the release in small intestine may increase absorption, therefore it may increase toxicity even though there is no report of toxicity in humans.

Table 9.9: Pediatric ulcerative colitis activity index (PUCAI)[26]		
	Items	*Points*
Abdominal pain:	No pain	0
	Pain can be ignored	5
	Pain cannot be ignored	10
Rectal bleeding	None	0
	Small amount only, in less than 50% of stools	10
	Small amount with most stools	20
	Large amount (50% of the stool content)	30
Stool consistency of most stools	Formed	0
	Partially formed	5
	Completely unformed	10
Number of stools per 24 hours	0–2	0
	3–5	5
	6–8	10
	>8	15
Nocturnal stools (any episode causing wakening)	No	0
	Yes	10
Activity level	No limitation of activity	0
	Occasional limitation of activity	5
	Severe restricted activity	10
Sum of PUCAI		**(0–85)**

The study indicates the good correlation of PUCAI and treatment decision making .The cut off score for remission is 10 points, more than 30 points is moderate disease and more than 65 points is severe disease (from Turner, Gastroenterology. 2007;133:423-32.)

The incidence of side effects is lower when administration of 5-ASA by oral or rectal route adjunct with sulfapyridine (as sulfasalazine). The actions of sulfasalazine and 5-ASA are inhibition of 5-lipoxygenase, and as a free radical scavenger being important in prevention of neutrophil-induced epithelial damage in IBD. Also sulfasalazine blocks NF-kB activatived by TNF-a and lipopolysaccharide where 5-ASA is ineffective.

The side effects of sulfasalazine are dose related toxicity and hypersensitivity.

5-ASA compounds can successfully treat mild to moderate acute UC as a single agent. The success rate depends on the dose given (4–8 g/day). To lower the toxicity the dose should be gradually increased. The clinical response often occurs after 2–4 weeks. In moderate to severe UC, combination of steroid and 5-ASA compounds have a better response of colitis. After the steroid has been tapered off, the patient must continue treatment with 5-ASA for the maintenance therapy.

The dose of 5-ASA to prevent relapsing in UC is also dose-response effect. If the patient is able to tolerate the high dose without any adverse effects, a higher dose is recommended for maintenance therapy.

Dosage for children older than 2 years is 25–40 mg/kg/day, which can be increased gradually to 75 mg/kg/day and the maintenance dose is 20 mg/kg/day.

(Folate deficiency should be considered when sulfasalazine has been used for long term).

Corticosteroid[28,34,41]

Steroids are highly effective in suppressing inflammation both in UC and CD. Corticosteroids block vascular proliferation, fibroblast activation, collagen deposition, neutrophil migration and cytokine production.

Oral prednisolone dose for induction is 1–2 mg/kg/day and the response usually occurs within 2 weeks.

Corticosteroid enemas are suitable to treat left-sided colitis. The clinical response and remission is 92% after 7 weeks of oral prednisolone in a dose of 1 mg/kg/day, although the endoscopic remission has a lower rate.

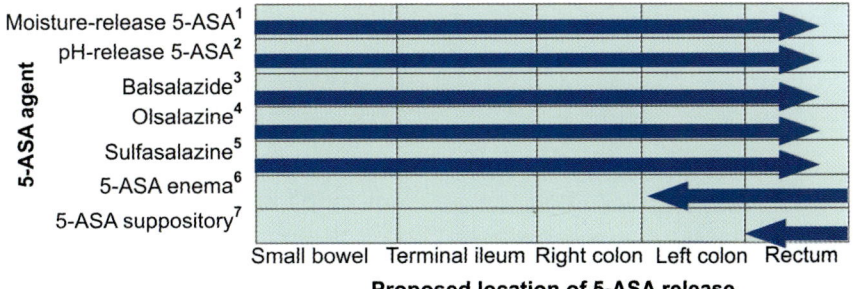

Fig. 9.1: Proposed location of release of 5-aminosalicylate (5-ASA; mesalamine) preparations 32 available in the United States. 1, Pentasa; 2, Asacol or Lialda, 3, Colazal; 4, Dipentum; 5, Azulfidine; 6, Rowasa; 7, Canasa

The parameters to monitor disease activity are pediatric Crohn disease index (PCDAI) or fecal calprotection and lactoferin.

The side effects of corticosteroids are dose dependent and the risk depends on plasma protein binding (hypoalbuminuria has higher risk). Gastric acid suppression with proton pump inhibitors (e.g. Omeprazole) may be required in the presence of gastritis.

With medical management, most children achieve remission within 3 months; however, 5–10% continue to have symptoms unresponsive to treatment beyond 6 months. Many children with disease requiring frequent corticosteroid therapy are started on immunomodulators such as azathioprine (2.0–2.5 mg/kg/day) or 6-mercaptopurine (1–1.5 mg/kg/day).

Immunomodulators

Azathioprine[36-37]

Azathioprine is a prodrug that is non-enzymatically converted to 6-MP. Because of its delay in efficacy, 6-mercaptopurine (6-MP) and azathioprine (AZA) are not used for induction of remission; however, they are often used in conjunction with corticosteroids or other therapy used to induce remission with the knowledge that by the time corticosteroids are weaned, 6-MP and AZA will be effective in maintaining remission. AZA also has a role in the maintenance of remission in moderate to severe pediatric UC. Azathioprine and 6-MP induce leukopenia in a dose-dependent manner, and patients who became leukopenic are more likely to go into remission. The patient is considered to be in remission induced by 6-MP or azathioprine if the disease activity does not flare as steroids are withdrawn. If the activity flares as steroids are withdrawn, the patient is considered to have failed to respond to 6-MP or azathioprine and the drug is withdrawn.

Methotrexate[37-40]

Methotrexate is another immunomodulator that has been used in IBD. Patients who achieve remission on methotrexate are likely to remain in remission on a low dose. But oral methotrexate is not effective as the parenteral route. Also methotrexate has a high incidence of side effects, including nausea, bone marrow suppression, and hepatic toxicity.

Cyclosporine: In children with steroid-refractory UC, intravenous or oral cyclosporine therapy has also successfully induced remission. Tacrolimus can also be used to induce remission in steroid refractory UC.

Antibiotics[15,16]

Intercurrent infections are thought to induce relapses by altering the colonic flora and thus altering the relationship between the mucosal immune system and the antigens in the lumen. For patients with ulcerative colitis with enteric infections, it is important to determine if the patient has only an enteric infection or an enteric infection plus a flare of UC. Antibiotics are typically used in perianal or enterocutaneous fistulas seen in CD, although there is little published literature regarding the topic. One study showed a benefit of combined therapy with metronidazole and ciprofloxacin in patients, who had perianal disease and received azathioprine. The dosage of metronidazole (7.5 mg/kg/dose tds) +/- Ciprofloxacin (5 mg/kg/dose twice daily) for perianal disease.

Biological Drugs[41-50]

Therapy with infliximab (chimeric monoclonal anti–tumor necrosis factor-α antibody) has resulted in clinical improvement in adults and children with UC.[41] In a larger, randomized, double-blind, placebo-controlled study of 43 adults with moderately active, glucocorticoid-resistant UC, there was no significant difference in remission rate or sigmoidoscopic score between the group treated with infliximab (5 mg/kg/dose at week 0 and 2) and the placebo group. Given the risk of infusion reactions, anti-nuclear antibody formation, and opportunistic infections and the unclear therapeutic benefit, the role of infliximab in the treatment of UC in children should be cautiously considered.

Surgery[51-54]

Surgery is indicated in patients with toxic megacolon, intractable UC unresponsive to medical treatment and intestinal fistula. Colectomy is the most common surgery to control intractable disease, complications of therapy, and fulminant disease. Parenteral nutrition is used to prepare patients for surgery when medical management fails.[55,56]

In UC total colectomy is the optimal approach to combine colectomy with an endorectal pull-through, which reserve a segment of distal rectum. The distal ileum is anastomosed with the internal anus above the rectal cuff distal to the created ileal pouch. The child can maintain the anal sphincter function and remains continence. Temporary ileostomy is done during this period to protect the anastomosis and the ileostomy is closed after several months. The ileostomy is usually closed within several months, restoring bowel continuity. The major complication of surgery[57] is *pouchitis* presented with bloody diarrhea and abdominal pain with low-grade fever. Pouchitis is seen in 30–40% of patients who have UC and responded well with antibiotics such as oral metronidazole or ciprofloxacin. Otherwise several probiotics have also been shown to the occurence of pouchitis. In CD, although bowel resection for the intestinal obstruction is to be done, the recurrence rate after bowel resection is high (>50% by 5 year).

Other Support

Psychological[22,58-61] support for the child with IBD is strongly needed because of the sense of being different, disfigured body appearance due to steroid therapy and ileostomy, limitation from age-appropriate activities, and family conflict of the burden of long-term disease. Social support and individual psychologic counseling are important in the adjustment to a difficult problem at any age.

REFERENCES

1. Shih DQ, Targan SR, McBovern D. Recent advances in IBD pathogenesis: genetics and immunobiology. Curr Gastroenterol Rep. 2008;10:568-75.
2. Kugathasan S, Amre D. Inflammatory bowel disease-environmental modification and genetic determinants. Pediatr Clin North Am. 2006;53:727-49.
3. Griffiths AM. Specificities of inflammatory bowel disease in childhood. Best Pract Res Clin Gastroenterolo. 2004;18:509-23.
4. Inflammatory bowel disease in Nelson Textbook of Pediatrics 19th Ed. In: Kliegman RM, Stanton BF, St. Game JW, Schor NF, Behrman RE (Eds). Elsevier Saunders 2011; United State: pp.1294-304.
5. Scherr R, Kugathasan S. Inflammatory bowel disease. In: Bishop WP (Ed). Pediatric practice gastroenterology. McGrawHill Medical: China. 2010;233-35.
6. C W Lees, J C Barrett, M Parkes, et al. New IBD genetics: common pathways with other diseases. Gut. 2011;60:1739-53.
7. Leena Halme, Paulina Paavola-Sakki, Ulla Turunen, et al. Family and twin studies in inflammatory bowel disease. World J Gastroenterol. 2006;12(23):3668-72.
8. Chassaing B, Darfeuille-Michaud A. The commensal microbiota and enteropathogens in the pathogenesis of inflammatory bowel disease. Gastroenterology. 2011;140:1720-28.
9. Lees CW, Barrett JC, Parkes M, et al. New IBD genetics: common pathways with other diseases. Gut. 2011;60:1739-53.
10. McCauley JL, Andrey MT. Genetics in diagnosing and managing inflammatory bowel disease. Gastroenterol Clin N Am. 2012;41:513-22.
11. Osterman MT, Lichtenstein GR. Ulcerative colitis in Sleisanger and Fordtrans's Gastrointestinal and Liver Disease, pathophysiology/diagnosis/management. 9th Ed. Feldman M, Friadman LS, Brandt LS (Eds). Saunders Elsevier. 2010. Canada. pp.1975-2015.
12. Surawicz CM, Belic L. Rectal biopsy helps to distinguish acute self-limited colitis from idiopathic inflammatory bowel disease. Gastroenterology. 1984;86:104.
13. Hoffenberg EJ, Fidanza S, Sauala A. Serologic testing for IBD. J Pediatr. 1999;130:447-52.
14. Mow WS, Vasilauskas EA, Lin YC et al. Associations of antibody responses to microbial antigens and complications of small bowel Crohn disease. Gastroenterology. 2004;126:414-24.
15. Hyam JS. Inflammatory bowel disease. Nelson's Textbook of Pediatrics. 18th Ed. pp.1579-80.
16. Griffiths AM, Hugot JP. Crohn's disease. In: Kleinman RE, Sanderseon IR, Goulet O, Sherman PM, Miele-Vergani G, Schneider BL (Eds). Walker's pediatric gastrointestinal disease, physiology, diagnosis, management. 5th ed. Hamilto: BC Decker. 2008 p.545-57.
17. Ruemmele FM, Targan SR, Levy G, et al. Diagnostic accuracy of serological assays in pediatric inflammatory bowel disease. Gastroenterology. 1998;115:822-9.
18. Dubinsky MC, Ofman JJ, Urman M, et al. Clinical utility of serodiagnostic testing in suspected pediatric inflammatory bowel disease. Am J Gastroenterol. 2001;96:758-65.
19. Peeters M, Joossens S, Vermeire S, et al. Diagnostic value of anti-Saccharomyces cerevisiae and antineutrophil cytoplasmic auto-antibodies in inflammatory bowel disease. Am J Gastroenterol. 2001;96:730.
20. Auvin S, Molinie F, Gower-Rousseau C, et al. Incidence, clinical presentation and location at diagnosis of pediatric inflammatory bowel disease: a prospective population-based study in northern France (1988–1999). J Pediatr Gastroenterol Nutr. 2005;41:49.184.
21. Truelove SC, Witts LJ. Cortisone in ulcerative colitis; final report on a therapeutic trial. BMJ. 1955;2(4947):1041.
22. Kim SC, Ferry GD. Inflammatory bowel diseases in pediatric and adolescent patients: clinical, therapeutic, and psychosocial considerations. Gastroenterology. 2004;126:1550.
23. Leach ST, Nahidi L, Tilakaratne S, Day AS, Lemberg DA. Development and Assessment of a Modified Pediatric Crohn Disease Activity Index J Pediatr Gastroenterol Nutr. 2010;51:232-6.
24. Best WR, Becktel JM. Singleton JW, et al. Development of a Crohn's disease activity index. National Cooperative Crohn's Disease Study Gastroenterology. 1976;70:439-44.
25. Best WR, Becktel JM, Singleton JW. Rederived values of the eight coeffits of the Crohn 's disease Acitivty Index (CDAI). Gastroenterology. 1979;77:83-6.
26. Turner D, Otley AR, Mack D, et al. Development, validation, and evaluation of a pediatric ulcerative colitis activity index: a prospective multicenter study. Gastroenterology. 2007;133:423-32.
27. Zachos M, Tondeur M, Griffiths AM. Enteral nutritional therapy for induction of remission in Crohn's disease. Cochrane Database Syst Rev. 2007;(1):CD000542. DOI: 10.1002/14651858.
28. Borrelli O, Cordischi L, Cirulli M, et al. Polymeric diet alone versus corticosteroids in the treatment of active pediatric Crohn's disease: a randomized controlled open-label trial. Clin Gastroenterol Hepatol. 2006;4:744-53.
29. Takagi S, Utsunomiya K, Kuriyama S, et al. Effectiveness of an 'half elemental diet' as maintenance therapy for Crohn's disease: a randomized-controlled trial. Aliment Pharmacol Ther. 2006;24:1333-40.

30. Akobeng AK, Thomas AG. Enteral nutrition for maintenance of remission in Crohn's disease. Cochrane Database Syst Rev 2007;(3):CD005984. DOI: 10.1002/14651858.

31. Sutherland L, Macdonald JK. Oral 5-aminosalicylic acid for induction of remission in ulcerative colitis. Cochrane Database Syst Rev (Online). 2006:CD000543.

32. Harrell LE, Hanauer SB. Mesalamine derivatives in the treatment of Crohn's disease. Gastroenterol Clin North Am. 2004;33:303.

33. Akobeng AK, Gardener E. Oral 5-aminosalicylic acid for maintenance of medically-induced remission in Crohn's Disease. Cochrane Database Syst Rev (Online). 2005:CD003715.

34. Griffiths A, Koletzko S, Sylvester F, et al. Slow-release 5-aminosalicylic acid therapy in children with small intestinal Crohn's disease. J Pediatr Gastroenterol Nutr. 1993;17:186-92.

35. Markowitz J, Grancher K, Kohn N, et al. A multicenter trial of 6- mercaptopurine and prednisone in children with newly diagnosed Crohn's disease. Gastroenterology. 2000;119:895.

36. Thomsen OO, Cortot A, Jewell D, et al. A comparison of budesonide and mesalamine for active Crohn's disease. International Budesonide-Mesalamine Study Group. N Engl J Med. 1998;339:370.

37. Ramakrishna J, Langhans N, Calenda K, et al. Combined use of cyclosporine and azathioprine or 6-mercaptopurine in pediatric inflammatory bowel disease. J Pediatr Gastroenterol Nutr. 1996;22:296-302.

38. Ei-Matary W, Vandermeer B, Griffiths AM. Methotrexate for maintenance of remission in ulcerative colitis. Cochrane Database Syst Rev. 2009;(3):CD007560. DOI:10.1002/14651858.

39. Ravikumara M, Hinsberger A, Spray CH. Role of methotrexate in the management of CD . J Pediatr Gastroenterol Nutr. 2007;44:427-30.

40. Bebb JR, Scott BB. How effective are the usual treatments for ulcerative colitis? Aliment Pharmacol Ther. 2004;20:143.

41. Rizzello F, Gionchetti P, D'Arienzo A, Mangusto F, Di Mateo G, Annesse V, et al. Oral beclomaethasone dipropionate in the treatment of acute ulcerative colitis: a double blind placebo controlled study. Aliment Pharmacol Ther. 2002;16:1109-16.

42. Su C, Salzberg BA, Lewis JD, et al. Efficacy of anti-tumor necrosis factor therapy in patients with ulcerative colitis. Am J Gastroenterol. 2002;97:2577-84.

43. Chey WY, Hussain A, Ryan C, et al. Infliximab for refractory ulcerative colitis. Am J Gastroenterol. 2001;96:2373-81.

44. Ahluwalia JP Immunotherapy in inflammatory bowel disease Med Clin N Am. 2012;96:525-44.

45. Hyams JS, Lerer T, Griffiths A. Long-term outcome of maintenance infliximab therapy in children with Crohn's disease. Inflammatory Bowel Dis. 2009;15:816-22.

46. Baldassano R, Braegger CP, Escher JC, et al. Infliximab (remicade) therapy in the treatment of paediatric CD. Am J Gastroenterology. 2003;98(4):833-8.

47. Markowitz J, Grancher K, Kohn N. Daum F. Immunomodulatory therapy for pediatric inflammatory bowel disease: changing patterns of use, 1990 –2000. Am J Gastroenterol. 2002;97:928.

48. Borrelli O, Bascietto C, Viola F, et al. Infliximab heals intestinal inflammatory lesions and restores growth in children with Crohn's disease. Dig Liver Dis. 2004;36:342-7.

49. Hyams J, Crandall W, Kugathasan S, Griffiths A, Olson A, Johanns J, et al. Induction and maintenance infliximab therapy for the treatment of moderate-to-severe Crohn's disease in children. Gastroenterology. 2007;132:863-73.

50. Hogenauer C, Wenzl HH, Hinterleitner TA, Petritsch W. Effect of oral tacrolimus (FK 506) on steroid-refractory moderate/severe ulcerative colitis. Aliment Pharmacol Ther. 2003;18:415.

51. Jacobstein DA, Mamula P, Markowitz JE, et al. Predictors of immunomodulator use as early therapy in pediatric Crohn's disease. J Clin Gastroenterol. 2006;40:145.

52. Ba'ath ME, Mahamalat MW, Kapur P, Smith NP, Dalzell AM, Casson DH, et al. Surgical management of inflammatory bowel disease. Arch Dis Child. 2007;92:312-6.

53. Polle SW, Slors JFM, Weverling GJ, Gouma DJ, Hommes DW, Bemelman WA. Recurrence after segmental resection for colonic Crohn's disease. Br J Surg. 2005;92:1143-9.

54. Bach SP, Mortensen NJ. Revolution and evolution: 30 years of ileoanal pouch surgery. Inflamm Bowel Dis. 2006;12:131-45.

55. Telander RL, Spencer M, Perrault J, et al. Long-term follow-up of the ileoanal anastomosis in children and young adults. Surgery. 1990;108:717.

56. Newby EA, Sawczenko A, Thomas AG, Wilson D. Interventions for growth failure in childhood Crohn's disease. Cochrane Database Syst Rev. 2005;CD003873.

57. Wesson DE, Shandling B. Results of bowel resection for Crohn's disease in the young, J Pediatr Surg. 1981;16:449.

58. Farmer RG, Hawk WA, Turnbull RB Jr. Clinical pattern in Crohn's disease : a statistical study of 615 cases. Gastroenterology. 1975;68:627.

59. Mawdsley JE, Rampton DS. Psychological stress in IBD: new insights into pathogenic and therapeutic implications. Gut. 2005;54:1481.

60. Maunder RG. Evidence that stress contributes to inflammatory bowel disease: evaluation, synthesis, and future directions. Inflammatory bowel diseases. 2005;11:600.

61. Mardini HE, Kip KE, Wilson JW. Crohn's disease: a two-year prospective study of the association between psychological distress and disease activity. Dig Dis Sci. 2004;49:492.

Chapter 10

Disorders of the Pancreas

A Riyaz

The pancreas is a retroperitoneal organ with four parts:
- Head, including uncinate process
- Neck
- Body
- Tail

The middle part of the body of the pancreas is pushed anteriorly by the bodies of L1 and L2 vertebrae and, therefore, lies closest to the anterior abdominal wall. Because of its prominence and restricted mobility in this region, this area of the pancreas is most vulnerable to blunt abdominal trauma.

The bodies of the first and second lumbar vertebrae push the middle part of the body of the pancreas anteriorly, which is thus closely related to the anterior abdominal wall. Hence, this part of the pancreas is highly vulnerable to blunt abdominal trauma due to its prominence and also limited mobility.

The pancreas has three primary functions:
- Production of a bicarbonate-rich fluid by the duct cells, which helps to neutralize gastric HCl entering the duodenum
- Synthesis of digestive enzymes, which play a very important role in digestion of complex nutrients
- Production of hormones like insulin and glucagon.

The main pancreatic duct of Wirsung extends from the tail of the pancreas to the major duodenal papilla. The sphincter of Oddi consists of circular smooth muscles that surround the common channel of the common bile duct and the main pancreatic duct at the ampulla of Vater.

The average diameter of the duct in the adult tapers from 4 mm to 2 mm, and it is widest in the head of the gland. The accessory pancreatic duct of Santorini, which is present in 40–70% of people, usually communicates with the main duct and passes transversely to the right in the upper part of the head of the pancreas. It usually opens into the proximal portion of the second part of the duodenum at the minor papilla.

The endocrine portion of the pancreas consists of about one million islets of Langerhans, which are distributed throughout the gland, but are relatively concentrated in the tail of the pancreas.

Pancreas has two ducts—the major duct of Wirsung and the accessory duct of Santorini. Most of the pancreatic secretions pass through the duct of Wirsung which joins the common bile duct to form the ampulla of Vater. It opens into the middle of the second part of duodenum through the major duodenal papilla, which is guarded by the sphincter of Oddi. Some people have an accessory pancreatic duct of Santorini which enters the duodenum more proximally at the minor papilla.

The pancreas has about 1 million islets of Langerhans scattered throughout the gland. They constitute only about 2% of the volume of the gland and are more abundant in the tail (Table 10.1).

CONGENITAL ANOMALIES

Pancreas Divisum

Pancreas divisum is the most common congenital anomaly of the pancreas, seen in 2–6% of otherwise healthy people. It results from a failure of the dorsal and ventral pancreatic ducts to fuse during the fifth and sixth weeks of gestation. Here, the ventral duct of Wirsung empties into the duodenum through the major papilla but drains only a small portion of the pancreas.

Table 10.1: Cells of islets of Langerhans		
Cells	Hormone	% of total cells
Beta cells	Insulin and amylin	70–80
Alpha cells	Glucagon	15–20
Delta cells	Somatostatin	3–10
PP cells/F cells	Pancreatic polypeptide	3–5
Epsilon cells	Ghrelin	< 1

Secretions from the tail, body, neck, and remainder of the head of the pancreas are drained into the duodenum by the duct of Santorini through the minor papilla.

Eventhough pancreas divisum may present at any age, it is usually asymptomatic in childhood. It may cause occasional postprandial epigastric pain. It may also cause severe acute pancreatitis due to a combination of pancreas divisum and stenosis at the level of the accessory papilla, with impediment of pancreatic secretory flow. Chronic pancreatitis with associated sequelae may also occur.

Endoscopic retrograde cholangiopancreatography (ERCP) is the gold standard for diagnosis of pancreas divisum. It demonstrates the reduced length and diameter of the duct of Wirsung. MR pancreatography is an emerging, noninvasive radiographic technique that helps to define ductal anatomy better.

Patients with mild symptoms can be managed conservatively, whereas those with recurrent episodes of acute pancreatitis or chronic pain require intervention to reduce accessory ductal stenosis. Surgical accessory duct sphincteroplasty is preferred in patients with recurrent episodes of acute pancreatitis.[1] Endoscopic therapy with a combination of minor duct sphincterotomy and stenting may also be tried.[2]

Annular Pancreas

This is due to the failure of complete rotation of the ventral pancreatic bud during development. Annular pancreas is a rare cause of duodenal obstruction in children and it is the most common gastrointestinal anomaly seen in Down Syndrome. Other associated anomalies include pancreas divisum, duodenal atresia, Meckel's diverticulum, malrotation of the intestine, bands, intestinal webs, tracheoesophageal fistula, imperforate anus, absence of the gallbladder, and congenital heart disease.[3] It is usually sporadic, although apparent autosomal dominant transmission has been noted.

The second part of the duodenum is completely encircled by a band of pancreatic tissue.[4] Neonates and infants develop bilious vomiting, upper abdominal distension and visible peristalsis.[5]

Upper GI bleeding, duodenal ulcer, and acute pancreatitis may be seen in older children. The stomach and duodenum may be markedly dilated resulting in a "double-bubble" sign in abdominal radiographs, which mimics duodenal atresia.

In older children, barium study may show a mid-duodenal stricture with proximal dilatation, constricting bands around the duodenum, and dilatation and reverse peristalsis of the proximal duodenum.[6] Endosonography may show a circumferential band-like structure with the same echo pattern as the pancreas, surrounding the duodenum.[7] Although ERCP, which helps to visualize the ductal system is diagnostic, CT and MRI may also help.[8]

The usual treatment is duodenoduodenostomy. If the disease presents as pancreatitis in later life, resection of the head of the pancreas is the preferable procedure. The annulus should not be divided as it may cause pancreatitis and pancreatic fistulae.

Ectopic Pancreas (Pancreatic Rests/Heterotopic Pancreas)

The term ectopic pancreas refers to segments of pancreatic tissue not in continuity with the main body of the pancreas. Seventy percent of this is found along the upper GIT, with the duodenum (27.7%), stomach (25.5%), and jejunum (15.9%) being the most frequent sites. Other intra-abdominal locations are the gallbladder, liver, small intestine, colon, appendix, omentum, and Meckel diverticulum.[9]

Treatment is required only if the child has significant symptoms or has developed complications like recurrent upper GI bleeding, and biliary or intestinal obstruction. Definitive treatment is surgical removal of the ectopic tissue. Asymptomatic subjects with incidental discovery of ectopic pancreas do not require further evaluation or treatment.[10]

GENETIC DISORDERS

Cystic Fibrosis[11]

Cystic fibrosis is one of the most common genetic diseases seen in Caucasians; it is relatively rare in our country. CF is an autosomal recessive disease, whose gene is located on 7q.

Exocrine pancreatic insufficiency is seen in almost 90% of patients with CF. It shows a distinct relationship to genotypes; 99% of patients who are homozygous for DF508 mutation and 70% of heterozygotes with other mutations have pancreatic insufficiency. The pancreas is shrunken, cystic, fibrotic and fatty. The pancreatic pathology is caused by obstruction of small ducts with thickened secretions and cellular debris. Calcification may be seen by plain X-ray or USG.

The child develops maldigestion of fats and proteins, resulting in failure to thrive. Recurrent pancreatitis is also an important complication.

Shwachman-Diamond Syndrome

Shwachman-Diamond syndrome (SDS) is the second most common inherited cause of pancreatic insufficiency in children after cystic fibrosis. This autosomal recessive disorder is due to mutations in the Shwachman-Bodian-

Diamond syndrome gene on 7q11. It is characterized by exocrine pancreatic insufficiency, hematologic abnormalities such as cyclic neutropenia, skeletal abnormalities and short stature.

The distinctive appearance of the pancreas on abdominal ultrasonography is due to pancreatic lipomatosis. CT helps to establish the diagnosis of SDS.

It causes steatorrhea and failure to thrive due to pancreatic insufficiency. A normal sweat chloride concentration or other normal measures of CFTR function distinguish SDS from CF. Pancreatic function and clinical tests of fat absorption are done serially, and pancreatic enzyme replacement therapy adjusted accordingly.

Johanson-Blizzard Syndrome (JBS)

This autosomal recessive disease is caused by mutations of the UBR1 gene. It is characterized by pancreatic exocrine insufficiency with hypoplasia of alae nasi or agenesis of the nasal cartilage. Other features include deafness, low birth weight, microcephaly, midline ectodermal scalp defects, psychomotor retardation, dwarfism, sparse dry hair and absent permanent teeth.

Endocrine abnormalities include hypothyroidism, growth hormone deficiency, diabetes, and panhypopituitarism.[12] Both JBS and SDS cause fatty replacement of the acini with relative sparing of other pancreatic structures. There is severe impairment of pancreatic enzyme secretion in both these disorders, with relative preservation of bicarbonate secretion.[13]

The treatment of pancreatic insufficiency in both conditions is similar.

Pearson's Marrow-Pancreas Syndrome

This is a rare autosomal dominant disease caused by large deletions or duplications of mitochondrial DNA. It causes refractory sideroblasticanemia and pancreatic insufficiency in infants.[14] The initial clinical presentation is with severe macrocytic anemia and lactic acidosis, which may even be fatal. The bone marrow appearance is characteristic, with severe hemosiderosis, vacuolization of bone marrow precursors and ringed sideroblasts. Ultimately, other blood cell lines may be involved. Pancreatic findings at autopsy include fibrosis rather than fatty replacement; pancreatic function testing shows abnormalities in both acinar and ductular secretions.[15]

Jeune's Syndrome (Asphyxiating Thoracic Dystrophy/Thoracic-Pelvic-Phalangeal Dystrophy)

This very rare multisystem autosomal recessive disorder, results in a constricted and narrow rib cage. It causes renal, hepatic, neurologic and retinal abnormalities as well as pancreatic insufficiency.

ACUTE PANCREATITIS

Acute pancreatitis is a disorder that can range in severity from a mild, self-limited illness in 75% to 80% of sufferers, to a potentially fatal illness with complications requiring intensive care or surgical intervention in 15% to 25% of patients. It may have a fatal outcome in approximately 1% of cases. Although pancreatitis has traditionally been considered a very rare disease in children, the diagnosis is being made more often over the past decade.

Acute pancreatitis is defined as a condition characterized by the sudden onset of abdominal pain and an increase in digestive enzymes in the blood or urine. There is varying involvement of other regional tissues or remote organ systems. The most important mechanism postulated is the premature activation of trypsinogen to trypsin within the pancreas, resulting in autodigestion of pancreas.[16]

Protective Mechanisms

❑ Prevention of trypsinogen activation in the acini
❑ Inhibition of active trypsin
❑ Destruction of trypsin
❑ Sweeping trypsin out of the pancreas
❑ Low calcium concentration, which minimizes trypsin activity
❑ Synthesis of trypsin in an inactive form (trypsinogen) with an activation site located in the target organ, which is the duodenal lumen.

Etiology

The etiology of acute pancreatitis in children is remarkably different from that in adults, in whom gallstones and alcohol are the most important causes, and include infections, trauma, drugs, systemic illnesses, and biliary disease. However, the cause is obscure in a large number of children.

Viral infections that can cause pancreatitis in children include mumps, varicella, rubella, measles, infectious mononucleosis and cytomegalovirus infection among others. Viral hepatitis and fulminant hepatitis, especially hepatitis A and B may also lead to pancreatitis.[17]

Several bacteria can cause acute pancreatitis including *Salmonella*, *Shigella*, *Campylobacter*, *Legionella*, *Leptospira*, and *Brucella* species, as well as enterohemorrhagic *Escherichia coli*.[18]

In developing countries, helminthic infections like *Ascaris lumbricoides* may result in pancreatitis.[19]

The most common systemic disease causing pancreatitis in children is hemolytic uremic syndrome. Others include sepsis, shock, collagen vascular disease, inflammatory bowel disease, Reye syndrome, Kawasaki disease and Henoch-Schonlein purpura.[20]

Although blunt accidental trauma like bicycle handlebar injury is a common cause of acute pancreatitis in children, accounting for nearly 20% of cases, child abuse should always be ruled out. It is vital to diagnose traumatic pancreatitis, as it may cause pancreatic duct transection, which may require surgical intervention.[16]

Drugs are an uncommon but important cause of acute pancreatitis (Table 10.2). Drug-induced pancreatitis can be diagnosed only after excluding other causes. There is usually an interval of 4–8 weeks between initiation of therapy and development of pancreatitis. Some drugs cause pancreatitis by a clear mechanism like inducing hypertriglyceridemia, which in turn, causes pancreatitis. Pancreatitis can be is reproduced on re-challenge with the same drug. One of the most commonly implicated drugs is valproic acid.

Atlanta Classification of Pancreatitis[21]

Based on clinical features, laboratory investigations and imaging, acute pancreatitis is classified into two types mild and severe. In the mild type, there are no complications and the child requires only symptomatic treatment. In the severe type, in which the child may develop local or systemic complications, the mortality is very high.

Clinical Presentation

The most common symptoms are upper abdominal pain and vomiting. The pain is sudden in onset, increases gradually in severity and reaches maximal intensity in a few hours. The most common site is the epigastrium,

followed by the right hypochondrium, periumbilical area, back and lower chest.

Some children may have fever, tachycardia, hypotension, jaundice, and abdominal signs like guarding, rebound tenderness, and a decrease in bowel sounds.[22] Children with severe systemic illnesses may develop feeding intolerance. Hence, pediatricians should rule out acute pancreatitis if a hospitalized child has worsening of clinical status or feeding intolerance. Jaundice or elevated transaminases should raise the possibility of biliary tract involvement. Rarely, patients present with ascites or an abdominal mass. Epigastric tenderness is a useful but nonspecific and unreliable sign.

Ecchymoses in the flanks (Grey-Turner sign) indicate retroperitoneal bleeding from hemorrhagic pancreatitis, whereas ecchymoses in the periumbilical region (Cullen sign), indicate intra-abdominal hemorrhage. These signs are seen in adults and are unusual in children (Table 10.3).

Diagnosis

As with most disease states, the most important and readily available diagnostic tools available to the clinician evaluating a patient with suspected acute pancreatitis are the clinical history and physical examination.

A high index of suspicion is essential as clinical features of acute pancreatitis are often nonspecific. The accepted clinical definition of acute pancreatitis in adults requires two of the following:
- Abdominal pain consistent with pancreatitis
- Serum amylase or lipase levels at least three times the upper limit of normal
- Radiologic evidence of pancreatitis.

Most children with acute pancreatitis will fulfil these criteria. However, many of them do not have abdominal pain.

Table 10.2: Drugs that cause pancreatitis	
• Acetaminophen overdose	• Mercaptopurine
• L-asparaginase	• Methyldopa
• Azathioprine	• Metronidazole
• Cimetidine	• Octreotide
• Carbamazepine	• Phenytoin
• Corticosteroids	• Pentamidine
• Enalapril	• Retrovirals: DDC, DDI, tenofovir
• Erythromycin	• Sulfonamides: Mesalamine, 5-aminosalicytates, sulfasalazine, trimethoprim/ sulfomethoxazole
• Estrogen	
• Furosemide	
• Isoniazid	
• Lamivudine	• Thiazides
• Lisinopril	• Vincristine

Table 10.3: Clinical features of acute pancreatitis		
	Common	*Rare*
Symptoms	Irritability in infants • Anorexia • Nausea • Vomiting • Abdominal pain	• Jaundice • Fever • Feeding Intolerance • Respiratory distress
Signs	• Dehydration • Abdominal distension • Abdominal tenderness	• Ascites • Pleural effusion • Grey-Turner sign • Cullen sign • Abdominal mass • Shock • Renal failure

Serum Lipase

Serum lipase level generally is the primary diagnostic marker for acute pancreatitis because of high sensitivity and specificity. It has become more reliable with the recent incorporation of co-lipase. Serum lipase will rise within 4 to 8 hours of onset, peak at 24 hours, and may remain elevated for 8 to 14 days before normalizing.[23] Lipase levels are more reliable indicators of pancreatitis in patients who are first seen several days after the onset of their illness.

Serum lipase estimation is more than 90% sensitive for the diagnosis of acute pancreatitis. However, in children with renal failure, renal excretion of lipase is impaired and hence serum lipase may increase up to two times above normal.[24]

Serum Amylase

Serum amylase continues to be the most common diagnostic test for pancreatitis. However, it is not very specific as amylase can be synthesized by many tissues other than pancreas, like salivary glands and fallopian tubes.

Amylase levels increase during acute pancreatitis due to leakage from the inflamed pancreas into the bloodstream and from decreased renal excretion. Serum amylase levels will rise within 2 to 12 hours of onset of pancreatitis, peak within the first 48 hours, and remain elevated for 3 to 5 days before returning to baseline. Hyperamylasemia is a very sensitive diagnostic test for pancreatitis, but its specificity is generally poor. Although many disorders cause mild to moderate hyperamylasemia, an amylase level > three times above normal is highly specific for pancreatitis.

Delay in presentation can result in missing the amylase peak and is one scenario in which AP may be diagnosed with a normal amylase. In comparison, most patients will have a selective elevation of either amylase or lipase at presentation. Hence ideally, both amylase and lipase should be measured in patients with suspected acute pancreatitis.[25]

Some drugs may cause low levels of amylase and lipase. These are given in Table 10.4.

An increase in the serum ALT level by three-fold or more suggests a biliary origin of acute pancreatitis. The combination of elevated amylase/lipase and ALT may be more predictive of pancreatitis than elevated amylase or lipase alone.

A fasting triglyceride value of >1,000 mg/dL or a persistent increase after the attack has resolved suggests hyperlipidemia as the cause rather than the effect of acute pancreatitis.

Several diseases other than pancreatitis can cause increased levels of amylase. These are given in Table 10.5.

It is essential to differentiate acute biliary pancreatitis from pancreatitis due to nonbiliary etiologies, as the former may require urgent ERCP, with biliary sphincterotomy and stone extraction. An elevated ALT leads to a suspicion of biliary pancreatitis. Fortunately, such cases are rare in children.

Other laboratory abnormalities that may occur in acute pancreatitis include leukocytosis, hyperglycemia, glucosuria, hypocalcemia, elevated γ-glutamyltranspeptidase, coagulopathy and hyperbilirubinemia.

A high hematocrit is an indicator of the severity of pancreatitis. It is secondary to hemoconcentration, which in turn, correlates with hypovolemia, reduced pancreatic perfusion, and higher risk of necrosis and organ failure.

The TAP (trypsinogen activation peptide) assay is an indirect measure of the amount of active trypsin. From a pathophysiological standpoint, this is an elegant measure

Table 10.4: Causes of low serum amylase and lipase values

Amylase	Lipase
• Citrates	• Calcium ions
• Oxalate	• Hydroxyurea
• Saquinavir	• Protamine
• Hypertriglyceridemia	• Somatostatin
	• 5-Aminosalicylates

Table 10.5: Non-pancreatitic causes of hyperamylasemia[26]

Diseases	Etiology	Differentiating features
Parotitis (mumps, *Staph aureus*, CMV, HIV, Epstein-Barr virus)	Salivary amylase increases because of inflammation of the salivary glands	Determination of isoenzymes and normal serum lipase help in the differentiation
Renal failure	Serum amylase increases due to decreased renal clearance	An amylase level >3 times normal is relatively specific for pancreatitis even in the presence of renal failure
Esophageal perforation	Extraesophageal leakage of salivary amylase	Hyperamylasemia may be a valuable clue to esophageal perforation
Macroamylasemia	IgA bound amylase is too large to be excreted by the kidneys	Amylase-to-creatinine renal clearance is <1% due to poor renal clearance of macroamylase
Pregnancy	Only mild rise of serum amylase in pregnancy	An amylase level >3 times normal is S/O pancreatitis in pregnancy also

of severity; the more the trypsin activation, the more the pancreatic damage. Rapid measurement of urinary trypsinogen-2 and urinary trypsinogen activating peptide is useful in the emergency department as a screening test for acute pancreatitis in patients with abdominal pain; a negative dipstick test rules out acute pancreatitis with a high degree of probability, whereas a positive test should prompt further evaluation.[27]

Blood urea nitrogen (BUN) is increased because of dehydration. Serial BUN measurements are the most valuable laboratory test for predicting mortality during the initial 48 hours.

Hyperglycemia in a previously normal patient correlates well with the degree of pancreatic malfunction and may be related to increased release of glycogen, catecholamines, and glucocorticoids and to decreased release of insulin.

Plain erect radiographs of the chest and abdomen are not diagnostic of acute pancreatitis, but are useful in ruling out other possibilities considered in the differential diagnosis (Table 10.6).

Role of Imaging

Abdominal ultrasonography and CT scans help to document pancreatitis, determine the severity and identify complications like pseudocysts. They also help in the diagnosis of any underlying chronic pancreatitis.

USG Findings

These include:
- Enlargement and altered echogenicity of the pancreas
- Dilated main pancreatic duct, common bile duct and intrahepatic bile ducts

- Gallstones
- Biliary sludge
- Pancreatic calcification
- Choledochal cysts
- Fluid collections—peripancreatic or cystic.

A CT scan will show similar findings. However, CT is usually done several days into a severe course of acute pancreatitis, when the patient fails to improve. CT contrast given early in the course of acute pancreatitis may diminish the already compromised blood flow to ischemic areas of the pancreas and thereby aggravate necrosis. Hence, most experts are of the opinion that a CT scan is not indicated in the early phase of acute pancreatitis.[16] The severity of pancreatitis detected on CT may be staged according to the Balthazar criteria.[28]

Nonstandard Imaging Tests

MRI has had limited application for diagnostic imaging of acute pancreatitis because it is more cumbersome and more expensive than CT. It is useful in pregnancy (because of the radiation teratogenicity of CT), those who are allergic to the contrast used for enhanced CT, and those who have renal insufficiency, that can be exacerbated by the iodinated contrast required for CT. It may prove to be superior to CT in the characterization of pancreatic fluid collections.

Magnetic resonance cholangiopancreatography (MRCP) delineates the bile and pancreatic ducts better than CT, and has a higher sensitivity in detecting choledocholithiasis, with up to 90% sensitivity and 95% specificity in a recent meta-analysis.[29] MRCP is used currently to detect choledocholithiasis before therapeutic ERCP (Table 10.7).

There is limited experience with ERCP in Indian children. In a study in 2004 on 70 children with pancreatitis, ERCP was useful in 17 out of 24 children for removing stones, dilating ductal strictures and placing stents for drainage and relieving pain.[30]

In contrast to trans-abdominal ultrasonography, endoscopic ultrasonography (EUS) picks up gallstones or

Table 10.6: Roentgenography

Chest radiographs	Abdominal radiographs
• Atelectasis • Basilar infiltrates • Elevation of the hemi-diaphragm • Left-sided pleural effusion (rarely right) • Pericardial effusion • Pulmonary edema • A diffuse alveolar interstitial shadowing may suggest acute respiratory distress syndrome	• A sentinel loop (an isolated dilated loop of small bowel overlying the pancreas) • Air in the right and transverse colon that abruptly terminates at the splenic flexure (colon cutoff sign) • Ileus • Pancreatic calcification (in recurrent pancreatitis) • Blurring of the left psoas margin • Pseudocyst • Diffuse abdominal haziness (ascites) • Peripancreatic extraluminal gas bubbles

Table 10.7: MRCP vs CT scan in pancreatitis

	MRCP	CT scan
Cost	More expensive	Cheaper
Pregnancy	Can be done	Contraindicated
Renal failure	Safe	Contrast enhanced CT contraindicated in renal failure
Detection of choledocholithiasis	High sensitivity and specificity	Poor sensitivity and specificity

sludge within the gallbladder and extrahepatic bile duct, regardless of obesity or gas.

EUS helps to detect additional abnormalities, such as pancreas divisum which may not be apparent with other imaging modalities.[31] However, there is limited experience with EUS in children.

Both sterile and infected acute necrotizing pancreatitis may cause fever, leukocytosis, and severe abdominal pain. Hence, it is difficult to distinguish between them. However, the distinction is important because without intervention, the mortality rate for patients with infected acute necrotizing pancreatitis is nearly 100%. CT-guided fine-needle aspiration and culture of pancreatic and peri-pancreatic tissue fluid help to identify the organism and to start appropriate antimicrobials. USG-guided aspiration has a lower sensitivity and specificity, but the advantage is that it can be performed at the bed side itself.

The bacteriologic status of the pancreas may be determined with CT-guided fine-needle aspiration of pancreatic and peri-pancreatic tissue or fluid. USG-guided aspiration may have a lower sensitivity and specificity, but it can be performed at the bedside.

Medical Management of Acute Pancreatitis

Treatment consists of supportive care to provide adequate intravenous hydration, to control pain, and to monitor for complications. Pancreatic rest or nothing by mouth is still practiced, but its use should be limited.

All children should be carefully monitored for any signs of early organ failure such as hypotension and pulmonary or renal insufficiency by close following of vital signs and urinary output. If the child has tachypnea, blood gas measurements and oxygen supplementation are mandatory. Any child showing signs of early organ dysfunction should be immediately transferred to ICU, since deterioration can be rapid and fatal. This may be one of the most important decisions the clinician must make.

Proper analgesia and intravenous fluids are the mainstays of management. Traditionally, opiates are used because of their potency. Morphine is avoided in acute pancreatitis because it increases the sphincter of Oddi pressure. Meperidine (1 to 2 mg/kg IM/IV) is the opioid of choice because it does not raise the sphincter pressure.

Nutritional Support

Previously, starvation was considered a mainstay of care of children with acute pancreatitis. However, recent clinical and experimental evidence strongly supports the role of early feeding of patients with pancreatitis. After fluid resuscitation and pain control are implemented, enteral nutrition should start within 24 hours of admission. In children with mild acute pancreatitis, a period of fasting may not be necessary, and they can be allowed to eat and drink as tolerated. Studies have shown that in severe acute pancreatitis, early enteral nutrition through nasogastric feeding is preferred to parenteral nutrition.[32]

The child should be closely monitored for complications.[17] Full attention must be paid to fluid balances because many patients are usually kept starving, and may lose fluids from the vascular compartment from a capillary leak syndrome and "third spacing." Fluid losses are exaggerated if a nasogastric tube is used to decompress the stomach. Volume expansion early in the course of acute pancreatitis is important for cardiovascular stability. It also helps to prevent development of pancreatic necrosis.

Antibiotics are usually unnecessary, except for the most severe cases, especially if significant pancreatic necrosis is present.

Metabolic Complications

Severe pancreatitis may cause hyperglycemia initially. However, it usually normalizes as the inflammatory process subsides, and blood sugar levels fluctuate widely.

Hypoalbuminemia may lead to hypocalcemia which is asymptomatic and does not require any specific therapy. However, reduced serum ionized calcium may cause neuromuscular irritability.

Late life-threatening complications of acute pancreatitis are related to infected pancreatic necrosis and multisystem organ failure, although pancreatic necrosis appears to be uncommon in children. Judicious use of antibiotics and attention to nutrition may help limit these late complications.[20]

Local Complications

These include:

❏ Fluid collections
❏ Pancreatic necrosis (sterile or infected)
❏ Pancreatic abscess
❏ Duct rupture
❏ Duct strictures
❏ Bleeding
❏ Pseudocyst formation.

Pancreatic necrosis is a segmental pancreatic infarction, which may result in serious complications. Fortunately, it is very rare, seen in <5% of adults and <1% of children. The combination of hypovolemia, inflammation, and high hematocrit decreases pancreatic blood flow, resulting in infarction. A contrast-enhanced CT helps in the diagnosis as it shows a segment of pancreatic gland without perfusion.

Pancreatic pseudocysts are rarely seen in children. They may resolve spontaneously or may require drainage. Both endoscopic internal drainage and external drainage by interventional radiologists are available.

Abscesses can be managed with intravenous antibiotics and external drainage. Surgical drainage is usually not necessary. Traumatic rupture of the duct may require surgery or endoscopic stenting.

Surgical Management of Acute Pancreatitis

The role of surgery is usually limited to debridement of infected pancreatic necrosis. Fine-needle aspiration for bacteriology helps to differentiate infected from sterile pancreatic necrosis. Necrosectomy for severe pancreatitis is usually deferred for at least 2 weeks, to permit proper demarcation of pancreatic and peri-pancreatic necrosis to occur, and to provide the optimal operative conditions.[33] This helps to decrease the risk of bleeding. It also helps to minimize surgery-related loss of vital tissue, and thus prevents endocrine and exocrine pancreatic insufficiency following surgery.

CHRONIC PANCREATITIS

Chronic pancreatitis is a painful, destructive, inflammatory condition of the pancreas, characterized by progressive fibrosis that leads to irreversible destruction of exocrine and endocrine tissue, resulting eventually in exocrine and endocrine insufficiency.[34] Histologic changes include irregular fibrosis, acinar cell loss, islet cell loss, and inflammatory cell infiltrates.[35]

Etiology of Chronic Pancreatitis

In children, chronic pancreatitis is usually associated with genetic diseases such as CF or hereditary pancreatitis or may be idiopathic. In adults, chronic pancreatitis is usually associated with chronic alcoholism (~ 70%) or is less often idiopathic (~ 20%).

There is an increase in the incidence of chronic pancreatitis in children. This may be due to better diagnostic tools or an apparent rise in recurrent acute pancreatitis.[36]

Genetic Causes

- Hereditary pancreatitis
- *CFTR* mutations
- *SPINK1* mutations
- Cationic trypsinogen (PRSS*1*) gene mutations
- Shwachman-Bodian-Diamond syndrome gene (*SBDS*) mutations

Metabolic Causes

- Types I, II, and V hyperlipidemia
- Hypercalcemia
- Chronic renal failure

Autoimmune

- Inflammatory bowel disease–associated chronic pancreatitis
- Isolated autoimmune chronic pancreatitis
- Sjögren syndrome-associated chronic pancreatitis

Obstructive

- Pancreas divisum
- Sphincter of Oddi disorders
- Duct obstruction (tumors)

Miscellaneous

- Juvenile tropical pancreatitis
- Fibrocalculous pancreatic diabetes
- Pancreatic divisum
- Post-irradiation
- Post-ERCP
- Idiopathic

Genetic Causes of Chronic Pancreatitis

Mutations of several genes can cause chronic pancreatitis. Hereditary pancreatitis is an autosomal dominant disease associated with mutations in the trypsinogen gene PRSS1 that promote premature conversion of trypsinogen to active trypsin resulting in pancreatic autodigestion. It leads to chronic pancreatitis at a very young age. There is a high risk of developing pancreatic cancer.[37]

Mutations in SPINK1, a gene that encodes for a pancreatic trypsin inhibitor, are associated with acute and chronic pancreatitis, resulting from an impaired ability to counteract the effects of activated trypsin within pancreatic acinar cells. These patients typically develop chronic pancreatitis in childhood.[38]

SPINK1 is a gene that encodes for a pancreatic trypsin inhibitor. Mutations of this gene may result in acute and chronic pancreatitis in childhood.[38]

Severe homozygote mutations of the *CFTR* gene cause cystic fibrosis. Patients who are compound heterozygotes for mild *CFTR* gene mutations have a 40- to 80-fold increased risk of developing chronic pancreatitis compared with the general population.[39] These patients do not develop other manifestations of cystic fibrosis, such as sinopulmonary disease, and have normal sweat chloride levels.

Cystic fibrosis may be caused by severe homozygote mutations of the CFTR gene. There is a 40–80 fold increased risk of developing chronic pancreatitis compared with the general population, if a child is a compound heterozygote for mild CFTR gene mutation.[39]

Patients who are compound heterozygotes for mild *CFTR* gene mutations have a 40- to 80-fold increased risk of developing chronic pancreatitis compared with the general population.[39] These patients do not develop other manifestations of cystic fibrosis, such as sinopulmonary disease, and have normal sweat chloride levels.

Clinical Features

Pain

The most common presenting symptom of chronic pancreatitis is abdominal pain, which is usually epigastric, dull and constant and characteristically radiates to the back. A distinctive feature is the almost instantaneous aggravation of pain by food ingestion. This should always raise the suspicion of pancreatic disease. Although food ingestion may aggravate the pain of other abdominal conditions also including peptic ulcer or irritable bowel syndrome, there is usually a much greater interval between the meal and the discomfort, than in pancreatic disease.

Weight Loss

Nausea, vomiting, anorexia, and weight loss are common in chronic pancreatitis. Weight loss is secondary to decreased caloric intake, owing to fear of aggravation of the abdominal pain. Malabsorption or uncontrolled diabetes may also contribute. Such severe weight loss is relatively unusual in other painful conditions like peptic ulcer. The combination of chronic upper abdominal pain and severe loss of weight should always alert the clinician to the possibility of pancreatic disease.

Malabsorption

Malabsorption does not occur until enzyme secretion is reduced to <10% of normal and so diarrhea and steatorrhea occur relatively late in the course of chronic pancreatitis. Patients may pass bulky, formed stool, as opposed to the frank watery diarrhea observed in other conditions like celiac disease. For a given degree of steatorrhea, the absorption of fat-soluble vitamins (A, D, E, and K) is much better in pancreatic insufficiency than in celiac sprue.

Diagnosis

The diagnosis of chronic pancreatitis can be made by histologic or morphologic criteria alone or by a combination of morphologic, functional, and clinical findings.[40]

Functional abnormalities alone are not diagnostic of chronic pancreatitis because these tests do not differentiate chronic pancreatitis from pancreatic insufficiency without pancreatitis. Pancreatic insufficiency should be considered as either an end stage of destructive chronic pancreatitis or as arising from an independent condition, such as Shwachman-Diamond syndrome.[41]

Management

Treatment depends upon the stage and etiology of chronic pancreatitis. It is identical to that for acute pancreatitis during the early phases, when discrete episodes of acute pancreatitis occur.

Pain Relief

Persistent, unrelenting pain dominates the clinical symptoms in many patients. Treatment begins with acetaminophen, but most patients will require narcotics. Patient comfort must take precedence over concerns for addiction, although it is important that a side effect of chronic narcotic use is abdominal pain, the narcotic bowel syndrome.[42]

In children with intractable pain, endoscopic sphincterotomy with stent placement and nerve block therapies have been tried. The individual anatomy guides surgical approaches. If the main duct is dilated, operations aimed at drainage or decompression of the duct are performed. Patients with more severe, localized disease may benefit from partial pancreatic resection. Multiple centers now offer total pancreatectomy with islet cell auto-transplantation.

Pancreatic Insufficiency

Pancreatic enzyme supplementation has been tried in the belief that it may reduce the cholecystokinin-mediated secretion of pancreatic enzymes. The goal is to restore digestive function as much as possible. Enzyme supplementation is most effective in patients with some pancreatic function and predominantly small-duct disease. As enzymes are proteins in nature, they may be destroyed by gastric HCl. This can be tackled by the addition of a PPI to the regime. Enzymes should be taken about 15 minutes before each meal or snack. For prolonged meals, additional enzymes should also be taken during the meal. Parents and adolescent patients should be taught to adjust the enzyme dosage according to the anticipated amount of fat in a meal.

In children or young adults with CF, pancreatic enzymes are given by units of lipase/kg/meal or in units of lipase/g of fat ingested. This translates into approximately 500 to 2000 units of lipase/kg/meal, or 500 to 4000 units of lipase/g of fat. Doses exceeding 10,000 units/kg/day are not recommended, and doses in excess of 6000 units/kg/meal have been associated with colonic strictures in children below 12 years.

Another major problem is the development of diabetes through destruction of the pancreatic islet cells. Although early surgical intervention with islet cell autotransplant is a consideration in these patients, the problem of islet yield, especially if delayed until chronic pancreatitis is advanced, and long-term benefit, remain important issues without clear answers.

Endoscopic and Surgical Treatment

Exploration of the pancreatic duct and removal of stones or endoscopic papillotomy and removal of stones are useful procedures. Abdominal pain can be intractable and difficult to manage. When there is no response to medical treatment, surgical intervention may be needed.

In patients with a dilated main pancreatic duct, ductal decompression and side-to-side pancreaticojejunostomy may be performed (Puestow-Gillesby operation). In Duval's procedure, distal pancreaticojejunostomy is done. The Whipple procedure and distal pancreatectomy have been used in the past for patients with small-duct CP. Newer resection techniques like Beger procedure and Frey procedure are useful in intractable pain.

Juvenile Tropical Pancreatitis[43]

Juvenile tropical pancreatitis (JTP) is a form of chronic calcific, non-alcoholic pancreatitis prevalent almost exclusively in the developing countries of the tropical world. In India, the highest incidence is in the south eastern part of Kerala, the prevalence being 125/100000 population. The exact pathogenesis is not known, but the following factors may predispose to it: PEM, free radicals and SPINK1 gene mutations. The toxiccyanogenic glycosides like linamarin and methyl linamarin present in cassava, which is the staple diet of these people, have also been blamed.

The clinical features of JTP were aptly summarized in the 1960s and 70s as recurrent abdominal pain in childhood, diabetes mellitus and pancreatic calculi by adolescence, and death in the prime of life, due to severe malnutrition, complications of uncontrolled diabetes and carcinoma of pancreas. However, the prognosis is much better now due to improved nutrition and better control of diabetes. Diabetes which is an inevitable consequence of JTP and occurs one or two decades after the first episode of abdominal pain, is referred to as fibrocalculous pancreatic diabetes (FCPD). One of the characteristic features of FCPD is that despite requiring insulin for control, patients rarely become ketotic on withdrawal of insulin unlike type I diabetes. Carcinoma of pancreas is the most sinister complication of JTP.

Autoimmune pancreatitis is an extremely rare condition of unknown pathogenesis in children. It presents with progressive weight loss, abdominal pain and jaundice. The pancreas is enlarged and hypodense on CT. Treatment is with steroids.

TUMORS OF PANCREAS

The most common secretory pancreatic tumor in children is insulinoma, which is relatively benign. Zollinger-Ellison syndrome associated with gastrinoma, Werner-Morrison syndrome (VIPoma), and multiple endocrine neoplasia (MEN) are rare in children and are more often malignant. Glucagonomas and somatostatinomas have not been reported in children.

VIPoma (Verner-Morrison syndrome/WDHA syndrome—watery diarrhea, hypokalemia and achlorhydria) is caused by a neuroendocrine tumor of pancreas that produces vasoactive intestinal polypeptide (VIP). 75% of VIPomas are malignant, and 50% have already metastasized at the time of diagnosis. It causes massive watery diarrhea which results in hypokalemia and severe dehydration. Stool volume may exceed 3 L/day. As the stools resemble those of cholera, the term pancreatic cholera is often used.

CT and MRI help to localize the tumor. Somatostatin receptor scanning and EUS also are are also effective for imaging these tumors. The first priority of treatment is to correct the dehydration and electrolyte abnormalities especially hypokalemia. Long-acting octreotide helps to control the diarrhea.

Surgical resection is curative in approximately 30% of patients.

Multiple Endocrine Neoplasia

This is of three types:
- MEN-I (Wermer's syndrome)
- MEN-IIA (Sipple's syndrome)
- MEN-IIB

MEN-I is associated with islet cell tumors of the pancreas, hyperparathyroidism, and nonfunctional adenomas of the pituitary.

The MEN-II syndromes are not associated with pancreatic tumors, but include thyroid (medullary carcinoma) and adrenal (pheochromocytoma) tumors. MEN-IIA, or Sipple's syndrome, is distinguished by its association with parathyroid hyperplasia, and MEN-IIB is associated with multiple mucosal and alimentary tract neuromas. Each of these syndromes has autosomal dominant inheritance.

MEN-I and -IIA usually occur in adults, whereas MEN-IIB may present in childhood.

Other Tumors

Pancreatoblastomas, pancreatic adenocarcinomas, cystadenomas, and rhabdomyosarcomas are rarely encountered in children.

Pancreatic lesions in von Hippel-Lindau disease are usually benign and cystic. Cystadenomas, familial adenocarcinomas, and islet cell tumors are less common.

Frantz tumor is a papillary cystic tumor usually found in girls and young women. Typical presenting symptoms are abdominal pain, mass, or jaundice. The treatment of choice is total surgical removal.[44]

REFERENCES

1. Bradley EL, Stephan RN. Accessory duct sphincteroplasty is preferred for long-term prevention of recurrent acute pancreatitis in patients with pancreas divisum. J Am Coll Surg. 1996;183:65.
2. Lehman GA, Sherman S, Nisi R, Hawes RH. Pancreas divisum: results of minor papilla sphincterotomy. Gastrointest Endosc. 1993; 39:1.
3. Stanley P, Law BS, Young LW. Down syndrome, duodenal stenosis/annular pancreas, and a stack of coins. Am J Dis Child. 1988;142:459.
4. Sternberg A, Zelikovski A, Abu-Dalu J, Urca I. Fibromuscular annular pancreas: a variant of pancreatic malformation? Int Surg. 1978;63:170.
5. Merrill JR, Raffensperger JG. Pediatric annular pancreas: twenty years' experience. J Pediatr Surg. 1976;11:921.
6. Lieber A, Schaefer JW, Belin RP. Hypotonic duodenography: diagnosis of annular pancreas in an adult. JAMA. 1968;203:425.
7. Chen YC, Yeh CN, Tseng JH. Symptomatic adult annular pancreas. J Clin Gastroenterol. 2003;36:446.
8. Chevillotte G, Sahel J, Raillat A, Sarles H. Annular pancreas: report of one case associated with acute pancreatitis and diagnosed by endoscopic retrograde pancreatography. Dig Dis Sci. 1984;29:75.
9. Wolloch Y. Heterotopic pancreatic tissue in the gallbladder. Acta Chir Scand. 1986;152:557.
10. Rohrmann C Jr, Delaney JH Jr, Protell RL. Heterotopic pancreas diagnosed by cannulation and duct study. Am J Roentgenol. 1977;128:1044.36516.
11. Riyaz A. Cystic fibrosis. In: Riyaz A (Ed.) Pediatric gastroenterology and Hepatology. 3rd ed. Paras Publishers, Hyderabad. 2008.pp. 569-72.
12. Gershoni-Baruch R, Lerner A, Braun J, Katzir Y, Iancu TC, Benderly A. Johanson-Blizzard syndrome: Clinical spectrum and further delineation of the syndrome. Am J Med Genet. 1990;35:546.
13. Zenker M, Mayerle J, Lerch MM, Tagariello A, Zerres K, Durie PR. et al. Deficiency of UBR1, a ubiquitin ligase of the N-end rule pathway, causes pancreatic dysfunction, malformations and mental retardation (Johanson-Blizzard syndrome). Nat Genet 2005;37:1345.
14. Rotig A, Bourgeron T, Chretien D, Rustin P, Munnich A. Spectrum of mitochondrial DNA rearrangements in the Pearson marrow-pancreas syndrome. Hum Mol Genet. 1995;4:1327.
15. Durie PR. Pancreatic aspects of cystic fibrosis and other inherited causes of pancreatic dysfunction. Med Clin North Am. 2000;84:609.
16. Werlin SL, Kugathasan S, Frautschy BC. Pancreatitis in children. J Pediatr Gastroenterol Nutr. 2003;37:591-5.
17. Lerner A, Branski D, Lebenthal E. Pancreatic diseases in children. Pediatr Clin North Am. 1996;43:125-56.
18. Renner F, Nimeth C, Demmelbauer N. High frequency of concomitant pancreatitis in Salmonella enteritis. Lancet. 1991;337:1611.
19. Das S. Pancreatitis in children associated with round worms. Indian Pediatr. 1977;14:81-3. 38.
20. DeBanto JR, Goday PS, Pedroso MR, Iftikhar R, Fazel A, Nayyar S, et al. Acute pancreatitis in children. Am J Gastroenterol. 2002;97:1726-31.
21. Bradley E. A clinically based classification system for acute pancreatitis. Arch Surg. 1993;128:586.
22. Benifla M, Weizman Z. Acute pancreatitis in childhood: analysis of literature data. J Clin Gastroenterol. 2003;37:169-72.
23. Smotkin J, Tenner S. Laboratory diagnostic tests in acute pancreatitis. J Clin Gastroenterol. 2002;34:459-62.
24. Smith RC, Southwell-Keely J, Chesher D. Should serum pancreatic lipase replace serum amylase as a biomarker of acute pancreatitis?. ANZ J Surg. 2005;75.(6):399-404.
25. Lowe ME. Pancreatitis. In: Wyllie R, Hyams JS, Kay M (Eds). Pediatric Gastrointestinal and Liver Disease, 4th edn, Saunders; 2011.
26. Cappell MS. Acute pancreatitis: Etiology, Clinical Presentation, Diagnosis, and Therapy. Med Clin N Am. WB. Saunders, 2008;92:4.
27. Werner J, Hartwig W, Uhl W, Muller C, Buchler MW. Useful markers for predicting severity and monitoring progression of acute pancreatitis. Pancreatology. 2003;3:115-27.
28. Balthazar E, Robinson D, Megibow A, Ranson J. Acute pancreatitis: value of CT in establishing prognosis. Radiology. 1990;174:331.
29. McMahon CJ. The relative roles of MRCP and endoscopic ultrasound in diagnosis of common bile duct calculi: a critically appraised topic. Abdom Imaging. 2008;33(1):6-9.
30. Mohan N, Bansal S, Arora A, Sud R. Role of endoscopic retrograde. cholangiopancreatography in the management of pancreatitis in children. J Pediatr Gastroenter and Nutr. 2004;39(Suppl 1):S44.
31. Coyle WJ, Pineau BC, Tarnasky PR, Knapple WL, Aabakken L, Hoffman BJ, et al. Evaluation of unexplained acute and acute recurrent pancreatitis using endoscopic retrograde cholangiopancreatography, sphincter of Odd imanometry and endoscopic ultrasound. Endoscopy. 2002;34:617-23.
32. Singh N, Sharma B, Sharma M, et al. Evaluation of early enteral feeding through nasogastric and nasojejunal tube in severe acute pancreatitis: a noninferiority randomized controlled trial. Pancreas. 2012;41(1):153-9.
33. Uhl W, Warshaw A, Imrie C, Bassi C, McKay CJ, Lankisch PG, et al. IAP guidelines for the surgical management of acute pancreatitis. Pancreatology. 2002;2:565-7.
34. Whitcomb DC. Value of genetic testing in management of pancreatitis. Gut; 2004.

35. Homma T, Harada H, Koizumi M. Diagnostic criteria for chronic pancreatitis by the Japan Pancreas Society. Pancreas. 1997;15:14-5.

36. Etemad B, Whitcomb DC. Chronic pancreatitis: diagnosis, classification, and new genetic developments. Gastroenterology 2001;120:682-707.

37. Teich N, Mossner J. Hereditary chronic pancreatitis. Best Pract Res Clin Gastroenterol. 2008;22(1):115-30.

38. Schneider A, Barmada MM, Slivka A. Clinical characterization of patients with idiopathic chronic pancreatitis and SPINK1 mutations. Scand J Gastroenterol. 2004;39.(9):903-4.

39. Fink EN, Kant JA, Whitcomb DC. Genetic counseling for nonsyndromic pancreatitis. Gastroenterol Clin North Am. 2007;36.(2): 325-33.

40. Lankish PG. Progression from acute to chronic pancreatitis: a physician's view. Surg Clin North Am. 1999;79:815-27.

41. Boocock GR, Morrison JA, Popovic M, et al. Mutations in SBDS are associated with Shwachman-Diamond syndrome. Nat Genet. 2003;33:97-101.

42. Applebaum SE, Kant JA, Whitcomb DC, Ellis IH. Genetic testing: counseling, laboratory and regulatory issues and the EUROPAC protocol for ethical research in multicenter studies of inherited pancreatic diseases. Med Clin North Am. 2000;82:575-88.

43. Riyaz A. Tropical pancreatitis. In: Riyaz A (Ed). Pediatric gastroenterology and Hepatology. 3rd ed. Paras Publishers, Hyderabad. 2008.pp.293-7.

44. Werlin SL. Pancreatic Tumors. In: Kliegman RM, Stanton BF, Geme JW, Schor NF, Behrman RE (Eds). Nelson Textbook of Pediatrics, 19th ed, Saunders 2011.pp.1374.

Chapter

11

Short Bowel Syndrome

Intestinal failure (IF) is commonly defined as a critical reduction of the gut mass or its function below the minimum needed to absorb nutrients and fluids required for adequate growth in children and weight maintenance in adults.[1,2] The short bowel syndrome (SBS) is the leading cause of IF in infants and children. The SBS is a disorder usually following extensive surgical resection leaving the bowel length below a critical value for adequate nutritional supply and requiring parenteral nutrition (PN).[2]

ETIOLOGY AND INCIDENCE

European data report an incidence of children on home PN to be 2–6.8 per million population.[3-5] Among these cohorts of pediatric home-PN, SBS accounts for 50–65%.

Using data from quality of life studies as a proxy, in 2002 in France, there were 104 children below 19 years of age on HPN for digestive diseases and cared for by the 5 French HPN centers (approx 1.7 per million).[6] In the mean time, 21 children below the age of 16 in Sweden were on home-PN (approx 2.4 per million).[7]

The SBS may be secondary to prenatal disease causing abnormal development of the GI tract (intestinal atresia, gastroschisis, extensive aganglionosis) or postnatal ischemia-related events such as mid gut volvulus, necrotizing enterocolitis (NEC), or trauma (Table 11.1).

Intestinal Atresia

Intestinal atresia is the most frequent congenital abnormalities that cause SBS. The classification of jejuno-ileal atresias delineates 4 different types (Fig. 11.1).[8] Atresia affecting the colon is, in most cases, a type IIIa defect according to this classification. The original cause for intestinal atresia remains debated: lack of revacuolization of the solid cord stage or a late intrauterine mesenteric vascular accident as a result of intestinal volvulus,

Table 11.1: Etiology of short bowel syndrome in children				
Syndrome	*USA**	*CANADA+*	*France°*	*International#*
Atresia (%)	30	30	39	23
Volvulus (%)	10	10	24	24
Gastroschisis (%)	17	12.5	14	14
NEC (%)	43	35	14	27

*Andorsky et al. J Pediatr. 2001;139:27-33.
+Wales et al. J PediatrSurg. 2004;39:690-95.
°Goulet et al. Eur J Pediatr Surg. 2005;15:95-101.
#Koffeman et al. BPRCG. 2003;17:879-93.

intussusception, internal hernia, or strangulation in a tight gastroschisis or omphalocele defect. Rare familial cases of jejunoileal and colonic atresia suggest that genetic factors may play a role.

Duodenal atresia is, in general, limited to the duodenum and is mostly associated with congenital anomalies, including those of the pancreas, intestinal malrotation, esophageal atresia, Meckel's diverticulum, variants of imperforate anus, congenital heart disease, central nervous system lesions, renal anomalies... . Down syndrome occurs in 25–30% of patients with duodenal atresia. Intestinal atresia isolated or multiple has been reported to be associated with severe combined immune deficiency.[9,10] The gene mutation of this familial disease has been recently evidenced.[11]

Prenatal ultrasonography may identify the presence of polyhydramnios and distention of the stomach and duodenum. At birth, there are signs of bowel obstruction, including bilious vomiting, abdominal distention, and failure to pass meconium. Surgery performing end-to-end anastomosis with or without enteroplasty, small bowel lengthening or jejunostomy, should be performed early and is highly dependent on the extent of atresia, the importance of the distention of the proximal small

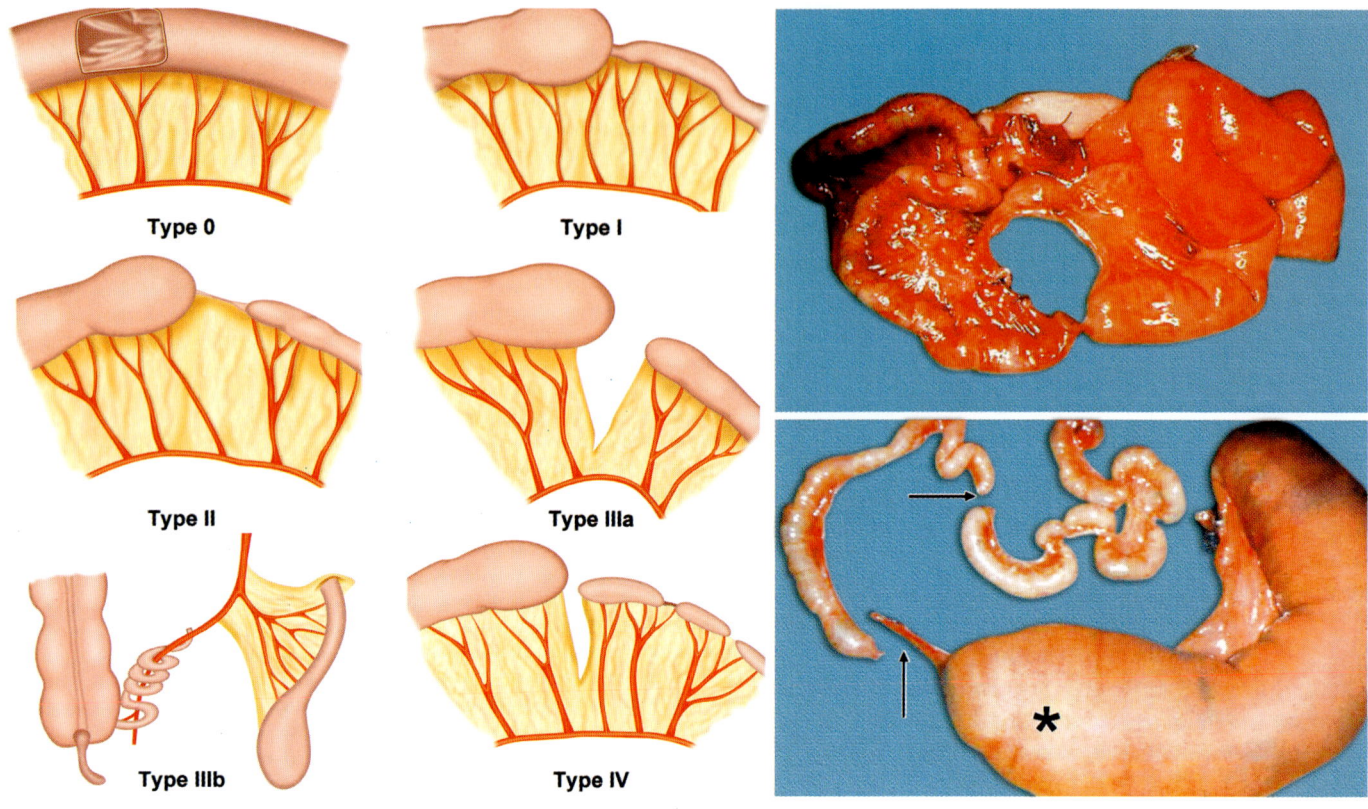

Fig. 11.1: Classification of intestinal atresia.
Type 0: luminal obstruction with intact mesentery; Type I: mucosal defect with an intact mesentery; Type II: fibrous cord connecting the atretic bowel ends; Type IIIa: atretic segment with a V-shaped mesenteric defect; Type IIIb: "apple peel syndrome", in which there is a proximal jejunal atresia and the distal bowel is supplied by a single retrograde blood vessel; Type IV: multiple atresias are present ("string of sausage" effect).

intestine, and the experience of the surgeon. Recent data have shown that experimental atresia in fetal rat induces differential myenteric plexus phenotypical as well as functional changes (motility and permeability) between the two sides of the obstruction. These changes might help identify markers predictive of motility dysfunction and define guidelines for postsurgical care.[12]

Gastroschisis

Gastroschisis is an abdominal wall defect characterized by an intact umbilical cord with evisceration of bowel through a defect in the abdominal wall, generally to the right of the cord, and without a covering membrane. European data covering over 4 million births, from 1999 to 2008, show incidence of 2.98 per 100,000 births with an increase of 6% over 2-year period.[13,14] The increasing incidence reported might result from unknown environmental factors.[15] Around 40% of babies with gastroschisis are born to mothers under the age of 20 years compared with only 9% of overall births. Genetic factors are supported by familial incidence and selected gene polymorphism.[15] An association between maternal

medication during pregnancy and an increased risk of gastroschisis has been suggested. Prenatal diagnosis is routinely performed allowing to choose delivery place and timing, thus, facilitating the neonatal surgery. Both the mode of delivery or the use of ward reduction of gastroschisis rather than performing this procedure under anesthesia in an operating room appears not to influence the outcome for infants with gastroschisis.[16,17] However, most clinicians agree on the need for C-section when the liver is outside the abdomen. Early surgical management aims to reduce meticulously the herniated viscera into the abdomen while avoiding high intra-abdominal pressure. When immediate reduction is not possible, the surgeon uses a prosthetic silo created from silastic or Teflon for protecting the bowel until it returns into the abdomen in the following days.

Long-term survival of neonates with gastroschisis is over 95%.[18] Most infants benefit from short-term PN associated with appropriate feeding and nursing. However, some cases may be more difficult because of a combination of factors, such as dysmotility caused by amniotic fluid peritonitis, intestinal atresia (10–20% of cases), perforation, perinatal bowel infarction, and the development of volvulus. Approximately 10–20% of infants with gastroschisis often require long-term PN.

Intestinal Aganglionosis

Hirschsprung's disease (HD), also known as aganglionic megacolon, derives from a congenital malformation of the enteric nervous system (ENS).[19,20] It displays an incidence of 1 in 5000 live births with a 4:1 male-to-female sex ratio. This severe congenital condition is caused by the absence of colonic neural ganglia and thus lack of intrinsic innervation of the colon due in turn to improper colonization of the developing intestines by ENS progenitor cells. These progenitor cells are derived from a transient stem cell population called neural crest cells. The disease has been linked to mutations in genes that encode the crucial signals for the development of the enteric nervous system, including the RET and EDNRB signaling pathways.[21] The genetics of HD is complex and can involve mutations in multiple genes. However, it is estimated that mutations in known genes account for less than half of the cases of HD observed clinically. In 80% of infants, the aganglionosis is confined to the rectum and sigmoid, but it may extend to encompass the entire colon (total colonic aganglionosis) or very rarely (less than 1% of HD) affect the entire intestine subtotal or total intestinal aganglionosis (TIA).

The TIA or sub-TIA is revealed early after birth with abdominal distention and bilious vomiting most of the time after delayed meconium passing. During surgery, the extent of the aganglionic segment of the small intestine and the appropriate placing of a stoma may be guided by perioperative histopathological examinations of biopsies. Because of the absence of functional colon (SBS type 1 from Table 11.2), infants with <50 cm of ganglionic small intestine are likely to have permanent IF requiring long-term PN. Although several surgical approaches, such as longitudinal myotomy-myectomy of the aganglionic small bowel or lengthening, tapering, STEP of the ganglionic segment have been attempted, there is no evidence to support any one approach. Recurrent surgery should be avoided, since these are likely to compromise any future intestinal transplantation procedure. An early referral to an expert intestinal failure unit should be made for the child with TIA to optimize nutritional management with a view to transplantation in the future.[22]

Malrotation and Midgut Volvulus

The incidence of malrotation in children 1–18 years of age is 5.3 per million population;[23] figures for prematures and infants are unavailable. Midgut volvulus (MGV) is one of the four most common conditions that lead to intestinal

Table 11.2: Type of diet to be used in SBS patients
Breast milk
• Contains lactose, oligosaccharides, growth factors, nucleotides, long chain fatty acids, glutamine, and other amino acids that promote mucosal trophicity and intestinal adaptation
• Promotes microbiota rich in lactobacilli and bifidobacteria
• Promotes or preserves mother–child interactions
• In infants with SBS it may reduce the duration of parenteral nutrition
• Should be used as much as possible in neonatal SBS
Enteral formulas
Carbohydrates
Oligo- and polysaccharides:
• Poorly tolerated by patients with limited mucosal absorptive surface area
• Broken down into small intestinal lumen in osmotically active organic acids
Lipids
Long chain triglycerides
• Poorly digested in case of SIBO because of bile acids changes
• Poorly absorbed in patients with severe malabsorption
• Have trophic effects on small intestinal mucosa
• Supplementation with n-3- or n-6- PUFA may enhance mucosal growth
Medium chain triglycerides (MCT)
• Rapidly hydrolyzed by pancreatic lipase
• Water soluble and absorbed intact, directly into the portal circulation
• Less dependent on an extensive absorptive surface for adequate absorption
• As part of lipid supply appropriate for most infants with SBS
• Excessive intake can cause diarrhea
• Do not provides essential fatty acids
• Recommended use of formulas containing MCT
Nitrogen
Extensively hydrolyzed protein formulas (EHPF)
• No demonstrated advantages in comparison with intact protein infant formula
• All formula commercially available EHPF are lactose free and contain 40–60% MCT as fat
• Recommended in SBS patients
Elemental amino acid-based formula
• Not yet established if this type of formula may influence outcome of SBS
Glutamine (Gln)
• Currently no benefit demonstrated

failure in infants. Any pediatrician should recognize in a newborn without any risk factor and normally orally fed, the sudden occurrence of clinical signs, including intermittent yellow or green bile stained vomiting together with abdominal distention and in some cases blood in the stool suggesting intestinal obstruction from MGV. Whatever, hemodynamic disorders are present or not,

MGV is a surgical emergency for avoiding extensive small bowel infarction.

Malrotation is caused by abnormal process occurring during the 5th gestational week when the fetal small intestine forms a loop which extrudes into the umbilical cord. The fetal gut subsequently undergoes enlargement, elongation, and return to the abdominal cavity with rotation and fixation.[24] The fixation of the intestine may be abnormal, with fibrous bands (Ladd's bands) forming between the duodenum and the right colon a short mesentery allowing the bowel to twist (volve) causing bowel obstruction and loss of blood supply. Intrauterine MGV is thought to be the cause of intestinal atresia type III b. An MGV in the newborn may develop as a result of malrotation but may also occur without, more often in premature infants with lax tissue. An MGV may occur later in life as a result of malrotation or as a complication of previous surgery. The symptoms of MGV are those of intestinal obstruction. Abdominal pain accompanied by bilious vomits is more commonly seen as a symptom of malrotation in children above one year of age.

As soon as the diagnosis is suspected, the surgeon should be involved while everything has to be done for avoiding any delay for the surgery. In that setting, investigations used to confirm the diagnosis, such as Doppler assessment of the superior mesenteric vessels, barium follow through and enema, may delay surgery.

Surgical management of MGV is an emergency involving detorsion of the volvulus, restoration of circulation, separation of adhesions between bowel loops and attempts to preserve bowel length. A conservative resection of only clearly necrotic tissue is recommended while bowel with questionable viability should be left *in situ* and re-evaluated 24–36 hours later during a "second look laparotomy".

Necrotizing Enterocolitis

Necrotizing enterocolitis (NEC) remains the leading cause of SBS, especially in premature infants. The incidence of NEC is inversely correlated with gestational age and birth weight. Incidence of NEC varies among areas around the world.[25,26] Whether NEC results from ischemic injury of the small bowel, which must often has to be resected remains debated.[26] Interestingly, the percentage of SBS caused by NEC range from 14 to 43% among the series.[25-28]

An NEC presents usually with variable symptoms: feed intolerance, gastric aspirates, abdominal distention, bilious vomiting, and blood in the stool. Local tenderness or an abdominal mass may be apparent on clinical examination and progression to pneumoperitoneum and sepsis with respiratory failure, shock, and death may follow very quickly.

Emergent treatment of NEC includes stopping feeds supported by TPN, nasogastric decompression, fluid and electrolyte resuscitation, broad-spectrum antibiotics and, in selected cases, respiratory support. Severity, whether mild or critical, determines the duration of medical therapy. Parenteral antibiotics and TPN are usually prescribed for 7–14 days. Surgery for NEC should be limited as it may lead to bowel resection. Nevertheless, surgery is indicated by (i) presence of pneumoperitoneum, indicating perforation of the intestine, (ii) clinical deterioration despite maximal medical treatment, (iii) abdominal mass with persistent intestinal obstruction or sepsis, and (iv) development of intestinal stricture. More or less extensive intestinal resection is too often performed involving most of the time ileum and proximal colon while function of the remnant small intestine may be compromised. Acute surgical management of NEC involves the often competing priorities of controlling sepsis and preserving bowel length. Bowel-preserving strategies for NEC, designed to limit SBS, are based on peritoneal drainage, venting ostomy, limited resection, or a combination of them. Drainage-based strategies are generally favored in smaller neonates, while laparotomy-based strategies are favored in larger patients, especially those with a more limited extent of intestinal injury. Comparisons of drainage-based and resection-based approaches are limited by confounding variables, and neither approach is clearly superior with regard to subsequent SBS.[28] Prevention of NEC has become an area of research priority. Prevention of NEC is debated, especially regarding the date and type of feeding.[29-33] Finally, the incidence of NEC has not changed significantly despite the dramatic advances in perinatal care. Given the role of inflammatory mediators in its pathogenesis, newer immune modulators are being studied as potential agents for prevention/treatment of NEC.[26] Recent data suggest that probiotics administration might be helpful in decreasing incidence of NEC in preterm infants.[34-38] The meta-analysis of Deshpande et al.[36] concludes on significant benefits of probiotic supplements in reducing death and disease in preterm neonates. He suggests that the dramatic effect sizes, tight confidence intervals, extremely low P values, and overall evidence indicate that additional placebo-controlled trials are unnecessary if a suitable probiotic product is available. Other authors consider that future clinical trials of any promising preventative agent(s), such as probiotics need to be designed carefully.[39,40]

PATHOPHYSIOLOGY

Consequences of Intestinal Resection

The SBS is characterized by a compromised bowel absorptive capacity due to a severely reduced mucosal surface resulting in diarrhea, fluid and electrolyte imbalance, and failure to thrive.[2] The functional consequences of SBS depend not only on the length, surface and site of the resected small intestine but also on the functional capacity of the remaining intestine. The cause of resection and age of the patient at the time at which surgery was carried out also influence the capacity of the remaining gut function and potential for adaptation. Term neonates have a small bowel length of 250 ±40 cm which doubles during the last trimester of gestation, suggesting that a short bowel remnant does not have the same prognosis in a preterm infant as in a full-term baby.[41] The same difference exists between neonates and older children. Thus, if the surgical resection occurs earlier, the opportunity for adaptive growth is greater.[2] According to the length of the small intestine measured along the antimesenteric border at surgery, short resection leaves more than 100–150 cm or small intestine, large resection leaves between 40 cm and 100 cm and massive resection less than 40 cm. The major determinants of IF in SBS are the age of the child at the time of resection, the extent and the portion of the small bowel resected (jejunum, ileum, ileocecal valve, colon, etc.) (Fig. 11.2), and the functional integrity of the residual intestine.[42-46] Pathophysiology of SBS, including the consequences of anatomical changes, has been extensively reviewed by Buchman et al.[47] and Goulet et al.[48,49]

Resection of the Jejunum

Both the transit time and the direct contact or intraluminal nutrients with the jejunal epithelium determine the malabsorption syndrome following extensive jejunal resection. The resulting malabsorption concerns all nutrients as well as minerals, electrolytes, trace elements and most the vitamins. Severe diarrhea following extensive jejunal resection is associated with steatorrhea and creatorrhea. Moreover, the resection of the jejunum reduces the secretion of cholecystokinin and secretin leading to a decrease in biliary and exocrine pancreatic secretions which may lead, in turn, to a reduction in nutrient absorptive capacity. The reduced production of cholecystokinin, vasoactive intestinal peptide (VIP), gastric inhibitory peptide, and serotonin may cause gastric hypersecretion seen more frequently after jejunal resection. The degree or malabsorption is proportional to the length or jejunum resected and will be compensated, to some extent, by the ileum and/or by the process or adaptation in response to loss or intestinal surface. The colon is also an important player in reducing the diarrhea and even the malabsorption syndrome (see below)

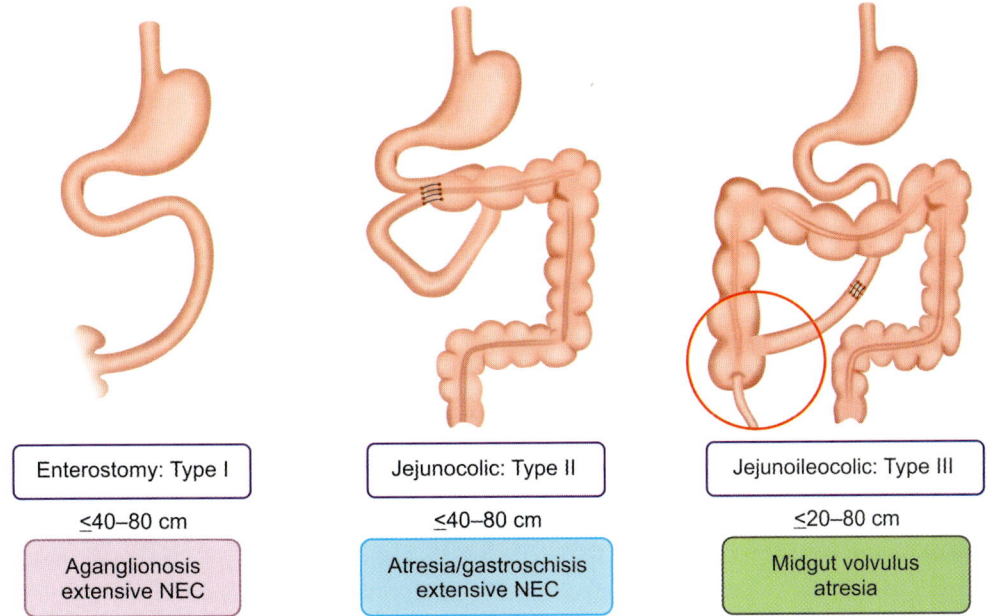

Fig. 11.2: Anatomy of short bowel according to the type of the remnant bowel. The most frequent cause of resection is mentioned for each type

Resection of the Ileum

Despite the fact that, normally, most nutrients are absorbed in the proximal jejunum, the residual ileum is able to adapt and to assume the role of macronutrient absorption. However, the specialized cells of the terminal ileum, where vitamin B_{12}/intrinsic factor receptors are located and where bile salts are reabsorbed, cannot be replaced by jejunal hypertrophy. Thus, the ileum has specific functions which the jejunum cannot substitute. In addition, resection of the distal ileum usually includes the ileocaecal valve (ICV). Finally, ileal resection impairs vitamin B_{12} absorption, which can cause macrocytic anemia and neuropathy. Malabsorption of bile salts is responsible for the following specific complications:

1. **The decrease of bile salt reabsorption** by the ileum reduces their circulating pool and leads to lipid malabsorption and steatorrhea. Unabsorbed fatty acids are then hydroxylated by colonic bacteria increasing mucosal injury and secretory diarrhea. The consequences are proportional to the concentration and dehydroxylation of bile salts into the lumen (deoxycholic and chenodeoxycholic acids). Because of the decreased pool of bile salts, fat soluble vitamins (A, D, E and K) are also prone to be malabsorbed.

2. **Cholelithiasis** seems to be the direct consequence of the reduced concentration of bile salts in bile. Resection of the terminal ileum by disrupting the enterohepatic circulation of biliary acids increases the lithogenicity of bile. Premature infants are especially exposed to cholelithiasis, because of their low production of conjugated bile acids.

3. **Hyperoxaluria** with formation of renal stones results from loss of the ileum and subsequent lipid malabsorption (long chain triglycerides). This complication became rare with the enlarged use of medium chain triglyceride rich diets (see below).

Finally, extensive loss of the ileum reduces transit time by suppressing the so-called "ileal brake". It has been shown that the ileum has a greater potential for adaptation than the jejunum. In addition, ileum is the site of enteric hormones release, such as enteroglucagon, which are essential in the process of adaptation after extensive resection (see below).

Ileocecal Valve Resection

The resection of the ileocecal valve (ICV) decreases transit time (ileocecal breake) and allows colonic bacteria to enter and populate the small intestine increasing the likelihood of the development of a severe form of SBS.[50-52] Bacterial overgrowth may negatively impact on digestion and nutrient absorption, as bacteria compete for nutrients with enterocytes. Thus, ICV resection represents an additional major cause of malabsorption of nutrients, water and electrolytes, dehydroxylation of bile salts, mucosal injury and motility disorders. The lack of the ICV appears to greatly influence the period required to achieve intestinal autonomy following efficient small bowel adaptation.[42-46] In addition, ICV resection increases the risk of sepsis of intestinal origin that occurred more frequently in infants without the ICV than in those with an intact cecum.[53]

Resection of the Colon

Colon is a crucial partner for small intestinal adaptation and function in SBS patients by involving fluid and electrolytes absorption, absorption of medium-chain triglycerides, and production of short-chain fatty acids for malabsorbed energy salvage.[50-52] The removal of both ileum and colon obviously drastically increases fluid loss, dehydration, volume depletion, and causes hypocalcemia, and hypomagnesemia. Preservation of the colon in cases of major small intestinal resection appears to lessen the severity of SBS. In experimental studies, increased enterocyte expression and function of apical membrane Na/H exchangers in regions distal to the anastomosis play a role in the adaptive process after massive small bowel resection. The increased luminal Na load to distal bowel regions after proximal resection may stimulate increases in apical membrane Na/H exchangers gene transcription and protein expression.[54] The colon may adapt after small intestinal resection, whereas it hosts the most important part of the intestinal microbiota, which plays a crucial role in intestinal function and health. Also, colon may be responsible for D-lactic acidosis as well, as it can be injured by noninfectious colitis.

Associated Disorders

Besides the anatomical impairment and its consequences, small bowel resection may be aggravated by several associated disorders.

1. **Gastric acid hypersecretion** occurs in 50% of pediatric patients with SBS while hypergastrinemia is inconstant.[47,55,56] Acid hypersecretion occurs early after resection and depends on the extent of the resection. Hypersecretion is transitory, but it increases with enteral feeding leading to a larger amount or intestinal fluid loss. Gastric acid hypersecretion, by reducing duodenal pH, decreases the activity of pancreatic enzymes, such as amylase and lipase, which in turn, increases fat malabsorption.

2. **Gastric emptying** of liquids is more rapid following jejunal resection, although intestinal transit may still remain normal because of the braking effect of the ileum.[57] The loss of inhibition on gastric emptying and intestinal transit in children without colon is related to a

significant decrease in peptide YY (PYY), glucagon-like peptide I (GLP-I), and neurotensin.[47] A PYY is normally released from L cells in the ileum and colon when stimulated by fat or bile salts. Rapid gastric emptying may contribute to fluid losses in children with SBS.

3. **Alteration in gut motor activity** may be observed especially in case of prenatal small bowel malformations (atresias) or severe postnatal pathology, such as extensive NEC. They contribute together with repeated surgical procedures, by increasing plastic peritonitis, to impair motor activity leading to bacterial overgrowth and the above-mentioned complications. These particular patients are at highest risk to develop rapid and severe liver disease that impairs intestinal adaptation process and may require combined liver-intestine transplantation (see below).

Adaptation after Extensive Intestinal Resection

Soon after small bowel resection, physiological process of adaptation of the remaining SB develop. Adaptation is a slow process accompanied by a gradual increase in absorption capacity of nutrients, electrolytes, and minerals.[47-49] This comprises muscular hypertrophy (increased bowel diameter and wall thickness) and hyperplasia of the intestinal mucosa (Figs 11.3 and 11.4). This mucosal hyperplasia is characterized by an increased number of enterocytes per unit of SB length, an increased rate of enterocyte proliferation, and an increased villous height and crypt depth. In animals, it was shown that epithelial hyperplasia following gut resection results in increased mucosal mass, including higher mucosal wet weight, higher protein content as well as higher DNA and RNA content per unit of bowel length. The complex regulation of gut mucosal growth involves a multitude of factors, including hormonal mediators, such as enteroglucagon, glucagon-like peptides neurotensine, peptide YY, growth hormone, and insuline-like growth factor. Additionally, oral or enteral feeding stimulate the release of enterotrophic hormones, such as gastrin, cholecystokinin, and neurotensine, which may further improve the process of gut adaptation.[57-62]

Intraluminal substrates and nutrients, stimulate the adaptation of intestinal mucosa through several mechanisms:

❑ Direct contact of intraluminal nutrients with intestinal cells
❑ Trophic effects of gastrointestinal secretions enhanced by food
❑ Release of several trophic hormones secreted by the gastrointestinal tract, mainly enteroglucagon.[57-62] The postulated influence of cholecystokinin (CCK) and secretin might an indirect action via the stimulation of pancreatic secretions that could lead to the release of enteroglucagon. In turn, enteroglucagon stimulates the cell turn over, motility and absorptive capacity of the small intestine.

• **Glutamine (Gln)** is the most important circulating amino acid, which plays a role for the metabolism of enterocytes.[63] In dogs, Gln perfusion increases the intestinal metabolism of this amino acid, suggesting

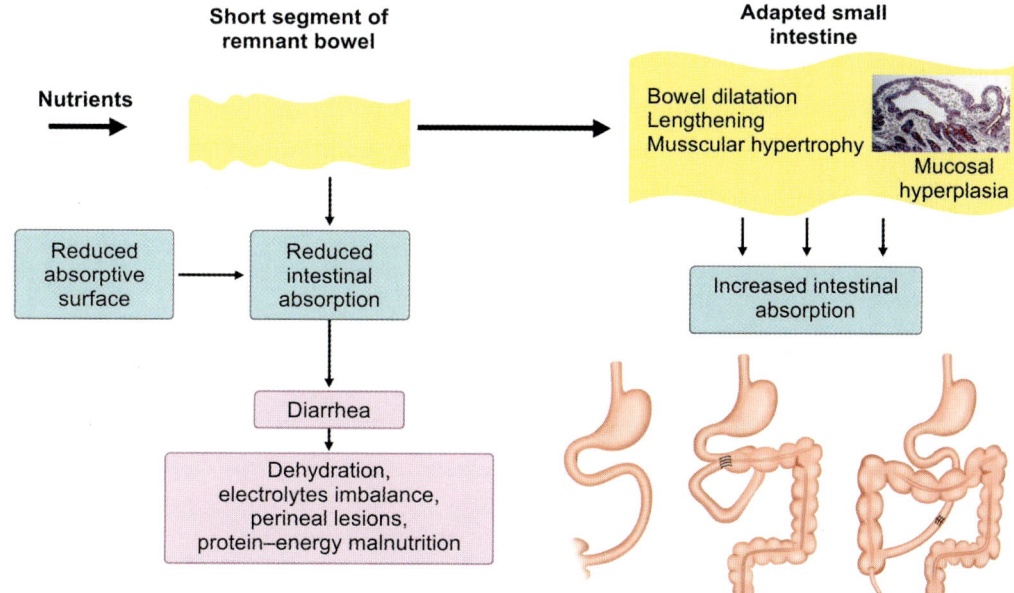

Fig. 11.3: Consequences of small intestinal resection and mechanisms of bowel adaptation

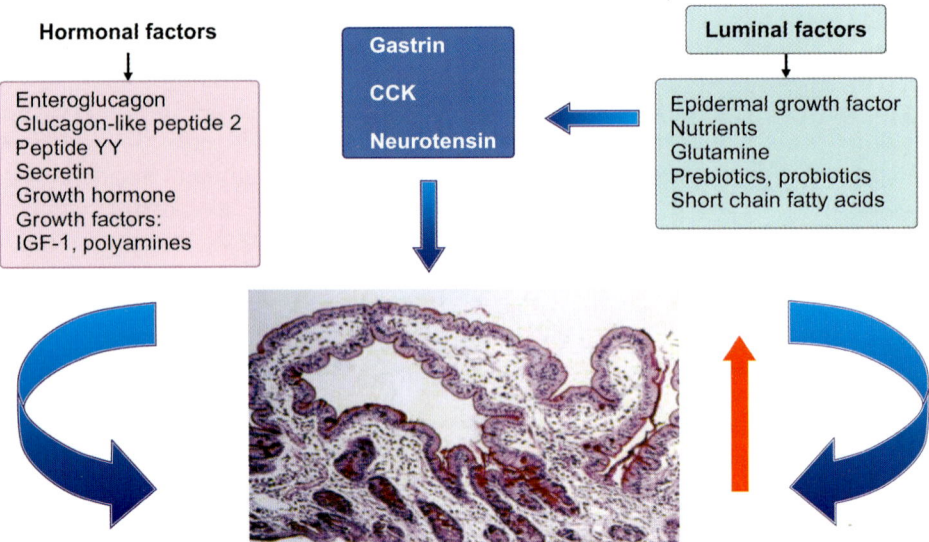

Fig. 11.4: Factors involved in the physiological process of intestinal adaptation

the importance of Gln as a substrate during PN in patients with SBS.[64]

- **Short-chain fatty acids (SCFA)** are produced from the fermentation of unabsorbed CHO by the colonic microbiota. The SCFA could be energetic substrates for the topical nutrition of intestinal cells.[66] Pectin, a water soluble, noncellulose dietary fiber, was shown to enhance jejunal and colonic mucosal adaptation when added to the enteral diet.[66,67]

Besides nutrients, other factors seem to play an important role in the mucosal adaptation process:

- **Epidermal growth factor (EGF)** present in human milk and produced in the salivary glands and duodenal cells is a trophic substance for the gastrointestinal tract.[68,69]
- **Polyamines (spermine, spermidine),** whose synthesis is dependent on ornithine decarboxylase activity, greatly enhance intestinal cell turnover and protein synthesis.[70,71]
- **Exogenous prostaglandin** (16,16-dimethyl prostaglandin E1) has been shown to stimulate mucosal hyperplasia in the gastric antrum and in the jejunum.[72,73]

Thus, adaptation of the remaining small bowel is dependent on exogenous and endogenous factors, emphasizing the usefulness of early enteral feeding after resection.

The goal of intestinal adaptation is to develop the ability to withdraw artificial nutrition thanks to a compensatory increase in the mucosal surface area and absorption capacity. The two indicators which have historically been used to predict weaning from PN in

children, residual bowel length measured at final surgery and serum citrulline, though helpful, have not proven to be highly reliable prognostic factors in SBS patients.[74-78] In clinical practice, the degree of intestinal insufficiency may be measured by the percentage of PN required for normal body weight gain and growth. PN requirements remain, therefore, the best measure of the degree of intestinal sufficiency in this setting.[2]

MANAGEMENT

Initial Surgery

Every time intestinal resection is performed for an acute event (MGV, NEC) or for a malformation (atresia, TIA, gastroschisis), the initial surgery aims at saving as much intestine as possible (see above). When small bowel resection includes the terminal ileum, it is suggested that a gallbladder resection be performed to prevent the occurrence of cholelithiasis.[79] The question as to whether a gastrostomy should be performed at the initial phase depends on the experience of the team. Nevertheless, if long-term enteral nutrition is planned, a gastrostomy is better for the patient's comfort. Extensive small bowel resection will require fluid replacement after surgery and in a number of patients long-term PN. Thus, a permanent indwelling cuffed central venous catheter (CVC) must be placed.

Medical Therapy

It is classical to consider three phases in the clinical course after small bowel resection. The first phase follows small

bowel resection and is associated with massive losses of water and electrolytes. Severe diarrea is increased by gastric hypersecretion. During this period, total PN is required in association with small amounts of substrates provided by the enteral route, orally, or by continuous gastric infusion as soon as intestinal transit has recovered. The second phase is marked by the initiation of enteral feeding by oral or tube feeding and the gradual cyclization of PN. As supported by the mechanisms of adaptation, there is a clear advantage in providing early gradual amounts of nutrients into the residual intestine for stimulating mucosal hyperplasia. In the mean time, PN allows the remaining bowel to develop and to become functional without exceeding its capacities. This period can take several months or years before maximal intestinal adaptation is reached. The third phase starts when intestinal function is sufficient to absorb nutrients enabling PN to be withdrawn. All calories are provided by the enteral route. Oral intake can then be further liberalized both in volume and variety, according to the tolerance of the patient. This long period requires special management and follow up.

Parenteral Nutrition

Excess fluid and electrolyte losses may complicate the management of SBS patients, particularly in patients with high output jejunostomies. Fluids with a sodium concentration of 75–90 mEq/L are typically used to replace jejunostomy. Replacement fluids intravenously may be adjusted based on electrolyte concentration of the lost fluids. Monitoring urine sodium concentration for excessive retention (<10 mEq/L) may indicate the need to provide more sodium, even if serum values are near normal. Excessive magnesium losses can occur with large ostomy volumes, and appropriate magnesium replacement may also improve calcium utilization. Zinc and selenium losses increase with watery diarrhea and high ostomy output. Zinc deficiency can lead to a decreased activity of zinc-dependent intestinal metalloenzymes, such as alkaline phosphatase, leucine aminopeptidase, and other intestinal disaccharidases and delay intestinal adaptation. Zinc supplements are often used empirically, given that serum values do not reliably reflect body stores.

Parenteral nutrition provides adequate nutritional supply to the child allowing optimal growth. Such nutritional support includes the use of 1.5–2.5 g/kg/day amino acids through a pediatric solution, a caloric intake consisting of 70–80% of nonprotein energy substrates, such as dextrose and 20–30% energy provided by a 20% intravenous fat emulsion.[80,81] Maintenance amounts of vitamins and trace elements are added to the PN solution by using commercially available preparations. Calcium,

phosphate, and magnesium are also added to the solution according to the patient needs and the stability of the solution.

During the early phases of therapy, serum electrolytes, glucose, urea and calcium should be measured daily. When the patient's condition and the intestinal losses become stable, blood monitoring can be less frequent.

During the early phase after resection, H_2-receptor blocking agents (ranitidine) should be given intravenously to inhibit gastric hypersecretion.[47,82] 15–20 mg/kg/day added to PN solution, the drug being delivered as a continuous infusion. H_2-blockers, by increasing duodenal pH, also improve the digestion and absorption of nutrients. The end of the phase of management is considered to be accomplished when the patient has recovered from the surgical procedure and is stable on PN with controlled intestinal losses and motility. Parenteral nutrition should ideally not be stopped until adequate intake, and growth can be achieved with oral and/or enteral feeding alone.

Enteral Feeding

When possible the GI tract should be used for feeding as it is the most physiological and safest way to provide nutrition. The optimal strategies for enteral feeding, including oral versus tube feeding and continuous versus bolus, remain a matter of debate. The advantages of oral feeding, when feasible, include the maintenance of sucking and swallowing functions along with the interest and enjoyment associated with eating, as well as the stimulation of growth factors and hormones released by the GI tract promoting adaptation. For example, oral feeding promotes the release of epidermal growth factor (EGF) from salivary glands, increases GI secretion of trophic factors, and helps prevent feeding disorders.[83] Sialoadenectomy in animals significantly attenuates ileal villus height, total protein, and DNA content after small bowel resection. Both systemic and oral EGF administration has been shown to reverse the effects of sialoadenectomy.[84]

Enteral or oral feeding should be started as soon as possible after surgery (Tables 11.2 and 11.3). In an infant, breastfeeding should be encouraged or when this is not possible an extensively hydrolyzed formula can be used.[85,86] Human milk may be considered the first choice in this setting, followed by whole protein feeds if tolerated.[87-91] Breast milk contains IgA, growth factors, nucleotides, long chain fatty acids, glutamine, and other amino acids that may promote intestinal adaptation. In addition, breastfeeding has been associated with improved immune function, as well as the genesis of a fecal microbiota rich in lactobacilli and bifidobacteria, both of which might improve SBS prognosis. On the other hand, breast milk

Table 11.3: Management of feeding in SBS

Mode of feeding

- Oral feeding (OF) is the most physiological and the most stimulating for promoting intestinal adaptation, psychological behavior and oral skills
- Oropharyngeal shunting suppresses the direct stimulation of salivary glands resulting in lower release of EGF that is an important intestinal mucosa trophic factor
- Enteral tube feeding (ETF) is beneficial in patients with SBS, by improving saturation of carrier transport proteins, thus taking full advantage of the available absorptive surface area as compared to bolus feeding
- Continuous infusion leads to the loss of self regulation of intake with subsequent vomiting, or intestinal stasis with increased risk of SIBO with subsequent mucosal injury, sepsis, and liver disease…
- In case of full ETF, small quantities of OF should be introduced in infants 2–4 times a day to stimulate sucking and swallowing and to minimize the chances of eating disorders in the future
- Nasogastric tube may impair normal acquisition of oral behavior and induces eating disorders
- Percutaneous gastrostomy is indicated for children who will require EF for >3 months
- Jejunal feeding
  - Whatever nasojejunal, gastrojejunal or jejunal, should be limited to special situations
  - Exposes to the risk of contaminating the intestine with subsequent SIBO and sepsis
  - Excessive infusion rate may be responsible for severe diarrhea and dehydration

Progression and monitoring of feeding program
- Intestinal transit must be well established by coloanal transit or ostomy
- Absence of contraindications:
  - Patient general condition (sepsis, bleeding, respiratory distress syndrome…)
  - High ostomy or stool output >3–5 mL/kg/hour or bloody stools
  - Bilious and/or persistent vomiting
  - Water-electrolytes imbalance

- **Quantify feeding tolerance**
  - Stool or ostomy output
  - Reducing substances in stools or ostomy output
  - Recurrent vomiting and abdominal distension
  - Perianal skin lesions

- **Ultimate goals**
  - Provide 150–200 mL/kg/day, 100–140 kcal/kg/day
  - If ostomy/stool output precludes advancement at 20 cal/oz for 7 days
  - Increasing caloric density of the formula can be performed
  - Isocaloric reductions in PN supply simultaneously with enteral feeding (OF or ETF) advancement according to an optimal body weight gain and growth

- **Warning**
  - Eating disorders are usually caused by missing early oral feeding, long-term or repeated bowel rest periods, long-lasting ventilation in NICU. Early attempts at oral feeding should be performed as much as possible while complementary feeding should be introduced on time
  - ETF can induce adverse effects related to intestinal overload of a poorly motile small intestine leading to intestinal distension, vomiting and child discomfort
  - Bacterial contamination with subsequent SIBO induces mucosal changes with increased permeability causing food sensitization and malabsorption as well as translocation, sepsis and liver disease (Fig. 11.5)

contains lactose, which is sometimes not well tolerated in patients with reduced intestinal surface area. In a population of 30 infants with SBS (defined as more than 90 days of dependency on PN), the percentage of days that infants received breast milk was strongly correlated with fewer days of PN use (r = –0.821, p <.03).[92] Human milk also contains glutamine and growth factors, such as epidermal growth factor, which possibly promote bowel adaptation. Extensively hydrolyzed formulas are mostly used when whole protein feeds are not tolerated, while amino acid-based formulas (AABF) have been used as a last resort. The AABF are generally used in the treatment of food allergies or in case of milk protein hydrolyzate intolerance.[93,94] True food allergies have been rarely documented in children with SBS. Andorsky reported less intestinal allergy by using AABF, without clearly defining the criteria for the diagnosis of allergy.[94] Two retrospective studies report that the use of an AABF was associated with earlier weaning

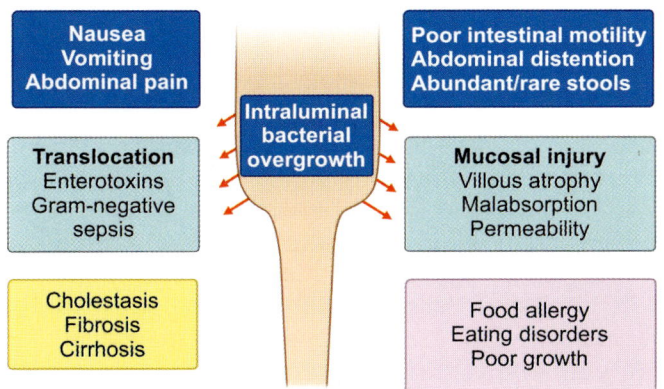

Fig. 11.5: Consequences of overfeeding a dilated intestine with subsequent intestinal stasis and small intestinal bacterial overgrowth (SIBO)

from PN and also a reduced rate of allergies.[95,96] However, the very small sample sizes and the lack of a control group in these studies limit the applicability of these findings to all children with SBS and IF.

The mode of feeding remains debated among the different centers.[85,86,97-99] It should always take into account the physiology, the psychological behavior of the infant (mother–child feeding relationships, acquisition of oral skills, abdominal and digestive comfort of the child), and finally, the nutritional efficiency. Oral feeding should always be promoted. ETF may be administered either continuously or in frequent small boluses, initially aiming at supplying a minimal enteral feeding (20–25 kcal/kg/day) and then increasing gradually as tolerated with larger boluses during the day and continuous feeding overnight. Continuous feeding appears to improve growth and adaptation through the optimization of absorption by challenging the enteral capacity. Complementary food can be started early. Tolerance is evaluated by measuring stool and by the observation of vomiting, irritability, intestinal distension and perinanal skin lesions. Stool output should be no more than 2/3 of feeding volume. Many factors can affect stool volume in SBS, including the length of the residual intestinal segment, the type of segment (the more proximal the resection the larger the fluid and sodium losses), the mucosal and endoluminal variables (residual enzymatic activity and absorptive capacity, bacterial overgrowth), the presence of the colon that can absorb large amounts of water, sodium, medium chain triglycerides (MCT) and peptides as well as carbohydrates metabolized to short chain fatty acid.[50,86] Enteral feeding is the most important factor to promote adaptation; nevertheless, it is important to avoid overfeeding which may worsen fluid, minerals and nutrients malabsorption and may result in severe

perianal skin lesions. Carbohydrate intolerance presents with frequent and liquid stools, the presence of reducing substances and with stool pH <6. Bile salts malabsorption should be suspected in children with no ICV and/or colon, high stool volume and perianal maceration, especially if there are no stool reducing substances. In these subjects a trial of cholestyramine (fractionated 4–8 g/day) should reduce the diarrhea.[100] Fluid losses in these patients are often accompanied by sodium loss and depletion; enteral sodium supplements should, therefore, be provided with the aim of maintaining urinary sodium above 20 mmol/L, with a sodium/potassium urinary ratio of at least 2:1.

Risks and Consequences of Microbiological Disorders

Small intestinal bacterial overgrowth (SIBO) is common especially in patients with no ICV and those having abnormal intestinal motility. A common finding in these patients include dilated loops of bowel containing residual nonabsorbed nutrients.[101-110] The SIBO can further cause mucosal inflammation and increased permeability that in turn may lead to sensitization and allergy as well as bacterial translocation, sepsis and cholestasis[111-114] (Fig. 11.5). It has been shown in experimental models that intestinal derived lipopolysaccharide (LPS) activates Kupffer cells through toll-like receptor 4 (TLR4) signaling.[111] Activated Kupffer cells are probably involved in the pathogenesis of intestinal failure associated liver disease (IFALD).[112-114] In some patients with dysmotile intestinal loops (intestinal atresia, gastroschisis, NEC) and liver disease, aggressive continuous tube feeding is often attempted with the aim of weaning a patient off of PN. This favors intestinal distention, stasis and SIBO which is considered as the main cause of liver injury. In these conditions, over-aggressive feeding leads to the loss of self-regulation of intake and results in abdominal discomfort, intestinal distention, SIBO with subsequent further mucosal and liver injury (Fig. 11.5). Surgical procedures (see below), such as longitudinal intestinal lengthening and tailoring (LILT) or serial transverse enteroplasty (STEP) aim not only to enhance the bowel length but also to reduce the diameter of dilated intestinal loops, thus, improving its motility and reducing the risk for developing SIBO.[115-117]

Clinical manifestations of feeding intolerance, such as abdominal distention, bloating, and nausea, due to colonic microbiological hypermetabolism.[118,119] D-lactic acidosis may occur in some children during the process of bowel adaptation and even long after weaning off PN. Indeed, *Lactobacillus* and other bacteria, including *Clostridium perfringens and Streptococcus bovis*, when present, may ferment nonabsorbed carbohydrate to D-lactic acid which cannot be metabolized by L-lactate dehydrogenase.[120-122] These microorganisms may proliferate in the acidic environment of the colon; that is the result of the metabolism of unabsorbed carbohydrate to SCFAs. D-lactic acidosis presents with encephalopathy (ataxia, blurred speech, decreased consciousness) and should be considered when there is a high anion gap metabolic acidosis in the setting of normal serum lactate levels. Preventive measures for D-lactic acidosis includes the reduction of carbohydrate intake, followed by antibiotics (such as metronidazole, bactrim, cotrimoxazole, rifaximine) when dietary changes fail.[123]

An other rare complication, which may be observed late after PN weaning, is intestinal ulcerations, usually close to intestinal anastomosis. They might be due to intestinal dysbiosis. They may cause chronic bleeding with hyposideremic anemia requiring iron IV supplementation or even blood transfusion. Acute bleeding may occur either with severe clinical condition. Treatment is difficult and includes attempts at bowel decontamination, probiotics and more recently we feel to have been successful in providing omega-3 fatty acids oral supplementation.

Hormonal Therapy and Other Adaptive Treatments

Recombinant human growth hormone (rhGH): It was used in adult patients with SBS in both, open and randomized clinical trials.[124-126] However, the use of rhGH treatment in adult remains controversial while the incidence rate of secondary effect is high.

Few studies have been currently reported in infants or children with SBS.[127-133] An open-labeled trial involved 8 PN-dependent children with neonatal SBS receiving >50% of their protein-energy requirements from PN.[130] They received 0.6 $IU.kg^{-1}.day^{-1}$ rhGH for 3 months. All were weaned from PN during the treatment period. However, only two children remained free of PN one year later. PN-dependent children with neonatal SBS received 0.14 $mg.kg^{-1}.day^{-1}$ and glutamine for 3 months.[128] Results suggested beneficial effect of rhGH by decreasing the need for PN but mild effects on body composition and gut mucosa. In addition, there was no apparent benefit from glutamine treatment. Two girls with neonatal SBS received exogenous GH (0.3 mg/kg per week subcutaneously) and concurrent glutamine supplementation, beginning at 6 and 1/2 years of age.[129] Both patients were weaned off PN, taking enteral nutrition alone. These data show that late exogenous treatment with rhGH and glutamine supplementation improved growth parameters in SBS children. Earlier use of rhGH in SBS infants or children might be helpful for future management.

Glucagon-like peptide-2 (GLP-2): The effect of GLP-2 analog on the gastrointestinal function was assessed in patients without a terminal ileum and colon who have functional short-bowel syndrome with severe malabsorption and no postprandial secretion of GLP-2.[134] Balance studies were performed before and after treatment with GLP-2, 400 µg subcutaneously twice a day for 35 days. Treatment with GLP-2 improved the intestinal absorption of energy and increased body weight. Thus, GLP-2 improves intestinal absorption and nutritional status in SBS patients with impaired postprandial GLP-2 secretion in whom the terminal ileum and the colon have been resected, based on the hypothesis that distal small bowel and cecal resection would decrease GLP-2 levels and reduce adaptation.[134-137] A recent European trial has shown that a GLP-2 analog teduglutide was successful in weaning off PN adult SBS.[136]

A study was performed in young infants correlating postprandial GLP-2 levels with intestinal length, nutrient absorption, and patient outcome.[60] These results suggest that in infants with intestinal dysfunction, GLP-2 levels are correlated with residual small bowel length and nutrient absorption, and may be predictive of outcome. GLP-2 might be the most logical medical approach for early management of SBS patients especially those with ileal resection. Further studies involving recombinant GLP-2 required to examine the ontogeny of the GLP-2 axis and the possible therapeutic role of GLP-2 supplementation. To date, no results of clinical trials involving infants or children are published in the literature.

Epidermal growth factor (EGF): It has been shown to have a role both in maintaining epithelial tissues as well as controlling intestinal adpatation.[91] An EGF and a bombesin (BBS) were compared in Sprague-Dawley male rats for achieving intestinal adaptation following massive intestinal resection. This study suggests that EGF and BBS act synergistically in facilitating the adaptive response of the remnant ileum to massive intestinal resection. In clinical setting, 5 SBS pediatric patients (<25% bowel length predicted for age) received 100 µg/kg per day given mixed with enteral feeds for 6 weeks.[138] All patients showed a significant improvement in carbohydrate absorption and improved tolerance of enteral feeds (enteral energy as percent of total energy, 25% ± 28% pretreatment vs 36% ± 24% post-treatment; mean ± SD; (P < .05). EGF treatment was not associated with significant changes in intestinal permeability, the rate of weight gain, or liver function tests. However, this study involving only 5 patients assessed with discussable parameters, does not allow to draw any conclusion.

Insulin: It has been shown to influence intestinal structure and absorptive function.[138] The effects of parenteral insulin on structural intestinal adaptation, cell proliferation, and apoptosis were shown in rats. This favorable effect of insulin is relevant and is now considered in SBS patients as well as others growth factors.[140]

Nontransplant Surgery

Nontransplant surgery (NTS) has been used in the last 3 decades to improve the intestinal function in children with SBS having rapid transit time, dilated bowel loops and insufficient absorptive capacity.[141-145] Early experience has been reported with the technique called longitudinal intestinal lengthening and tailoring (LILT), and more recently with the serial transverse enteroplasty technique (STEP)[61,62] (Fig. 11.6). Indications for bowel-lengthening surgery include the presence of a large intestinal diameter (>3 cm) for at least 20 cm of small bowel and a minimum total bowel length of 40 cm.[145-154]

The LILT operation involves the longitudinal resection of a dilated loop of the small bowel between the peritoneal leaves of the mesentery; this gives origin to two hemiloops each having its own blood supply. These are sutured longitudinally and anastomosed sequentially, doubling the length and halving the diameter of the operated loop (Fig. 11.6). The advantages of the LILT procedure include the maintenance of the normal orientation of the muscular fibers allowing more physiological peristaltic contractions, and the possibility to further perform a STEP procedure on the lengthened segments. The disadvantages are represented by the risks of vascular complications during the procedure making LILT more technically demanding as compared to the STEP procedure.[148]

The STEP operation involves the use of a surgical stapler applied sequentially, from alternating and opposite directions to the dilated loop, in a transverse, partially overlapping fashion creating a zigzag–like channel of approximately 2–2.5 cm in diameter (Fig. 11.6). This operation has the great advantage of being simple and reproducible. These techniques also alleviate the consequences of severe bowel dilatation with subsequent intestinal stasis and SIBO in children with SBS.

A recent review of the literature (39 publications) aimed to compare LILT and STEP.[152] For both procedures, the main indication is failure to achieve intestinal autonomy by conservative therapy while end-stage liver disease is the main contraindication. Both procedures have a similar extent of intestinal lengthening (approximately 70%) and result in improvement of enteral nutrition and reversal of IF related complications. STEP seems to have a lower mortality and overall progression to transplantation. STEP and LILT are both accepted procedures for management of SBS in children. However, the outcome after STEP seems to be more favorable. The International STEP Registry was analyzed to identify preoperative factors that are significantly associated with transplantation or death or attainment of enteral autonomy after STEP.[148]

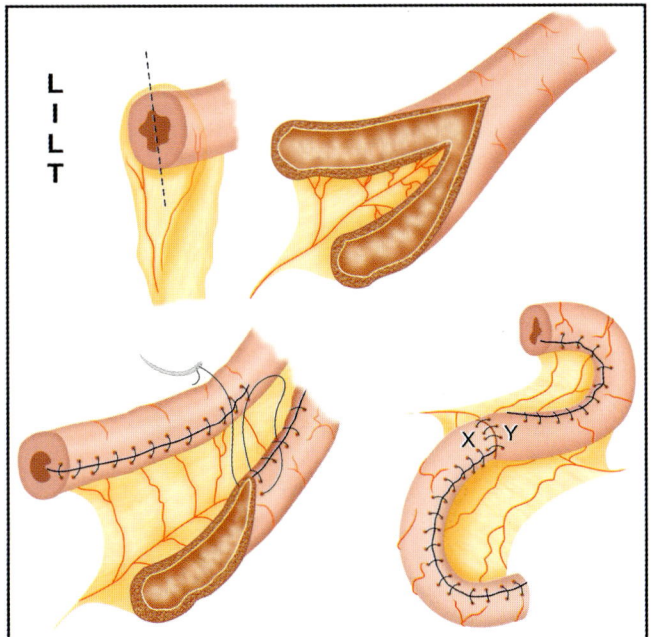
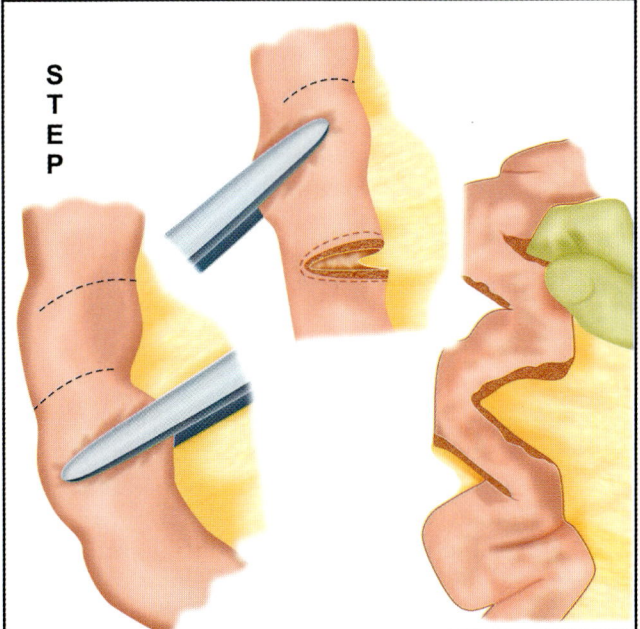

Fig. 11.6: Nontransplant surgery in the short bowel syndrome
Abbreviations: LILT, longitudinal intestinal lengthening and tailoring; STEP, serial transverse enteroplasty.

Table 11.4: Intestinal bacterial overgrowth

- Several factors intrinsic to SBS predispose to small intestinal bacterial overgrowth (SIBO) and explain its high prevalence in SBS patients
- Poorly motile segments of small intestine in close proximity to colon are common in patients with SBS and dysmotility. Intestinal stasis and bacterial contamination promote abnormal growth of bacteria in the small intestine
- The link between SIBO, translocation, cholestasis, portal fibrosis and cirrhosis is now clearly established
- SIBO may significantly compromise digestive and absorptive functions and may delay or prevent weaning from PN
- Clinical as well as biological tests for documenting SIBO may be unreliable
- Intestinal microbiota plays an important role in intestinal adaptation and should be preserved as much as possible
- Antibiotic therapy should be used very carefully to avoid bacterial selection and resistance
- The use of probiotics offers potential based on experimental evidence, but there is lack of sufficient data from human studies
- Management of SIBO may include nontransplant surgery (SITL or STEP) surgery, if advocated
- D-lactic acidosis is secondary to bacterial hypermetabolism, especially in the preserved colon, as a consequence of small intestine malabsorption

Definition
Colonies forming units (CFUs) per mL of bacteria in the proximal small bowel
- overgrowth of >105 CFUs per mL
- overgrowth of >103 CFUs per mL provided that the species of bacteria isolated from the jejunal aspirate are those that normally colonize the large bowel or providing that the same species are absent from saliva and gastric juice
- Breath hydrogen testing by using lactulose

Caused by small intestine stasis from:
- Intestinal obstruction (e.g. stenosis, narrowed anastomosis)
- Blind loop from terminolateral anastomosis
- Dilated and poorly motile segments of small bowel in close proximity to colon

Consequences (Fig. 11.5)
- Small intestine mucosal injury with villous atrophy and subsequent malabsorption
- Increased small intestinal mucosal permeability
- IgE- or non-IgE-mediated sensitization and allergic enteritis
- Gram-negative sepsis from bacterial translocation
- Portal inflammation, cholestasis, fibrosis and end-stage liver disease (cirrhosis)

Management
- Reversal or removal of any predisposing condition(s)
  - Redo-anastomosis
  - Enteroplasty (Fig. 11.6)
    - Longitudinal intestinal lengthening and tapering (LILT)
    - Serial transverse enteroplasty (STEP procedure)
- Appropriate nutritional support and feeds replacement whenever possible
- Suppression or eradication of the contaminating bacteria (used but not validated approaches)
  - Intermittent bowel decontamination with antibiotics
  - Use of probiotics (*Lactobacillus* GG, *Saccharomyces boulardii*....)

Data were collected from September 2004 to January 2010 with 97 patients being analyzed. Eleven patients died and 5 progressed to intestinal transplantation. On multivariate analysis, higher direct bilirubin and shorter pre-STEP bowel length were independently predictive of progression to transplantation or death (p = 0.05 and p < 0.001, respectively). Of the 78 patients who were 7 days of age or older and required PN at the time of STEP, 37 (47%) achieved enteral autonomy after the first STEP. Longer pre-STEP bowel length was also independently associated with enteral autonomy (p = 0.002). Median time to reach enteral autonomy was 21 months (95% CI, 12–30). Patients with longer pre-STEP bowel length were significantly more likely to achieve enteral autonomy. STEP is a safe, well tolerated procedure, which has definitive benefit in reducing PN calorie requirements over the first year following the procedure. It has an important role in achieving enteral independence in children with SBS.[146]

Table 11.5: Outcome of neonatal short bowel syndrome according to anatomical characteristics

The SBS is a very variable condition which can be as mild as that following terminal ileal resection to a very debilitating condition which follows total jejuno- ileal and colonic resection. Management and outcome vary according to the cause, the extent and site of resection and the degree of adaptation of the remaining bowel. Patients with dilated, poorly motile segments of SB (gastroschisis, atresia, NEC) should benefit from an approach aiming in reducing bowel dilatation and small intestinal bacterial overgrowth (SIBO), since they may develop progressive liver disease. Parenteral nutrition (PN) should be delivered, as soon as tolerance permits, by cyclical infusion. Early oral feeding (OF) should be promoted while the benefits of continuous enteral feeding (CEF) should be balanced in combination with PN, the risk of "intestinal overload" with subsequent SIBO and the tube feeding induced food aversion and eating disorders.

- **SBS with small bowel length (SBL) <40 cm with loss of the ileocecal valve (ICV) and associated partial or large colectomy:**
  Patients need very long-term home-PN. The indication to wean PN is appropriate weight gain and tolerance to other feeds, including ETF if needed. Ileum resection requires vitamin B_{12} supplementation

- **SBS with SBL <40 cm or only duodenum with totally or largely intact colon:**
  Patients need long-term home-PN. However many infants and children, may have a degree of adaptation and require less PN and benefit from orally and/or enterally administered nutrients. Some of them may be progressively weaned from PN. Infants with duodeno-right colon anastomosis have no chance to be weaned from PN and should receive oral feeding to promote optimal psychological behavior. These patients are at risk of developing D-lactic acidosis. They may become candidates for intestinal transplantation

- **SBS with SBL (40–100 cm) with loss of the ileocecal valve (ICV) and associated partial or large colectomy:**
  Patients require mid-term home-PN and can be fed orally immediately. Combination of CEF and oral feeding may help in reducing the PN duration. Bile salt-induced diarrhea may impede rapid PN weaning. Ileum resection requires vitamin B_{12} supplementation

- **SBS with SBL (40–100 cm) with terminal ileum and the entire colon:**
  In general, patients require short-term PN and can be fed orally immediately. ETF in combination with oral feeding may help in reducing PN duration. These patients are at risk of developing D-lactic acidosis, because of intestinal malabsorption and colonic bacterial hypermetabolism

- **SBS with terminal ileum resection:**
  Patients have a bile salt-induced diarrhea, and benefit from the administration of 1–2 g of cholestyramine 3 times a day to bind bile salts left unabsorbed by the resected ileum. Vitamin B_{12} plasma levels should be measured and if low, supplemental vitamin B_{12} should be provided by intramuscular injection in a dose of 100–150 μg per month or 1000 mg every 6 months

LONG-TERM OUTCOME AND GROWTH OF PATIENTS

When oral feeding and home PN are commenced in combination, amounts and/or rate of PN infusion are progressively decreased.[147] In our experience, the combination of oral feeding and cyclic PN allows home PN to be achieved in the best conditions.[44] The combination of CTF and cyclic PN seems to us less logical since nutritional support would only take place during the nocturnal period. If not, the patient would be dependent on an artificial nutritional support for 24 hours a day. In the last 20 years we have treated, in hospital followed by home PN, more than 300 patients, mainly infants, with SBS. Time for PN weaning depends on several factors which include the length of the remaining total intestine, lack of the ICV, and the functional capacity of the remaining small intestine. The slow transition from PN to full oral feeding requires time during which nutritional status has to be maintained at the optimal level. Trying to wean from PN to rapidly an infant with neonatal SBS lead to the risk of failure to thrive and metabolic complications (Table 11.6).

Special care should be taken to monitor children with SBS who are weaned off PN. They should be screened from time to time for nutritional deficiencies. Hyperphagia should be considered a sign of intestinal insufficiency and supported by feeding optimization.

During the long-term follow-up, weight and height growth must be regularly monitored. Dietary intake should be adapted to digestive tolerance, the child's preference and growth. Whenever a growth failure occurs, it is important to perform a dietetic evaluation of the nutrient intake, stool balance studies and investigations for bacterial overgrowth. Long-term growth has been reported in several studies.[44,155-157]

In case of failure to thrive, one should discuss the opportunity for restarting nutritional support by enteral feeding or in some case using parenteral nutrition. A retrospective study was carried out in 87 children, born

Table 11.6: The main causes of failure to thrive in SBS patients

- Insufficient and/or unadapted parenteral nutrition intake*
- Trace elements deficiencies (especially zinc)
- Sodium depletion from high stomy output
- Inefficient enteral tube feeding (malabsorption, SIBO)
- Gut mucosal inflammation from bacterial overgrowth
- Chronic metabolic acidosis (D-lactic acidosis)
- Repeated sepsis (catheter related, translocation)
- Intestinal failure associated liver disease (IFALD)

* The sum of PN and EN even if fitting the RDA may be not sufficient for growth because of intestinal malabsorption. PN intake should be increased for achieving optimal growth and nutrition

between 1975 and 1991 who had undergone extensive neonatal small bowel resection, followed up over a mean 15 years-period.[44] The overall survival was 89.7% depending on the date of birth. The duration of PN-dependency varies according to the intestinal length and the presence of the ICV. All patients who remain PN dependent had less than 40 cm of small bowel and/or the absence of ICV. Those who were weaned off PN grow up normally with normal puberty and final height as expected from genetic target height. Initial PN require careful monitoring of growth and may sometimes require nutritional support to be restarted.

Patients on long-term PN are at significantly increased risk for the development of metabolic bone disease. This condition is characterized by incomplete mineralization of osteoid with consequent disturbances ranging from osteopenia to severe bone disease with fractures. Bone mineral mass has to be assessed by dual-X-ray absorptiometry. However, few data are available in children.[158-160] Micronutrients deficiencies have been reported in children after weaning off PN.[161,162]

CONCLUSION

Long-term PN exposes to the risk of sepsis from both the central line and the digestive tract. There is a link between the onset of sepsis and liver disease.[163] Current practice of catheter care and prevention of sepsis, including ethanol locks, have decreased the rate of catheter-related infections.[164-168] Intestinal failure associated liver disease (IFALD) may be predicted in patients with SBS.[169-172] The link between lipid emulsions and liver disease has been pointed,[173] while fish oil based lipid emulsions are considered today as nutritionally efficient and able to reverse or prevent IFALD.[174-179]

Current pediatric intestinal failure (IF) is a multifaceted condition requiring the competent contributions of several medical and allied health professionals both for inpatient and outpatient care. Therefore, the formation of a multidisciplinary team is vital to achieve optimal results.[180-184] The intestinal failure team should ideally include a staff specialized in surgery, gastroenterology and nutrition, a pediatric dietician and a nurse experienced in central venous catheters handling and parenteral nutrition infusion. Special consideration should be given to the link between the hospital team and the homecare team. Fostering coordination of surgical, medical, and nutritional management is vital to provide high quality, integrated care of patients with IF, thus, improving remarkably the survival of these patients. The three most important issues in the management of children with IF include a good and early link between primary care givers and intestinal failure programs, the presence in the program of both intestinal rehabilitation and intestinal transplantation expertise and

participation in the network of the organisations providing home PN solutions. Collaborative strategies must be developed in order to reduce mortality and morbidity in patients with IF, especially for those who are referred for permanent IF or intestinal transplantation.

Although a large percentage of children with IF can survive with long-term PN, a proportion of patients eventually develop life-threatening complications, such as severe septic episodes, fluid and electrolytes imbalance, loss of venous access for PN and end-stage liver disease. In these patients nutrition has failed both in the enteral and the parenteral routes and may be called "nutritional failure".[2] These patients should be referred for transplantation.

Advances have been achieved in the field of intestinal and multivisceral transplantation in the last 10 years with significant improvement in the long-term patient and graft survival. According to the intestinal transplant registry, approximately 2500 intestinal transplants have been carried out so far in 79 worldwide transplant centers, of whom half are alive.

There is probably a different threshold for intestinal transplantation on the two sides of the Atlantic ocean. In accordance with the European approach, the European teams are more reluctant to refer a child for ITx and are inclined to support long-term home PN, which is cost effective and which to provides a better quality of life. Support for this view comes from Pironi et al. who have recently performed a 3-year prospective study (including both adults and children) on long-term PN for IF, and compared 'non-candidates' for ITx (no indications nor contraindications), with 'candidates' (who had an indication according to the USA Center for Medicare and Medicaid Services definitions, and a high risk of death or morbidity according to the American Society of Transplantation position paper).[4] The results showed that only patients with nutritional failure due to IFALD or major catheter complications had an increased risk of death on home PN, thus, supporting its use as the primary treatment for IF. Therefore, it was suggested that ITx should be used only as a lifesaving procedure. Home PN is the treatment of choice for IF in adults as well as in children.[1-5]

REFERENCES

1. Goulet O, Ruemmele F. Causes and management of intestinal failure in children. Gastroenterology. 2006;130 (2 Suppl 1): S16-28.
2. D'Antiga L, Goulet O. Intestinal failure in children: the European view. J Pediatr Gastroenterol Nutr. 2013;56:118-26.
3. Colomb V, Dabbas-Tyan M, et al. Long-term outcome of children receiving home parenteral nutrition: a 20-year single-center experience in 302 patients. J Pediatr Gastroenterol Nutr. 2007;44:347-53.

4. Pironi L, Joly F, Forbes A, et al. Long-term follow-up of patients on home parenteral nutrition in Europe: implications for intestinal transplantation. Gut. 2011;60:17-25.

5. Beath S Gowen H, Puntis JW. Trends in paediatric home parenteral nutrition and implications for service development. Clin Nutr. 2011;30:499-502.

6. Gottrand F, Staszewski P, Colomb V, et al. Satisfaction in different life domains in children receiving home parenteral nutrition and their families. J Pediatr. 2005;146:793-7.

7. Engstrom I, Bjornestam B, Finkel Y. Psychological distress associated with home parenteral nutrition in Swedish children, adolescents, and their parents: preliminary results. J Pediatr Gastroenterol Nutr. 2003;37:246-50.

8. Martin LW, Zerella JT. Jejunoileal atresia: a proposed classification. J Pediatr Surg. 1976;11:399-403.

9. Moreno LA, Gottrand F, Turck D, Manouvrier-Hanu S, Mazingue F, Morisot C, et al. Severe combined immunodeficiency syndrome associated with autosomal recessive familial multiple gastrointestinal atresias: study of a family. Am J Med Genet. 1990;37:143-6.

10. Gilroy RK, Coccia PF, Talmadge JE, Hatcher LI, Pirruccello SJ, Shaw BW, Jr., et al. Donor immune reconstitution after liver-small bowel transplantation for multiple intestinal atresia with immunodeficiency. Blood. 2004;103:1171-4.

11. Chen R, Giliani S, Lanzi G, et al. Whole-exome sequencing identifies tetratricopeptide repeat domain 7A (TTC7A) mutations for combined immunodeficiency with intestinal atresias. J Allergy Clin Immunol. 2013;132:656-64.

12. Khen-Dunlop N, Sarnacki S, Victor A, et al. Prenatal intestinal obstruction affects the myenteric plexus and causes functional bowel impairment in fetal rat experimental model of intestinal atresia. PLoS One. 2013;8(5):e62292.

13. Rankin J, Pattenden S, Abramsky L, Boyd P, Jordan H, Stone D, et al. Prevalence of congenital anomalies in five British regions, 1991-99. Arch Dis Child Fetal Neonat. 2005;90:F374-9.

14. Loane M, Dolk H, Kelly A, Teljeur C, Greenlees R, Densem J, et al. Paper 4: EUROCAT statistical monitoring: identification and investigation of ten year trends of congenital anomalies in Europe. Birth Defects Res A Clin Mol Teratol. 2011;91(Suppl 1):S31-43.

15. Torfs CP, Christianson RE, Iovannisci DM, Shaw GM, Lammer EJ. Selected gene polymorphisms and their interaction with maternal smoking, as risk factors for gastroschisis. Birth Defects Res A Clin Mol Teratol. 2006;76(10):723-30.

16. Segel SY, Marder SJ, Parry S, Macones GA. Fetal abdominal wall defects and mode of delivery: a systematic review. Obstetrics and gynecology. 2001;98(5 Pt 1):867-73.

17. Davies MW, Kimble RM, Woodgate PG. Ward reduction without general anaesthesia versus reduction and repair under general anaesthesia for gastroschisis in newborn infants. Cochrane database of systematic reviews (Online). 2002(3):CD003671.

18. van Manen M, Hendson L, Wiley M, Evans M, Taghaddos S, Dinu I. Early childhood outcomes of infants born with gastroschisis. J Pediatr Surg. 2013;48:1682-7.

19. Kenny SE, Tam PK, Garcia-Barcelo M. Hirschsprung's disease. Semin Pediatr Surg. 2010;19:194-200.

20. Bergeron KF, Silversides DW, Pilon N. The developmental genetics of Hirschsprung's disease. Clin Genet. 2013;83:15-22.

21. Butler Tjaden NE, Trainor PA. The developmental etiology and pathogenesis of Hirschsprung disease. Transl Res. 2013;162:1-15.

22. Sauvat F, Grimaldi C, Lacaille F, et al. Intestinal transplantation for total intestinal aganglionosis: a series of 12 consecutive children. J Pediatr Surg. 2008;43:1833-8.

23. Lee HC, Pickard SS, Sridhar S, Dutta S. Intestinal malrotation and catastrophic volvulus in infancy. J Emerg Med. 2012;43: e 49-51.

24. Millar AJ, Rode H, Cywes S. Malrotation and volvulus in infancy and childhood. Semin Pediatr Surg. 2003;12:229-36.

25. Luig M, Lui K; NSW and ACT NICUS Group. Epidemiology of necrotizing enterocolitis--Part I: Changing regional trends in extremely preterm infants over 14 years. J Paediatr Child Health. 2005;41:167-73.

26. Patole S. Prevention of necrotising enterocolitis: year 2004 and beyond. J Matern Fetal Neonatal Med. 2005;17:69-80.

27. Neu J, Walker WA. Necrotizing enterocolitis. N Engl J Med. 2011;364:255-64.

28. Operative strategies for necrotizing enterocolitis: The prevention and treatment of short-bowel syndrome. Semin Pediatr Surg. 2005;14:191-8.

29. Patole SK, de Klerk N. Impact of standardised feeding regimens on incidence of neonatal necrotising enterocolitis: a systematic review and meta-analysis of observational studies. Arch Dis Child Fetal Neonatal Ed. 2005;90: F147-51.

30. Berseth CL. Feeding strategies and necrotizing enterocolitis. Curr Opin Pediatr. 2005;17:170-3.

31. Smith JR. Early enteral feeding for the very low birth weight infant: the development and impact of a research-based guideline. Neonatal Netw. 2005;24:9-19.

32. Tyson JE, Kennedy KA. Trophic feedings for parenterally fed infants. Cochrane Database Syst Rev. 2005;20:CD000504.

33. Tubman TR, Thompson SW, McGuire W. Glutamine supplementation to prevent morbidity and mortality in preterm infants. Cochrane Database Syst Rev. 2005;25:CD001457.

34. Bin-Nun A, Bromiker R, Wilschanski M, Kaplan M, Rudensky B, Caplan M, Hammerman C. Oral probiotics prevent necrotizing enterocolitis in very low birth weight neonates. J Pediatr. 2005;147:192-6.

35. Lin HC, Su BH, Chen AC, Lin TW, Tsai CH, Yeh TF, Oh W. Oral probiotics reduce the incidence and severity of necrotizing enterocolitis in very low birth weight infants. Pediatrics. 2005;115:1-4.

36. Deshpande G, Rao S, Patole S, Bulsara M. Updated meta-analysis of probiotics for preventing necrotizing enterocolitis in preterm neonates. Pediatrics. 2010;125:921-30.

37. Mihatsch WA, Braegger CP, Decsi T, et al. Critical systematic review of the level of evidence for routine use of probiotics for reduction of mortality and prevention of necrotizing enterocolitis and sepsis in preterm infants. Clin Nutr. 2012;31:6-15.

38. Hall NJ, Eaton S, Pierro A. Necrotizing enterocolitis: Prevention, treatment, and outcome. J Pediatr Surg. 2013;48(12):2359-67.

39. Janvier A, Malo J, Barrington KJ. Cohort Study of Probiotics in a North American Neonatal Intensive Care Unit. J Pediatr. 2014 Jan 7. [Epub ahead of print]

40. Ofek Shlomai N, Deshpande G, Rao S, Patole S. Probiotics for preterm neonates: what will it take to change clinical practice? Neonatology. 2014;105:64-70.

41. Touloukian RJ, Smith GJ. Normal intestinal length in preterm infants. J Pediatr Surg. 1983;18:720-3.

42. Quiros-Tejeira RE, Ament ME, Reyen L, et al. Long-term parenteral nutritional support and intestinal adaptation in children with short bowel syndrome: a 25-year experience. J Pediatr. 2004;145:157-63.

43. Spencer AU, Neaga A, West B, et al. Pediatric short bowel syndrome: redefining predictors of success. Ann Surg. 2005;242:403-9.

44. Goulet O, Baglin-Gobet S, Talbotec C, et al. Outcome and long-term growth after extensive small bowel resection in the neonatal period: a survey of 87 children. Eur J Pediatr Surg 2005;15:95-101.

45. Infantino BJ, Mercer DF, Hobson BD, et al. Successful rehabilitation in pediatric ultrashort small bowel syndrome. J Pediatr. 2013; 163:1361-6.

46. Diamanti A, Conforti A, Panetta F, et al. Long-Term Outcome of Home Parenteral Nutrition In Patients With Ultra-Short Bowel Syndrome. J Pediatr Gastroenterol Nutr. 2013 Nov 13. [Epub ahead of print]

47. Buchman AL, Scolapio J, Fryer J. AGA technical review on short bowel syndrome and intestinal transplantation. Gastroenterology. 2003;124:1111-34.

48. Goulet O. Short bowel syndrome in pediatric patients. Nutrition. 1998;14:784-7.

49. Goulet O, Sauvat F. Short bowel syndrome and intestinal transplantation in children. Curr Opin Clin Nutr Metab Care. 2006;9:304-13.

50. Jeppesen PB, Mortensen PB. Colonic digestion and absorption of energy from carbohydrates and medium-chain fat in small bowel failure. J Parent Enteral Nutr. 1999;23(5 Suppl): S101-5.

51. Goulet O, Colomb-Jung V, Joly F. Role of the colon in short bowel syndrome and intestinal transplantation. J Pediatr Gastroenterol Nutr. 2009;48(Suppl 2):S66-7.

52. Joly F, Mayeur C, Bruneau A, et al. Drastic changes in fecal and mucosa-associated microbiota in adult patients with short bowel syndrome. Biochimie. 2010;92:753-61.

53. Cole CR, Ziegler TR. Small bowel bacterial overgrowth: a negative factor in gut adaptation in pediatric SBS. Curr Gastroenterol Rep. 2007;9:456-62.

54. Musch MW, Bookstein C, Rocha F, Lucioni A, Ren H, Daniel J, et al. Region-specific adaptation of apical Na/H exchangers after extensive proximal small bowel resection. Am J Physiol Gastroint Liver Physiol. 2002;283: G975-85.

55. Jeppesen PB, Staun M, Tjellesen L, Mortensen PB. Effect of intravenous ranitidine and omeprazole on intestinal absorption of water, sodium, and macronutrients in patients with intestinal resection. Gut. 1998;43:763-9.

56. Kato J, Sakamoto J, Teramukai S, Kojima H, Nakao A. A prospective within-patient comparison clinical trial on the effect of parenteral cimetidine for improvement of fluid secretion and electrolyte balance in patients with short bowel syndrome. Hepatogastroenterology. 2004;51:1742-6.

57. Holst JJ. Glucagon-like peptide-1: from extract to agent. The Claude Bernard Lecture, 2005. Diabetologia. 2006;49:253-60.

58. Vegge A, Thymann T, Lund P, et al. Glucagon-like peptide-2 induces rapid digestive adaptation following intestinal resection in preterm neonates. Am J Physiol Gastrointest Liver Physiol. 2013;305: G277-85.

59. Litvak DA, Evers BM, Hellmich MR, Townsend CM Jr. Enterotrophic effects of glucagon-like peptide 2 are enhanced by neurotensin. J Gastrointest Surg. 1999;3:432-39.

60. Botsios DS, Vasiliadis KD. Factors enhancing intestinal adaptation after bowel compensation. Dig Dis. 2003;21:228-36.

61. Zhang W, Li N, Zhu W, Shi Y, Zhang J, Li Q, Li J. Peptide YY induces enterocyte proliferation in a rat model with total enteral nutrition after distal bowel resection. Pediatr Surg Int. 2008;24:913-9.

62. Bortvedt SF, Lund PK. Insulin-like growth factor 1: common mediator of multiple enterotrophic hormones and growth factors. Curr Opin Gastroenterol. 2012;28:89-98.

63. Gouttebel MC, Astre C, Briand D, Saint-Aubert B, Girardot PM, Joyeux H. Influence of N-acetylglutamine or glutamine infusion on plasma amino acid concentrations during the early phase of small-bowel adaptation in the dog. JPEN J Parenter Enteral Nutr. 1992;16:117-21.

64. Mok E, Hankard R. Glutamine supplementation in sick children: is it beneficial? J Nutr Metab. 2011;Epub 2011 Nov. 14.

65. Koruda MJ, Rolandelli RH, Settle RG, Saul SH, Rombeau JL. Harry M. Vars award. The effect of a pectin-supplemented elemental diet on intestinal adaptation to massive small bowel resection. JPEN Journal of parenteral and enteral nutrition. 1986;10:343-50.

66. Koruda MJ, Rolandelli RH, Settle RG, Zimmaro DM, Rombeau JL. Effect of parenteral nutrition supplemented with short-chain fatty acids on adaptation to massive small bowel resection. Gastroenterology. 1988;95(3):715-20.

67. Jeppesen PB, Mortensen PB. Colonic digestion and absorption of energy from carbohydrates and medium-chain fat in small bowel failure. JPEN Journal of parenteral and enteral nutrition. 1999; 23 (5 Suppl): S101-5.

68. Sigalet DL, Martin GR, Butzner JD, Buret A, Meddings JB. A pilot study of the use of epidermal growth factor in pediatric short bowel syndrome. Journal of pediatric surgery. 2005;40:763-8.

69. Sukhotnik I, Mogilner JG, Shaoul R, et al. Responsiveness of intestinal epithelial cell turnover to TGF-alpha after bowel resection in a rat is correlated with EGF receptor expression along the villus-crypt axis. Pediatr Surg Int. 2008;24:21-8.

70. Guo M, Li Y, Li J. Role of growth homone, glutamine and enteral nutrition in pediatric short bowel syndrome: a pilot follow-up study. Eur J Pediatr Surg. 2012;22:121-6.

71. Zaouche A, Loukil C, De Lagausie P, et al. Effects of oral Saccharomyces boulardii on bacterial overgrowth, translocation, and intestinal adaptation after small-bowel resection in rats. Scand J Gastroenterol. 2000;35:160-5.

72. Buts JP, De Keyser N, Marandi S, et al. Saccharomyces boulardii upgrades cellular adaptation after proximal enterectomy in rats. Gut. 1999;45:89-96.

73. Kollman-Bauerly KA, Thomas DL, Adrian TE, Lien EL, Vanderhoof JA. The role of eicosanoids in the process of adaptation following massive bowel resection in the rat. JPEN J Parenter Enteral Nutr. 2001;25:275-81.

74. Crenn P, Coudray-Lucas C, Thuillier F, Cynober L, Messing B. Postabsorptive plasma citrulline concentration is a marker of absorptive enterocyte mass and intestinal failure in humans. Gastroenterology. 2000;119:1496-505.

75. Rhoads JM, Plunkett E, Galanko J, Lichtman S, Taylor L, Maynor A, et al. Serum citrulline levels correlate with enteral tolerance and bowel length in infants with short bowel syndrome. The Journal of pediatrics. 2005;146:542-7.

76. Jianfeng G, Weiming Z, Ning L, Fangnan L, Li T, Nan L, et al. Serum citrulline is a simple quantitative marker for small intestinal enterocytes mass and absorption function in short bowel patients. The Journal of surgical research. 2005;127:177-82.

77. Pappas PA, A GT, Gaynor JJ, Carreno MR, Ruiz P, Huijing F, et al. An analysis of the association between serum citrulline and acute rejection among 26 recipients of intestinal transplant. American journal of transplantation : official journal of the American Society of Transplantation and the American Society of Transplant Surgeons. 2004;4:1124-32.

78. Bailly-Botuha C, Colomb V, Thioulouse E, et al. Plasma citrulline concentration reflects enterocyte mass in children with short bowel syndrome. Pediatr Res. 2009;65:559-63.

79. Thompson JS. The role of prophylactic cholecystectomy in the short-bowel syndrome. Arch Surg. 1996;131:556-9.

80. Koletzko B, Goulet O, Hunt J, et al. Guidelines on Paediatric Parenteral Nutrition of the European Society of Paediatric Gastroenterology, Hepatology and Nutrition (ESPGHAN) and the European Society for Clinical Nutrition and Metabolism (ESPEN), Supported by the European Society of Paediatric Research (ESPR). J Pediatr Gastroenterol Nutr. 2005; 41(Suppl 2): S1-S87.

81. Goulet O, Joly F, Corriol O, et al. Some new insights in intestinal failure-associated liver disease. Curr Opin Organ Transplant. 2009;14:256-61.

82. Hyman PE, Everett SL, Harada T. Gastric acid hypersecretion in short bowel syndrome in infants: association with extent of resection and enteral feeding. J Pediatr Gastroenterol Nutr. 1986;5:191-7.

83. Parvadia JK, Keswani SG, Vaikunth S, et al. Role of VEGF in small bowel adaptation after resection: the adaptive response is angiogenesis dependent. Am J Physiol Gastrointest Liver Physiol. 2007;293:G591-8.

84. Helmrath MA, Shin CE, Fox JW, et al. Adaptation after small bowel resection is attenuated by sialoadenectomy: the role for endogenous epidermal growth factor. Surgery. 1998;124:848-54.

85. Olieman JF, Penning C, Ijsselstijn H, et al. Enteral nutrition in children with short-bowel syndrome: current evidence and recommendations for the clinician. J Am Diet Assoc. 2010;110:420-6.

86. Goulet O, Olieman J, Ksiazyk J, et al. Neonatal short bowel syndrome as a model of intestinal failure: physiological background for enteral feeding. Clin Nutr. 2013;32:162-71.

87. Donovan SM. Role of human milk components in gastrointestinal development: Current knowledge and future Needs. J Pediatr. 2006;149:S49-S61.

88. Vanderhoof J. Hydrolyzed versus nonhydrolyzed protein diet in short bowel syndrome in children. J Pediatr Gastroenterol Nutr. 2004;38:107-8.

89. Cummins AG, Thompson FM. Effect of breast milk and weaning on epithelial growth of the small intestine in humans. Gut. 2002;51:748-54.

90. Playford RJ, Macdonald CE, Johnson WS. Colostrum and milk-derived peptide growth factors for the treatment of gastrointestinal disorders. Am J Clin Nutr. 2000;72:5-14

91. DiBaise JK, Young RJ, Vanderhoof JA. Intestinal rehabilitation and the short bowel syndrome: part 1. Am J Gastroenterol. 2004;99:1386-95.

92. Andorsky DJ, Lund DP, Lillehei CW, et al. Nutritional and other postoperative management of neonates with short bowel syndrome correlates with clinical outcomes. J Pediatr. 2001;139:27-33

93. de Boissieu D, Dupont C. Allergy to extensively hydrolyzed cow's milk proteins in infants: safety and duration of amino acid-based formula. J Pediatr. 2002;141:271-3.

94. Berni Canani R, Nocerino R, Terrin G, et al. Formula selection for management of children with cow's milk allergy influences the rate of acquisition of tolerance: a prospective multicenter study. J Pediatr. 2013;163:771-7.

95. Bines J, Francis D, Hill D. Reducing parenteral requirement in children with short bowel syndrome: impact of an amino acid-based complete infant formula. J Pediatr Gastroenterol Nutr. 1998;26:123-8.

96. De Greef E, Mahler T, Janssen A, et al. The Influence of Neocate in Paediatric Short Bowel Syndrome on PN Weaning. J Nutr Metab. 2010;2010. pii: 297575.

97. Gupte GL, Beath SV, Kelly DA, et al. Current issues in the management of intestinal failure. Arch Dis Child. 2006;91:259-64.

98. Joly F, Dray X, Corcos O, et al. Tube feeding improves intestinal absorption in short bowel syndrome patients. Gastroenterology. 2009;136:824-31.

99. Javid PJ, Malone FR, Reyes J, et al. The experience of a regional pediatric intestinal failure program: Successful outcomes from intestinal rehabilitation. Am J Surg. 2010;199:676-9.

100. Barkun AN, Love J, Gould M, Pluta H, Steinhart H. Bile acid malabsorption in chronic diarrhea: pathophysiology and treatment. Can J Gastroenterol. 2013;27:653-9.

101. Quigley EM. Bacteria: a new player in gastrointestinal motility disorders--infections, bacterial overgrowth, and probiotics. Gastroenterol Clin North Am. 2007;36:735-48.

102. Olieman JF, Poley MJ, Gischler SJ, et al. Interdisciplinary management of infantile short bowel syndrome: resource consumption, growth, and nutrition. J Pediatr Surg. 2010;45: 490-8.

103. Cole CR, Frem JC, Schmotzer B, et al. The rate of bloodstream infection is high in infants with short bowel syndrome: relationship with small bowel bacterial overgrowth, enteral feeding, and inflammatory and immune responses. J Pediatr. 2010;156:941-7.

104. O'Keefe SJ. Bacterial overgrowth and liver complications in short bowel intestinal failure patients. Gastroenterology. 2006; 130(2 Suppl 1): S67-9.

105. Geier A, Fickert P, Trauner M. Mechanisms of disease: mechanisms and clinical implications of cholestasis in sepsis. Nat Clin Pract Gastroenterol Hepatol. 2006;3:574-85.

106. Fuchs M, Sanyal AJ. Sepsis and cholestasis. Clin Liver Dis. 2008;12: 151-72.

107. Wagner M, Zollner G, Trauner M. New molecular insights into the mechanisms of cholestasis. J Hepatol. 2009;51:565-80.

108. Copple BL, Jaeschke H, Klaassen CD. Oxidative stress and the pathogenesis of cholestasis. Semin Liver Dis. 2010;30:193-202.

109. Zhu Q, Zou L, Jagavelu K, Simonetto DA, Huebert RC, Jiang ZD, et al. Intestinal decontamination inhibits TLR4 dependent fibronectin-mediated cross-talk between stellate cells and endothelial cells in liver fibrosis in mice. J Hepatol. 2012;56:893-9.

110. Hartmann P, Haimerl M, Mazagova M, Brenner DA, Schnabl B. Toll-like receptor 2-mediated intestinal injury and enteric tumor necrosis factor receptor I contribute to liver fibrosis in mice. Gastroenterology. 2012;143:1330-40.

111. El Kasmi KC, Anderson AL, Devereaux MW, et al. Toll-like receptor 4-dependent Kupffer cell activation and liver injury in a novel mouse model of parenteral nutrition and intestinal injury. Hepatology. 2012;55:1518-28.

112. Fouts DE, Torralba M, Nelson KE, Brenner DA, Schnabl B. Bacterial translocation and changes in the intestinal microbiome in mouse models of liver disease. J Hepatol. 2012;56:1283-92.

113. Bhogal HK, Sanyal AJ. The molecular pathogenesis of cholestasis in sepsis. Front Biosci (Elite Ed). 2013;5:87-96.

114. Schnabl B. Linking intestinal homeostasis and liver disease. Curr Opin Gastroenterol. 2013;29:264-70.

115. Ching YA, Fitzgibbons S, Valim C, et al. Long-term nutritional and clinical outcomes after serial transverse enteroplasty at a single institution. J Pediatr Surg. 2009;44:939-43.

116. Thompson J, Sudan D. Intestinal lengthening for short bowel syndrome. Adv Surg. 2008;42:49-61.

117. Modi BP, Javid PJ, Jaksic T, et al; International STEP Data Registry. First report of the international serial transverse enteroplasty data registry: indications, efficacy, and complications. J Am Coll Surg. 2007;204:365-7.

118. Jeppesen PB, Mortensen PB. The influence of a preserved colon on the absorption of medium chain fat in patients with small bowel resection. Gut. 1998;43:478-83.

119. Joly F, Mayeur C, Bruneau A, et al. Drastic changes in fecal and mucosa-associated microbiota in adult patients with short bowel syndrome. Biochimie. 2010;92:753-61.

120. Mayne AJ, Handy DJ, Preece MA, George RH, Booth IW. Dietary management of D-lactic acidosis in short bowel syndrome. Archives of disease in childhood. 1990;65:229-31.

121. Uchida H, Yamamoto H, Kisaki Y, et al. D-lactic acidosis in short-bowel syndrome managed with antibiotics and probiotics. J Pediatr Surg. 2004;39:634-6.

122. Abeysekara S, Naylor JM, Wassef AW, Isak U, Zello GA. D-Lactic acid-induced neurotoxicity in a calf model. American J Physiol. 2007;293:E558-65.

123. Gutierrez IM, Kang KH, Calvert CE, et al. Risk factors for small bowel bacterial overgrowth and diagnostic yield of duodenal aspirates in children with intestinal failure: a retrospective review. J Pediatr Surg. 2012;47:1150-4.

124. Scolapio JS. Effect of growth hormone, glutamine, and diet on body composition in short bowel syndrome: a randomized, controlled study. JPEN Journal of parenteral and enteral nutrition. 1999;23(6):309-12; discussion.

125. Szkudlarek J, Jeppesen PB, Mortensen PB. Effect of high dose growth hormone with glutamine and no change in diet on intestinal absorption in short bowel patients: a randomised, double blind, crossover, placebo controlled study. Gut. 2000;47:199-205.

126. Seguy D, Vahedi K, Kapel N, Souberbielle JC, Messing B. Low-dose growth hormone in adult home parenteral nutrition-dependent short bowel syndrome patients: a positive study. Gastroenterology. 2003;124:293-302.

127. Socha J, Ksiazyk J, Fogel WA et al. Is growth hormone a feasible adjuvant in the treatment of children after small bowel resection. Clin Nutr. 1996;15:185-8.

128. Lifschitz C, Duggan C, Lazngston C, Vanderhoof J, Shulman RJ. Growth Hormone (GH) therapy in children with short bowel syndrome (SBS): a randomized, placebo controlled study. Digestive Disease Week; Orlando. 2003: A100.

129. Ladd AP, Grosfeld JL, Pescovitz OH, Johnson NB. The effect of growth hormone supplementation on late nutritional independence in pediatric patients with short bowel syndrome. J Pediatr Surg. 2005;40:442-5.

130. Goulet O, Dabbas-Tyan M, Talbotec C, et al. Effect of recombinant human growth hormone on intestinal absorption and body composition in children with short bowel syndrome. JPEN J Parent Enter Nutr. 2010;34:513-20.

131. Peretti N, Loras-Duclaux I, Kassai B, et al. Growth hormone to improve short bowel syndrome intestinal autonomy: a pediatric randomized open-label clinical trial. J Parenter Enteral Nutr. 2011;35:723-31.

132. Guo M, Li Y, Li J. Role of growth hormone, glutamine and enteral nutrition in pediatric short bowel syndrome: a pilot follow-up study. Eur J Pediatr Surg. 2012;22:121-6.

133. Wales PW, Nasr A, de Silva N, et al. Human growth hormone and glutamine for patients with short bowel syndrome. Cochrane Database Syst Rev. 2010;6:CD006321.

134. Jeppesen PB, Sanguinetti EL, Buchman A et al. Teduglutide (ALX-0600), a dipeptidyl peptidase IV resistant glucagon-like peptide 2 analogue, improves intestinal function in short bowel syndrome patients. Gut. 2005;54:1224-31.

135. Wallis K, Walters JR, Gabe S. Short bowel syndrome: the role of GLP-2 on improving outcome. Curr Opin Clin Nutr Metab Care. 2009;12:526-32.

136. Jeppesen PB, Gilroy R, Pertkiewicz M, et al. Randomised placebo-controlled trial of teduglutide in reducing parenteral nutrition and/or intravenous fluid requirements in patients with short bowel syndrome. Gut. 2011;60:902-14.

137. Sigalet DL, Martin G, Meddings J, Hartman B, Holst JJ. GLP-2 levels in infants with intestinal dysfunction. Pediatr Res. 2004;56:371-6.

138. Sigalet DL, Martin GR, Butzner JD, Buret A, Meddings JB. A pilot study of the use of epidermal growth factor in pediatric short bowel syndrome. J Pediatr Surg. 2005;40:763-8.

139. Sukhotnik I, Mogilner J, Shamir R, Shehadeh N, Bejar J, Hirsh M, Coran AG. Effect of subcutaneous insulin on intestinal adaptation in a rat model of short bowel syndrome. Pediatr Surg Int. 2005;21:132-7.

140. McMellen ME, Wakeman D, Longshore SW, et al. Growth factors: possible roles for clinical management of the short bowel syndrome. Semin Pediatr Surg. 2010;19:35-43.

141. Bianchi A. Intestinal loop lengthening—a technique for increasing small intestinal length. J Pediatr Surg. 1980; 15: 145-51.

142. Bianchi A. Intestinal lengthening: an experimental and clinical review. J R Soc Med. 1984;77(Suppl 3):35-41.

143. Kim HB, Lee PW, Garza J, et al. Serial transverse enteroplasty for short bowel syndrome: a case report. J Pediatr Surg. 2003;38: 881-5.

144. Sudan D, Thompson J, Botha J, et al. Comparison of intestinal lengthening procedures for patients with short bowel syndrome. Ann Surg. 2007;246:593-601.

145. Khalil BA, Ba'ath ME, Aziz A, et al. Intestinal Rehabilitation And Bowel Reconstruction Surgery: Improved Outcomes In Children With Short Bowel Syndrome. J Pediatr Gastroenterol Nutr. 2011 [Epub ahead of print].

146. Javid PJ, Sanchez SE, Horslen SP, Healey PJ. Intestinal lengthening and nutritional outcomes in children with short bowel syndrome. Am J Surg. 2013;205:576-80.

147. Pakarinen MP, Kurvinen A, Koivusalo AI, Iber T, Rintala RJ. Long-term controlled outcomes after autologous intestinal reconstruction surgery in treatment of severe short bowel syndrome. J Pediatr Surg. 2013;48:339-44.

148. Jones BA, Hull MA, Potanos KM, Zurakowski D, Fitzgibbons SC, Ching YA, Duggan C, Jaksic T, Kim HB; International STEP Data Registry. Report of 111 consecutive patients enrolled in the International Serial Transverse Enteroplasty (STEP) Data Registry: a retrospective observational study. J Am Coll Surg. 2013;216:438-46.

149. Almond SL, Haveliwala Z, Khalil B, Morabito A. Autologous intestinal reconstructive surgery to reduce bowel dilatation improves intestinal adaptation in children with short bowel syndrome. J Pediatr Gastroenterol Nutr. 2013;56:631-4.

150. Millar AJ. Non-transplant surgery for short bowel syndrome. Pediatr Surg Int. 2013;29:983-7.

151. Frongia G, Kessler M, Weih S, Nickkholgh A, Mehrabi A, Holland-Cunz S. Comparison of LILT and STEP procedures in children with short bowel syndrome—a systematic review of the literature.. J Pediatr Surg. 2013;48:1794-805.

152. Bhalla VK, Pipkin WL, Hatley RM, Howell CG. The use of multiple serial transverse enteroplasty (STEP) procedures for the management of intestinal atresia and short bowel syndrome. Am Surg. 2013;79:826-8.

153. Mercer DF, Hobson BD, Gerhardt BK, et al. Serial transverse enteroplasty allows children with short bowel to wean from parenteral nutrition. J Pediatr. 2014;164:93-8.

154. Norman JL, Crill CM. Optimizing the transition to home parenteral nutrition in pediatric patients. Nutr Clin Pract. 2011;26:273-85.

155. Olieman JF, Tibboel D, Penning C. Growth and nutritional aspects of infantile short bowel syndrome for the past 2 decades. J Pediatr Surg. 2008;43:2061-9.

156. Olieman JF, Penning C, Spoel M, et al. Long-term impact of infantile short bowel syndrome on nutritional status and growth. Br J Nutr. 2012;107:1489-97.

157. Pichler J, Chomtho S, Fewtrell M, Macdonald S, Hill SM. Growth and bone health in pediatric intestinal failure patients receiving long-term parenteral nutrition. Am J Clin Nutr. 2013;97:1260-9.

158. Diamanti A, Bizzarri C, Basso MS, et al. How does long-term parenteral nutrition impact the bone mineral status of children with intestinal failure? J Bone Miner Metab. 2010;28:351-8.

159. Mutanen A, Mäkitie O, Pakarinen MP. Risk of metabolic bone disease is increased both during and after weaning off parenteral nutrition in pediatric intestinal failure. Horm Res Paediatr. 2013;79:227-35.

160. Pichler J, Chomtho S, Fewtrell M, Macdonald S, Hill S. Body composition in paediatric intestinal failure patients receiving long-term parenteral nutrition. Arch Dis Child. 2014;99:147-53.

161. Yang CF, Duro D, Zurakowski D, et al. High prevalence of multiple micronutrient deficiencies in children with intestinal failure: a longitudinal study. J Pediatr. 2011;159:39-44.e1.

162. Miyasaka EA, Brown PI, Kadoura S, et al The adolescent child with short bowel syndrome: new onset of failure to thrive and need for increased nutritional supplementation. J Pediatr Surg. 2010;45:1280-6.

163. Hermans D, Talbotec C, Lacaille F, et al. Early central catheter infections may contribute to hepatic fibrosis in children receiving long-term parenteral nutrition. J Pediatr Gastroenterol Nutr. 2007;44:459-63.

164. Pittiruti M, Hamilton H, Biffi R, et al. ESPEN Guidelines on Parenteral Nutrition: Central Venous Catheters (access, care, diagnosis and therapy of complications). Clinical Nutr. 2009;28:365-77.

165. Greenberg RG, Moran C, Ulshen M, et al. Outcomes of catheter-associated infections in pediatric patients with short bowel syndrome. J Pediatr Gastroenterol Nutr. 2010;50:460-2.

166. Kim JS, Holtom P, Vigen C. Reduction of catheter-related bloodstream infections through the use of a central venous line bundle: Epidemiologic and economic consequences. Am J Infect Control. 2011;39:640-6.

167. Miller SJ. Bloodstream Infections Associated With Parenteral Nutrition Preparation Methods in the United States: A Retrospective, Large Database Analysis. J Parenter Enteral Nutr 2011. Sep 30. [Epub ahead of print].

168. Wales PW, Kosar C, Carricato M, et al. Ethanol lock therapy to reduce the incidence of catheter-related bloodstream infections in home parenteral nutrition patients with intestinal failure: preliminary experience. J Pediatr Surg. 2011;46:951-6.

169. Willis TC, Carter BA, Rogers SP, et al. High rates of mortality and morbidity occur in infants with parenteral nutrition-associated cholestasis. J Parenter Enteral Nutr. 2010;34:32-37.

170. Kaufman SS, Pehlivanova M, Fennelly EM, et al. Predicting liver failure in parenteral nutrition-dependent short bowel syndrome of infancy. J Pediatr. 2010;156:580-5.

171. Duro D, Kalish LA, Johnston P, et al. Risk factors for intestinal failure in infants with necrotizing enterocolitis: a Glaser Pediatric Research Network study. J Pediatr. 2010;157:203-8.

172. Hsieh MH, Pai W, Tseng HI, et al. Parenteral nutrition-associated cholestasis in premature babies: risk factors and predictors. Pediatr Neonatol. 2009;50:202-7.

173. Colomb V, Jobert-Giraud A, Lacaille F, et al. Role of lipid emulsions in cholestasis associated with long-term parenteral nutrition in children. J Parenter Enteral Nutr. 2000;24:345-50.

174. Gura KM, Duggan CP, Collier SB, et al. Reversal of parenteral nutrition- associated liver disease in two infants with short bowel syndrome using parenteral fish oil: implications for future management. Pediatrics. 2006;118:e197-e201.

175. Koletzko B, Goulet O. Fish oil containing intravenous lipid emulsions in parenteral nutrition-associated cholestatic liver disease. Curr Opin Clin Nutr Metab Care. 2010;13:321-6.

176. Tomsits E, Tolgysi A, Fekete G, et al. Safety and efficacy of a lipid emulsion containing a mixture of soybean, olive, coconut and fish oils: a randomized double blind trial in premature infants requiring parenteral nutrition. J Pediatr Gastroenterol Nutr. 2010;51: 514-21.

177. Goulet O, Antebi H, Wolf C, et al. A new intravenous fat emulsion containing fish oil: a single center, double-blind randomized study on long-term efficacy and safety in pediatric patients. J Parenter Enteral Nutr 2010;34:485-95.

178. Le HD, de Meijer VE, Robinson EM, et al. Parenteral fish-oil-based lipid emulsion improves fatty acid profiles and lipids in parenteral nutrition-dependent children. Am J Clin Nutr. 2011;94:749-58.

179. Premkumar MH, Carter BA, Hawthorne KM, King K, Abrams SA. Fish oil-based lipid emulsions in the treatment of parenteral nutrition-associated liver disease: an ongoing positive experience. Adv Nutr. 2014;5:65-70.

180. Sudan D, Dibaise J, Torres C, et al. A multidisciplinary approach to the treatment of intestinal failure. J Gastrointest Surg. 2005;9:165-76.

181. Modi BP, Langer M, Ching YA, et al. Improved survival in a multidisciplinary short bowel syndrome program. J Pediatr Surg. 2008;43:20-4

182. Beath S, Pironi L, Gabe S, et al. Collaborative strategies to reduce mortality and morbidity in patients with chronic intestinal failure including those who are referred for small bowel transplantation. Transplantation. 2008;85:1378-84.

183. Miller M, Burjonrappa S. A Review of Enteral Strategies in Infant Short Bowel Syndrome: evidence-based or NICU Culture? J Pediatr Surg. 2013;48:1099-112.

184. Stanger JD, Oliveira C, Blackmore C, Avitzur Y, Wales PW. The impact of multi-disciplinary intestinal rehabilitation programs on the outcome of pediatric patients with intestinal failure: a systematic review and meta-analysis. J Pediatr Surg. 2013;48: 983-92.

185. Wales PW, Christison-Lagay ER. Short bowel syndrome: epidemiology and etiology. Semin Pediatr Surg. 2010;19:3-9.

Chapter 12

Surgical Disorders of the Gastrointestinal Tract

Rajeev Redkar, Parag Karkera

The disorders of the gastrointestinal tract have been discussed under three broad headings:

1. Congenital disorders like esophageal atresia, pyloric stenosis, intestinal atresia, malrotation of gut, meconium ileus, Hirschsprung's disease and anorectal malformations.
2. Acute emergencies like appendicitis, intussusceptions and intestinal obstruction.
3. Rarer issues and recent advances like pancreatic disorders, gastroesophageal reflux disease and bariatric surgical procedures.

CONGENITAL ANOMALIES

ESOPHAGEAL ATRESIA AND TRACHEOESOPHAGEAL FISTULA

Esophageal atresia (EA) is a congenital malformation in which there is, defect in the continuity of the esophagus with or without a fistula with the trachea. It usually consists of a blind upper oesophageal pouch, with a lower oesophageal segment that bears communication with the trachea through a distal tracheoesophageal fistula (TEF).

It is seen in 1 per 3500 live births with a male predominance.[1,2]

Classification (Gross 1953)[3] (Fig. 12.1)

- Type A: Pure esophageal atresia (6%)
- Type B: Esophageal atresia with proximal TE fistula (4%)
- Type C: Esophageal atresia with distal TE fistula (84%)
- Type D: Esophageal atresia with fistula to both pouches (1%)
- Type E: Tracheoesophageal fistula without esophageal atresia (5%)
- Type F: Esophageal stenosis

Clinical Presentation[1]

- Excessive salivation—first clinical sign
- Coughing, choking during feeding
- Respiratory distress due to:
  - Recurrent aspiration of saliva and gastric fluid regurgitation leading to chemical pneumonitis
  - Abdominal distension due to passage of air through the fistula into the stomach.

Associated Anomalies[4-6]

It is seen in 50–70% of patients, e.g. VACTERL association (3 or more):

- **V**ertebral anomalies (i.e. hemivertebrae, spina bifida)
- **A**norectal malformations

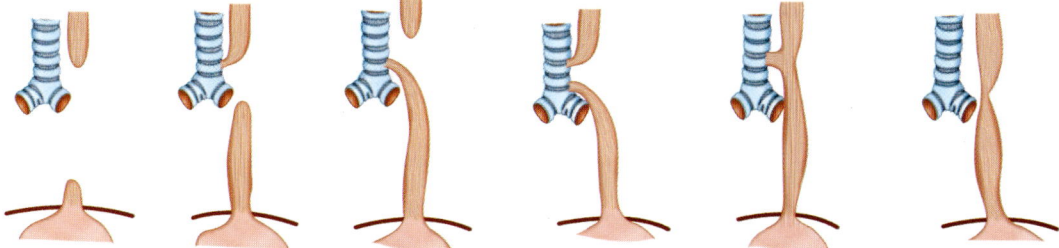

Fig. 12.1: Anatomical classification of esophageal atresia (Gross)

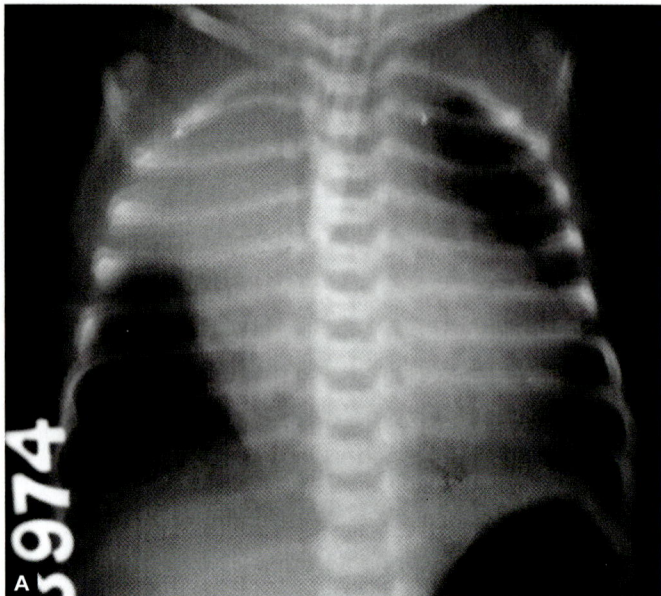
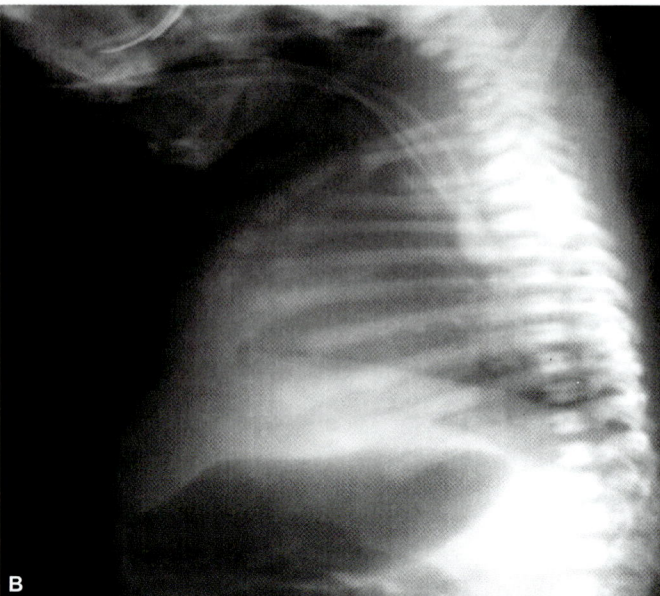

Figs 12.2A and B: Plain X-ray chest—AP and lateral showing an infant feeding tube coiled in the upper esophageal pouch in a case of esophageal atresia

- ❏ **C**ardiac malformations (i.e. VSD, ASD, tetralogy of Fallot)
- ❏ **T**racheoesophageal fistula
- ❏ **R**enal Deformities (i.e. renal agenesis, horseshoe kidney, hypospadias)
- ❏ **L**imb dysplasia.

Diagnosis[1]

Resistance on passage of a firm orogastric catheter or a coiled flexible catheter in the proximal pouch seen in chest and neck radiograph are diagnostic. When in doubt, thin, small amount of barium instilled in proximal pouch may help in diagnosis.

Presence of air in the stomach and bowel suggests EA with distal TEF, while its absence is suggestive of pure EA (Figs 12.2A and B).

Treatment[1,6]

Preoperative Management

- ❏ Upper pouch secretion aspiration with Replogle (double lumen) tube or by frequent oral suctioning
- ❏ Vigorous chest physiotherapy

Operative Management

A posterolateral thoracotomy, usually right thoracotomy, and extrapleural division and closure of the tracheaesophageal fistula with primary end-to-end esophageal anastomosis without undue tension is performed (Fig. 12.3).

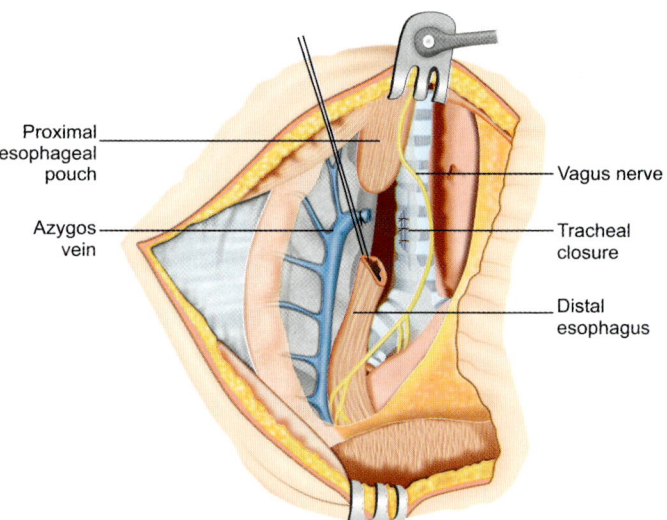

Fig. 12.3: Operative representation of esophageal atresia repair

In pure EA, long gap EA, premature infants, a delayed anastomosis or esophageal replacement with stomach or colon may be considered.

Outcome[7,8]

Predictors of adverse outcome are: low birth weight, prematurity, severe pulmonary dysfunction, and presence of major congenital cardiac disease.

Complication after Surgery[1]

Anastomotic leak, stricture, gastroesophageal reflux, tracheomalacia and recurrent TEF.

INFANTILE HYPERTROPHIC PYLORIC STENOSIS

Infantile hypertrophic pyloric stenosis (IHPS) is a common cause of gastric outlet obstruction in infants. It commonly occurs in the first 3–6 weeks of life, although rarely may be present at birth.[9]

Epidemiology

- ❑ 1.5–4.0 in 1000 live births in whites[10]
- ❑ More common in first born males[10]
- ❑ First reported by Hirschsprung in 1888.[11]
- ❑ Occurrence is associated with environmental and familial factors with a genetic predisposition.[9]

Pathogenesis

The appearance of the pylorus in IHPS is that of an enlarged, pale muscle mass usually measuring 2–2.5 cm in length and 1–1.5 cm in diameter. Pronounced muscle hypertrophy and hyperplasia primarily involving the circular layer produces partial or complete luminal occlusion.[12,13]

Clinical Presentation[9]

Nonbilious, projectile vomiting is a characteristic feature of IHPS, which over a period of days become more frequent and more forceful. Untreated cases may present with severe dehydration and electrolyte disturbances (hypokalemic, hypochloremic metabolic alkalosis) (Fig. 12.4).

Diagnosis

- ❑ A gastric peristaltic wave going from left to right may be visible
- ❑ Palpation of the pyloric olive in the midline in the epigastrium below the edge of the liver. It is usually palpable when the child is calm, cooperative (with the help of a small feed or a pacifier) in a nondistended stomach and relaxed abdominal musculature[9]
- ❑ Upper GI contrast study shows a distended stomach with an elongated and narrowed pyloric canal—the "string" and the "double tract" sign[14]
- ❑ Ultrasonography is investigative modality of choice. The most commonly used criteria are a pyloric muscle thickness of 4 mm or more and pyloric channel length of 16 mm or more[15] (Fig. 12.5).

Treatment

Preoperative Management[9]

Preoperative care consists of correction of dehydration and electrolyte imbalance (usually with 5% dextrose in 0.45% normal saline with 20–40 m eq/L of potassium at 1.25–2 times the maintenance dose) before surgical intervention.

Surgical Management

Ramstedt's pyloromyotomy: It involves making a serosal incision on the antero-superior aspect of the pylorus beginning approximately 1–2 mm proximal to the duodenum and extended into the nonhypertrophied antrum (Fig. 12.6).

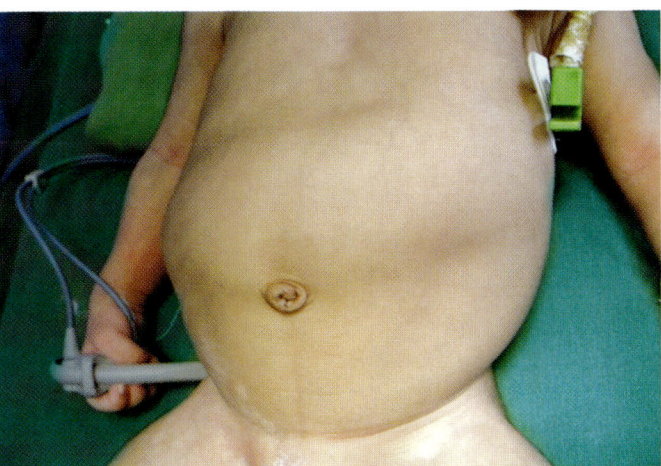

Fig. 12.4: Gastric wave of peristalsis in IHPS

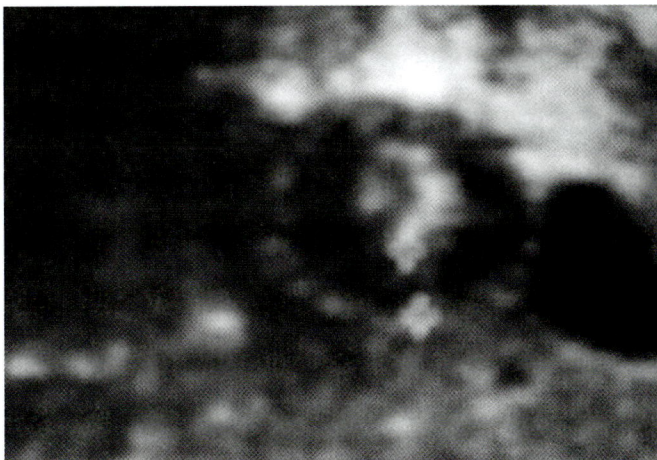

Fig. 12.5: Ultrasonography demonstrating a hypertrophied pylorus

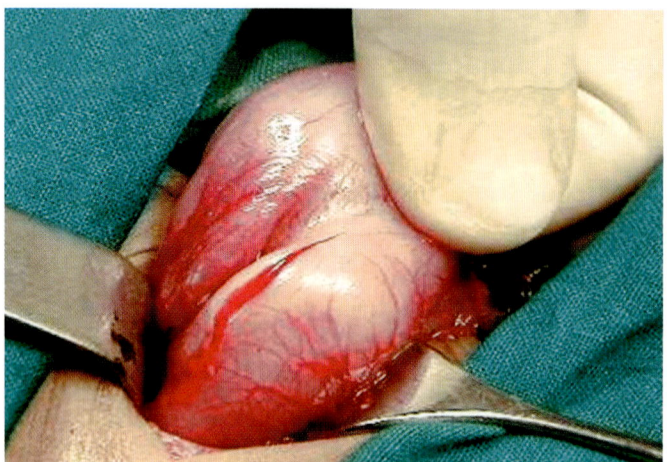

Fig. 12.6: Ramstedt's pyloromyotomy on IHPS

The hypertrophied circular muscle is spread and further disrupted till the mucosa pouts.[16]

DUODENAL ATRESIA

Etiology

The condition is probably the result of failure of canalization.[17]

Incidence

Incidence: 1 in 6000–10,000 live births.[18]

Location: Most common site of obstruction is just distal to the ampulla of Vater.[19]

Associated Conditions

Low birth weight, Down syndrome and other major anomalies (up to 50%) [annular pancreas, malrotation, congenital heart disease, esophageal atresia, genito-urinary and anorectal malformations].[20]

Clinical Presentation[21,22]

❑ Maternal polyhydramnios in 50% of cases
❑ Prenatal USG shows double bubble obstructive pattern with a dilated, fluid-filled stomach, and duodenum
❑ Repeated bilious vomiting within few hours of birth
❑ Fullness in the epigastrium with rest of the abdomen being scaphoid.

Diagnosis[23]

Abdominal radiographs show a "double bubble" with gas in a dilated stomach and duodenum without any gas distally

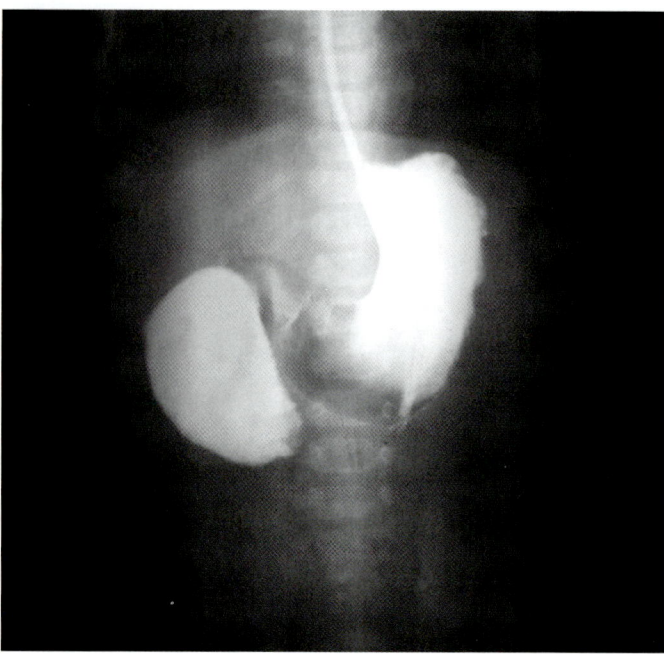

Fig. 12.7: Contrast study showing a duodenal atresia and no dye in distal intestines

in the abdomen. Occasionally, an upper gastrointestinal contrast series may be required to differentiate intrinsic duodenal obstruction from midgut volvulus (Fig. 12.7).

Management[24]

Duodenoduodenostomy

It involves bypass of the obstruction and a simple side to side or Kimura's diamond (proximal transverse and distal longitudinal) anastomosis.

ILEAL AND JEJUNAL ATRESIA

Small bowel atresias are the most common intestinal anomalies and frequent cause of neonatal intestinal obstruction. It usually results due to a late intrauterine mesenteric vascular accident (i.e. internal hernia, intrauterine volvulus, and intussusception).[25,26]

Classification of Intestinal Atresia (Grosfeld)[26] [Fig. 12.8]

❑ Type I (20%): A mucosal (septal) atresia with an intact bowel wall and mesentery
❑ Type II (30%): Two atretic blind ends connected by a band of fibrous tissue (cord) and an intact mesentery
❑ Type IIIa: Two ends of atretic bowel separated by a gap (V-shaped defect) in the mesentery

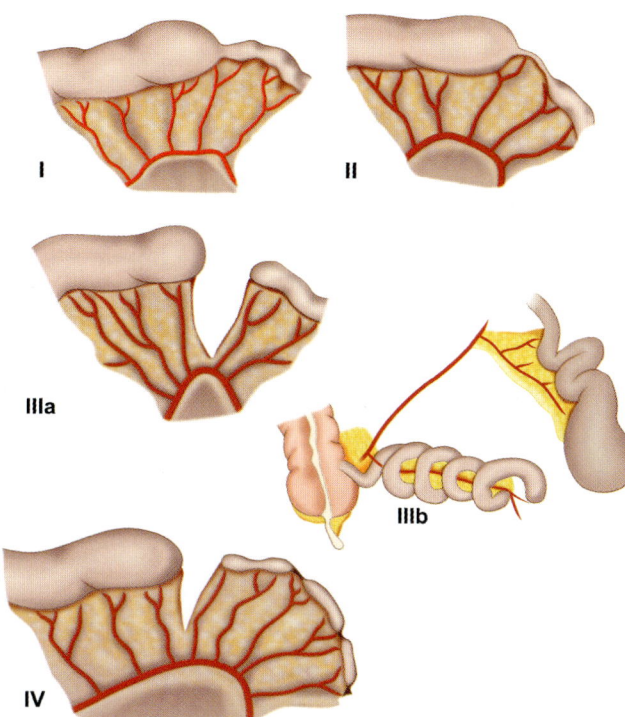

Fig. 12.8: Classifications of intestinal atresia (Grosfeld)

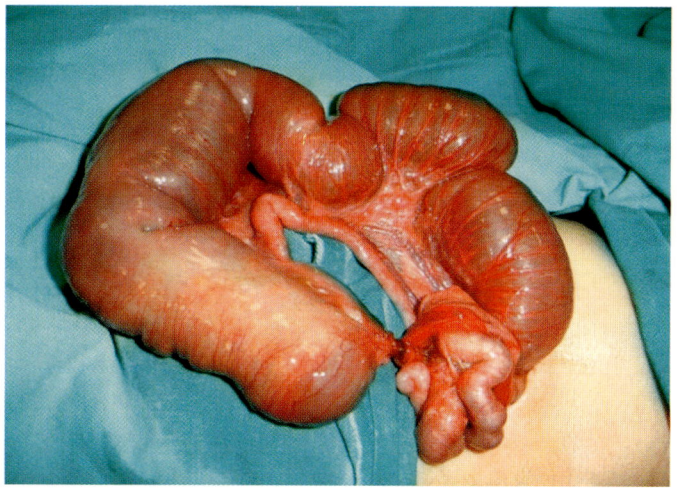

Fig. 12.9: Jejunal atresia

❑ Type IIIb: Apple-peel atresia presents with jejunal atresia near the ligament of Treitz, foreshortened bowel and a large mesenteric gap
❑ Type IV (6–20%) (String-of-sausages appearance): Multiple atresias.

Associated Conditions

Low birth weight (40%).

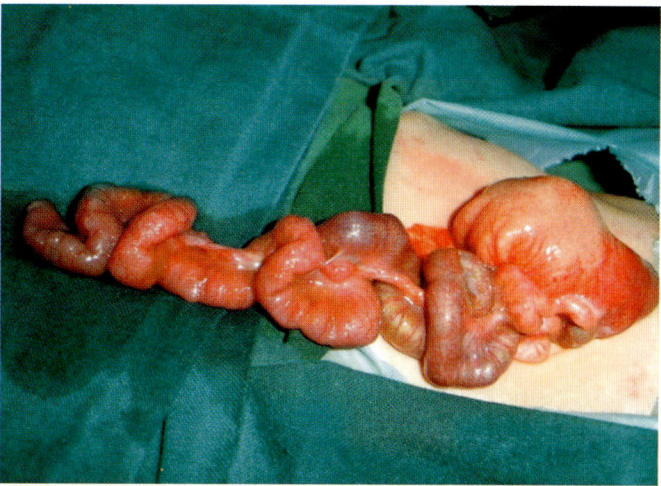

Fig. 12.10: Ileal atresia with a distal apple peel deformity

Clinical Presentation[27,28]

The most common clinical features include bilious vomiting, abdominal distension, failure to pass meconium on the first day of life, maternal polyhydramnios, and indirect jaundice.

Diagnosis[29]

Plain abdominal radiographs show many dilated bowel loops with air-fluid levels. High jejunal atresia may present with a few air fluid levels while ileal atresias are associated with multiple levels and no further gas beyond that.

Management[26]

Laparotomy with resection of the proximal dilated end with primary end-to-end anastomosis is usually possible. In certain cases like atresia with volvulus where there is vascular compromise and severe meconium peritonitis, temporary enterostomy followed by delayed anastomosis after 3–12 weeks is performed (Figs 12.9 and 12.10).

▌MECONIUM ILEUS

This disorder causes obstruction of the small bowel with inspissisated meconium and is seen in approximately 15% of infants with cystic fibrosis.[30]

Clinical Presentation[31]

Family history of cystic fibrosis and maternal polyhydramnios is present in almost 20% of patients.

In uncomplicated cases, abdominal distension at birth, bilious vomiting, and failure to pass meconium are seen.

Doughy bowel loops with indentation on palpation—the so called putty sign may be noticed.

Complicated meconium ileus will present with evidence of bowel obstruction complicated by evidence of previous intestinal perforation and/or necrosis: clinically evident as peritonitis including an erythematous or edematous abdominal wall and/or demonstrable abdominal tenderness.

Imaging Studies

Plain abdominal radiograph demonstrates:
- Disparity in size of bowel loops, no or few air-fluid levels, a granular 'soap bubble or ground glass 'appearance[31-33]
- Cresecents or speckles of intra-abdominal calcifications in complicated meconium peritonitis[28]
- Contrast enema demonstrates a microcolon, which may be empty or with pellets of inspissated meconium.[34]

Management

Nonoperative Treatment

Gastrograffin (meglumine-diatrizoate) with polysorbate 80 (tween 80) enemas to dissolve the meconium.[35]

Surgical Treatment

Surgery is indicated:
- In uncomplicated meconium ileus that have failed to respond to nonoperative treatment with enema solubilizing agents
- Meconium ileus complicated with intestinal atresia, volvulus, perforation, meconium cyst formation with peritonitis, intestinal gangrene, or combinations of these events.

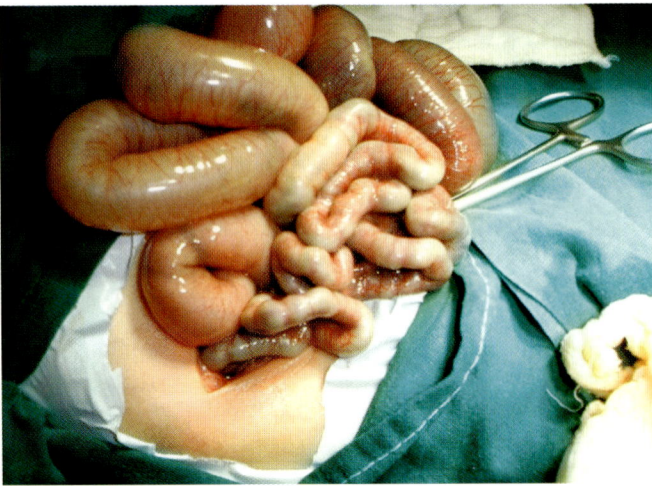

Fig. 12.11: Pellets of inspissated meconium seen in distal ileum in meconium ileus

The goal of operation is the relief of intraluminal ileocolonic obstruction by either the evacuation of the adherent intraluminal meconium or by resection of the portion of bowel filled with inspissated material[36] (Fig. 12.11).

Postsurgical Management[31]

- N-acetyl cysteine instillation through nasogastric tube to dissolve residual meconium
- Early enteral or parenteral nutrition with vigorous pulmonary therapy
- Sweat test (pilocarpineiontophoresis) to confirm a diagnosis of cystic fibrosis.

MALROTATION OF GUT

Normal rotation and fixation involves the two ends of intestinal tract, proximal duodenojejunal loop, and distal cecocolic loop around an axis formed by superior mesenteric artery, a total arc of 270°. The term malrotation refers to all abnormalities of intestinal position and attachment.

Malrotation of gut is a common cause of neonatal intestinal obstruction, failure or delay in diagnosis of which may prove fatal when associated with midgut volvulus.[37,38]

In the classic form of malrotation, the cecum lies in the epigastrium while the duodenojejunal(DJ) flexure lies inferiorly and to the right of the midline. Peritoneal bands pass from the right upper quadrant lateral to the duodenum to the cecum and ascending colon (Ladd's bands). Midgut volvulus occurs when there is incomplete malrotation of the midgut between the cecum and the DJ flexure around a narrow pedicle. Duodenal obstruction can occur either due to Ladd's bands or midgut volulus.

Clinical Presentation[39]

- Sudden onset of bilious emesis is the primary presenting sign
- Scaphoid abdomen soon after vomiting
- Bleeding per rectum, abdominal tenderness, and signs of peritonitis are seen in cases with vascular compromise.

Diagnosis[37,40]

- Plain abdominal radiographs are nondiagnostic, but may show 'double bubble 'sign in duodenal obstruction or gasless abdomen in midgut volvulus (Fig. 12.12)
- Ultrasound abdomen with color Doppler or CT scan abdomen may show the 'whirlpool' flow pattern of superior mesenteric vein around the superior mesenteric artery in midgut volvulus

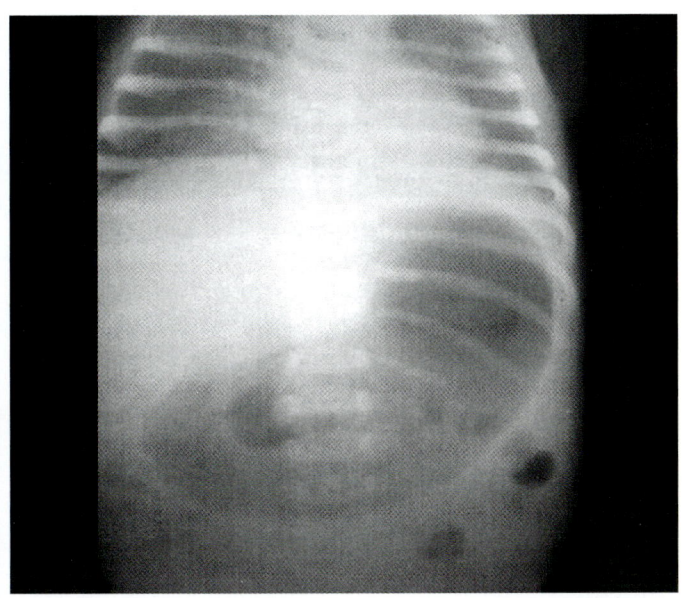

Fig. 12.12: Plain X-ray abdomen showing a distended stomach and scanty gas in small intestines suggestive of malrotation

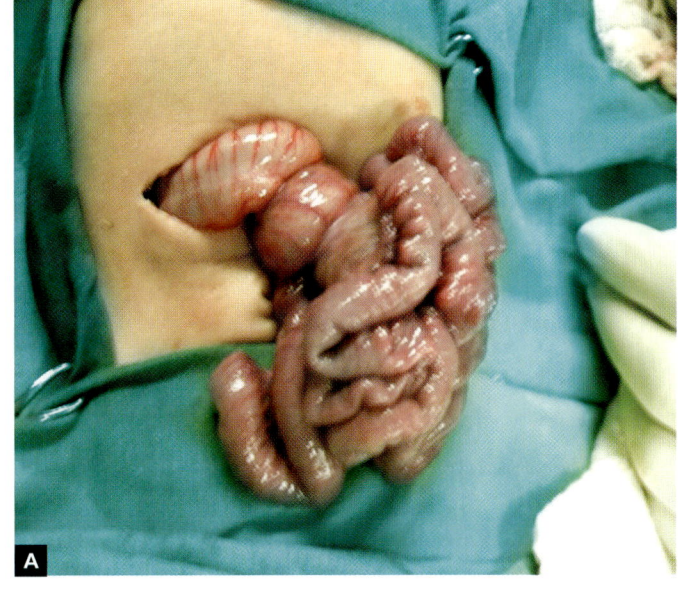

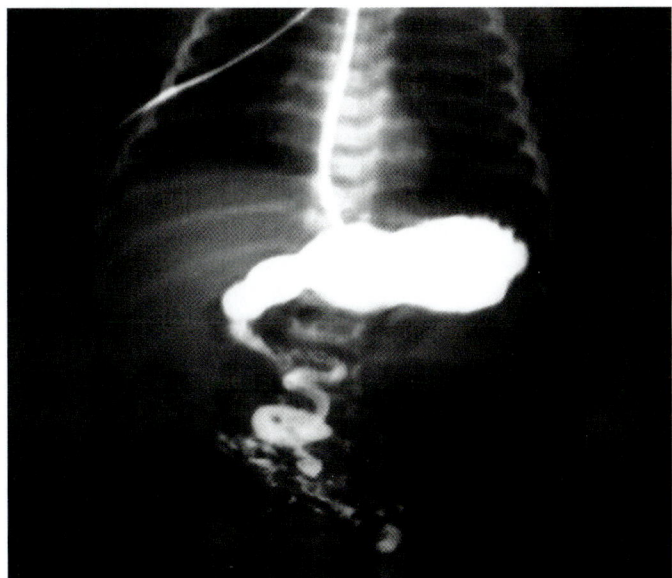

Fig. 12.13: Upper GI contrast study showing a jejunal twisting with the duodenojejunal junction on the right side of the spine indicative of malrotation of gut

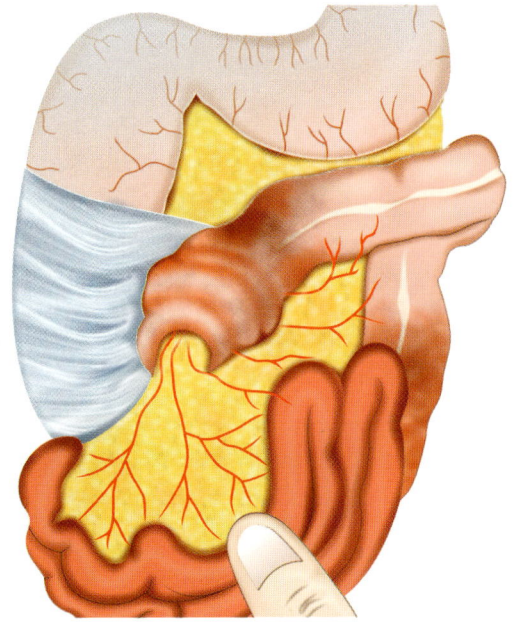

Figs 12.14A and B: Volvulus of small intestines in malrotation with a diagrammatic representation

❑ Upper gastrointestinal contrast study—the DJ junction is found in the midline or on the right side and below the level of the gastric outlet instead of being on the left side and at the level of the gastric outlet (Fig. 12.13).

Surgical Management[41]

Ladd procedure which incorporates the following steps (Figs 12.14A and B):

❑ Evisceration of midgut and inspection of root of mesentery
❑ Counterclockwise derotation of a midgut volvulus
❑ Lysis of Ladd's peritoneal bands (Peritoneal folds passing from the ascending colon to the duodenum and into the right lateral gutter) and straightening of duodenum along the right abdominal gutter
❑ Appendectomy—conventional or by inversion technique
❑ Placement of the cecum in the left lower quadrant.

ABDOMINAL WALL DEFECTS (OMPHALOCELE AND GASTROCHISIS)

Omphalocele

Omphaloceles are central abdominal defects resulting from failure of infolding of the body wall . They are covered by a sac of amnio-peritoneal membrane, usually more than 4 cm. The umbilicus is attached to the summit of the sac which contains intestines in smaller defects (<4 cm) and the liver and occasionally, the spleen and gonad in larger defects (Fig. 12.15).

Gastroschisis

Gastroschisis is generally a small defect (<4 cm) to the right of the umbilicus without a sac covering it. The umbilicus is normally placed and the midgut herniates through the defect.

The bowel loops become thick, matted, edematous and covered by a fibrinous, exudative peel due to the irritating effect of the amniotic fluid , which contains fetal urine and various growth factors.[42]

Embryology[43]

The anterior abdominal wall is formed by fusion of two lateral, one caudal, and one cephalic abdominal folds.

Omphalocele is a result of failure of these folds to fuse along with failure of the midgut to return to the abdominal cavity.

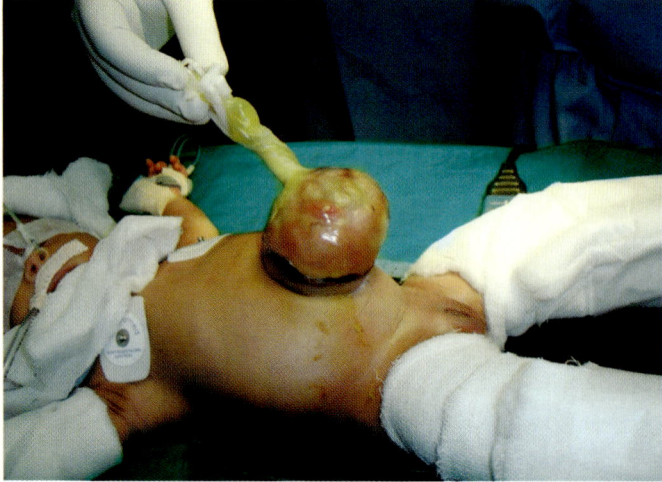

Fig. 12.15: Exomphalus with a sac cover and the umbilical cord attached to its summit

Gastroschisis is due to the failure of the umbilical celom to develop. Abnormal involution of right umbilical vein results in a mesenchymal defect to the right of umbilicus and the intestines rupture out through that defect.

Associated Anomalies[42]

Omphalocele

They are usually macrosomic and may be associated with cardiac defects, chromosomal anomalies, musculoskeletal defects, neural tube defects, gastroesophageal reflux, and undescended testes.

Gastroschisis

Intestinal atresia, gastroesophageal reflux, and cryptorchidism.

Management

Prenatal ultrasound and elevated maternal serum alpha-fetoprotein levels are useful for antenatal diagnosis.

Treatment begins immediately following delivery and consists of nasogastric tube aspiration, intravenous fluid resuscitation. Body temperature, serum electrolytes, blood glucose and hematocrit are monitored. Broad-spectrum antibiotics are started and complete examination done to rule out associated anomalies, including echocardiogram and ultrasonography for urinary anomalies.

The sac or exposed intestines should be covered by a barrier-type dressing. The bowel should be supported to prevent strangulation.

Surgical Treatment[42,44,45]

Omphalocele Small defects are managed by primary closure. It consists of excision of the sac, reduction of the viscera, i.e. intestines and liver, raising skin flaps, full thickness muscular closure and skin closure.

If fascial closure is deemed tight so as to increase the intra-abdominal pressure, only skin flaps are close with repair of postoperative hernia later at 1 year of age. If even skin closure is not possible, viscera is covered in a silastic silo, which allows slow reduction over a 1 week period.

Giant omphaloceles may require skin flaps with or without prosthetic mesh underneath for closure of the defect with skin grafts on the residual area.

In poor surgical candidates, such as premature infants, those with chromosomal abnormalities, cardiac disease, or lung hypoplasia, topical agents, e.g. mercurochrome, iodine, silver sulfadiazine can be used to promote granulation and epithelialization.

Gastroschisis: Immediate operative reduction and surgical repair is the method of choice. The closure can be facilitated by extending the defect superiorly, decompressing the intestinal contents either retrograde into the stomach or prograde into the colon and stretching the abdominal wall. When primary closure is not possible, Dacron reinforced silastic silo can be sewn to the fascial defect with staged reduction of the herniated contents into the abdominal cavity (Fig. 12.16).

HIRSCHSPRUNG'S DISEASE

Hirschsprung disease (HD) is a developmental disorder of the intrinsic component of the enteric nervous system in which the myenteric and submucosal plexuses of the distal intestine are devoid of ganglion cells. Ganglion cells are responsible for normal peristalsis; hence, patients with HD present with functional intestinal obstruction at the level of aganglionosis. Aganglionosis mostly involves the rectum or rectosigmoid, but it can extend for varying lengths, and in 5% to 10% of cases can involve the entire colon or varying lengths of small intestine. The incidence of Hirschsprung's disease is approximately 1 in 5000 live-born infants.[46,47]

Etiology[46,48]

In infants with HD, the process of migration of ganglion cells derived from the neural crest cells is disturbed, so the ganglion cells are absent in the distal bowel. This may be because they mature into ganglion cells early or fail to survive or proliferate.

Clinical Presentation

Neonatal Obstruction

Abdominal distension, bilious vomiting, and feeding intolerance are the presenting features in most cases. Ninety percent of the children have delayed passage of meconium beyond the first 24 hours. Cecal or appendiceal perforation may be an initial event[46,49] (Fig. 12.17).

Chronic Constipation

Some patients present later in childhood, with chronic constipation, most commonly breastfed infants, at the time of weaning. Clinical features that point to this diagnosis include failure to pass meconium in the first 48 hours of life, failure to thrive, gross abdominal distension, and dependence on enemas without significant encopresis.[46,50]

Enterocolitis

About 10% of children present with fever, abdominal distension, and diarrhea due to Hirschsprung-associated enterocolitis. It occurs due to stasis caused by functional obstruction by the aganglionic bowel permitting bacterial overgrowth, most commonly *Clostridium difficile*.[46,51]

Diagnosis

Radiological Examination

❑ Plain abdominal radiograph—dilated bowel loops all over the abdomen, paucity of gas in the pelvis (Fig. 12.18).

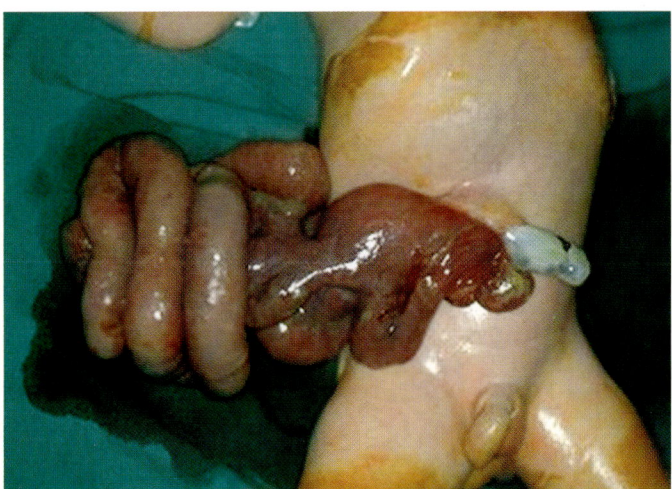

Fig. 12.16: Gastroschisis with the defect on the right side of a normally placed umbilicus

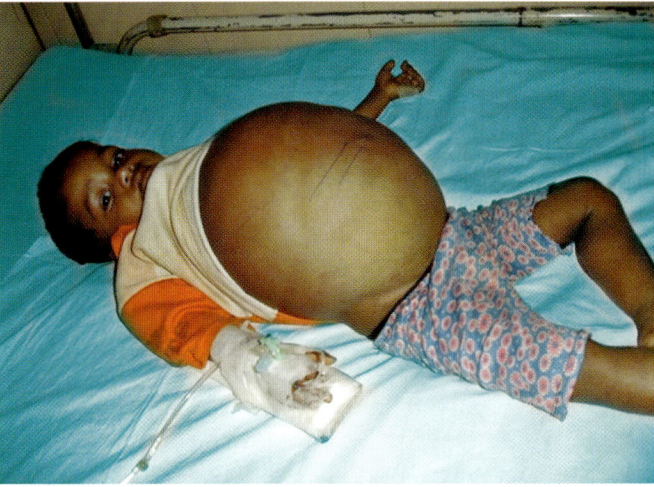

Fig. 12.17: Abdominal distension caused by chronic constipation due to Hirschsprung's disease

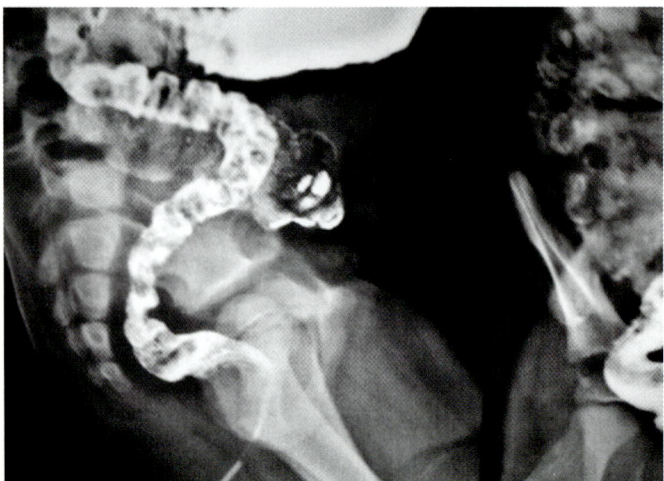

Fig. 12.18: Contrast enema showing a collapsed rectum and a dilated sigmoid colon with a zone of coning suggestive of Hirschsprung's disease

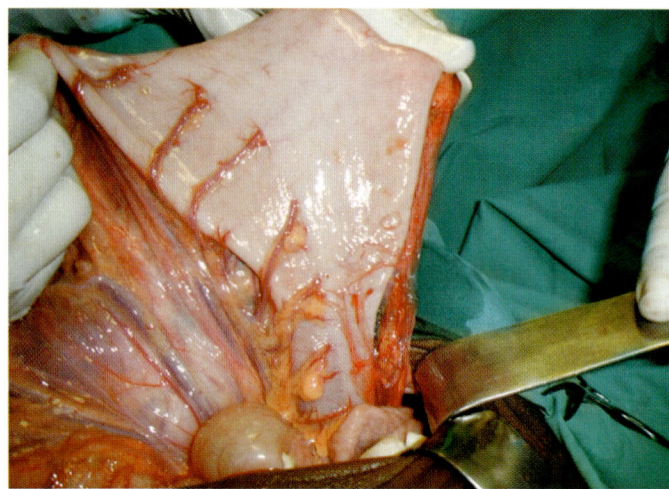

Fig. 12.19: Dilated colon with the zone of coning in Hirschsprung's disease

❑ Contrast enema delineates a transition zone between the ganglionic (dilated) and aganglionic (collapsed) bowel, although 10% of neonates and older children with a short aganglionic segment may not show radiologic transition zone. Other findings include a reversed rectosigmoid index and retention of contrast in the colon on a 24-hour postevacuation film.[46,52]

Rectal Biopsy

Diagnosis is confirmed by rectal muscle biopsy (suction mucosal or full-thickness) showing an absence of ganglion cells in the submucosal plexus and hypertrophied nerve bundles.[46]

Management[46]

In neonatal intestinal obstruction or enterocolitis, resuscitation with intravenous fluids, broad-spectrum antibiotics and nasogastric tube decompression are commenced. Decompression of the colon using digital rectal stimulation, irrigations, or occasionally an emergency stoma may be needed.

Definitive Treatment

The goals of surgery in HD are to remove the aganglionic bowel and reconstruct the intestinal tract by bringing the normally innervated bowel down to the anus while preserving normal sphincter function (Fig. 12.19).

Definitive surgical management may consist of:
❑ Single-stage pull through with preoperative washouts
❑ Two-stage procedure (leveling colostomy followed by pull through procedure), or

❑ Three-stage procedures (diverting colostomy, pull-through, colectomy closure).
   The most commonly performed operations are the Swenson, Duhamel, and Soave procedures.
❑ Swenson's procedure: A two-layered circumferential colorectal anastomosis performed as low as possible to anocutaneous junction is done, thereby, excising the aganglionic segment nearly completely.
❑ Modified Duhamel's procedure: Pull through of ganglionic colon through an incision made in posterior rectal wall about 1 cm from anal (margin) orifice using linear cutter stapler. Final outcome is the creation of bowel, anterior wall made up of aganglionic rectum and posterior wall made up of pulled through ganglionic colon
❑ Soave's endorectal pull through: Removal of mucosa and submucosa of rectum and pulling of ganglionic intestine through the aganglionic muscular cuff and an anastomosis at the anus (Fig. 12.20).

Complications of the Disease and Treatment

Postoperative intestinal obstruction, enterocolitis, anastomotic disruption, fecaloma, incontinence, enterocutaneous fistula, stenosis-constipation, fecal soiling, etc.

■ ANORECTAL MALFORMATIONS

Incidence

The average incidence worldwide is 1 in 5000 live births with a male preponderance.[53,54]

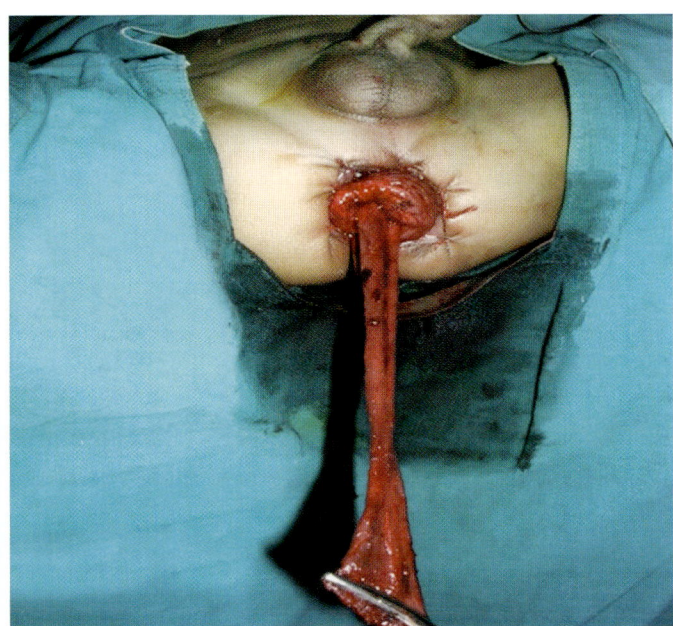

Fig. 12.20: Soave's pull-through procedure

Table 12.1: Krickenbeck classification of anorectal malformation	
Standards for diagnostic procedures: International classification (Krickenbeck)	The international grouping (KRICKENBECK) of surgical procedures for follow-up
Major clinical groups • Perineal (cutaneous) fistula • Rectourethral fistula • Bulbar • Prostatic • Rectovesical fistula • Vestibular fistula • Cloaca • No fistula • Anal stenosis	*Operative procedures* • Perineal operation • Anterior sagittal approach • Sacroperineal procedure • Posterior sagittal anorectoplasty(PSARP) • Abdomino-sacroperineal pull-through • Abdomino-perineal pull-through • Laparoscopically assisted pull-through
• Rare/regional variants • Pouch colon • Rectal atresia/stenosis • Rectovaginal fistula • H type fistula • Others	

Associated Malformations (50–60%)[55]

The most common being urological followed by cardiac, vertebral, gastrointestinal, gynecological, and chromosomal anomalies. It may be a part of *VACTREL* syndrome.

Classification

The key difference between the different types of anomaly lies in the relationship of the terminal bowel to the pelvic floor muscles and the levator ani muscle and presence or absence of fistula to the urogenital tract or the skin.

Anorectal malformations (ARM) have been popularly classified as high (supralevator), intermediate (partially translevator), and low (translevator).[56]

The current international classification of Krickenbeck is shown in Table 12.1.[57] It has therapeutic and prognostic implications.

Male Defects[58](12.21)

❑ *Cutaneous fistula:* It is a low defect, with the fistulous tract extending into the midline perineal raphe, scrotum or base of penis. It may present as meconium pearls, e.g. covered anus incomplete, anal membrane stenosis, bucket handle malformation
❑ *Rectourinary fistulae*: Rectourethral (rectoprostatic or rectobulbar) is more common than rectovesical fistula. It may present as meconuria
❑ *Anorectal agenesis without fistula:* Common in trisomy 21
❑ *Rectal atresia:* It has a dilated blind upper pouch of rectum and a lower small anal canal and has an excellent prognosis.

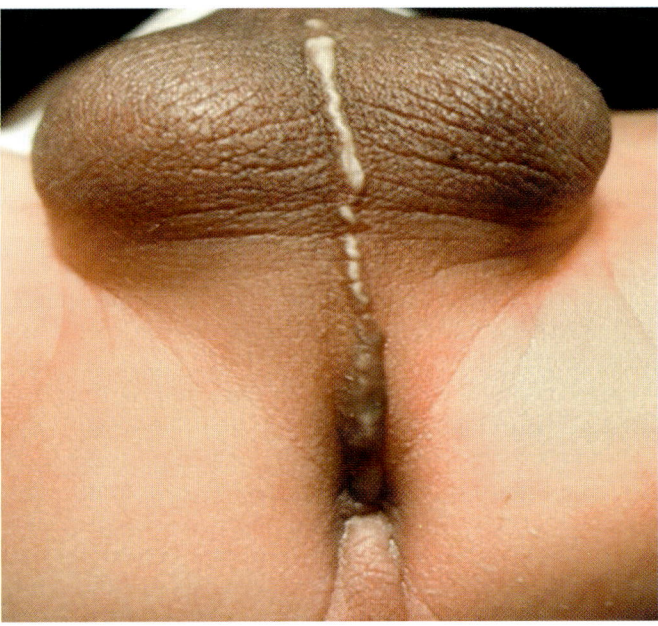

Fig. 12.21: Male child with imperforate anus

Female Defects[58] (Fig. 12.22)

❑ *Perineal fistulae*
❑ *Vestibular fistulae:* The rectum opens immediately behind the hymen in the vestibule. Clinically, there are 3 openings in the vestibule
❑ *Persistant cloaca:* Defect in which rectum, vagina and urinary tract meet and fuse into a single common channel the length of which varies from 1 to 7 cm.

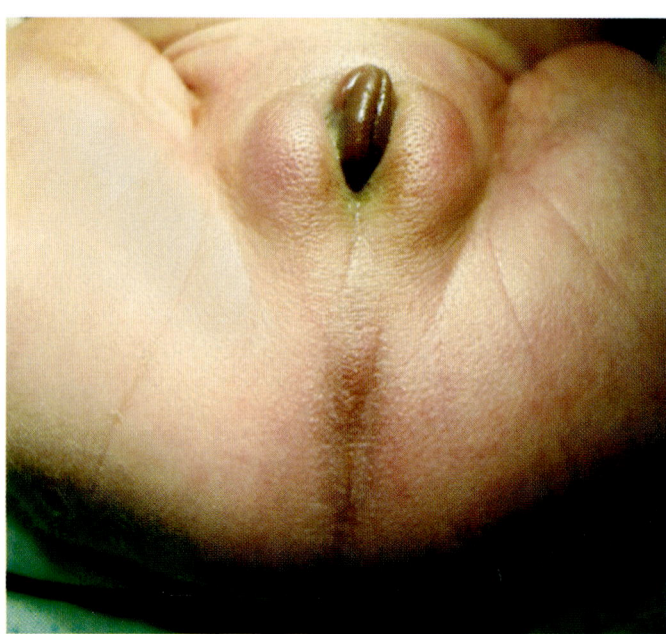

Fig. 12.22: Female child with imperforate anus

Imaging[59]

- ❏ To determine the relationship of the rectum to the anorectal sphincter muscles and demonstrate associated anomalies
- ❏ The lateral decubitus X-ray/inversion radiograph, done after 18–24 hours after birth, uses bowel gas as contrast to measure the position of the terminal bowel against the bony landmarks (pubococcygeal line, ischial spine), to determine its relation to the sphincter muscles
- ❏ To detect associated anomalies: X-rays of the spine and chest, ultrasound abdomen and spine, 2D-echocardiography
- ❏ To plan a definitive procedure, the following are required:
  - Micturating cystourethrogram—to look for rectourinary fistula (in addition to vesicoureteric reflux)
  - Pressure augmented distal cologram—to look for the anatomy of the terminal colon and fistula.

Management

Colostomy[60]

In the neonatal age, high sigmoid or a descending divided colostomy is recommended in males with high or intermediate defects and in females with cloacas and high defects without a perineal opening. High stoma offers adequate distal rectal length for definitive procedure and divide stoma offers complete diversion of stools for optimal definitive repair.

Perineal Procedures[58]

It includes anal cutback and V-Y anoplasty for low ARMs like anocutaneous fistula, covered anus, anal stenosis. It is now superseded by limited PSARP procedure, which provides better results in terms of incontinence.

Definitive Surgery

The cardinal principles of all definitive procedures are as follows:
- ❏ Identification of the blind atretic pouch of the rectum
- ❏ Identifying and isolating the fistula with the urogenital tract
- ❏ Adequate mobilization of the rectum
- ❏ Pulling the rectum through the sphincter muscle complex to the anal verge.

Posterior Sagittal Anorectoplasty[61]

It is the most popular definitive procedure in male ARMs and occasionally in female ARMs. It is generally done after a colostomy, but primary neonatal PSARP have been performed lately by experienced surgeons with encouraging results. Occasionally, in high male ARMs and in cloacas, an additional abdominal approach may be required to mobilize the rectum.

Anterior Sagittal Anorectoplasty[62]

It is usually used to correct female ARMs, such as rectovestibular fistula, perineal canal, and anterior perineal anus. In this procedure, the patient is placed in the lithotomy position and the approach is anterior. Its advantage in female ARMs is better visualization of the vagina and fistula with better cosmesis and is usually done as a primary procedure without a protective colostomy.

Sacroperineal Pull-through[63]

This procedure is also performed in the prone position, but the muscles are not divided in the midline. The mobilized rectum is pulled through the puborectalis sling instead.

Laparoscopic-assisted Pull-through[64]

This procedure is considered anatomically sound and leaves the external sphincter intact. It allows centrality of the pullthrough which leads to less scarring of pelvic floor and better rectal compliance.

Complications[65]

Complications associated with anorectal malformations are divided into three groups as follows:

Group A (Patients with fecal incontinence)—These patients typically have an abnormal sacrum, flat perineum, and poor sphincters.

Group B (Perioperative complications)—Wound infection, rectal problems (dehiscence, retraction), rectourinary fistula, rectovaginal fistula, acquired vaginal/urethral atresia, neurogenic bladder.

Group C (Complications from mismanagement of constipation)—It may lead to overflow pseudoincontinence. Complications of incontinence and constipation require a bowel mangement program of an appropriate diet, laxatives, enema therapy, etc.

ACUTE EMERGENCIES

APPENDICITIS

Appendicitis is the most common surgical condition of the abdomen with an incidence of 1 in 1000. About one-third of patients are younger than 18 years, with a peak incidence between 11 years and 12 years.[66]

Pathophysiology[66]

Appendicitis results due to infection following luminal obstruction, most commonly caused by fecaliths or lymphoid hyperplasia. Lymphoid hyperplasia may be caused by bacterial infection (*Yersinia*, *Shigella*, *Salmonella*), parasitic infestations (*Entamoeba*, *E. vermicularis*, *Ascaris*), and viral infections.

Appendix—luminal obstruction (fecolith/lymphoid hyperplasia)

⇓

Increased mucus secretion, inflammatory exudation

⇓

Increased intaluminal pressure + decreased lymphatic drainage

⇓

Increase in edema + decrease in venous drainage

⇓

Ischemia, gangrene

⇓

Perforation

⇙ ⇘

Localized abscess   Generalized peritonitis

Clinical Features[66]

Early complaints include dull central abdominal pain around the umbilicus along with anorexia and nausea.

This is visceral pain due to appendicular distention that causes early, visceral pain in the periumbilical region (T-10 dermatome). A few episodes of vomiting usually follow the pain. Later, inflammation of the parietal peritoneum leads to severe pain in the right lower quadrant, most typically at the McBurney point. Systemic complaints, such as fever, tachycardia, and leukocytosis accompany due to bacteremia.

Clinical Examination[66]

Localized tenderness is noted on palpation or percussion most commonly at the McBurney point. Rebound tenderness may be present. Localized abscess may be palpable as a tender boggy mass. Generalized peritonitis may progresses from simple involuntary guarding to generalized rigidity of the abdomen. Deep palpation in the left lower quadrant may cause tenderness in the right lower quadrant (Rovsing sign), indicating peritoneal irritation.

Investigations

Hematological tests usually reveal **leukocytosis with neutrophilic predominance**.

Plain radiography[67] may show nonspecific features like-fecoliths (10–20% cases).

Abnormal gas pattern in the right lower quadrant, lumbar scoliosis away from the right lower quadrant and obliteration of the psoas shadow (Figs 12.23A and B).

Barium enema or follow-through series[67] may show—Nonvisualization of appendix, appendiceal filling defects or luminal irregularity and extrinsic mass effect on the cecum or terminal ileum are suggestive of appendicits.

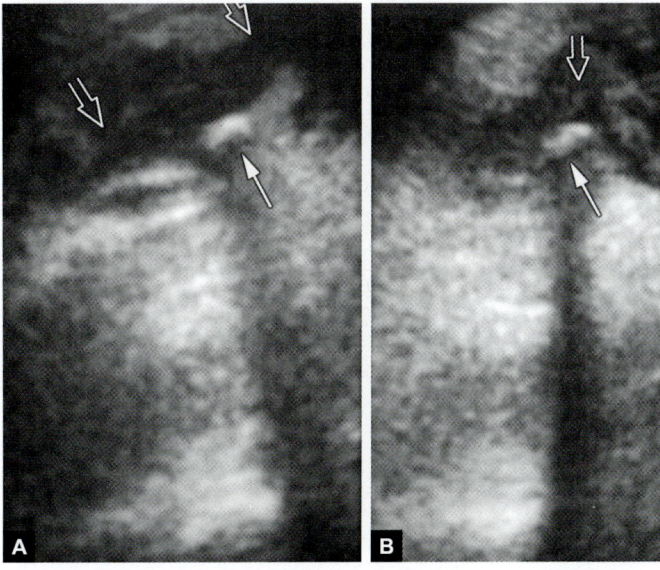

Figs 12.23A and B: USG showing an inflamed appendix

Ultrasonography[68]

A noncompressible appendix that is 7 mm or larger in anteroposterior diameter is suggestive, and the visualization of an appendicolith may help in diagnosis.

Computed Tomography (CT)[69]

Enlarged appendix (>6 mm), appendiceal wall thickening (>1 mm), periappendiceal fat stranding, and appendiceal wall enhancement are useful diagnostic criteria.

Treatment

Appendectomy—Open or Laparoscopic[70]

Open appendectomy involves making a transverse or oblique right lower quadrant incision through the McBurney point[71] (Fig. 12.24).

Laparoscopic appendectomy can be done by a laparoscope-assisted technique in which the appendix is mobilized laparoscopically using one or two ports and is drawn through a small abdominal opening and removed by standard open technique.[72] Alternatively, the appendix can be removed entirely laparoscopically.

Complications[66]

Wound infection (the most common), intra-abdominal abscess formation, postoperative intestinal obstruction, prolonged ileus, and rarely, enterocutaneous fistula.[66]

■ INTUSSUSCEPTION

The word intussusception is derived from the Latin words 'intus' (within) and 'suscipere' (to receive). It involves telescoping of one segment of intestine into an adjacent segment, most probably proximal into distal.

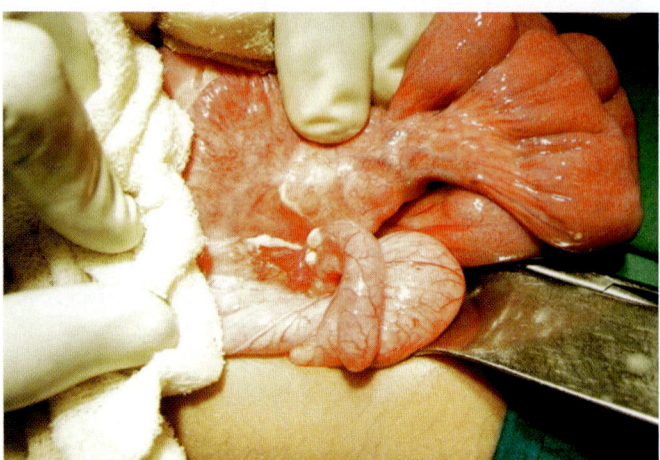

Fig. 12.24: Early acute appendicitis

An intussusception involves three parts, i.e the inner or entering tube, the middle or returning tube (both of them together form the intussusceptum), and the outer tube or receiving sheath (intussuscipiens).

Intussusception is one of the most frequent causes of acute bowel obstruction in infants and toddlers.[73,74]

Incidence and Demographics[75,76]

It occurs in 1 to 4 in 2000 infants and children, with a male predominance. Although intussusception can be seen in all pediatric ages, 90% in children within 3 years of age with more than 40% are seen between 3 months and 9 months of age. The frequency of intussusception displays a seasonal variation that usually correlates with viral infections (respiratory, gastrointestinal, or both), with most cases seen in May, June, and July.

Types[77]

Intussusception can be categorized anatomically into ileo-colic (85%); ileoileocolic (10%), appendicocolic, ceco-colic, or colocolic (2.5%); jejunojejunal, ileoileal (2.5%); and those occurring around indwelling tubes.

Although the majority of the cases are fixed and permanent, transient (spontaneous reduction) intussusceptions occur in almost 20% of the cases.

Lead Points

All intussusceptions have a lead point. In most cases, peyer patches which enlarge with respiratory or gastrointestinal viral infections (rota virus or adenovirus) acts as a lead point causing idiopathic intussusception. The rest of the cases have pathological lead points such as Meckel's diverticulum, polyps, duplications, appendix, carcinoid etc.[78,79]

Clinical Findings and Physical Examination[80-82]

Two classic symptoms of intussusceptions are abdominal pain or vomiting while two classic signs are abdominal mass or rectal bleeding.

Episodes of screaming and drawing up of the legs in a previously well infant is the most common classic symptom of pediatric intussusceptions. The attacks last for a few minutes and recur repeatedly. In between episodes the child may lie listless. Vomiting may not occur at the outset but may be bile-stained later. There may be history of passage of blood with mucus per rectally—the' red currant jelly' stool.

On abdominal examination, a sausage-shaped lump with its concavity towards the umbilicus, which hardens on palpation may be palpable. It may be associated with a feeling of emptiness in the right iliac fossa (the sign of Dance). On rectal examination, blood-stained mucus, and occasionally, the apex of the intussusceptum may be palpable or even visible. The child may be febrile, dehydrated and in shock in cases of bowel ischemia.

Diagnostic Evaluation

Plain abdominal radiographs are not diagnostic. It may reveal multiple air fluid levels suggesting intestinal obstruction.

Ultrasonography (US)[83]

It is often diagnostic with high accuracy rates.

It reveals the characteristic "target sign", seen as two rings of low echogenicity with an intervening hyperechoic ring similar to a doughnut. The pseudo-kidney sign is also described because the edematous walls of the intussusception appear as superimposed hyperechoic and hypoechoic layers.

Contrast Enema[84]

Before ultrasound, barium contrast study of the colon (BE) was considered the gold standard to diagnose intussusception. It is quick, most cost-effective, and if positive, it becomes therapeutic if used for hydrostatic reduction. The 'meniscus' sign, the 'coiled spring' sign, and 'pincer claw' signs are suggestive of intussusception on contrast enema (Fig. 12.25). Its disadvantages are that it is an invasive procedure and requires radiation.

Treatment

Definitive treatment options include radiologic reduction or surgical reduction

Radiological Reduction

Contraindications to attempted enema reduction include clinical evidence of dehydration, shock, peritonitis, or radiographic evidence of perforation with free air.[85]

Currently used techniques include pneumatic or hydrostatic pressure enemas under fluoroscopy or ultrasound guidance.

Pneumatic Reduction:[86] In this procedure, air is insufflated into the rectum under fluoroscopic guidance, with pressures not exceeding 120 mm Hg.
- *Advantages:* Quicker, less messy, and decreases radiation exposure time
- *Drawbacks:* Possibilty of tension pneumoperitoneum, poor visualization.

Hydrostatic Reduction[87,88]

Saline or barium is allowed to flow in the rectum from a height of not more than 3 feet above the patient and signs of reduction are looked for which include:

Fluid entering small bowel-terminal ileum, disappearance of previously palpable mass, passage of flatus and contrast through anus, and the child becomes quiet and falls asleep.

The clear advantage of ultrasound is that it avoids radiation and has higher accuracy and reliability for monitoring the reduction process and postreduction follow-up. Barium is no longer the choice for hydrostatic reduction, because if a perforation occurs, it causes intense inflammatory reaction in the peritoneal cavity.[89]

Operative Management[81,86]

Indications for surgical intervention include contraindications for radiographic reduction, failure of or incomplete radiological reduction, presence of peritonitis, pneumoperitoneum, or a pathologic lead point (Fig. 12.26).

Manual reduction requires slow constant pinching and squeezing of the most distal part of the intussusceptum toward its origin, just like squeezing a tube of toothpaste. In patients, with unviable bowel post-reduction, or unsuccessful manual reduction, or pathologic lead point, a primary end-to-end anastomosis, after resection of the ischemic bowel, is performed.

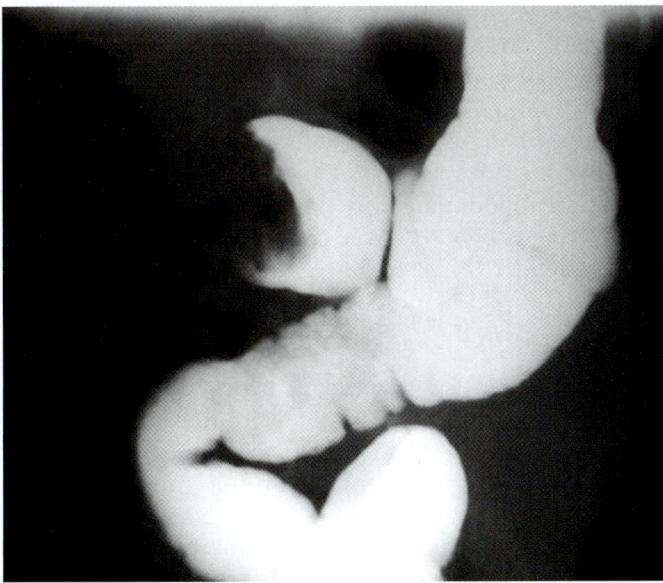

Fig. 12.25: Barium enema showing a 'pincer claw' sign of intussusception

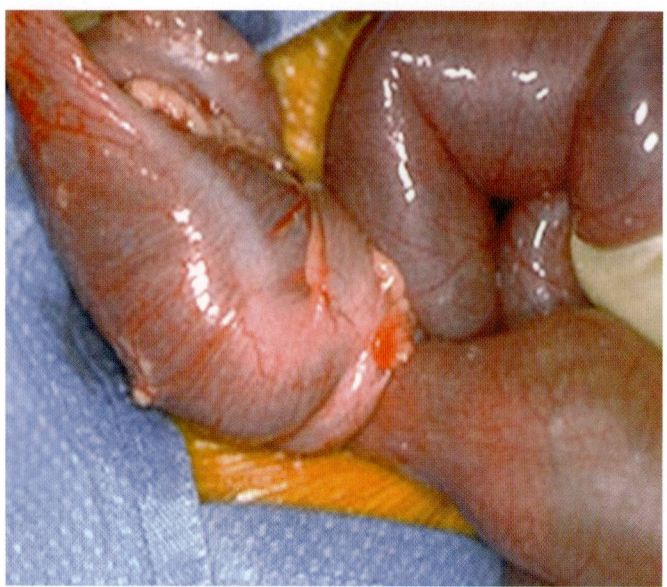

Fig. 12.26: Operative picture of ileocolic intussusception

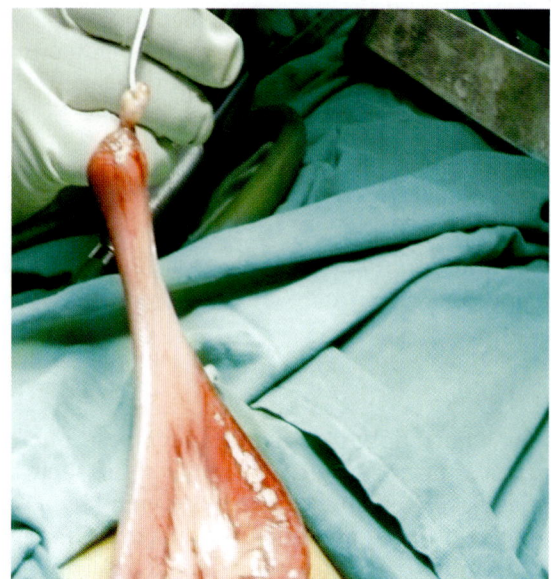

Fig. 12.27: Meckel's diverticulum

■ MECKEL'S DIVERTICULUM

Meckel's diverticulum is the most common congenital anomaly of the gastrointestinal tract. This is a true diverticulum with all normal intestinal layers. The diverticulum usually presents by one of its complications. Embryologically, it is caused by a failure of regression of the vitelline duct, a process that normally occurs between the fifth and seventh weeks of fetal life. [90,91]

Features ("Rule of 2")[92]

- ❑ Present in 2% of population
- ❑ 2 in in length and 2 cm in diameter
- ❑ Twice as common in males
- ❑ Approximately 2 feet away from ileocecal junction
- ❑ Blood supply from 2 vitelline arteries, of which left involutes
- ❑ Two types of mucosa: gastric (65–90%) and pancreatic (5%)
- ❑ Usually symptomatic before 2 years of age.

Clinical Features[92]

Meckel's diverticulum may present with:
- ❑ Lower gastrointestinal bleeding which can be painless, episodic, and massive
- ❑ Intestinal obstruction due to intussusception, volvulus, vitelline bands, herniation of diverticulum (Littre's hernia)
- ❑ Inflammation resulting in Meckel's diverticulitis
- ❑ Neoplasia include benign lesions like leiomyomas, lipomas, angiomas, and neurofibromas and malignant lesions like leiomyosarcoma, carcinoids, adenocarcinoma, villous adenoma, and gastrointestinal stromal tumors.

Investigations

- ❑ 99m technetium scan (Meckel's scan) is useful in detecting heterotopic gastric mucosa. 99m technetium isotope is stored and secreted into the lumen of the bowel by mucinous surface cells of the gastric mucosal type[93]
- ❑ CT abdomen may detect Meckel's diverticulum as a fluid-filled tubular structure arising from a small bowel loop. It may also detect complications like free fluid in abdominal cavity is seen in case of perforation or intussusception can be detected with signs of obstruction.[94]

Management[95]

The treatment of a symptomatic Meckel diverticulum is resection, open, or laparoscopic techniques (Fig. 12.27).

A Meckel's diverticulum can be removed by either simple resection of the diverticulum and transverse closure across the base, or resection of a short segment of ileum containing the diverticulum with reanastomosis.

INTESTINAL OBSTRUCTION

Intestinal obstruction can occur at any age from newborn infants to adults. Small bowel obstruction in infants and children is more common than large bowel obstruction. The most common causes are:

- Congenital malformations:
  - Intestinal atresias and stenoses (including imperforate anus and pyloric atresia)
  - Anomalies of rotation and fixation (including midgut volvulus)
  - Hirschsprung's disease
  - Meconium diseases: meconium ileus, meconium plug, pseudocyst, etc.
- Other causes include:
  - Adhesive small bowel obstruction
  - Tumors
  - Inflammatory bowel disease: abscess or adhesions from peritonitis
  - Peritoneal bands
  - Segmental volvulus
  - Incarcerated hernia (inguinal, internal or diaphragmatic).[96]

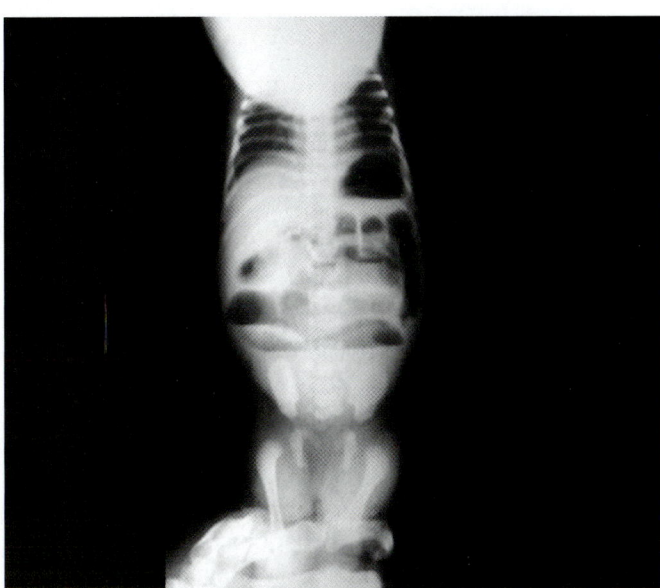

Fig. 12.28: Plain X-ray abdomen (erect) showing multiple air-fluid levels in small intestines suggestive of intestinal obstruction

Clinical Features[97]

Cardinal clinical features of acute obstruction are as follows:

- Vomiting: bilious vomiting is always abnormal
- Distension (scaphoid abdomen may be seen in duodenal atresia, malrotation)[22,39]
- Delayed, scanty or no passage of meconium in neonates or constipation in older children[27,31]
- Abdominal pain: With increasing distension, initial colicky pain is replaced by mild constant diffuse pain. Severe pain may be suggestive of bowel ischemia.

Diagnosis

Radiological Imaging

Abdominal radiographs: Obstruction is manifested by dilated bowel loops with air-fluid levels (Fig. 12.28).

- Duodenal atresia—'double bubble'[23]
- Jejunal atresia—triple bubble/few gas filled loops beyond duodenum
- Ileal atresia/distal ileal obstruction—many gas filled loops (requires 24 hours)[29]
- No gas in distal small bowel—diagnostic in complete high obstruction
- Hirschsprung's disease/meconium plug syndrome—dilated bowel loops all over, paucity of gas in pelvis[51]
- Malrotation of the gut—nonspecific findings, double bubble, gasless abdomen.[40]

Contrast enhanced computed tomography: In older children, it may help to rule out other diagnoses and may identify an abnormal vascular course or a transition zone of the obstruction.[98]

Contrast Enema[99]

To differentiate the various types of low intestinal obstruction:

- *Microcolon:* Complete obstruction of the small bowel
- *Meconium plug syndrome:* Colon dilated proximal to an intraluminal mass
- *Hirschsprung's disease:* Proximal dilation with transitional zone and distally narrow segment
- *Small left colon syndrome:* Colon dilated to the splenic flexure, then becomes narrow.

Upper gastrointestinal contrast series: Procedure of choice in diagnosing malrotation of the intestines.[40]

Treatment of Acute Intestinal Obstruction[96]

- Gastrointestinal drainage
- Fluid and electrolyte replacement
- Relief of obstruction.

Surgical treatment is necessary for most cases of intestinal obstruction but should be delayed until resuscitation is complete, provided there is no sign of strangulation or evidence of closed-loop obstruction.

Principles of Surgical Intervention for Obstruction

Management of:
- ❑ The segment at the site of obstruction
- ❑ The distended proximal bowel
- ❑ The underlying cause of obstruction.

▌INFLAMMATORY BOWEL DISEASE

Crohn's disease (CD) and ulcerative colitis (UC) comprise a wide spectrum of clinical pathology under the broad heading of inflammatory bowel disease (IBD).

Crohn's disease is a debilitating chronic inflammatory bowel disorder, which can affect any part of the gastrointestinal tract from the lips to the anal margin, but ileocolonic disease is the most common presentation.[100,101] Operative interventions should be reserved for (i) failure of medical therapy, (ii) complications of the disease, (iii) severe dysphagia, (iv) cancer and (v) stagnated growth and development.[102]

Surgical Options

Ileocecal resection is the usual procedure for ileocaecal disease with a primary anastomosis between the ileum and the ascending or transverse colon depending on the extent of the disease.[103]

Resection: It can be *segmental resection* for short segments of small or large bowel involvement eg: stricture or *total abdominal colectomy with ileorectal anastomosis, and proctocolectomy with end ileostomy* for extensive colonic involvement.[104]

Stricturoplasty: Multiple strictured areas of CD can be treated by a local widening procedure, stricturoplasty, to avoid excessive small bowel resection.[105]

Anal disease: It is usually treated conservatively by simple drainage of abscesses, placing setons around any fistulae. Occasionally in patients with inactive disease, primary repair of a rectovaginal or high fistula-*in-ano* may be attempted.[106]

Ulcerative Colitis

UC is a chronic inflammatory disease of the rectal and colonic mucosa.

Indications for Surgery[107]

The need for surgery is highest in the first year after the disease onset for:
- ❑ Severe or fulminating disease failing to respond to medical therapy
- ❑ Chronic disease with anaemia, frequent stools, urgency and tenesmus

- ❑ Steroid-dependent disease—here, the disease is not severe but remission cannot be maintained without substantial doses of steroids
- ❑ The risk of neoplastic change—patients who have severe dysplasia on review colonoscopy
- ❑ Extraintestinal manifestations.

Operations

Total abdominal colectomy and ileostomy is a first aid procedure in an emergency situation. The rectal stump is left long but runs the risk of on-going hemorrhage. Advantages include faster recovery, the histology of the resected colon can be checked, and restorative surgery can be done later.[105]

Proctocolectomy and Ileostomy[108]

Although with the lowest complication rate, it is indicated in patients who are not candidates for restoration. The disadvantages of permanent ileostomy are the psychological and social impact on life.

Ileostomy with a Continent Intra-abdominal Pouch (Kock's Procedure)[109]

The Kock continent ileal reservoir with a nipple valve obviates the need for wearing an ileostomy drainage bag and an alternative to permanent ileostomy. Because of the need for multiple drainages each day, need for frequent reoperation, and pouch complications related to the nipple valve and stagnant loop syndrome, it has been superceded by the ileoanal pull-through procedure.

Restorative Proctocolectomy with an Ileoanal Pouch (Parks)[108]

In this operation, a pouch is made out of ileum as a substitute for the rectum and sewn or stapled to the anal canal. It is reserved for patients with adequate anal sphincters. Four pouch configurations which have been used clinically are the lateral and S-, J-, and W-shaped pouches. Complications include pelvic sepsis, small bowel obstruction, pouchitis and pouch vaginal fistula. This is the operation of choice in younger patients as it avoids a permanent stoma

Colectomy and ileorectal anastomosis:[109] It may be considered in minimal rectal inflammation. Advantages include avoidance of stoma and minimal risk to sexual function, but there is a persistent risk of inflammation and malignancy.

RARER ISSUES AND RECENT ADVANCES

ANNULAR PANCREAS

This condition is due to normal pancreatic tissue encircling the duodenum. Abnormal rotation of the developing ventral pancreatic bud and when the ventral bud splits into two with part rotating posteriorly and the remainder rotating anteriorly to form a complete or incomplete ring of pancreatic tissue.

This anomaly occurs in 1 in 20,000 births and is more frequent in males than females with a ratio of 2:1.

Clinical Presentation

It may be completely asymptomatic or incidentally detected during laparotomy or symptomatic due to complete or incomplete duodenal obstruction.

Complete duodenal obstruction may present within hours after birth and may or may not be associated with duodenal atresia, while incomplete obstructions have a delayed presentation later in life (Fig. 12.29).

Prenatal hydramnios, bilious vomiting ' double bubble' on abdominal radiographs are characteristic features.

Treatment

Duodenoduodenostomy—a procedure to bypass the obstruction without damaging the pancreas.[110,111]

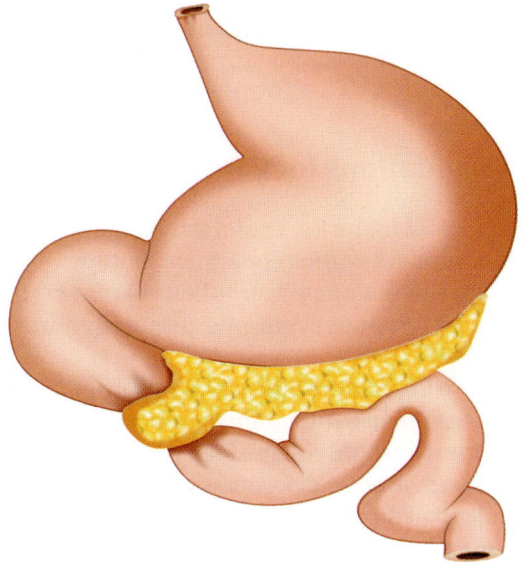

Fig. 12.29: Annular pancreas around the duodenum

PANCREAS DIVISUM[112-114]

It is the most common congenital malformation of the pancreas due to the failure of the vental and dorsal ducts to fuse when the two pancreatic buds unite. As a result, the duct of Wirsung is small, while duct of the dorsal bud, the duct of Santorini becomes the major ductal system and drains through the minor papilla the minor papilla.

Incidence

Pancreas divisum, seen in 4% to 11% of all patients, is found in 25% of the patients with recurrent pancreatitis.

Investigations

Magnetic resonance cholangiopancreatography is a useful and noninvasive modality, while *endoscopic retrograde cholangiopancreatography (ERCP)* although invasive, may be used as a therapeutic option.

An ERCP may show the extension of the duct of Santorini along the the entire length of the body and tail of the pancreas.

Pathology

Impaired drainage of the minor papilla due to a stenotic orifice may result in pancreatitis.

Treatment

Primary aim is to establish adequate drainage of the duct of Santorini to relieve symptoms and to prevent pancreatitis and pancreatic insufficiency .

Sphinteroplasty or endoscopic sphincterotomy help to achieve drainage.

For chronic pancreatitis, pancreatic resection or Puestow's longitudinal pancreaticojejunostomy are considered.

GASTROESOPHAGEAL REFLUX DISEASE

Gastroesophageal reflux is the undetected backflow of the gastric contents into the oesophagus, rarely mouth or pharynx causing regurgitation.

Gastroesophageal reflux disease (GERD) is a situation in which reflux causes major symptoms and complications such as failure to thrive, disturbance of sleep, recurrent aspiration in very young infants, epigastric or retrosternal pain, heartburn, esophagitis, stenosis, or Barrett esophagus.[115]

Risk Factors

Neurologically impaired children
Congenital problems: Esophageal atresia, Congenital diaphraghmatic hernia, gastroschisis, omphalocele

Clinical History[116]

Patients may present with failure to thrive, primary aspiration, coughing, stridor, apneoa, recurrent pneumonia, irritability, heartburn, dysphagia, abdominal pain.

Investigations[116]

Upper gastrointestinal contrast series: To see the anatomy, hiatal hernia, esophageal stricture, malrotation, pyloric stenosis.

Esophageal pH monitoring: Measures duration and frequency of acid reflux episodes.

Nuclear scintigraphy: Technetium–labeled formula is ingested and patients are scanned for GER. Lack of standardization, short duration limits its value.

Esophageal manometry: Used more commonly for primary and secondary esophageal motility alterations, and infrequently to diagnose GER.

Endoscopy and biopsy: To detect presence of esophagitis, strictures, webs, infections, etc.

Treatment

Medical Therapy

Aim of treatment is control of symptoms; prevent complications and facilitate healing of oesophagitits.
Two main categories:
❑ Acid suppressants: Antacids, histamine H_2 receptor antagonists, proton pump inhibitors.
❑ Prokinetics: Erythromycin, cisapride.

Surgical Treatment[117-119]

Indications:
❑ Failure of medical therapy
❑ Anatomical defect: Hiatal hernia, malrotation, diaphragmatic hernia
❑ Esophageal stricture secondary to GERD
❑ Neurologically impaired children.

Surgical Technique

❑ Aim to prevent reflux and avoid complications like dysphagia.

❑ Currently, the most popular procedure is laparoscopic fundoplication:
  • Nissen's procedure with a 360° wrap is most common amongst all the fundoplication techniques.
❑ Others include Toupet technique with a semicircular dorsal wrap
❑ Thal procedure—semicircular ventral wrap

Complications[116]

Recurrent GERD, dysphagia, wrap herniation

▌BARIATRIC SURGERY

Obesity is the second most common cause of premature death after smoking. Most cases are due to many genetic factors interacting with environmental ones.[120,121]

Definition

In adults, Body mass index greater 25 kg/m² and 30 kg/m² are the cut-offs for overweight and obesity respectively.

In children, BMI >85th percentile signifies overweight while BMI. >95th percentile signifies obesity.[122]

Low birth weight, Diabetic mother increases the risk of obesity while prolonged breast feeding and later onset of adiposity reduces the risk.[122-125]

Bariatric surgery, at present, is considered most efficient in achieving consistent, durable weight loss and to resolve most of the comorbidities. Candidates for surgical therapy must be willing to comply with postoperative dietary recommendations, exercise, and follow-up requirements for long term success.[126]

Bariatric surgery is considerd in adolescents who have failed 6 months of attempts at professionally supervised weight loss.

Recommendations for Patient Selection[127]

❑ Psychological maturity: Understands nature of surgery and is compliant with preoperative therapy.
❑ BMI ≥ 35 with major co-morbidities like type 2 diabetes mellitus, sleep apnea syndrome, pseudotumour cerebri, severe NASH.
❑ BMI ≥ 40 with comorbidities like hypertension, insulin resistance, glucose intolerance, impaired quality of life or activities, dyslipidemias, sleep apnea.
❑ Patients with mental disorders, syndromic obesity, and psychological disorders should be evaluated on case by case basis.
❑ When medical, nutritional and behavioural changes are ineffective.

Surgical Options

Roux-en-Y Gastric Bypass[128,129]

It is mainly a restrictive procedure and modestly malabsorptive. It combines limitation of oral intake, by creating a small stomach pouch, with some malabsorption and appetite suppression by construction of the Roux limb and gastrojejunostomy. It leads to 40% weight loss over 1–2 years. Complications include dumping syndrome, internal hernias, marginal ulcers, stomal stenosis, etc.

Vertical-banded Gastroplasty and Adjustable Gastric Banding[130]

These are restrictive procedures. Vertical banded gastroplasty, a small gastric pouch which is in continuity with the remaining stomach was created near the gastroesophageal junction with a narrowed outlet. The adjustable gastric banding procedures position an adjustable inflatable bandlike device near the gastric cardia to limit oral intake. Though designed for laparoscopic purpose, a traditional open approach can also be used to place the band. Complications include gastric prolapse, stoma obstruction and band erosion into the stomach. There may be 25–30% weight loss over 3 years.

Sleeve Gastrectomy[131]

It involves surgical removal of a large portion of the stomach along the greater curvature resulting a sleeve or tube like structure. The resection extends from just proximal from pylorus to the angle of his, creating the sleeve along the lesser curve. The procedure permanently reduces the size of the stomach, although there could be some dilatation of the stomach later on in life. About 33–83% weight loss is expected over 3 years.

Biliopancreatic Diversion with or without Duodenal Switch[132]

This operation disrupts intestinal absorptive capacity by short-circuiting a portion of the small intestine. A subtotal gastrectomy is performed leaving a gastric remnant around 200 mL in size. The small intestine is divided into a long enteric limb anastomosed to a long biliopancreatic limb and a common channel 50–150 cm is created from the ileocecal valve. The duodenal switch modification was introduced in an effort to minimize the risk of dumping syndrome and marginal ulceration by preserving the antrum, pylorus, and duodenum. Although weight loss is greater,complications are most in this procedure. Complications include vitamin, nutrient and protein deficiencies.

REFERENCES

1. Harmon CM, Coran AG. Congenital anomalies of the esophagus. In: Coran AG. Pediatric Surgery, 7th edition. Philadelphia: Elsevier Saunders. 2012.p.893-918.
2. Torfs CP, Curry CJ, Bateson TF. Population-based study of tracheoesophageal fistula and esophageal atresia. Teratology. 1995;52:220-32.
3. Gross RE. The Surgery of Infancy and Childhood. Philadelphia, WB Saunders. 1953.
4. Leonard H, Barrett AM, Scott JE, Wren C. The influence of congenital heart disease on survival of infants with oesophageal atresia. Arch Dis Child Fetal Neonatal Ed. 2001;85:F204-6.
5. Beasley SW, Phelan E, Kelly JH, et al. Urinary tract abnormalities in association with oesophageal atresia: Frequency, significance and influence on management. Pediatr Surg Int. 1992;7:94.
6. Spitz L, Kiely E, Brereton RJ, Drake D. Management of esophageal atresia. World J Surg. 1993;17:296-300.
7. Poenaru D, Laberge JM, Neilson IR, Guttman FM. A new prognostic classification for esophageal atresia. Surgery. 1993; 113:426-32.
8. Spitz L, Kiely EM, Morecroft JA, Drake DP. Oesophageal atresia: At-risk groups for the 1990s. J Pediatr Surg. 1994;29:723-25.
9. 9.Schwartz MZ. Hypertrophic pyloric stenosis. In: Coran AG. Pediatric Surgery,7th edn. Philadelphia: Elsevier Saunders; 2012.p.1021-28.
10. Mitchell LE, Risch N: The genetics of infantile hypertrophic pyloric stenosis. Am J Dis Child. 1993;147:1203.
11. Hirschsprung H. Falle von angeborener Pylorus Stenose. J Kinderheilk. 1888;27:61.
12. Oue T, Puri P. Smooth muscle cell hypertrophy versus hyperplasia in infantile hypertrophic pyloric stenosis. Pediatr Res. 1999; 45:853.
13. Hernanz-Schulman M, Lowe LH, Johnson J, et al. In vivo visualization of pyloric mucosal hypertrophy in infants with hypertrophic pyloric stenosis: Is there an etiologic role?. AJR Am J Roentgenol. 2001;177:843.
14. Keller H, Waldermann D, Greiner P. Comparison of preoperative sonography with intraoperative findings in congenital hypertrophic pyloric stenosis. J Pediatr Surg. 1987;22:950.
15. Haran P, Darling D, Sciammas F. The value of the double track sign as a differentiating factor between pylorospasm and hypertrophic pyloric stenosis in infants. Radiology. 1966; 86:723-25.
16. Ramstedt C. Zur Operation der angeborenen Pylorus Stenose. Med Klin. 1912;8:1702.
17. Tandler J. Zur Entwicklungsgeschichte des menschlichen duodenums im fruhen Embryonal stadium. Gegenbaurs Morphologisches Jahrbuch. 1900;29:187-216.
18. Fonkalsrud EW, DeLorimier AA, Hays DM. Congenital atresia and stenosis of the duodenum: A review compiled from the members of the Surgical Section of the American Academy of Pediatrics. Pediatrics. 1969;43:79-83.
19. Boyden EA, Cope JG, Bill AH. Anatomy and embryology of congenital intrinsic obstruction of the duodenum. Am J Surg. 1967;114:190-202.

20. Sweed Y. Duodenal obstruction. In: Puri P (Ed.) Neonatal Surgery, 2nd ed, London: Arnold. 2003:423-33.

21. Merrill JR, Raffensperger JG. Pediatric annular pancreas: twenty years' experience. J Pediatr Surg. 1976;11:921-5.

22. Norton KI, Tenreiro R, Rabinowitz JG. Sonographic demonstration of annular pancreas and a distal duodenal diaphragm in a newborn. Pediatr Radiol. 1992;22:66-7.

23. Mikaelsson C, Arnbjornsson E, Kullendorff CM. Membranous duodenal stenosis. Acta Paediatr. 1997;86:953-5.

24. Escobar MA, Ladd AP, Grosfeld JL, et al. Duodenal atresia and stenosis. Long-term follow-up over 30 years. J Pediatr Surg. 2004;39:867-71.

25. Louw JH, Barnard CN. Congenital intestinal atresia; observations on its origin. Lancet. 1955;269:1065-7.

26. Grosfeld JL, Ballantine TV, Shoemaker R. Operative management of intestinal atresia and stenosis based on pathologic findings. J Pediatr Surg. 1979;14:368-75.

27. DeLorimier AA, Fonkalsrud EW, Hays DM. Congenital atresia and stenosis of the jejunum and ileum. Surgery. 1969;65:819-27.

28. Grosfeld JL. Alimentary tract obstruction in the newborn. Curr Probl Pediatr. 1975;5:3-47.

29. Berdon WE, Baker DH, Santulli TV, et al. Microcolon in newborn infants with intestinal obstruction. Its correlation with the level and time of onset of obstruction. Radiology. 1968;90:878-85.

30. Kerem E, Corey M, Kerem B, et al. Clinical and genetic comparisons of patients with cystic fibrosis, with or without meconium ileus. J Pediatr. 1989;114:767-73.

31. Ziegler MM, Meconium Ileus, Coran AG. Pediatric Surgery, 7th edn. Philadelphia: Elsevier Saunders. 2012.p.1073-83.

32. Henson RE. Meconium ileus. Radiology. 1957;68:568-71.

33. White H. Meconium ileus: A new roentgen sign. Radiology. 1956;66:567.

34. Lillie JG, Chrispin AR. Investigation and management of neonatal obstruction by Gastrografin enema. Ann Radiol. 1972;15:237.

35. Rowe MI, Furst AJ, Altman DH, et al. The neonatal response to Gastrografin enema. Pediatrics. 1971;48:28-35.

36. O'Neill JA, Grosfeld JL, Boles Jr ET, et al. Surgical treatment of meconium ileus. Am J Surg. 1970;119:99-105.

37. Dassinger MS, Smith SD. Disorders of intestinal rotation and fixation. In. Coran AG. Pediatric Surgery, 7th edn. Philadelphia: Elsevier Saunders. 2012.p.11;11-25.

38. Estrada. Anomalies of intestinal rotation and fixation. Springfield, Ill, Charles C. Thomas. 1958.

39. Powell DM, Othersen HB, Smith CD. Malrotation of the intestines in children: The effect of age on presentation and therapy. J Pediatr Surg. 1989;24:777.

40. Pracros JP, Sann L, Genin G, Tran-Minh VA, Morin de Finfe CH, Foray P, Louis D. Ultrasound diagnosis of midgut volvulus: the "whirlpool" sign. Pediatr Radiol. 1992;22(1):18-20.
Ablow RC, et al. Z-shaped duodenojejunal loop: Sign of mesenteric fixation anomaly and congenital bands. Am J Radiol. 1983;141:461.

41. Ladd WE, Gross RE. Abdominal Surgery of Infancy and Childhood. Philadelphia, WB Saunders. 1941.

42. Klein MD. Congenital defects of the abdominal wall. In: Coran AG. Pediatric Surgery, 7th edition. Philadelphia: Elsevier Saunders; 2012.p.893-918.

43. Duhamel B. Embryology of exomphalos and allied malformations. Arch Dis Child. 1963;38:142.

44. Schlatter M, Norris K, Uitvlugt N, et al. Improved outcomes in the treatment of gastroschisis using a preformed silo and delayed repair approach. J Pediatr Surg. 2003;38:459.

45. van Eijck FC, de Blaauw I, Bleichrodt RP, et al. Closure of giant omphaloceles by the abdominal wall component separation technique in infants. J Pediatr Surg. 2008; 43:246.

46. Langer JC. Hirschsprung Disease. In: Coran AG (Ed.) Pediatric Surgery, 7th edn. Philadelphia: Elsevier Saunders. 2012.p.1265-78.

47. Orr J, Scobie W. Presentation and incidence of Hirschsprung's disease. BMJ. 1983;287:1671.

48. Gariepy C. Developmental disorders of the enteric nervous system: Genetic and molecular bases. J Pediatr Gastroenterol Nutr. 2004;39:5-11.

49. Newman B, Nussbaum A, Kirkpatrick Jr JA. Bowel perforation in Hirschsprung's disease. AJR Am J Roentgenol. 1987;148:1195-7.

50. Lewis NA, Levitt MA, Zallen GS, et al. Diagnosing Hirschsprung's disease: Increasing the odds of a positive rectal biopsy result. J Pediatr Surg. 2003; 38:412-416.discussion 6.

51. Wilson-Storey D, Scobie WG, McGenity KG. Microbiological studies of the enterocolitis of Hirschsprung's disease. Arch Dis Child. 1990;65:1338-9.

52. Smith GHH, Cass D. Infantile Hirschsprung's disease—is barium enema useful? Pediatr Surg Int. 1991;6:318-21.

53. Brenner E. Congenital defects of the anus and rectum. Surg Gynecol Obstet. 1975.579-98.

54. Falcone Jr R, Levitt M, Peña A, et al. Increased heritability of certain types of anorectal malformations. J Pediatr Surg. 2007;42:124-7. discussion.127-8.

55. Smith E, Saeki M. Associated anomalies. Birth Defects Orig Artic Ser. 1988;24:501-49.

56. Stephens FD, Smith ED. Anorectal Malformation in Children, Year Book Medical Publications, Chicago. 1971.

57. Holschneider, et al. Preliminary report on the International Conference for the Development of Standards for the Treatment of Anorectal Malformations. J Pediatr Surg. 2005;40:1521-6.

58. Smith DE, Yokoyama J, Saeki M. Procedure for identification and management of anorectal anomalies in the newborn infant. In: F Douglas Stephens, E Durham Smith (Eds). Anorectal Malformations in children: Update. Alan R. Liss INC: New York; 1988.p1-10.

59. Bekhit E, Murphy F, Puri P, Hutson JM. The Clinical Features and Diagnostic Guidelines for Identification of Anorectal Malformations. In: Holschneider AM, Hutson AM (Eds). Anorectal malformations in children. Springer New York. p.185-200.

60. Wilkins S, Peña A. The role of colostomy in the management of anorectal malformations. Pediatr Surg Int. 1988;3:105-9.

61. DeVries PA, Peña A. Posterior sagittal anorectoplasty. J Pediatr Surg. 1982;17:638-43.

62. Okada A, Kamata S, Imura K, Fukuzawa M, Kubota A, Yagi M, et al. Anterior sagittal anorectoplasty for rectovestibular and anovestibular fistula. J Pediatr Surg. 1992 Jan;27(1):85-8.

63. de Vries PA, Dorairajan T, Guttman FM, Kottmeir PK, del Campo NM, Nixon HH, et al. Operative management of high and intermediate anomalies in males. In: Stephens DF, Smith DE. (Eds) Anorectal malformations in children. Update. Alan R. Liss INC: New York. 1988.p-317-402.

64. Georgeson K, Inge T, Albanese C. Laparoscopically assisted anorectal pull-through for high imperforate anus—a new technique. J Pediatr Surg. 2000;35:927-30.discussion 930-21.

65. Levitt MA, Pena A. Complications after the Treatment of Anorectal Malformations and Redo Operations. In: Holschneider AM, Hutson AM (Eds). Anorectal malformations in children. Springer New York. p.319-28.

66. Addis DG, Shaffer N, Fowler BS, Tauxe RV. The epidemiology of appendicitis and appendectomy in the United States. Am J Epidemiol. 1990;132:910.

67. Dunn JYC. Appendicitis. In: Coran AG (Ed). Pediatric Surgery, 7th edn.Philadelphia: Elsevier Saunders. 2012.p.1255-64.

68. Sarfati MR, Hunter GC, Witzke DB, et al. Impact of adjunctive testing on the diagnosis and clinical course of patients with acute appendicitis. Am J Surg. 1993;166:660.

69. Wade DS, Marrow SE, Balsara ZN, et al. Accuracy of ultrasound in the diagnosis of acute appendicitis compared with the surgeon's clinical impression. Arch Surg. 1993;128:1039.

70. Choi D, Park H, Lee YR, et al. The most useful findings for diagnosing acute appendicitis on contrast-enhanced helical CT. Acta Radiol. 2003;44:574-82.

71. Muehlstedt SG, Pham TQ, Schmeling DJ. The management of pediatric appendicitis: A survey of North American Pediatric Surgeons. J Pediatr Surg. 2004;39:875-9.

72. Feigin E, Carmon M, Szoid A, Seror D. Acute stump appendicitis. Lancet. 1993;341:757.

73. Esposito C. One-trocar appendectomy in pediatric surgery. Surg Endosc. 1998;12:177-8.

74. Hamby LS, Fowler CL, Pokorny WJ. Intussusception. In: Donnellan WL (Ed.) Abdominal Surgery of Infancy and Childhood, Australia: Harwood. 1996:1.

75. Swenson O. Pediatric Surgery. 2nd ed. New York, Appleton-Century-Crofts. 1962.

76. Blanch AJ, Perel SB, Acworth JP. Paediatric intussusception: epidemiology and outcome. Emerg Med Australas. 2007;19:45.

77. Ein SH, Stephens CA. Intussusception: 354 cases in 10 years. J Pediatr Surg. 1971;6:16.

78. Columbani PM, Scholz S. Intussusception. In: Coran AG. Pediatric Surgery, 7th edition. Philadelphia: Elsevier Saunders; 2012.p.1093-110.

79. Bines JE, Liem NT, Justice FA, et al. Risk factors for intussusception in infants in Vietnam and Australia: Adenovirus implicated, but not rotavirus. J Pediatr. 2006;149:452.

80. Mulcahy DL, Kamath KR, de Silva LM, et al. A two part study of the aetiological role of rotavirus in intussusception. J Med Virol. 1982;9:51.

81. DiFiore JW. Intussusception. Semin Pediatr Surg. 1999; 8:214.

82. Gross RE. Intussusception. The Surgery of Infancy and Childhood, Philadelphia: WB Saunders; 1953:281

83. Ravitch MM. Intussusception. In: Welch KJ, Randolph JG, Ravitch MM, et al (Eds). Pediatric Surgery, 4th ed. Chicago: Year Book; 1986:868.

84. Harrington L, Connolly BL, Hu X, et al. Ultrasonographic and clinical predictors of intussusception. J Pediatr. 1998;132:836.

85. Hryhorczuk AL, Strouse PJ. Validation of US as a first-line diagnostic test for assessment of pediatric ileocolic intussusception. Pediatr Radiol. 2009;39:1075.

86. Daneman A, Navarro O: Intussusception Part 2: An update on the evolution of management. Pediatr Radiol. 2004; 34:97.

87. Stringer DA, Ein SH. Pneumatic reduction: Advantages, risks and indications. Pediatr Radiol. 1990;20:475.

88. Ko HS, Schenk JP, Tröger J, et al. Current radiological management of intussusception in children. Eur Radiol. 2007;17:2411.

89. Daneman A, Alton DJ, Ein S, et al. Perforation during attempted intussusception reduction in children—a comparison of perforation with barium and air. Pediatr Radiol. 1995;25:81.

90. Albu I, Munteanu V, Florescu P, et al. The ileal diverticulum. Morpho-clinical and epidemiological study. Rom J Morphol Embryol. 1993;39:37-42.

91. Skandalakis J, Gray S, Ricketts R. The small intestines. Embryology for Surgeons, 2nd ed. Baltimore: Williams & Wilkins. 1994:213-25.

92. Snyder CL. Meckel's Diverticulum. In: Coran AG (Ed). Pediatric Surgery,7th edn. Philadelphia: Elsevier Saunders. 2012.p.1085-92.

93. Ford PV, Bartold SP, Fink-Bennett DM, et al. Procedure guideline for gastrointestinal bleeding and Meckel's diverticulum scintigraphy. Society of Nuclear Medicine. J Nucl Med. 1999; 40:1226-32.

94. Olson DE, Kim Y, Donnelly LF. CT findings in children with Meckel diverticulum. Pediatr Radiol. 2009;39:659-63.

95. Chan KW, Lee KH, Mou JWC, et al. Laparoscopic management of complicated Meckel's diverticulum in children: A 10-year review. Surg Endosc. 2008;22:1509-12.

96. Angood PB, Gingalewski CA, Andersen DK. Surgical complications. In: Townsend C (Ed). Sabiston's Textbook of Surgery, 16th edn. Philadelphia: WB Saunders. 2001:189-225.

97. Winslet MC. Intestinal obstruction. In: Williams NS, Bulstrode CJK, O'Connell PR (Eds). Bailey and Love's Short practice of surgery, 25th edition. London: Haddor Arnold; 2008.p.1188-203.

98. Sebastian VA, Nebab KJ, Goldfarb MA. Intestinal obstruction and ileus: Role of computed tomography scan in diagnosis and management. Am Surg. 2007;73:1210-14.

99. Anderson N, Malpas T, Robertson R. Prenatal diagnosis of colon atresia. Pediatr Radiol. 1993;23:63-64.

100. Crohn BB, Yunich AM. Ileojejunitis. Ann Surg. 1941;113:371-80.

101. Auvin S, Molinie F, Gower-Rousseau C, et al. Incidence, clinical presentation and location at diagnosis of pediatric inflammatory bowel disease: A prospective population-based study in northern France (1988–1999). J Pediatr Gastroenterol Nutr. 2005;41:49-55.

102. Alos R, Hinojosa J. Timing of surgery in Crohn's disease: A key issue in the management. World J Gastroenterol. 2008;14:5532-39.

103. Diefenbach KA, Breuer CK. Pediatric inflammatory bowel disease. World J Gastroenterol. 2006;12:3204-12.

104. Fichera A, McCormack R, Rubin MA, et al. Long-term outcome of surgically treated Crohn's colitis: A prospective study. Dis Colon Rectum. 2005; 48:963-9.

105. Yamamoto T, Fazio VW, Tekkis PP. Safety and efficacy of strictureplasty for Crohn's disease: A systematic review and meta-analysis. Dis Colon Rectum. 2007;50:1968-86.

106. Sandborn WJ, Fazio VW, Feagan BG, et al. AGA technical review on perianal Crohn's disease. Gastroenterology. 2003;125:1508-30.

107. Mortensen NJM, Ashraf S. The small and large intestines. In: Williams NS, Bulstrode CJK, O'Connell PR (Eds). Bailey and Love's Short practice of surgery, 25th edition. London: Haddor Arnold. 2008.p.1154-87.

108. Orkin BA, Telander RL, Wolff BG, et al. The surgical management of children with ulcerative colitis. The old vs. the new. Dis Colon Rectum. 1990; 33:947-55.

109. Aylett SO. Three hundred cases of diffuse ulcerative colitis treated by total colectomy and ileo-rectal anastomosis. Br Med J. 1966;1:1001-5

110. Rogers JC, Harris DJ, Holder T. Annular pancreas in a mother and daughter. Am J Med Genet. 1993;45:116.

111. Jimenez JC, Emil S, Podnos Y. et al. Annular pancreas in children: A recent decade's experience. J Pediatr Surg. 2004;39:1654-7.

112. Warshaw AL. Pancreas divisum: A case for surgical treatment. Adv Surg. 1987;21:93.

113. Warshaw AL, Richter J, Schapiro RH. The cause and treatment of pancreatitis associated with pancreas divisum. Ann Surg. 1983; 198:443.

114. Neblett III WW, O'Neill Jr JA. Surgical management of recurrent pancreatitis in children with pancreas divisum. Ann Surg. 2000; 231:899.

115. Vandenplas Y, Hassal E. mechanisms of gastroesophageal reflux and gastresophageal reflux disease. J Pediatr Gastroenterol Nutr. 2002;39:119.

116. Hollwarth ME. Gastroesophageal reflux disease. In: Coran AG (Ed). Pediatric Surgery, 7th edn. Philadelphia: Elsevier Saunders. 2012.p.947-58.

117. Fonkalsrud AW. Nissen fundoplication for pediatric gastroesophageal reflux disease. Semin Pediatr Surg. 1998;7:110.

118. Toupet A. Technique d'eosophago-gastroplastie avec phreno-gastropexie dans la cure radicals des hernies hiatales et comme complement de l'operation de Heller dans les cardiospasmes. Mem Acad Chir (Paris). 1963;89:394-9.

119. Thal AP, Hatafuku T, Kurtzman R. New Operation for Distal Esophageal Stricture. Arch Surg. 1965; 90:464-72.

120. Must A, Jacques PF, Dallal GE, et al. Long-term morbidity and mortality of overweight adolescents. A follow-up of the Harvard Growth Study of 1922 to 1935. N Engl J Med. 1992;327:1350-5.

121. Ben-Shlomo Y, Kuh D. A life course approach to chronic disease epidemiology: Conceptual models, empirical challenges and interdisciplinary perspectives. Int J Epidemiol. 2002;31:285-93.

122. Freedman DS, Mei Z, Srinivasan SR. et al. Cardiovascular risk factors and excess adiposity among overweight children and adolescents: The Bogalusa Heart Study. J Pediatr. 2007;150:12-7.

123. Byberg L, McKeigue PM, Zethelius B, Lithell HO. Birth weight and the insulin resistance syndrome: Association of low birth weight with truncal obesity and raised plasminogen activator inhibitor-1 but not with abdominal obesity or plasma lipid disturbances. Diabetologia. 2000;43:54-60.

124. Silverman BL, Rizzo TA, Cho NH, Metzger BE. Long-term effects of the intrauterine environment. The Northwestern University Diabetes in Pregnancy Center. Diabetes Care. 1998;21:B142-B149.

125. Gillman MW, Rifas-Shiman SL, Camargo Jr CA, et al. Risk of overweight among adolescents who were breastfed as infants. JAMA. 2001; 285:2461-7.

126. Whitaker RC, Deeks CM, Baughcum AE, Specker BL. The relationship of childhood adiposity to parent body mass index and eating behavior. Obes Res. 2000;8:234-40.

127. Pratt JS, Lenders CM, Dionne EA, et al. Best practice updates for pediatric adolescent weight loss surgery. Obesity (Silver Spring). 2009;17;901-10.

128. Schauer PR, Ikramuddin S. Laparoscopic surgery for morbid obesity. Surg Clin North Am. 2001;81:1145-79.

129. Pories WJ, Swanson MS, MacDonald KG, et al. Who would have thought it? An operation proves to be the most effective therapy for adult-onset diabetes mellitus. Ann Surg. 1995;222:339-50. discussion 350-2.

130. Chapman AE, Kiroff G, Game P, et al. Laparoscopic adjustable gastric banding in the treatment of obesity: A systematic literature review. Surgery. 2004;135:326-51.

131. Clinical Issues Committee: Sleeve gastrectomy as a bariatric procedure. Surg Obes Relat Dis. 2007;3:573-6.

132. Papadia FS, Adami GF, Marinari GM, et al. Bariatric surgery in adolescents: A long-term follow-up study. Surg Obes Relat Dis. 2007;3:465-8.

Section 2

Nutrition

Chapter 13

Nutritional Assessment in Health and Disease

K Vijayaraghavan

INTRODUCTION

Nutrition is the foundation for human health and development. Access to an affordable diet containing adequate amounts of all the nutrients, adoption of right practices of maternal and childcare and provision of healthy environment supported by adequate health services are essential for good nutrition. Proper nutrition in early life, particularly during the 1000 days between mother's pregnancy and her child's 2nd birthday would help healthy growth and normal cognitive development. During this period, the child's nutritional needs for normal growth and development are increased and the child is completely dependent on mother for nutrition and care. In malnutrition, an individual's performance with respect to pregnancy, lactation, physical growth and development, resistance to infections, the ability to recover from disease and physical work output are suboptimalpoor maternal nutrition retards fetal development leading to low birth weight, subsequent stunting and other forms of undernutrition. Apart from dietary deficiency, childhood morbidity also contributes to nutritional deficiencies either by causingimpaired absorption of nutrients or reduced appetite or dietary restriction due to several food taboos observed due to ignorance of care provider. Undernutrition in children manifests as growth retardation expressing as underweight, stunting and wasting. Undernutrition weakens immune system, and to gether with infection potentiates the lethal cycle of worsening illness, deteriorating nutritional status and may increase mortality risk.[1] For example, astunted or severely underweight child is about 5–10 times higher risk of deathdue to diarrhea than a child who is not. There is, therefore, a need for regular screening and monitoring of vulnerable communities through early detection of nutrition problems and effective management of malnutrition and associated health problems during illnessto promote appropriate nutrition.

GOALS

To start with, the goal of the nutrition assessment should be clear. The main aim, whether it is in a hospital or at the community level, will be to identify particularly children with poor nutritional status using appropriate parameters, to assess the need for any special dietary supplements, and evaluate influence of any cultural practices on diet so as to plan nutrition counseling on proper dietary practices and to develop plan for nutrition care. In the case of hospital cases, the main aim of the pediatrician should be to assess nutritional status so as to decrease the incidence of morbidity and mortality associated with nutritional problems among the children, and to provide timely, optimum, safe and cost-effective nutrition to improve clinical outcomes.

GUIDING PRINCIPLES

Nutrition assessment involves team work, the team consisting of clinician for clinical examination, anthropometrist for nutritional anthropometry and nutritionist/dietician for dietary assessment and biochemistfor biochemical assessment. In the case of population studies, to help in fixing sample size and representativeness of the selected groups a statistician should be consulted. Adequate attention should be given to the anthropometric equipment and adoption of standard methods. It should be ensured that the weighing scales are tested regularly with known standard weights and any zero error is adjusted regularly. The quality assurance should receive adequate attention, particularly in population studies. This involves ensuring interindividual (between measurements taken by two individuals) and intra-individual variation (agreement between duplicates) is in the accepted rangewith reference to data, by intensive training of the team members in different techniques. Quite often, the tasks are allotted to some junior nursing staff, particularly in hospitals, without emphasis on training. The subjects should be explained clearly the purpose and the methods of data collection.

The clinicians pay far too little attention to the underlying nutritional status despite its role on prognosis and outcome disease, and are not adequately oriented in screening of children for nutritional risk. It is important to pay particular attention to children as they are also in the processes of growth and development. The child cannot achieve the growth potential determined by his/her genetic makeup in the presence of constraints of either nutrition or disease. In the case of hospital settings, it should be kept in mind that the illness *per se* could influence the body weight and cause wasting, which can be identified by weight for height. Biochemical parameters like serum vitamin A could be lowered in fever, infections and infestations like ascariasis, over and above the changes due to the vitamin deficiency. Infections could increase serum ferritin making interpretation difficult. In certain diseases, restriction of diet is more of a rule than exception. This should be kept in mind during the dietary assessment of the individual. As hospital atmosphere could vitiate the results of dietary assessment, it should preferably be done at the patient's residence.

METHODS OF NUTRITION ASSESSMENT

The methods of direct assessment can be summarized as ABCD:
- **A**nthropometry
- **B**iochemical assessment
- **C**linical examination
- **D**ietary assessment

CLINICAL EXAMINATION

Clinical examination is quick and easy, inexpensive and more importantly noninvasive, and is considered the most practical and the simplest method of nutrition assessment of individuals. Inability to detect early cases is its major limitation. It involves identification of accepted, specific and relevant clinical signs of macro and micronutrient deficiencies. Physical examination should be carried out from head to toe in adequate light, paying particular attention to hair, particularly the angles of the mouth, tongue, palate, gums, nails, skin, eyes and thyroid gland. Complete nutritional history, including particularly the feeding practices with respect to breastfeeding and introduction of complementary foods is essential. Careful enquiry should be done about previous illnesses, particularly fever, measles and frequent diarrhoeal attacks, as these generally precede protein energy malnutrition. Subjective grading of clinical signs (mild or severe)

condition should be avoided. The ***clinical manifestations associated with common nutritional deficiency disease***s are discussed below.

Protein–Energy Malnutrition (PEM)

The term PEM covers a wide spectrum of severe clinical conditions of kwashiorkor and marasmus and milder forms of different grades of undernutrition exhibiting growth retardation, identifiable mostly by anthropometry.

Kwashiorkor

The term is derived from Ghana language, meaning 'the disease of a displaced child', reflecting the development of the disorder in an older child who is weaned from the breast when a younger sibling comes. The children are usually between 1 and 3 years of age. The three cardinal signs are:
- Edema
- Growth retardation (stuntingand underweight), and
- Mental changes (irritability and loss of interest in surroundings).

Other manifestations,though not required for makingthe diagnosis, are generally seen. The cheeks may appear to be swollen with either fatty tissue or fluid giving an appearance of moon face. The hair may be discolored and coppery redin color, and is easily pluckable (hair falls off with merepassing the hands through the hair) leading to sparseness. On the skin, dark pigmented patches may be present, which peel off or desquamate, resembling old sun-baked paint patches and, hence, referred as flaky-paint dermatosis. When some of the patches peel off there may be raw patches. In the initial stages, the child may have diarrhea or respiratory infection (Fig. 13.1A).

Marasmus

Nutritional marasmus, much more common than kwashiorkor, perhaps, can be considered as a form of starvation, mostly due to inadequate quantities of breast milk (often lactation failure). The precipitating causes are childhood infections and infestations. It is characterized extreme muscle wasting and severe underweight. The children are stunted and usually much below the reference standards—<60% or <3 SD of body weight for expected age. The face has typical simian ormonkey likelook. The extremities are so emaciated with so little subcutaneous tissue that the child appears to be 'skin and bones', with very prominent ribsand loose skin-folds hanging over the buttocks. The child may also have chronic infection like tuberculosis. As compared to kwashiorkor, the marasmic children appear much more alert and are less miserable.

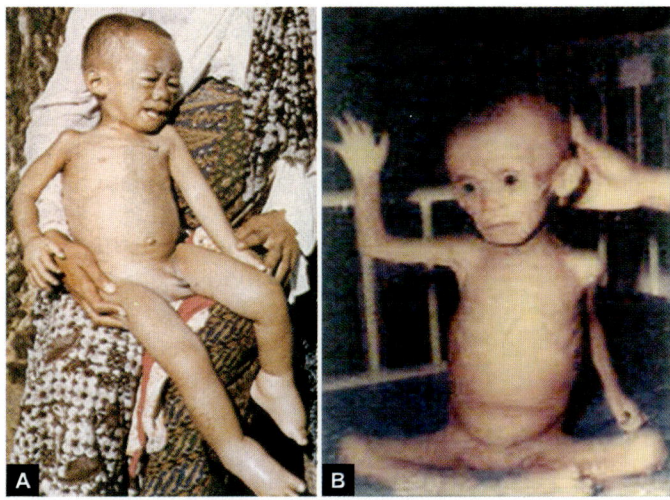

Figs 13.1A and B: (A) Kwashiorkor; (B) Marasmus
(*Courtesy*: NIN, Hyderabad)

Other nutritional deficiency signs, particularly anemia are usually present (Fig. 13.1B).

Marasmic Kwashiorkor

Children with marasmic kwashiorkor present with features of both kwashiorkor (edema) and marasmus (extreme muscular wasting). They will be emaciated, weighing <60% expected weight for age, and stunted. There may be skin and hair changes. Like in kwashiorkor or marasmus, the patients may have diarrhea and respiratory infections.

Vitamin A Deficiency

Vitamin A deficiency, main cause of nutritional blindnessamong young children, is animportant micronutrient deficiency in India. It is also referred as xerophthalmia, which encompasses all the ocular manifestations of vitamin A deficiency affecting conjunctiva, cornea and occasionally retina.The examination of eyes of the children should be carried out in good light, preferably with a loupe. Vitamin A is a component of rhodopsin, the pigment present in rods (photoreceptor cells) in retina, concerned with vision in dark and dim light. In vitamin A deficiency, since rhodopsin will not be formed, the patients cannot see in dim light, leading to night blindness (*rathaundi* in Hindi). In young children, it will be difficult to assess night blindness. However, an observant mother may complain that her child cannot see the plate of food in front in dim light or fumbles frequently at dusk or dawn. This can be tested by asking the mother to bring her child into a dark room from bright light and asking the child to pick a coin dropped on the floor. The child with night blindness cannot locate the coin. On examination of the eyes, there

may be *conjunctival xerosis*, which manifests as dry patches of nonwettable conjunctiva. When the eye is exposed for about 30 seconds, and when the child ceases to cry, the tears appear to emerge like "sand bank at receding tide". Conjunctival xerosis is subject to considerable investigator bias, making it absolutely necessary for standardization by proper training. Later, the child develops *Bitot's spot,* an extension of conjunctival xerosis. These are raised, muddy, and dry triangular patches on the temporal side of the cornea. The spots become prominentin girls applying *Kajal* (Eyetex). Bitot spot is considered an objective sign particularly in 1–5-year-old children (Fig. 13.2A). The next stage iscorneal xerosis, characterized by the presence of haziness or dryness of cornea giving it a groundglass appearance and may progress tocorneal ulcers, which are characteristically circular and sharply demarcated, and may leave scars (leucoma) on healing. Depending on location in relation to pupil of the eye there may be partial blindness. The final manifestation of vitamin A deficiency is the dreaded *Keratomalacia*, which represents rapidly progressive necrosis and death of tissue affecting the full thickness of the cornea leading to irreversible blindness. This may end up in extrusion of intraocular contents or complete atrophy of the eye (Fig. 13.2B).

Nutritional Anemia

Nutritional anemia affects up to three quarters of children of 1–5 years and is widely prevalent among older children as well. Anemia is defined as reduction of hemoglobin levels in circulation. The most common cause is inadequate consumption of the micronutrient iron. Folic acid deficiency and vitamin B_{12} deficiency may also contribute, less frequently. The clinical manifestations are due to low hemoglobin and the consequent reduction in capacity of the blood to transport oxygen. On examination, there may be pallor of the mucosa in the mouth, conjunctiva and the nail beds. Trained clinician canidentify pallor of conjunctiva and soft palate. The examiner can compare the redness below nail with his/her own nails. In severe anemia, the nails may be concave and spoon-shaped, known as koilonychia. The child may have difficulty in

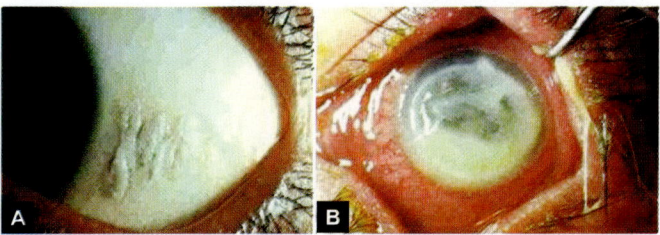

Figs 13.2A and B: (A) Bitot spot; (B) Keratomalacia
(*Courtesy*: NIN, Hyderabad)

breathing on exertion even in moderate anemia. Easy fatigability and lassitude are common. In very severe cases, there may be edema as well. Since diagnosis is subject to examiner bias, anemia is confirmed by hemoglobin estimation of a finger prick blood sample.

Iodine Deficiency Disorders (IDD)

The typical signs of endemic iodine deficiency disorders are goitre and cretinism. Goitre is noninflammatory and nontoxic enlargement of thyroid gland. Normal thyroid gland is not palpable. When the volume of thyroid lobes is larger than the subject'sterminal phalanx of thumb, it is diagnosed as goiter (Fig. 13.3). The WHO recommends the following grading of goiter:
- Grade 0: No palpable or visible goitre
- Grade 1: Palpablethyroid and not visible in normal position of the neck (not visiblyenlarged)
- Grade 2: A clearly visible swelling of thyroid gland when the neck is in normal position, which corresponds to enlarged thyroid found on palpation.

In IDD endemic areas, there will be growth retardation and also of retardation of intellectual development. Endemic cretinism occurs when there is severe iodine deficiency during intrauterine life. It includes a range of mental deficiency, deaf-mutism and spastic paralysis. At two years of age, the child may still be unable to walk unassisted, and at three years, he or she may not be able to talk or understand simple commands. Cretinism may occur in two forms. In neurological cretinism, more predominant in Asian and South American countries, there will be severe mental retardation, squint, deaf-mutism and spastic rigidity of lower limbs and inability to walk or shuffling gait. In contrast, in myxodematous cretinism, mostly seen in Zaire, there is evidence of hypothyroidism, the child is retarded in growth and mental development. The child may have deep hoarse voice and apathy.

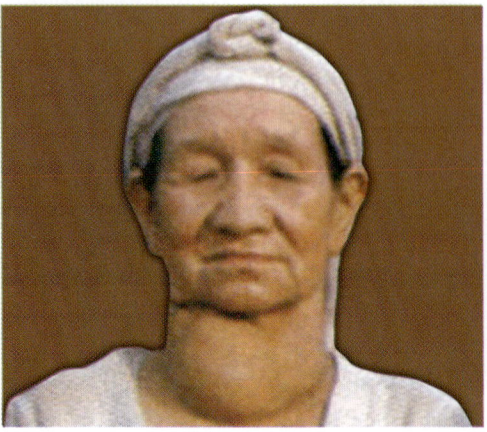

Fig. 13.3: Goiter (*Courtesy*: NIN, Hyderabad)

Vitamin B Complex Deficiency

Riboflavin Deficiency

It is characterized by orolingual lesions, sometimes associated with photophobia (intolerance to bright light) and dermal lesions. Angular stomatitis (cracks and fissures in the angles at the mucocutaneous junctions of the mouth) is the most common manifestation of riboflavin deficiency. The lesions on the tongue are referred to as glossitis, when the tongue is inflamed and appears red and raw. The papillae gradually progress from hypertrophy to atrophy, depending on the duration and the severity of deficiency. Hypertrophic papillae produce the typical magenta red tongue. When atrophy progresses, denudation, and baldness occur.

The mucous membrane of the lips becomes red and may get denuded, particularly along the line of closure. It may lead to cheilosis, characteristic of chronic deficiency, in which the lips have dry and chapped appearance with ulceration in severe deficiency. Sometimes on the face, seborrheic dermatitis in the nasolabial regions is seen known as nasolabial dyssabacia. Plugs of yellowish keratin standing out from the follicles are usually seen on each side of the nose extending sometimes to other parts of the face.

Thiamine Deficiency and Beriberi

Beriberi, due to deficiency of thiamine (vitamin B_1), is rare in India. It occurs in otherwise normal breastfed infants between 2 and 6 months of age, due mainly to inadequate thiamine in breast milk. The mother may not have any signs of beriberi. In its acute form, there is breathlessness, often associated with cyanosis, and invariably is fatal due to cardiac failure. In chronic forms, the infants develop aphonia (no sound while crying). It may simulate meningitis and the infant may even develop convulsions.

Pellagra

Pellagra—deficiency of dietary niacin—is generally associated with a maize diet in the Americas, and with *jowar* consumption in India. It is common in undernourished and middle-aged adults. It is characterized by 3 'D's—**D**ermatitis, **D**iarrhea and **D**ementia.

Dermatitis is typically present on the skin exposed to sunlight, like face, neck, back of the hands, forearm and the legs. Pellagrous skin is hyperpigmented, dry due to the loss of oily sheen, rough and scaly, with a clear demarcation between the lesions and the normal skin. With further progress, there may be cracking and fissuring. The lesions on the neck are described as Casal's necklace because of its typical shape, and on the face it is butterfly shaped on each side of the nose.

Diarrhea: Due to inflammation of the mucous membrane of the gastrointestinal tract, pellagrous patients present with bloody diarrhea, particularly very common in jowar eaters. Typically glossitis will be present.

Dementia: Mental functions are affected. In fact, in a number of them, it may be the presenting symptom seeking admission in institutions of mental health. The common manifestations are insomnia, irritability, anxiety and loss of memory. There may be disorientation and delirium. Some patients may develop tremors and paresthesia.

Rickets

It is a disease of growing children due to vitamin D deficiency. The child may appear miserable and the muscles may be flabby and without tone. The main feature is swelling of growing (epiphyseal) ends of the long bones like the radius bone. On the chest, the swelling at the junction of costal cartilage and ribs is referred to as 'rickety rosary' due to shape of the lesion. There is delay in achieving the milestones. The child may have bossing of the frontal bone. There may be craniotabes, seen mostly in the occipital and parietal bones, in which the bones collapse underneath with pressure and usually snap back into place when released. Once the child starts to stand and walk, and as the bones are soft and weak, the child will develop deformities, such as bow legs, knock-knees and spinal deformitiesin severe cases.

Scurvy

Scurvy, due to vitamin C deficiency, is rare. The common manifestations are spongy bleeding gums, which bleed painlessly easily at the base of the teeth, tiredness and weakness, bleeding points on the skin, nose-bleeds, and delayed wound healing and even anemia.

Fluorosis

In children, dental fluorosis, due to excessive consumption of fluorides in water and food, is seen on permanent teeth. It manifests as mottling of teeth, characterized by abnormal white flecks, yellowish spots scattered irregularly on the surface of the tooth. Sometimes, there may be pitting on the teeth. Skeletal fluorosis is noticed only in adults.

■ NUTRITIONAL ANTHROPOMETRY

Nutritional anthropometryis defined as measurement of human body at different ages and different levels of nutritional status.[2] While clinical examination reveals the anatomical changes that can be diagnosed by naked eye, anthropometry helps in the assessment of subclinical stages of malnutrition. It is acknowledged as a reliable tool to identify nutritionally vulnerable children; for monitoring changes in the extent of malnutrition; to select beneficiaries for nutrition intervention and to evaluate its impact. In clinical practice, it is also used to assess an individual's response to nutritional rehabilitation. Monitoring of weight and height of a child would help take the action against pooror no growth, weight loss, and to restore proper growth.

Anthropometric Measurements

The measurements should be the simplest and quickest to measure with easy reproducibility, providing maximum information about undernutrition. The most commonly used measurements are:
- Body weight,
- Standing height or crown-heel length.

Mid-upper arm circumference (MUAC) and fat fold at triceps are also usually taken in routine community nutrition surveys.

Body Weight

Body weight is the most extensively used and the simplest reproducible measurement for evaluatingthe nutritional status of children. It is a composite of all body constituents like water, minerals, fat, protein, bone, etc. Repeated measurements of weight, rather than a single measurement, are a sensitive index to changes in nutritional status. A reduction in growth velocity (gain in weight), as determined byserial measurementsis an early and more sensitive index of growth failure. Hence, in the largest national program, Integrated Child Development Services (ICDS), growth monitoring is an important component. Body weight is measured with regularly calibrated electronic or beam weighing scales, with an accuracy of 100 g, which are morer eliable and accurate than the commonly used bath room scales or spring balances. In the case of birth weights, which should be taken within 48 hours of birth, weighing scales with an accuracy of 10 g are recommended. Certain precautions should be taken before the measurement. The zero error of the weighing scale should be checked and corrected (if necessary) before taking the weight. The subject should wear minimum clothing and be without shoes, and should not lean against or hold anything, while recording the weight. In very cold weather, weight of warm clothing should be subtracted.

Height

Stunted linear growth (short stature) is now considered the main indicator of childhood undernutrition, because of its significant consequences for health and development. A severely stunted child has four times higher risk of death. In older children and adults, standing height is measured with a vertical measuring rod (anthropometer), while in children below the age of two years, who cannot stand properly, recumbent length (crown–heel length) is measured with an infantometer. The measurements of standing height and recumbent length are recorded in centimetres up to the nearest 1 millimeter (0.1 cm).

Measurement of Standing Height

Older children (>2 years of age) should stand erect with heels together on a levelled surface without shoes and looking straight. The investigator stands on the left side of the child and will place the anthropometer rod behind in the center of the heels perpendicular to the ground, firmly holding the child's chin with his/her left hand and the occiput of the subject with his right little finger to maintain the Frankfurt horizontal plane (an imaginary line joining the tragus of the ear and infraorbital margin of the eye) parallel to the ground. The moving head piece of the anthropometer should be slid down in the sagittal plane over the head of the subject, applying only slight pressure to reduce the thickness of hair, and the reading taken with the anthropometer rod still in position. Preferably, an average of three successive measurements is taken as the final measurement.

Measurement of Recumbent Length

The 'recumbent length' is measured by placing the child (<2 years) flat on its back on an infantometer, with head touching the fixed head board and legs toward the movable sliding board. A helper holds the infant's head firmly against the fixed head board. The investigator holds the infant's knees, gently pressed down, against the board with his left hand and moves the foot board with the right hand so that it comes in contact with the soles of the infant at right angles.

Mid-upper Arm Circumference

The mid-upper arm circumference (MUAC) indicates the status of muscle development. When measured along with fat fold at triceps, one can calculate mid arm muscle circumference on the assumption that the cross-section of the mid-upper arm circumference approximates a circle, and that the adipose tissue is evenly distributed around the area. The MUAC is measured on the left hand at the mid-point as a majority are right handed and with constant use the circumference may be higher. At the outset, midpoint between the tip of the acromion of scapula and the tip of the olecranon process of the forearm bone ulna is, marked with the arm flexed at right angle at the elbow. The MUAC is taken with the arm hanging freely, with a fiber glass tape placed gently embracing the arm without exerting too much pressure on the soft tissues. The reading is taken with the tape still in position, to the nearest millimeter.

Fat Fold at Triceps

Subcutaneous fat constitutes the body's main store of energy reserves and, the thickness of which is significantly reduced due to wasting in protein energy malnutrition. It is measured with fat fold callipers, at the same point on the dorsal side of the forearm where MUAC was taken. The skinfold is picked up between the thumb and the forefinger, about one centimetre above the mid-point, without including the underlying muscle. The tips of the skinfold callipers (Harpenden or Lange's callipers) are applied at the mid-point at a depth equal to the skinfold. The subcutaneous fat gets compressed if the callipers is kept for a longer time. The skinfold should be held gently in the left hand throughout the measurement.

Age Assessment

Since body weight and height are influenced by age, it is important to assess the correct ages of the children. In the urban areas and among literate communities, they have documentary evidence of date of birth. However, illiterate mothers in rural and tribal areas may not have any documentary evidence of birth dates. However, since the rural folk are familiar with festivals and other local events related mainly to agriculture or other important events, age assessment can be done accurately in relation to these local events. The mother is encouraged to recall child's birth in relation to any of the festivals/local events by enquiring whether the child was born around any festival or agriculture related event, and count the number of such events since the child's birth. Generally, a calendar based on local events can be prepared based on the dates of occurrence of these events during the previous five or six years. The age is assessed in completed years or months.

Reference Standards

The heights and weights of children have to be compared with reference growth standards to determine whether the children are growing normally or not. The growth standards are the values of weight and height for different ages of well-nourished and healthy children, and who were predominantly exclusively breastfed for the first six months. Currently, the standards obtained in a WHO multicenter growth reference study[3] are used. An individual child's growth pattern could be compared using a growth chart based on these standards. For detailed data for reference standards and charts for height and weight refer http://www.who.int/childgrowth/standards/en/.

Anthropometric Indicators

Body weight and height/length and derived parameters are used to assess nutritional status of individuals.

Underweight

Itis based on weight for age of the child and is a composite form of undernutrition which includes both stunting and wasting. A child whose weight for age is below minus two standard deviations (-2 Z) from median of the WHO child growth standards is underweight. This includes both moderate and severe undernutrition. Children whose weights are between median -2 Z and Median -3 Z are considered as moderately underweight and those with weights below median -3 Z are severely underweight.

Low birthweight is defined as a weight of less than 2,500 grams at birth. The following classification is accepted for birth weight:

Small for date: Born after completing 37 weeks of gestation with birth weight <2500 g.

Premature: Born before completing 37 weeks of gestation.

Stunting

Stunting signifies slowing in linear skeletal growth, and is indicated by low height for age (<Median -2 Z of expected height for age). It is an index of long duration malnutrition representing the accumulated consequences of retarded growth. Stunting, especially mild-to-moderate degree, is frequently associated with poor overall economic conditions, chronic or repeated infections, as well as inadequate nutrient intake. Stunting occurs more over time up to the age of 24 or 36 months. Children whose heights are between median -2 Z and median -3 Z of expected height for age are considered as moderately stunted and the heights below median -3 Z indicate severe stunting.

Wasting

Weight for height is anindex of wasting of children, and indicates the current nutritional and health status of children. Wasting indicates a reduction in muscle and fat as compared to the expected in a normal child of the same height or length. It may happen due either to failure to gain weight or from weight loss. Other precipitating factors are infections or some other household crisis and usually low dietary intake among children. Wasting can develop very rapidly, and can be restored as rapidly under favorable conditions. Using the reference values of height and weight, tables for expected weights for different heights/lengths are prepared. Employing the weight for height tables, the nutritional status of individuals can be assessed by expressing the weight as a percentage of the expected weight for the child's height or length or in terms of standard deviations or Z scores. Weight for height below minus two standard deviations from the median of the WHO child growth standards is considered as wasted. Children whose weight for height is between median -2 Z and median -3 Z of expected height for age are considered as moderately wasted and the values below median -3 Z indicate severe wasting.

Overweight

Childwith weight for height is above two standard deviations (overweight/obese) from the median of the WHO child growth standards. Those above 3 standard deviations are considered as obese).

Body Mass Index

Body mass index (BMI) is an anthropometric index derived from weight and height. It is defined asbody weight in kilograms divided by height in meters squared (BMI = weight (kg) ÷ height (meters).[2] Like weight-for-height, BMI is a screening tool for identifying individuals who are underweight or overweightand can be considered a proxy for measures of body fat.Unlike in adults, where one value (Asians: Overweight: >23) is recommended irrespective of age, in the case of children, BMI is gender specific and age specific. International Taskforce on obesity[4] recommends the use of BMI-for-age for children aged 2 years and older. BMI <5th percentile is considered to indicate underweight BMI-for-age at or above the 95th percentile indicates overweight and between the 85th and 95th percentile as at risk of overweight. BMI is an index of current nutritional status, energy deficit, particularly in the Indian context. Recent analysis of NFHS data, using WHO growth standards, indicates that at birth BMI for age is low, and the children appear normal between 9 and 23 months, due actually to poor linear growth as a result of energy deficit and consequent higher rates of stunting. If energy deficit is quickly corrected, wasting is reversed and the linear growth of children continues normally.Early detection of low BMI for age and expeditious correction of the same is likely to be the most effective intervention to prevent stunting.[5]

Interpretation of Data

All anthropometric data on children should be presented for separate age groups. Individual's nutritional status is determined by comparing the individual's measurement with the reference standards.

Percentile Chart

Simplest method is to plot the measured value on a percentile chart of reference values, for the age of the child. The values below 3rd percentile are considered to indicate underweight or stunting. A percentile is the number of a particular value in a set of 100 values arranged either ascending or descending order. The 3rd percentile is the 3rd value in a set of 100 arranged in ascending order and 3% of children are below that value and 97% are above that value. In other words, it represents the lowest 3% of reference population. Median (corresponding to average) or 50th percentile means that equal number of children is either above or below that number.

Z-scores

The World Health Organization (WHO)[6] recommends, particularly in community surveys, use of Z -scores taking into consideration the distribution of the reference values. The Z -score for a measure (e.g. height or weight) indicates how far and in what direction (positive vs. negative) a measured value deviates from the reference mean/median, expressed statistically in units of the population standard deviation (SD).

$$\text{Z-score} = \frac{\text{(Observed value)} - \text{(Median reference value)}}{\text{Standard deviation of reference population}}$$

All the children between –2 Z scores are considered as malnourished and among those less than –3 Z are severely malnourished. If the distribution of reference values follows a normal distribution, percentiles and Z scores are related through a mathematical transformation.

Percent of Expected Measurement

Another simple way is to express the measurement of individual as percent of median. Depending on the child's age, 80% of the median weight expected for age might be used as a cutoff and usually corresponds to below –2 Z score; and can help in identification of risk. Cutoff points for percent of reference are different for the different anthropometric indices.

▌BIOCHEMICAL ASSESSMENT

During the progress of deficiency biochemical changes precede clinically detectable (anatomical) changes. Bio-chemical assessment,[7] thus, helps in identifying subclinical status of nutritional deficiency. It involves measurement of the particular nutrient or its metabolite in blood or urine orestimation of an enzyme in RBC that is dependent on the nutrient or measurement of accumulated metabolite the disposal of which depends on a vitamin or mineral dependent enzyme.

An ideal biochemical test should be specific, sensitive and should indicate tissue depletion. Laboratory tests which can be conducted on easily accessible body fluids like blood and urine are preferred. For proper interpretation of the biochemical tests, qualified technicians should be involved in conducting laboratory tests. The biochemical tests for the common nutritional disorders are discussed below.

PEM

Serum albumin is the indicator of choice. Serum albumin >3 g/100 mL is considered as normal. In infants <2.5 g/100 mL is considered as high risk and in children between 1 and 5 years, albumin < 2.8 g/100 mL is indicative of severe deficiency. As total serum proteins are elevated in infections, which is common in PEM, are not considered as of diagnostic importance.

Vitamin A Deficiency

Estimation of serum vitamin A is done, generally using HPLC, to assess the subclinical status of vitamin A deficiency, particularly in children. However, these are not reliable estimates of liver stores. The WHO recommends the following guidelines:
- Deficient: <20 µg/dL (0.7 µmol/L)
- High risk: 20–30 µg/dL (0.7–1.05 µmol/L)
- Acceptable: >30 µg/dL (>1.05 µmol/L).

In the recent past, relative dose response (RDR) is considered to be a better indicator. RDR works on the principle that as vitamin A liver reserves become low as in deficiency, retinol binding protein (RBP) accumulates. When a challenge dose of vitamin A (retinyl ester) is administered, the retinol binds to this accumulated RBP and is rapidly released into the serum. RDR involves measurement of percent increase in serum retinol 5 hours after an oral dose of 450–1000 µg of vitamin A. Two blood samples are collected, the first at baseline and the second 5 hours after dosing. The post-dose increase is negatively related to vitamin A status and RDR >20% is indicative of deficiency.

Vitamin D

Estimation of serum vitamin D metabolite, 25-hydroxy cholecalciferol (25 HCC), is the acceptable indicator of vitamin D status. Low and also high levels predispose to osteoporosis. The cutoff levels suggested are:

- Deficient: <20 nmol/L (<8 ng/mL)
- Insufficient: 20–50 nmol/L (8–20 ng/mL)
- Optimal: 50–150 nmol/L (20–60 ng/mL)
- High: 150–225 nmol/L (60–90 ng/mL)
- Toxic: >225 nmol/L (90 ng/mL).

Thiamine

Earlier urinary thiamine estimation, either by fluorimetry or HPLC was relied upon. However, during the last 4 or 5 decades, transketolase test has been the accepted method. Transketolase, an enzyme that requires thiamine pyrophosphate (TPP), catalyzes reactions in the pentose phosphate pathway. So the level of transketolase activity in the red blood cell (*erythrocyte transketolase activity*) is a reliable diagnostic indicator of thiamine status. The enzyme transketolase is measured in erythrocyte hemolysate, in the absence and presence of in vitro added TPP. In thiamine deficiency, the enzyme's basal activity decreases, and the ratio of stimulated activity to that of basal, referred to as activation coefficient (ETK-AC), increases. The following are the guidelines for interpretation of *ETK-AC*:

- Acceptable: <1.15
- Medium risk: 1.15
- High risk: >1.25.

Riboflavin

Urinary riboflavin (normal: 80 µg/g of creatinine) was being used earlier. Currently, the most accepted method is *erythrocyte glutathione reductase activation test*. The test provides a measure of tissue saturation and long-term riboflavin status. *In vitro* enzyme activity in terms of activity coefficients (AC) is determined both with and without the addition of FAD to the medium. The AC represents a ratio of the enzyme's activity with FAD to the enzyme's activity without FAD. An AC < 1.2 is acceptable, while the AC of 1.2 to 1.4 is low and>1.4 is indicative of deficiency.

Folic Acid

Folic acid can be measured in serum or the red blood cells. To measure the amount of folic acid stored in the body, *RBC folate* estimation, however, is more accurate than the plasma folate. This is not usually influenced by the amount of folic acid in daily diet.
The suggested cut-offs are:

- High risk: <140 ng/mL
- Medium risk: 140–159 ng/mL
- Acceptable: 160 ng/mL.

In the case of *serum folate,* the following criteria may be used: Acceptable: >6.0 ng/mL; high risk: <3.0 ng/mL and 3.0–5.9 ng/mL is indicative of medium risk.

Vitamin B_{12}

Serum B_{12} levels are often reduced to assess B_{12} deficiency. The estimation is done using microbiological assay. Any value <150 picomol/liter is indicative of deficiency.

Iron Nutritional Status

In iron deficiency there are no mobilizable iron stores and there are signs of a reduced supply of iron to the tissues. Severe stages of iron deficiency are associated with anemia, in which hemoglobin concentrations are reduced to below-optimal levels. Hence, hemoglobin is the most common indicator to screen for iron deficiency. The following are the reference ranges of hemoglobin to diagnose anemia.

Age/physiological group	Hemoglobin (g/L)
Children (6 months to 59 months	110
Children (5–11 years)	115
Adolescents (12–14 years)	120
Non-pregnant women (above 15 years of age)	120
Pregnant women	110
Men (above 15 years of age)	130

Iron status can be characterized using the biochemical parameters of *serum ferritin, serum iron, transferrin and total iron-binding capacity*).

The *serum ferritin* level is the most specific biochemical test of relative total body iron stores, and low levels indicate depleted iron stores, in the absence of infection. The interpretation poses problems in the presence infections as the levels are elevated in infections or inflammation. Serum ferritin <15 µg/L is the generally accepted cut-off to indicate depleted iron stores in individuals of >5 years of agewhereas in children <5 years of age <12 µg/L is indicative depleted iron stores.

The levels of *erythrocyte protoporphyrin* (precursor of haem) >100 µg/dL indicate iron deficiency. A simplified and relatively inexpensive haematofluorometer that directly measures erythrocyte protoporphyrin fluorescence is now available.

In iron deficiency, there is a reduction in serum iron, transferrin saturation (serum iron ÷ total iron binding capacity). However, the diurnal variation both in serum iron and transferrin saturation is considerable. The following are indicative of iron deficiency:

❑ Transferrin saturation <15%
❑ Serum iron <60 µg/dL
❑ Total iron binding capacity of >300 µg/dL.

Iodine Status

Urinary iodine concentration is currently the most practical biochemical marker for iodine nutrition. Urinary iodine concentration of 100 µg/L indicates adequate iodine nutrition. In community surveys at least 50% of the sample should be above100 µg/L. In addition, not more than 20% of samples should be <50 µg/L.

Zinc Status

To date, *serum zinc* is the only biochemical indicator of zinc status. It should be recognized that serum zinc does not necessarily reflect individualzinc status. The recommended cut-offs for children <10 years of age are 65 µg/dL (9.9 µmol/L). Leukocyte zinc is considered a better indicator than serum levels. The normal range is 80-130 µg per 10^{10} WBC.

DIETARY ASSESSMENT

Diet being the primary determinant of individual's nutrition, nutrition deficiency is initiated by inadequate dietary consumption either as a primary cause or secondary to disease. **Dietary assessment** would help in finding out both the quantitative and qualitative aspects of diet. An understanding of any gap in nutrient intakes would help in planning diets to manage dietary deficiencies or even excesses. Dietary assessment can be done at the household level and more importantly at the individual level. At the outset, diet surveys require complete cooperation of the families. Therefore, the investigator should develop good rapport with the respondent. The investigators should also be aware of the local conditions and thoroughly trained.

Household Level

Weighment Method

Weighment of raw foods over a period of seven consecutive days (because of variation in daily diets) is the preferred method for assessing household diets. The results can be expressed either per person per day or per consumption unit (CU) per day. The consumption units are the calorie coefficients that have been arbitrarily assigned based on energy requirements for different age groups and each sex. The energy requirements of a sedentary adult male (2400 kcal) represent one CU. For other age and physiological groups, CUs are calculated by dividing the respective requirements by that of sedentary adult male. Thus, for the

sedentary adult female it will be 0.8 (1900 ÷ 2400). The CUs are not strictly applicable to other nutrients.

The method involves visiting the selected house, twice in a day, for 7 consecutive days, before the food is actually cooked, and weighing all the edible portion of raw foodstuffs that will go into each meal. The details, particularly the physical activity, age and physiological status (pregnancy/lactation) of all the members, including that of guests, partaking in the meal should be recorded. Avoid festival days, as generally families prepare special foods on these days. Intake of each food item is calculated by: Total raw food consumed for 7 days ÷ (Total CUs in the family × number of days of survey). The Nutrient content is calculated using the food composition tables (Nutritive Value of Indian Foods).[8]

Family Questionnaire Method

Same information can be collected by questioning the lady of the house, avoiding any weighment. It is not as accurate as the weighment since it is purely based on the information provided by housewife, whichcould be subjective. The remaining steps are same as in the weighment method.

Individual Label

Individual's dietary intake is assessed by 24 hours dietary recall. It involves assessing intakes of cooked food. The information is obtained by questioning the woman who actually cooks and distributes food. She is shown standardised cups, suited to the local conditions to help her assess the volumes of food cooked/consumed. A set of 12–14 cups of different volumes and spoons of different measurements are used. To start with, she is asked to list all the preparations (breakfast, lunch, midday, and supper) consumed on the previous day. For each meal, the total amounts of raw ingredients (TR) in each preparation for the total family are noted. The total cooked amount (volume/weight) of each preparation (TC) is assessed with the help of the standardised cups. The consumption of cooked quantities by the specific individual (IC) is assessed in terms of the cups. It is generally recommended to collect information for all the members of the family, as it helps in simultaneously verifying the accuracy of information. To help the respondent, it would be advantageous to fill the vessel used by the woman corresponding to the quantity of the total cooked quantity with water, and measure out the amounts consumed by each individual, so that any wrong assessment by the woman can be corrected on the spot. In the case of foods like butter milk or even milk, dilution factor should be noted. In the case of *rotis* or pancakes, edible portion of the total cooked as well as the individual cooked is assessed in terms of numbers. With respect to green leafy vegetables, it is preferable to standardise the weight of the bundles by collecting samples from different markets or weigh the raw quantities used for the family.

The individual intake in terms of raw foodstuffs is calculated as follows:

Individual intake (raw)

$$= \frac{\text{Total raw (TR) Volume (mL)}}{\text{Total cooked (TC) volume (mL)}} \times \text{Individual cooked intake (IC)}.$$

The nutritive value of each raw food consumed by individuals according to age is calculated using the food composition tables as described for the household weighment method.

It will be possible to improve the quality of the data; if in addition, information on the frequency of consumption of the foods (daily, alternate day, weekly, fortnightly, etc.) is also collected for the previous week/fortnight using a food frequency questionnaire. This would also help in assessing the consumption of foods that are not daily consumed like meat/chicken.

Duplicate Sample or Chemical Analysis

Generally, this method is adopted when the accurate nutrient consumption needs to be assessed like in research studies. In this method, the individual keeps aside in a separate plate the foods consumed equal to the amounts consumed. For example if 2 *roties* are consumed, 2 *roties* are kept separately in the plate. This is done for each and every preparation for the whole day. These are then mixed thoroughly in a laboratory andactual chemical analysis (estimation) of each nutrient is carried out. This, therefore, requires good laboratory support.

REFERENCES

1. Latham MC. Human nutrition in the developing world. Food and Nutrition Series. No.29, FAO,1997.
2. Jeliffe DB. The assessment of the nutritional status of the community (with special reference to field surveys in developing regions of the world) World Health Organization. 1966.
3. WHO child growth standards: methods and development: length/height-for-age, weight-for-age, weight-for-length, weight-for-height,bodymassindex-for-age. Geneva. WHO, 2006. Online: http://www.who.int/childgrowth/publications. Access. 06/07/2009.
4. International Obesity Task Force. Assessment of childhood and adolescent obesity. Am J ClinNutr. 1999;70:117S-75S.
5. Ramachandran P, Gopalan HS. Assessment of nutritional status in Indian Preschool children using WHO growth Standards, Ind J Med Res. 2011;134:47-53.
6. WHO Working Group. Use and interpretation of anthropometric indicatorsof nutritional status, Bulletin of the World Health Organization. 1986;64:929-41.
7. Bamji MS, Krishnaswamy K, Brahmam GNV. Textbook of Human Nutrition, 2nd Edition. Oxford & IBH Publishing House, New Delhi. 2003.
8. Gopalan C, Rama Sastri BV, Balasubramanian SC. (Revised and updated by Narasinga Rao BS, Deosthale YG. Pant KC). Nutritive Value of Indian Foods, Hyderabad, Revised Edition. Hyderabad: National Institute of Nutrition. 1995.

Chapter 14

Food Allergy

S Srinivas

INTRODUCTION

Adverse reactions to foods have been reported for the last 2000 years. Writings from ancient Rome indicate that Romans understood that food consumed safely by most people could provoke adverse reactions in others.

'Ádverse food reactions' is the umbrella term referring to any untoward reaction following ingestion of a food. These may include true *food allergies* (immune mediated reaction to food proteins) and food intolerance (non-immune-mediated reactions to food). True food allergy (FA) is an adverse immune response to food proteins.[1] Although 25–30% of the general population believe that they have a FA it may not be true. The incidence of FA in the United States confirmed by history and food challenges suggest a prevalence rate of 6% in children and 3.5% in adults.[2] FA is also being reported from developing countries though robust data is not available.[3]

The task faced by the pediatrician is to recognize the clinical features of food allergy and differentiate it from a wide spectrum of non immunologic adverse food reactions. This may be sometimes difficult in clinical practice since there is often a time delay between ingestion and symptoms and insufficient diagnostic tools. Further since there is no definite therapy except to avoid the food allergen this problem poses a great challenge to the parent and the pediatrician.

TERMINOLOGY AND DEFINITIONS

An adverse food reaction is an abnormal response to an ingested food, regardless of the pathophysiology. These may be divided into toxic and nontoxic adverse reactions. Toxic reactions (e.g. food poisoning) may occur in any individual if a sufficient dose of the toxin is ingested. Nontoxic reactions are more individual based and may be immune reactions (allergy/hypersensitivity) or nonimmune (intolerance) reactions (carbohydrate malabsorption).

The European Academy of Allergy and Clinical Immunology Task Force in 2001 proposed that all adverse reactions to foods should come under an "umbrella" term called ***food hypersensitivity*** which is defined as follows. *Hypersensitivity causes objectively reproducible symptoms or signs, initiated by exposure to a defined stimulus at a dose tolerated by normal subjects.*

This does not accommodate classical responses to infections, autoimmunity or toxic reactions. When immunological mechanisms are triggered by food proteins, the appropriate term to be used is ***food allergy***. When immunological mechanisms are not involved as in adverse reactions to substances other than food proteins, they proposed the term ***nonallergic hypersensitivity,*** e.g. hypersensitivity to aspirin, lactose intolerance, alcohol intolerance, pharmacological reactions like jitteriness to caffeine, migraine following ingestion of aged cheese containing tyramine.

INCIDENCE

About 6–8% of children younger than 3 years experience documented adverse reactions to foods. In adults, it is less than 3–4% though the perceived FA in adults may be as high as 25–30%. The peak incidence is seen around 1–2 years of age since most of FA is acquired at this age. The incidence falls progressively until late childhood and then remains stable. The reasons hypothesized for the increase in incidence in infants are the immature gut barrier, damage to the gut mucosa following diarrhea and early introduction of food by over enthusiastic parents.

IMMUNOLOGICAL BASIS OF FOOD ALLERGY

Food proteins are broken down into small peptides and aminoacids by digestive enzymes. In a normal situation, these food particles are prevented from entering the tissues by physiological and immunological barriers in the gut.

Table 14.1: Food allergies based on immunopathology

Immunopathology	Disorder	Typical age
I. IgE-mediated	Urticaria, angioedema	Children > adults
	Rhinoconjunctivitis/Asthma	Infant/child > adult
	Anaphylaxis	Any age
	Food dependent, exercise–induced anaphylaxis	Onset in late childhood/adulthood
	Oral allergy syndrome	Onset after pollen allergy established (adult > young child)
II. Mixed IgE and cell-mediated	Atopic disorders	Infant > child > adult
	Eosinophilic gastrointestinal disorders	Any age
III. Cell-mediated	Dietary protein–induced proctitis/proctocolitis	Infancy
	Food protein-induced enterocolitis syndrome	Infancy
	Celiac disease	Children and adults

However, sometimes small amounts of intact food proteins may be absorbed through the gastrointestinal tract and elicit an immunological response when presented to the T cells. This could either lead to stimulation of Th1 cells (non-IgE-mediated allergies) or Th2 cells (IgE-mediated allergies), depending upon a number of factors, such as the genetic make-up of the host, the characteristics of the food protein and the effect of the microenvironment. These lead to the development of food intolerance in most subjects, and the development of new allergies in some subjects. The Gell-Coombs' classification recognizes four distinct types of hypersensitivity reactions. While type I (IgE-mediated response) can manifest as urticaria, angioedema and anaphylaxis and type IV (T-cell mediated delayed hypersensitivity) can manifest as food protein enterocolitis and eczema, type II and III reactions for some reason are not known to play a role in food-related reactions (Table 14.1).

PATHOPHYSIOLOGY OF FOOD ALLERGY

Most of the food that is ingested does not cause any allergy because of "oral tolerance". Delivery of antigen to the small intestine: The dietary proteins undergo digestion by the enzymes in the saliva and gastric acid which reduces the immunogenicity. However, proteins with physiochemical features such as small molecular weight less than 70 kD, abundant source of the relevant antigen, glycosylation residues and resistance to heat/digestion may retain the allergenic potential when they reach the small intestine.

Gastrointestinal complex barrier: The gastrointestinal mucosal barrier uses both physiologic and immunologic barriers to prevent the penetration of foreign proteins. The physiologic barrier comprises of the intestinal epithelial cells (IEC), glycocalyx, intestinal microvillous membrane, tight junctions which block the penetration of antigens and the salivary amylases, gastric acid, pepsin, pancreatic and intestinal enzymes and epithelial lysozymes which break down the ingested antigens. The immunologic barriers comprise of antigen specific IgA and IgG which blocks and clears the penetration of ingested antigens.

Fate of food antigens that cross the barrier: The mature GALT, therefore, functions as a very complex integrated network of tissues and cells performing the daunting task of protection. Developmental immaturity of various components of the intestinal barrier and immune system reduces the efficacy of the complex barrier and plays a role in the high prevalence of FA seen in the first few years of life. About 2% of ingested food antigens are absorbed and transported throughout the body in an "immunologically" intact form or recognizable antigen even through the normal mature intestine. However, tolerance is the dominant response of GALT and is maintained by various antigen presenting cells (APC), such as IEC, dendritic cells and regulatory T cells. Commensal bowel flora and Langerhans cells in the oral mucosa also plays a role in oral tolerance. In young infants physiologic and immunologic barriers may allow increased penetration of food antigen and the GALT appears less capable of tolerance compared with the mature system and therefore food allergy or hypersensitivity occurs during this susceptible age.

IMMUNOPATHOGENESIS OF FOOD ALLERGIES

IgE-mediated Reactions

During a classic IgE mediated allergic response, food proteins (antigens) enter through the lung mucosa or gastrointestinal mucosa. Antigen-presenting cells engulf the antigen and present them to Th0 cells. In atopic individuals, the process stimulates th production of Th2 cells, which stimulate B cells to produce IgE-food specific antibodies to the protein encountered. IgE antibodies in plasma have a very short half-life but once bound to mast cells can remain in the tissues for months waiting to come into contact with the allergen. This is called sensitization.

On subsequent exposure to the allergen, the specific IgE antibodies recognize certain areas on the food protein called epitomes, which allows the protein to bind with the antibody, leading to degranulation of the mast cells and release of histamine and other mediators, which cause increased vascular dilation and permeability leading to inflammation. A few hours after the initial reaction, a more pronounced late phase reaction may be experienced mainly initiated by eosinophils; though other cells may also be involved.

In children the first exposure can be in utero or through breast milk. Subsequent exposure in the sensitized host can lead to an immediate hypersensitivity reaction in varying target organs. A breakdown in mucosal integrity caused by infection or inflammation can also cause sensitization due to increased permeability.

Non-IgE-mediated (T Cell-mediated) Reactions

Many research studies on the immunological basis of gastrointestinal non IgE-mediated allergies have clearly indicated the involvement of T-cells (mainly Th1) and cells such as eosinophils. T cells become sensitized at the initial exposure. On subsequent contact, the epitope combines with the sensitized T cells and releases their cytokines, which leads to chronic inflammation. In most cases, biopsies will be needed for a formal diagnosis. However diagnostic difficulties remain in non-IgE mediated food allergies (Table 14.2).

SYMPTOMS ASSOCIATED WITH FOOD HYPERSENSITIVITY

Symptoms most commonly associated with food hypersensitivity (FHS) can be systemic, gastrointestinal, skin or respiratory in nature. They may occur within minutes, hours or days of ingestion. They may be IgE-mediated, non-IgE mediated, or mixed reactions.

In non-IgE-mediated food allergy, though the symptoms tend to develop more slowly (over months), larger amounts of food are needed and anaphylactic reactions are not seen with non-allergic FHS.

CLINICAL PHENOTYPES/REACTIONS SEEN IN FOOD ALLERGY

Skin manifestations
- Acute urticaria and angioedema.
- Chronic urticaria and angioedema
- Atopic dermatitis
- Contact dermatitis
- Dermatitis herpetiformis

Respiratory manifestations
- Allergic rhinoconjunctivitis
- Asthma
- Heiner's syndrome

Food protein enteropathy as in celiac disease shall be covered separately and is beyond the purview of this chapter. Gastrointestinal manifestations in food allergy is presented in Table 14.3.

FOOD ALLERGY TO SPECIFIC FOODS

The common foods in infancy are cow's milk, egg, peanuts and soy. In younger children, the common food allergens are cow's milk, egg, peanuts, soy, wheat, tree nuts and shell fish. Food allergy (FA) in older children and adults is primarily caused by peanut, tree nuts, and seafood. Allergy to fruits and vegetables may be significant but usually not severe. Population-based studies in children

Table 14.2: Non-immunologic adverse food reactions which are not food allergies	
I. Toxic reactions	Shell fish: Saxitoxin Fish: Ciguatera poisoning Bacterial and fungal toxin: *C. botulinum*, ergot, aflatoxin Flavoring and preservatives: Sodium metabisulfite Dyes: Tartrazine Contaminants: Heavy metals, pesticides
II. Metabolic	Carbohydrate malabsorption (e.g. lactase deficiency, sucrose-isomaltase deficiency), Pancreatic insufficiency: Cystic fibrosis, Galactosemia Phenylketonuria
III. Pharmacologically active food component	Scombroid poisoning (fish: tuna, mackerel, sardines) tyramine (cheeses, pickled fish) Theobromine, caffeine
IV. Infections	Parasitic: *Giardia* Bacterial: *Salmonella* Viral: Hepatitis
V. Neurological	Auriculotemporal syndrome Gustatory rhinitis

Table 14.3: Clinical presentations of gastrointestinal allergies

Disorder	Charecteristics	Symptoms
Oral allergy syndrome	caused by sensitisation to aeroallergens (birch, ragweed or mugworth) which cross react with fruit, vegetable and nut proteins	Symptoms include mild itching, tingling and/or angioedema of the lips, tongue, mouth and throat
Gastrointestinal anaphylaxis		Quick onset of nausea/vomiting, abdominal pain/cramps, with or without diarrhea. Skin or respiratory symptoms are often present
Food protein-induced proctocolitis	Common in infancy. Usually caused by cow's or soy milk formula or these protein are passed by mother to infant through breast milk. An 80% resolve within 72 hr on extensively hydrolyzed formula and elemental aminoacid formula is rarely needed. Usually become tolerant by 1 yr	Specks of blood in stool, occasionally anemic. Hypoalbuminemia is rare
Allergic eosinophilic esophagitis	Infiltration of esophagus by eosinophils, basa zone hyperplasia, papillary elongation, absence of vasculitis and peripheral eosniphilia in some patients. Though prevalence of other allergic diseases is common; food allergy is usually non-IgE-mediated	Gastroesophageal reflux, vomiting and dysphagia—children typically complain of food sticking in the throat
Allergic eosinophilic gastroenteritis	May present in any age group, even infants. Often presents as pyloric stenosis with outlet obstruction. There is inflammation of stomach and intestines in response to milk, soy, egg, wheat and fish. Endoscopy and biopsy remain the gold standard. Resolutions of symptoms are seen within 6 weeks of removal of foods. Does respond to steroids as well	
Food protein-induced enterocolitis	Most commonly seen in infants under 3 months of age, but may be delayed in breastfed infants. The term "enterocolitis" implies both small and large bowel involvement	Protracted vomiting and diarrhea, often getting dehydrated—sometimes even hypotension

have documented cow's milk allergy at a prevalence rate of 2.5%, egg allergy in 1.5%, and peanut allergy in 1%.[4] FA is no longer a health problem confined to the West but also reported from Asia and depends on the culture and food habits. In Japan, the most common allergens causing FA were milk, egg, wheat, peanut and soy beans followed by sesame and buckwheat.[5] In Singapore, cow's milk and egg white are an important cause of anaphylaxis.[6] A report from Hyderabad has stated beans, mustard, cardamom and cashewnut as causative allergens in urticaria.[7]

COW'S MILK ALLERGY/COW'S MILK PROTEIN ALLERGY (CMA/CMPA)

CMPA is the most common food allergy in children with a documented prevalence of 0.3–3.5% in children less than 5 years of age and 1% in older children.[8] The incidence in breastfed infants is 0.5%. In India of 137 children with chronic diarrhea CMPA was seen in 6% and in children <2 years it was 13%.[9] CMPA can be IgE mediated or T cell mediated or both. The clinical manifestations that result from (IgE-mediated reactions) are systemic anaphylaxis, urticaria, angioedema, nausea, vomiting, diarrhea, abdominal pain, rhinoconjunctivitis, wheeze, and those

from (IgE and T cell mediated) are Heiner syndrome, atopic dermatitis, proctitis, enteropathy, proctocolitis, enterocolitis, eosinophilic esophagitis, and gastroenteritis. The other gastrointestinal manifestations are reflux like-vomiting, FTT in infants, constipation in older child-refractory to usual medications but responsive to milk withdrawal and abdominal pain in older children (2.2%).

High index of suspicion—based on medical history and physical examination and diagnosis based on a period of milk protein elimination resulting in cure of symptoms followed by a standardized positive oral challenge test.[14] Endoscopy with biopsies help in cases when there is often confusingly overlapping symptomatology with other conditions or in the setting of non-IgE-mediated milk protein allergy.

NATURAL HISTORY OF FOOD ALLERGY

Childhood food allergies are dynamic with spontaneous resolution of many but not all food allergies. Allergy to milk and egg usually resolves by third year of life whereas allergy to peanuts, seafood, and tree nuts are not lost over time and persist until adulthood.[4] Clinical reactivity is lost more quickly than the loss of food specific IgE measured by prick skin testing or RAST. Children who initially develop an allergy to a single agent, as, for example, IgE mediated, may subsequently develop other allergies. The process of outgrowing food allergies varies among individuals and with different foods. Children with food allergy need to be followed up at regular intervals with appropriate oral challenges to determine when they outgrow their food sensitivity. Strict avoidance may help in development of tolerance.

Diagnosis of Food Allergy Presenting with Gastrointestinal Manifestations

History

History is still the most important tool for the diagnosis of FA. The characteristics of food allergy are persistent symptoms occurring in relation to food involving two or more different organs and an allergic predisposition. Symptoms should follow contact with a food substance that is innocuous to most people. Immune mechanisms should be evident in the pathogenesis, other pathogenic mechanisms should be absent and lesions or functional abnormalities of the gut should be demonstrable.

Clinical scenarios which would raise suspicion of food allergy[12]

- ❏ Oral pruritus, vomiting, diarrhea immediately after ingestion of a particular food
- ❏ Mucus/blood in stools in an infant
- ❏ Malabsorption/failure to thrive
- ❏ Chronic vomiting/diarrhea/dysphagia
- ❏ Gastroesophageal reflux disease/chronic constipation recalcitrant to typical therapy
- ❏ Infantile colic not responding to behavioral intervention
- ❏ Gastrointestinal symptoms in a patient with atopy

Some descriptive case scenarios shall be elaborated further in this chapter.

Laboratory Tests[12]

Peripheral eosinophilia and elevated total IgE levels may be present in children with FA but are neither essential nor diagnostic when present. The tests which are included in the diagnostic panel are as follows:

- ❏ **Immunologic tests**: Specific IgE antibody to particular foods and RAST (Radio allegro sorbent test). These are used as indicators of sensitization and quantitative measurement is preferred. RAST has a high false positivity especially in young infants. Though measurement of specific IgG and IgG4 has been marketed it is not indicated in suspected or proven FA
- ❏ **Skin tests**: Skin prick tests (SPTs), Prick prick test, scratch test and Patch test: These skin tests evaluate

sensitization by re exposing the individual to a minute quantity of antigen. These tests though widely used are not universally accepted. Children with IgE mediated FA are likely to have positive results however false-negativity may be seen in children <3 years. Defined and standardized food antigens should be used for testing to avoid nonspecific reactions.

- ❏ **Adjunctive tests**: Endoscopy with biopsy, absorption studies and stool analysis (RBC, leukocytes, eosinophils) help in the diagnosis of the non-IgE-mediated, and mixed forms of FA and to differentiate it from other causes of esophagitis, enterocolitis, enteropathy and colitis.

A Practical and Simple Diagnostic Approach to Gastrointestinal Allergy

- ❏ If an IgE-mediated disorder is suspected, quantification of food specific IgE antibodies followed by an appropriate exclusion diet and blinded oral food challenge (OFC) are warranted. Selected prick tests may prove useful in older children.
- ❏ If a non-IgE-mediated GI hypersensitivity disorder is suspected laboratory and endoscopic studies (with or without OFC) are required for a diagnosis.

Management

Strict dietary elimination of the offending allergen is the only proven therapy. Growth of the child should be properly monitored.

Medical Position Paper by the Espghan on Diagnosis and Management of CMPA[14]

Breastfed infants: Mothers are encouraged to continue breastfeeding while avoiding all milk and milk products from their own diet.

Nonbreastfed infants: Extensively hydrolysed protein-based formula with proven efficacy in appropriate clinical trials. Amino acid based formula if children fail extensively hydrolysed formula. Soy protein formula if tolerated is an option for children more than 6 months of age.

Educating and instructing parents and children regarding reading of labels and introduction of a new food forms an important protocol of therapy. In children with documented FA, it is preferable to delay the introduction of one new solid food every 5–7 days. Drugs, such as H_1 and H_2 antihistamines and glucocorticoids modify symptoms to FA but overall have minimal efficacy or unacceptable side effects.

Knowledge of the natural history of FA helps in selecting the time of challenging or eliminating the specific allergen in the diet. The rule of 1,2,3 is a simple guideline where the least allergenic food is introduced at 6 months of age, cow's milk at 1 year, egg at 2 years, fish, nuts and peanuts at 3 years of age. New immune modulatory therapies, such as anti-IL-5 have shown promise in eosinophilic disorders. The emerging modalities are food allergen nonspecific and food allergen-specific therapies which are indicated in those with severe anaphylaxis and those who are unlikely to outgrow the allergy. Food allergen nonspecific therapy under evaluation includes monoclonal anti-IgE antibodies. The food allergen specific therapies include oral immunotherapy (OIT), sublingual immunotherapy (SLIT) and epicutaneous immunotherapy (EPIT) with native allergens and mutated recombinant proteins.

A recent review concluded that current management relies heavily on avoidance and emergency preparedness, and recent studies, guidelines, and resources provide insight into improving the safety and well-being of patients and their families. Incorporation of extensively heated (heat-denatured) forms of milk and egg into the diets of children who tolerate these foods, rather than strict avoidance, represents a significant shift in clinical approach. Recommendations about the prevention of food allergy and atopic disease through diet have changed radically, with rescinding of many recommendations about extensive and prolonged allergen avoidance. Numerous therapies have reached clinical trials, with some showing promise to dramatically alter treatment. Ongoing studies will elucidate improved prevention, diagnosis, and treatment (Table 14.4).[13]

Prevention of Food Allergy

Primary prevention: This strategy is to prevent the onset of IgE sensitization in high risk infants with a significant positive family history. Exclusive breastfeeding offers some protection against eczema and asthma but not food allergy when compared with cow's milk protein formulas. Wherever possible, exclusive breastfeeding should be encouraged till the age of 6 months. Complementary feeds with hydrolyzed infant formula may protect high risk infants when breast milk is not sufficient. There is little evidence to suggest that manipulation of the maternal diet during pregnancy and/or lactation has any protective effective on FA. Observational studies suggest that early complementary feeding of solids may increase the risk of allergic diseases but not FA. Dietary interventions, such as long chain polyunsaturated fatty acids, antioxidants, prebiotics, probiotics and vitamin supplementation have shown inconsistent results and not broadly recommended.

Secondary prevention: This step is necessary to interrupt the development of food allergy in IgE sensitized children and prevent progression of "atopy march".

Tertiary prevention: This important step is to reduce the expression of end organ allergic disease in children with food allergy by avoiding allergens and using medications.

DESCRIPTIVE CASE SCENARIOS IN FOOD ALLERGY

CASE SCENARIO 1

A two and a half month old boy was brought to the doctor with persistent diarrhea along with loss of weight and FTT.

Dietary history: Exclusively breastfed until twenty days of life but had inadequate weight gain. Supplemental normal formula was introduced and the child developed diarrhea the very next day, which resolved after stopping formula feeds. Normal formula was reintroduced after a gap of twenty days but he developed vomiting and diarrhea the same day with perianal excoriation. Lactose intolerance was suspected and lactose free soy milk based formula was introduced but the child continued to have diarrhea leading to dehydration. He was admitted and evaluated.

Complete blood count: Stool microscopy revealed 8–10 pus cells/HPF and 5–6 RBCs/HPF. Stool rotavirus Ag-negative. Serum IgE antibodies to cow's milk and soy milk tested high positive and a diagnosis of food protein- induced allergic enterocolitis was made. He was started on hypoallergenic elemental amino acid formula and he improved very well

Table 14.4: Cutaneous, respiratory and GI manifestations of food allergy

System	IgE-mediated acute/onset	Cell-mediated Chronic/delayed	Mixed Chronic/delayed
Cutaneous	Urticaria, angioedema, morbiliform rash, flushing	Contact dermatitis, dermatitis herpetiformis	
Respiratory	Acute rhinoconjuctivitis bronchospasm	Food-induced pulmonary hemosiderosis	Asthma
Gastrointestinal	Oral allergy syndrome GI anaphylaxis	Food protein-induced proctitis, enterocolitis, enteropathy syndrome	Eosinophilic esophagitis/ gastroenteritis

CASE SCENARIO 1 (CONTD....)

with complete resolution of diarrhea and excellent weight gain. He was subsequently put on a diet with strict exclusion of animal milk protein/ soy protein and remained well until one year of age. He underwent milk challenge at one year of age and seemed to tolerate it well from the standpoint of development of gastrointestinal manifestations but developed severe eczema and wheeze.

Discussion: This case illustrates IgE-mediated allergic enterocolitis to both cow's milk and soy milk. The reaction is usually immediate after ingestion of milk protein. Almost 30% of children with IgE-mediated cow's milk protein allergy may cross react with soy protein. IgE-mediated allergy is often associated with other allergies like skin and respiratory tract.

CASE SCENARIO 2

An eight-month-old girl was brought with a history of recurrent diarrhea and colitis.

Dietary history: Exclusively breastfed until five months of age and remained well. Rice powder based milk cereal introduced

CASE SCENARIO 2 (CONTD....)

at five months of age and she developed diarrhea, intermittently, from five and a half months of age. Supplemental formula introduced at six months of age and the diarrhea worsened with severe perianal excoriation. She was thought to have lactose intolerance and started on lactose free soy milk formula and did well. Biscuits were introduced at 7 months of age and she developed bloody diarrhea 10 days later.

LABS: CBC revealed a mild hypochromic microcytic anemia. Stool microscopy revealed 8–10 pus cells/ HPF and 5–6 RBCs/HPF. Serum total IgE was WNL and serum Ige antibodies to cow's milk and soy milk tested negative. Proctoscopy revealed multiple tiny aphthoid ulcers surrounded by normal looking mucosa and lymphonodular hyperplasia (Figs 14.1A to F). Histopathology revealed >20 eosinophils/HPF (Fig. 14.2).

A diagnosis of non-IgE-mediated cow's milk protein allergy was made and the child improved on dietary exclusion of milk protein. She could tolerate soy milk formula very well.

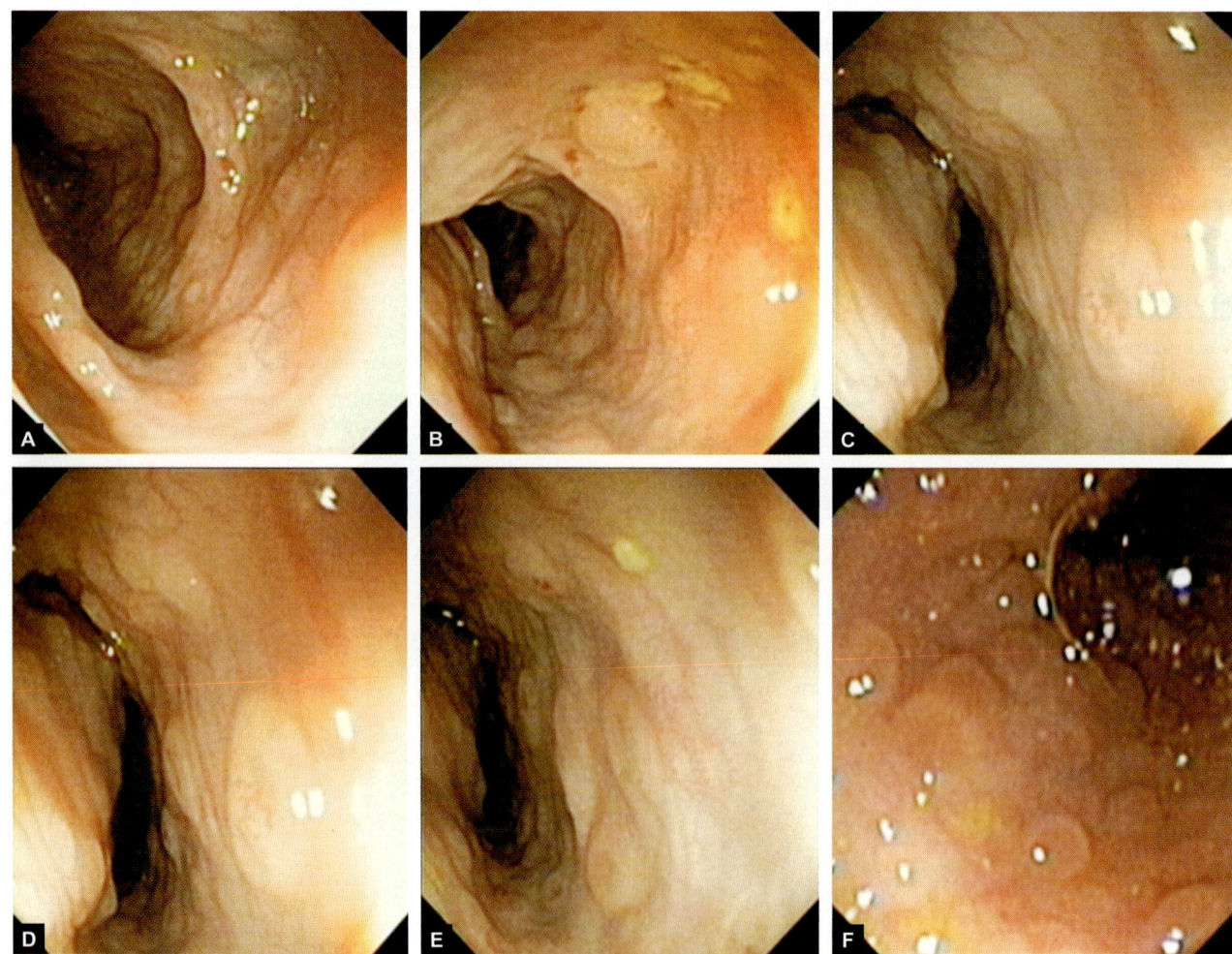

Figs 14.1A to F: Colonoscopy showing lymphonodular hyperplasia

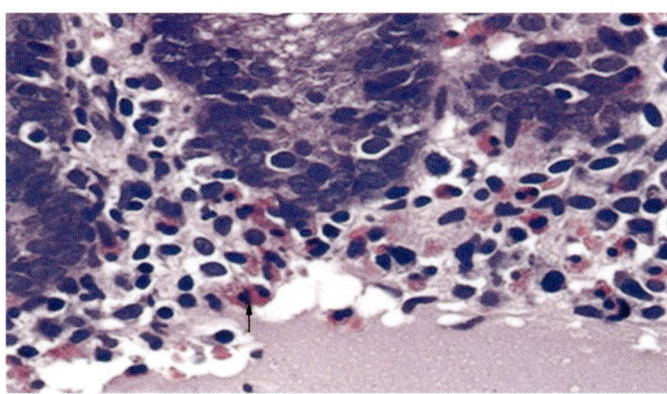

Fig. 14.2: HPE showing numerous eosinophils/HPF on rectal mucosal biopsy

CASE SCENARIO 2 (CONTD....)

Discussion: History is very important in suspecting food allergy. The elicitation of a temporal association between introduction of the milk protein and the reaction (which might be delayed as much as 15 days) and similarly exclusion of milk protein followed by resolution of symptoms should make us strongly suspect food allergy.

CASE SCENARIO 3

A two-months-old exclusively breastfed infant brought with a history of excessive cry, irritability and frequent passage of small specks of blood in stools. Abdominal ultrasound examination ruled out an intussusception. Stool microscopy and cultures were negative. IgE antibodies to cow's milk and soy milk protein tested negative.

Exclusion of cow's milk protein from the mother's diet resolved the symptoms.

Discussion: Milk protein allergy can occur in exclusively breast fed children through sensitization of animal milk protein introduced into the infant during breastfeeding.

CONCLUSION

Food allergy should be considered in children with reproducible signs and symptoms in relation to a specific food allergen. In many children the symptoms may be transient, mild and may be lost with age but in some, the reaction is severe and permanent. Elimination of the specific allergen without compromising the nutrition is the best therapeutic option. History is still an excellent tool in the IgE-mediated disorders. Endoscopy and histology are useful in a select group of children with FA and should be recommended. Recommendations about the prevention of food allergy and atopic disease through diet have changed radically, with rescinding of many recommendations about extensive and prolonged allergen avoidance.

REFERENCES

1. Johansson SG, Bieber T, Dahl R, Friedmann PS, Lanier BQ, Lockey RF, et al. Revised nomenclature for allergy for global use: Report of the Nomenclature Review Committee of the World Allergy Organization, October 2003. J Allergy Clin Immunol. 2004;113(5):832-6.
2. Sampson HA. Food allergies. Sleisenger and Fordtran's Gastrointestinal and liver disease.Pathophysiology/Diagnosis/Management. Feldman, Friedman and Brandt (Eds). Elsevier; 2010;1:139-48.
3. L van der Poel, J Chen, M Penagos. Food allergy epidemic-Is it only a western phenomenon? Current Allergy and Clinical Immunology. 2009;22:121-6.
4. Sampson HA, Leung DYM. Adverse reactions to foods. Nelson text book of Pediatrics.19 th edition. Elsevier. Kliegman, Stanton, St. Geme, Schor and Behrman (Eds). Philadelphia. 2011;pp:820-24.
5. Imamura T, Kanagawa Y, Ebisawa M. A survey of patients with self-reported severe food allergies in Japan. Pediatr Allergy Immunol. 2008; 19(3):270-4.
6. Khoo J, Shek L, Khor ES, Wang DY, Lee BW. Pattern of sensitization to common environmental allergens amongst atopic Singapore children in the first 3 years of life. Asian Pac J Allergy Immunol. 2001;19(4):225-9.
7. Priya V, Hari Sai, B Anuradha, VV Vijayalakshmi, Suman G Latha, KJR Murthy. Profile of food allergens in urticaria patients in Hyderabad. 2006;51:111-4.
8. Kattan JD, Cocco RR, Jarvinen KM. Milk and soy allergy. Pediatr Clin N Am. 2011;58:407-26.
9. Poddar U, Yachha SK, Krishnani N, Srivastava A. Cow's milk protein allergy: an entity for recognition in developing countries. J Gastroenterol Hepatol. 2010;25(1):178-82.
10. Brandtzaeg P. Current Understanding of Gastrointestinal Immunoregulation and its Relation to Food Allergy. Ann N Y acad Sci.2002;964:13-45.
11. Mansoor DK, Sharma HP. Clinical presentations of food allergy. Pediatr Clin N Am. 2011;58:315-26.
12. Sicherer SH. Clinical aspects of gastrointestinal food allergy in childhood. Pediatrics. 2003;111:1609-16.
13. Sicherer SH, Sampson HA. Food allergy: Epidemiology, pathogenesis, diagnosis, and treatment. J Allergy Clin Immunol. 2014;133(2):291-307.e5.
14. Koletzko S, et al. European Society of Pediatric Gastroenterology, Hepatology, and Nutrition. Diagnostic approach and management of cow's-milk protein allergy in infants and children: ESPGHAN GI Committee practical guidelines. J Pediatr Gastroenterol Nutr. 2012;55(2):221-9.

Chapter

15

Childhood Malnutrition

Md Iqbal Hossain, Tahmeed Ahmed

■ INTRODUCTION

Protein–energy malnutrition (PEM) remains one of the world's most serious health problems and the single biggest contributor to child morbidity and mortality. PEM is the syndrome that usually results from poor diets and/or illnesses (commonly infectious diseases) and leads to growth deficits observed particularly among under-5 years old children in the world's less developed countries.[1] It is often associated/complicated by micronutrient deficiencies. For detecting PEM status anthropometry is the widely used method. Three anthropometric indices are commonly used: weight-for-age (WA), height-for-age (HA) and weight-for-height (WH) (in the case of height, the recumbent length is generally used for children less than two years). A deficit (Z-score below –2) in any one of these indices reflects malnutrition and Z-score below –3 reflects a severe form of that index. In 2011, globally, more than 100 million under-5 children were underweight (WAZ-score <–2), 165 million were stunted (HAZ-score <–2) and 52 million were wasted (WHZ-score <–2).[2]

These 34 countries account for 90% of the global burden of malnutrition (Fig. 15.1).[3]

Malnutrition results in lower mental development or cognitive outcomes in children and reduced work productivity of adults. The social and economic costs of malnutrition burden to the individual, family and country are high. The etiology of childhood malnutrition is complex, involving interactions of multiple determinants that include biological, cultural and socioeconomic

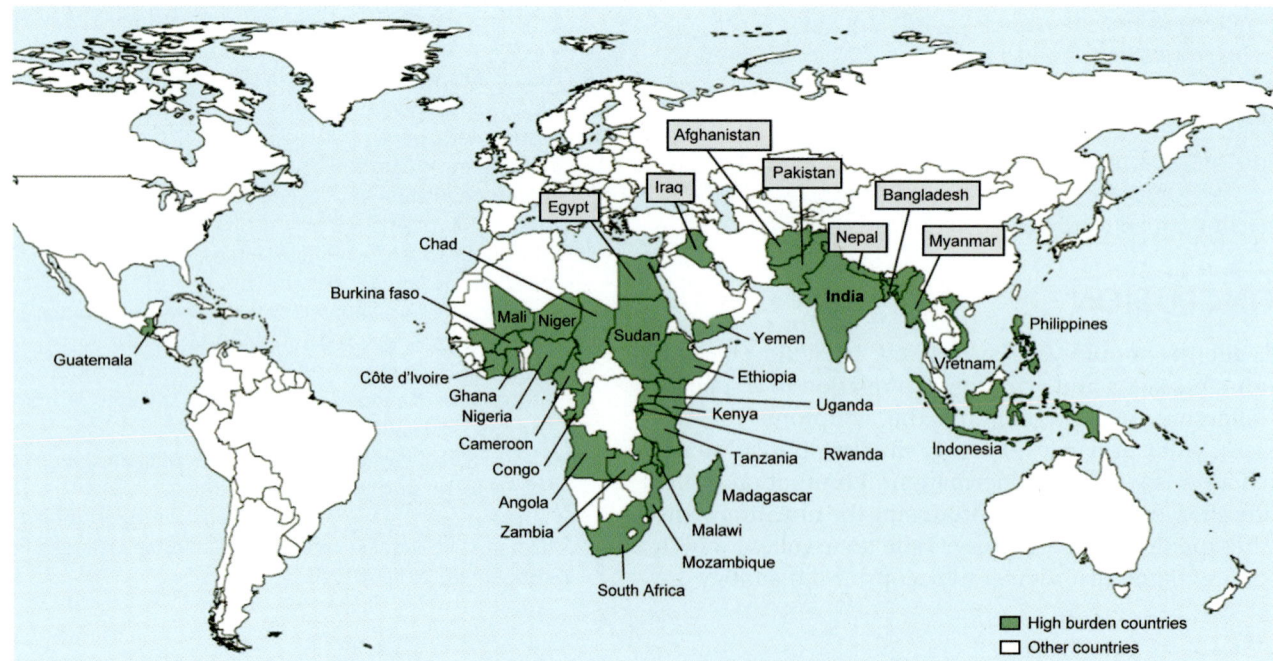

Fig. 15.1: Countries with the highest burden of malnutrition

influences. PEM and micronutrient deficiencies leading to early growth failure often can be traced to poor maternal nutritional and health care before and during pregnancy, resulting in intrauterine growth retardation and children born with low birth weight. The underlying causes of malnutrition vary across regions. In most Asian and African countries poverty, the low status of women, poor care during pregnancy, high rates of low birth weight, high population densities, unfavorable child caring practices, and poor access to health care are underlying causes of PEM.[4]

Children who are affected by moderate or severe PEM during the critical stage of life between conception and 24 months postnatal, if not provided with timely and quality care, will find it difficult to achieve their full potential. This period, known as the first 1000 days, has now attracted great attention for scaling up effective nutrition interventions. Scientific evidence has shown that beyond the age of 2–3 years, many effects of PEM are not readily amenable to treatment (for example, stunting) and can be irreversible. This means that to break the intergenerational transmission of poverty and undernutrition, children at risk must be reached during their first two years of life.

While children suffering from severe PEM need meticulous care, children with mild and moderate PEM are managed at the household and community levels. The major focus of management is on counseling of parents on health and nutrition education so that the diet of the child is improved, care during common illnesses, including diarrhea and/or respiratory tract infection, micronutrient supplementation, routine immunization, and 6 monthly deworming. A commonly used strategy in developing countries is growth monitoring and promotion (GMP) where under-5 children are weighed at regular intervals and a package of interventions provided at the contacts. Potential strengths of GMP are that it provides frequent contacts with health workers and a platform for child health interventions if it is sincerely carried out by respective health/nutrition workers. Food supplementation through large scale programs has been tried with limited success. Children with moderate acute malnutrition (wasting, WHZ between –2 and –3) should be given 25 kcal/kg per day on top of what is given to healthy peers, and their diet should contain animal source food.

Clinically there are three categories of severe PEM: marasmus or wasting, kwashiorkor or edematous malnutrition, and marasmic kwashiorkor (features of marasmus and kwashiorkor together). Functional definitions of PEM are now preferred. For example, severe acute malnutrition (SAM) is defined by severe wasting (i.e. weight for height Z score (WHZ) <–3 or mid-upper arm circumference (MUAC) <115 mm or the presence of nutritional edema. Until the end of the 20th century, the median under-5 case-fatality rate for SAM was 30% to 50%.[5] Nearly 20 million under-5 children are affected by SAM globally, and the vast majority is located in Asia and Africa. India alone is the home of more than 8 million children with SAM[6] whereas Africa has 5.6 million children with SAM. SAM has a >9-fold risk of death compared with well-nourished peers.[7] The United Nations has set the Millennium Development Goals (MDG) to be achieved by the year 2015. The fourth MDG is to reduce the mortality rate among under-5 children by two-thirds.[8] And to achieve it, the crucial component is proper management of SAM in regions where prevalence and incidence of SAM is high. The important reasons for the high death rates among SAM children are believed to be faulty case-management, considering management and control of severe acute malnutrition as a less important area, and faulty health systems. Appropriate feeding, micronutrient supplementation, broad-spectrum antibiotic therapy and judicious use of rehydration fluids (particularly intravenous fluids) are factors that can reduce death, morbidity and cost of treatment of these children.[9]

According to the World Health Organization, a death rate of >20% is unacceptable in the management of children suffering from SAM, 11–20% is poor, 5–10% is moderate, 1–4% is good, and <1% is excellent.[10] SAM in children can

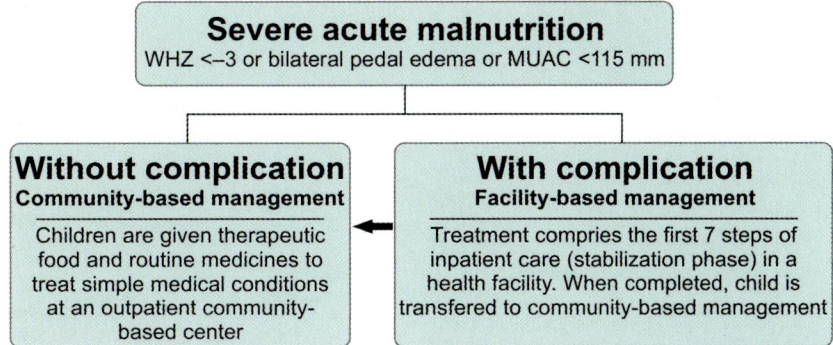

Fig. 15.2: Management of severe acute malnutrition with and without complications

be successfully treated by standard guidelines[9, 10] that have been shown to be feasible and sustainable even in small district hospitals with limited resources. Described below are guidelines in a structured approach to care taking into account the profound physiological changes that exist in SAM.

Management of Severe Acute Malnutrition: Combining Facility-based and Community-based Care

Facility-based inpatient care is essential when SAM children have medical complications. There is universal consensus that SAM without complications does not require inpatient treatment and can be effectively managed at the community level. But where there is no provision of community-based management of SAM, children should be managed in a facility (Fig. 15.2).

GUIDELINES FOR THE MANAGEMENT OF CHILDREN WITH SAM

The guidelines include:
- Assessment of SAM and admission criteria
- General principles for management (the '10 steps')
- Treatment of associated conditions and complications
- How to address failure to respond to treatment
- Guidelines for discharge before recovery is complete
  A child aged 6–59 months is classified as SAM if s/he has one or more of the following:
- Mid-upper arm circumference <115 mm
- Weight-for-height Z-score (WHZ) <–3
  (Annexure 1 and Annexure 2)
- Bilateral pedal edema (kwashiorkor and marasmic kwashiorkor are 'edematous malnutrition').
  Edema is usually seen in the feet and lower legs and arms. In severe cases it may also be seen in the upper limbs and face. To check for edema, grasp the foot so that it rests in your hand with your thumb on top of the foot. Press your thumb gently for ~ 3 seconds. The child has edema if a pit

(dent) remains in the foot when you lift your thumb. To be considered a sign of SAM, edema must appear in both feet. If the swelling is only in one foot, it may just be a sore or infected foot. Edema in all children is graded using the classification below and presented in Figure 15.3:
- Grade + (Mild): both feet/ankles
- Grade ++ (Moderate): both feet, plus lower legs, hands or lower arms
- Grade +++ (Severe): generalized edema including feet, legs, hands, arms and face.
  Till now there is lack of unified consensus regarding the classification of children aged <6 months as severely malnourished.[11] As long as newer information and agreement becomes available, a child aged <6 months should be classified as suffering from SAM if she/he has one or more of the followings:
- Visible wasting
- Weight-for-length Z-score <–3
- Bilateral pedal edema

Admission Criteria for Facility-based (Inpatient) or Community-based (Outpatient) Care

Children with one or more of the above criteria should be admitted to inpatient care, where only facility-based inpatient care is available. In areas where both facility-based and community-based cares are available: SAM children without medical complications should be treated through community-based care; but children with medical complications should be admitted in a facility for therapeutic care as inpatient until medical complications are controlled.

Evaluation of the SAM children: If the child with SAM is acutely ill and requires immediate treatment, details of the history and physical examination should be delayed. Laboratory tests are not essential for management. The following tests can be done if facilities are available:
- Blood glucose if the child is not alert
- Hemoglobin if the child is severely pale
- Urine for pus cells if urinary tract infection is suspected

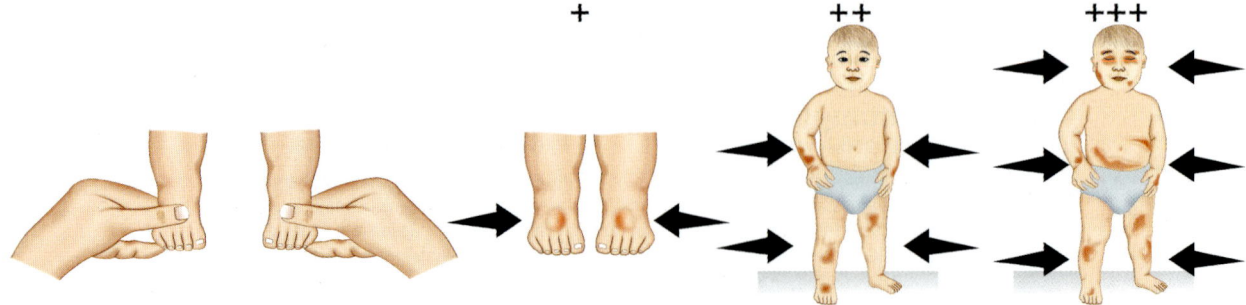

Fig. 15.3: Grading of edema in children

❑ X-ray chest if *severe* pneumonia, or if tuberculosis (TB) is suspected

❑ Mantoux test if TB is suspected (an induration of >5 mm indicates a positive test in a child with SAM), but in non-SAM child the cut-off of induration is >10 mm

❑ Serum electrolytes if the child is hypotonic, lethargic or irritable.

Reductive adaptation in SAM: Children with SAM undergo physiological and metabolic changes to conserve energy and preserve essential processes. This is known as reductive adaptation. If these changes are ignored during treatment, hypoglycemia, hypothermia, heart failure, untreated infection can cause death. Also due to this reductive adaptation high-energy diet and heavy fluid load are not tolerated by a child with SAM in the first few days (acute phase) of treatment. This can be illustrated further by the reasons for not giving iron during the initial acute phase treatment of SAM. The child with SAM makes less hemoglobin than usual. Giving iron early in treatment leads to 'free iron' that can cause free radical injury and promotes bacterial growth. Therefore, iron should not be given during the acute phase of management of SAM.

Phases of Management of SAM

The management of children with severe acute malnutrition can be divided into three phases:

Acute Phase

Problems that endanger life, such as hypoglycemia, hypothermia, water-electrolyte imbalance, and infection are identified and treated. Feeding and correction of micronutrient deficiencies are initiated during this phase. Broad-spectrum antibiotics are started. Small, frequent feeds are given with the objective to stabilize the child. Case fatality is highest during this phase especially within the first 1–2 days of admission. This phase, applicable for children with SAM and complications, usually takes about 3–7 days.

Nutritional Rehabilitation Phase

The aim of this phase is to recover lost weight by intensive feeding gradual increase of calorie and protein. The child is stimulated emotionally and physically, and the mother is trained to continue care at home. Micronutrients, including iron, are continued. Treatment remains incomplete without health and nutrition education of the mothers. This phase takes 2–4 weeks.

Follow-up

Follow-up is done to prevent relapse of SAM, and to ensure proper physical growth and mental development of the child. The likelihood of relapse into SAM is more within one month of discharge. Follow-up visits should be fortnightly initially and then monthly until the child has achieved WHZ >–1. Nutritional status and general condition are assessed and the caregivers counseled. Commonly occurring illnesses are treated and health and nutrition education for the caregivers reinforced.

These phases of management can be carried out through the following 10 steps of treatment:

Step 1: treat/prevent hypoglycemia: Hypoglycemia in SAM children is defined as a blood glucose level <3 mmol/L or 54 mg/dL. The child should be tested for hypoglycemia on admission or whenever lethargy, convulsions or hypothermia are present. If the child is conscious and hypoglycemia is diagnosed/suspected, give 50 mL bolus of 10% glucose/sucrose solution orally or by nasogastric (NG) tube. Then feed starter diet F-75 (see step 7). If the child is unconscious, lethargic or convulsing give IV sterile 10% glucose (5 mL/kg), followed by 50 mL of 10% glucose/sucrose by NG tube or orally (to prevent rebound hypoglycemia).

Step 2: Treat/prevent hypothermia: If the axillary temperature is <35°C (95°F) or the rectal temperature (preferable) is <35.5°C (95.5°F) start feeding right away (or start rehydration if needed). Re-warm the child by clothing (including head), covering with a warm blanket or placing the child on the mother's bare chest (skin to skin, Kangaroo care) and covering both of them. A heater or lamp may be placed nearby. During re-warming rectal temperature should be monitored frequently. Maintain room temperature between 25 to 30°C (77 to 86°F) if possible.

Step 3: Treat/prevent dehydration: The WHO-ORS (75 mmol sodium/L) contains comparatively high sodium and less potassium than needed for severely malnourished children. The SAM children should be given the special Rehydration Solution for Malnutrition (ReSoMal) (Tables 15.1 and 15.2).

Table 15.1: Recipe for ReSoMal from WHO-ORS*	
Ingredient	*Amount*
Water (boiled and cooled or safe-drinkable)	850 mL
WHO-ORS (75 mmol sodium/L)	1 (500 mL) sachet
Sugar	20 g
Electrolyte/mineral solution**	16.5 mL

*Note: If you have ORS with 3.5 g sodium chloride (previous WHO–ORS), with 500 mL sachet add 1 L of water, 25 g sugar and 20 ml electrolyte/mineral solution.
ReSoMal contains approximately Na <45 mmol/L, K 40 mmol, and Mg 3 mmol/L

Table 15.2: **Recipe for electrolyte/mineral solution

Ingredient	Amount in g	Molar content of 20 mL
Potassium chloride	224 g	24 mmol
Tri-potassium citrate	81 g	2 mmol
Magnesium chloride	76 g	3 mmol
Zinc acetate	8.2 g	300 µmol
Copper sulfate	1.4 g	45 µmol
Water up to	2500 mL	-

Note: Add selenium if available and if the small amounts can be measured locally (sodium selenate 0.028 g) and iodine (potassium iodide 0.012 g) per 2500 mL.

Preparation: Dissolve the ingredients in cooled boiled water. Store the solution in sterilized bottles in the refrigerator to retard deterioration. Make fresh each month and discard if it turns cloudy. If the preparation of this electrolyte/mineral solution is not possible and if premixed sachets are not available, give K, Mg and Zn separately.

It is difficult to estimate dehydration status in a severely malnourished child. Wasted/marasmic children are sometimes over-diagnosed and edematous (kwashiorkor) children may be under-diagnosed for dehydration. All children with watery diarrhea should be assumed to have dehydration and given:

❑ Every 30 minutes for first 2 hours, ReSoMal 5 mL/kg/wt orally/NG tube, then
❑ Alternate hours for up to 10 hours, ReSoMal 5–10 mL/kg/hr (the amount to be given should be determined by how much the child wants, and stool loss and vomiting). F-75 is given in alternate hours during this period until the child is rehydrated.

If the child has continuing diarrhea, offer ReSoMal (50–100 mL if aged <2 years, 100–200 mL if aged ≥2 years) between feeds to replace losses from stools. The amount given in this range should be based on the child's willingness to drink and the amount of ongoing losses in the stool.

If diarrhea is severe then WHO-ORS (75 mmol sodium/L) may be used because loss of sodium in stool is high, and symptomatic hyponatremia can occur with ReSoMal.[12] Severe diarrhea is usually defined as stool output >5 mL/kg/hr. Return of tears, moist mouth, eyes and fontanel appearing less sunken, and improved skin turgor, are signs that rehydration is proceeding. It should be noted that many SAM children would not show these changes even when fully rehydrated. Continuing rapid breathing and pulse during rehydration suggest coexisting infection or over hydration. Signs of excess fluid (over hydration) are increasing respiratory rate (>5/min) and pulse rate (>25/min), increasing edema and puffy eyelids.

If these signs occur, fluids are stopped immediately and the child reassessed after one hour. Intravenous rehydration should be used only in case of shock, infusing slowly to avoid overloading the heart.

Step 4: Correct electrolyte imbalance: All SAM children have excess body sodium even though serum sodium may be low. Deficiencies of potassium and magnesium are also present and may take at least two weeks to correct. Edema is partly due to these imbalances and must never be treated with a diuretic. Give extra potassium 4 mmol/kg/day for 5–7 days, 50% magnesium sulfate 0.1 mL/kg/day of for 3–5 days. Prepare food without salt.

Step 5: Treat/prevent infection: In children with SAM the usual signs of infection, such as fever, are often absent, and infections often hidden. Therefore give broad-spectrum antibiotics routinely on admission:

❑ If the child appears to have no complications give: oral amoxicillin 25 mg/kg 12-hourly for 5 days.
❑ If the child is sick looking or lethargic or has complications (hypoglycemia, hypothermia, skin lesions, respiratory tract or urinary tract infection) give:
  • Ampicillin 50 mg/kg IV/IM 6-hourly for 1 to 2 days, then oral amoxicillin 25 mg/kg 12-hourly for 5 days
  • Gentamicin 7.5 mg/kg IV/IM once daily for 7 days.
❑ If the child fails to improve clinically by 48 hours or deteriorates after 24 hours ceftriaxone 75–100 mg/kg/day IV once daily may be started with gentamicin. Ceftriaxone should also be given in case of septic shock or meningitis. Where specific infections are identified, add specific antibiotics as appropriate.

Table 15.3: Use of vitamins, electrolytes and minerals in different conditions

	CMV available	Combined electrolyte/mineral solution available	Neither combined electrolyte/ mineral solution nor CMV available
Vitamin A on day 1	–	√	√
Daily for at least 2 weeks			
Multivitamin	–	√	√
Folic acid 1 mg/d (give 5 mg on day 1)	√	√	√
Zinc 2 mg/kg/d	–	–	√
Potassium 4 mmol/kg/d for ~ 5 days	–	–	√
Injection magnesium sulfate (50%) 0.3 mL/ kg (total dose ≤2 mL) intramuscular single dose	–	–	√
Copper 0.3 mg/kg/d	–	–	√
Elemental iron 3 mg/kg/d when gaining weight during rehabilitation phase	√	√	√

Step 6: Correct micronutrient deficiencies: All severely malnourished children have vitamin and mineral deficiencies. Although anemia is common, do not give iron initially but wait until the child has a good appetite and starts gaining weight (usually by the second week). Give vitamin A orally on day 1 (for age >12 months, give 200,000 IU; for age 6–12 months, give 100,000 IU; for age 0–5 months, give 50,000 IU) unless there is definite evidence that a dose has been given in the last month.

Give daily the followings for the entire period of nutritional rehabilitation (at least 4 weeks):
❏ Multivitamin supplements
❏ Folic acid 1 mg/day (5 mg on day 1)
❏ Zinc 2 mg/kg/day
❏ Copper 0.3 mg/kg/day
❏ Iron 3 mg/kg/day but only when gaining weight (start after the stabilization phase is over).

A combined electrolyte/mineral/vitamin (CMV) mix for severe malnutrition is available commercially. This can replace the electrolyte/mineral solution and multivitamin supplements mentioned in steps 4 and 6, (i.e. no need for extrapotassium, magnesium, copper vitamin A, and multivitamin) but still give folic acid on day 1, and iron daily after weight gain has started (Table 15.3).

Step 7: Start cautious feeding: During the stabilization phase a cautious approach is required because of the child's fragile physiological state and reduced capacity to handle large feeds. Feeding should be started as soon as possible after admission. Starter formula, F-75, contains 75 kcal/100 mL and 0.9 g protein/100 mL (Annexure 1). It is best to feed the child with a cup and a saucer. Very weak children may be fed by spoon, dropper or syringe. Do not use a feeding bottle. Never leave the child alone to feed. Spend time with the child, hold the child, and encourage him to eat. Breastfeeding is encouraged between the feeds of F-75. A recommended schedule in which volume is gradually increased, and feeding frequency gradually decreased is given in Table 15.4.

Criteria for increasing volume/decreasing frequency of F-75 feeds: If vomiting, lots of diarrhea, or poor appetite, continue 2-hourly feeds. If the child is finishing most feeds with little or no vomiting and diarrhea decreasing, change to 3-hourly then 4-hourly.

If the child keeps vomiting, offer half the amount of feed twice as often. If the child is very weak, has mouth ulcers that prevent drinking or intake does not reach 80 kcal/kg/day despite frequent feeds, coaxing and re-offering, give the remaining feed by nasogastric (NG) tube. Do not plunge F-75 through the NG tube; let it drip in, or use gentle pressure. The NG tube can be removed when the child takes 80% of the day's amount orally or two consecutive feeds fully by mouth. Avoid withdrawal of NG tube at night hours or when staff coverage is less or there is lack of experienced staff who applies NG tube.

In case of SAM infants less than 6 months old, breast-feeding is continued and invariably needs technical help for re-lactation using breastfeeding supplementer. If there is no or insufficient breast milk feeding should be with F-75 (non-cereal based).

Table 15.4: Recommended schedule for brestfeeding

Days	Frequency	Volume/kg/feed	Volume/kg/24 hours
1–2	2-hourly	11 mL	130 mL
3–5	3-hourly	16 mL	130 mL
6+	4-hourly	22 mL	130 mL

Step 8: Achieve catch-up growth: During the nutritional rehabilitation phase feeding is gradually increased to achieve a rapid weight gain of >10 g gain/kg/day. The recommended milk-based F-100 contains 100 kcal and 2.9 g protein/100 mL (Annexure 1). Readiness to enter the rehabilitation phase is signaled by a return of appetite, finishes all F-75 feeds, in case of edematous child edema is reducing, and it usually takes about 5–7 days after admission. A gradual transition is recommended to avoid the risk of heart failure, which can occur if children suddenly consume huge amounts.

To change from starter to catch-up formula: Replace F-75 with the same amount of catch-up formula F-100 every 4 hours for 48 hours. During these 48 hours even the child is hungry do not increase the amount of F-100. *Until this period use the initial weight (without dehydration) to calculate the 4hourly ration of F-100.* After these 48 hours, increase each successive feed by 10 mL until some feed remains uneaten. The point when some remains unconsumed after most feeds is likely to occur when intakes reach about 30 mL/kg/feed. From now the child can feed freely on F-100 to an upper limit of 220 kcal/kg/day (equal to 220 mL/kg/day). *During these period consider the child's current (each day's) weight to calculate the acceptable range of the daily amount of feeds.* Gradual replacement of F-100 with the alternate low-cost food containing the equivalent amount of kilocalories, e.g. halwa, khichuri (recipes are given in Annexure 2 and Annexure 3) can be done provided they have comparable energy and protein concentrations.

Monitor the child carefully during transition: Every 6–8 hours check the child's respiratory and pulse rate. If F-100 is introduced carefully and gradually, problems are unlikely; however, increasing respiratory rate (>5/min) and pulse rate (>25/min) may signal heart failure. Call a physician for help.
If weight gain is:
❑ Poor (<5 g/kg/day), the child requires full reassessment for other underlying illnesses
❑ Moderate (5–10 g/kg/day); check whether intake targets are being met, or if infection has been overlooked
❑ Good (>10 g/kg/day), continue to praise staff and mothers.

Formula for calculating weight gain:

$$\text{Weight gain in g/kg/day} = \frac{(W2 - W1) * 1000}{(W1 * \text{number of days from W1 to W2})}$$

where W1 = initial or lowest weight in kg; W2 = weight in kg on the day of calculation

Step 9: Provide sensory stimulation and emotional support: In SAM there is delayed mental and behavioral development. Just giving diets will improve physical growth but mental development will remain impaired. This is improved by providing tender loving care and a cheerful, stimulating environment. The play sessions should make use of toys made of discarded material. Since psychosocial stimulation is an important aspect of rehabilitation, mothers are encouraged to engage the children in playing with toys and listening to songs meant for children. As physical activity promotes growth during rehabilitation, limbs of the immobile child are passively moved by the mother. Mobile children are encouraged to do activities like walking, rolling on the mat, kicking or tossing a ball, etc. To reduce the cost, the playing materials can be made by several discarded materials (with minor modification) those are safe for the children.

Step 10: Prepare for follow-up after recovery: Any in-patient stay in a severe malnutrition unit/ward/hospital should be as short as possible to avoid cross infection and defaulting. So discharge mothers and babies as soon as it is safe to do so. A child whose all infections and/or other medical complications/illnesses have been treated, and achieved WHZ ≥–2 SD (without edema) can be considered to have improved. At this point, the child is still likely to have a low weight-for-age because of stunting. Good feeding practices and sensory stimulation should be continued at home. Parents or caregivers should be counseled on:
❑ Feeding energy- and nutrient-dense foods
❑ Providing structured plays to the children
❑ To bring the child back for regular follow-up checks
❑ Ensure that booster immunizations are given
❑ Ensure that vitamin A (every six months) and antihelminthic drugs (every 3 months) are given.

Treatment of Complications/Associate Illnesses

Shock in SAM children: Shock may be due to severe dehydration or sepsis, which can coexist and difficult to distinguish from one another. Children with dehydration will respond to iv fluids while those with septic shock and no dehydration may or may not. The SAM child is considered to have shock if he/she:
❑ Is *lethargic or unconscious* and
❑ Has *cold hands*
plus either:
❑ *Slow capillary refill** (> 3 seconds) *or weak or fast pulse***
   *To check capillary refill: press the nail of the thumb or big toe for 2 seconds to produce blanching of the nail bed. Count the seconds from release until return of the pink color. If it takes longer than 3 seconds, capillary refill is slow.

**For a child 2 months up to 12 months of age, a fast pulse is ≥160/minute. For a child 12 months to 5 years of age, a fast pulse is ≥140/minute.

Emergency treatment of shock

- Oxygen inhalation
- Sterile 10% glucose (5 mL/kg) IV
- Infusion of an isotonic fluid at 20 mL/kg over 1 hour. The suitable isotonic fluid for SAM is Ringer's lactate solution with 5% glucose, if not available give 0.45% (i.e. half-normal) saline with 5% glucose (if possible add sterile potassium chloride 20 mmol/L). *If there is history of diarrhea then cholera saline with 5% glucose is the best choice for treatment of shock or severe dehydration.*
- Measure and record pulse and respiration rates every 15–30 minutes
- Give broad-spectrum antibiotics (step 5) if there are signs of improvement (pulse and respiration rates fall):
- Repeat infusion 20 mL/kg over 1 hour; then
- Switch to oral or nasogastric rehydration with ORS/ReSoMal, 5–10 mL/kg/h for 4–10 hours. Give feeding in every 2 hourly, i.e. in alternate hours.

If the child fails to improve (pulse and respiration rates fall) after the first hour of treatment with an infusion 20 ml/kg, assume that the child has septic shock. In this case:

- Give maintenance IV fluids (3 mL/kg/hour) while waiting for blood
- When blood is available transfuse fresh whole blood at 10 mL/kg *slowly* over 3 hours.

Very severe anemia in SAM children: A blood transfusion is required if:

- Hb is less than 4 g/dL or packed cell volume/hematocrit <12%
- Or if there is respiratory distress and Hb is below 6 g/dL. The child is given whole blood 10 mL/kg slowly over 3 hours and furosemide 1 mg/kg IV at the start of the transfusion. If the severely anemic child has signs of cardiac failure, transfuse packed cells (5–7 mL/kg) rather than whole blood. In all cases of anemia, oral iron (elemental iron 3 mg/kg/day) should be given for 2–3 months to replenish iron stores. This should not be started until the child has begun to gain weight.

Congestive heart failure: When heart failure is caused by fluid overload, *stop all IV fluids and be very cautious even in giving food.* Small amounts of 10% sugar water can be given orally if there is a concern about hypoglycemia. Give a furosemide (1 mg/kg). In rare cases, a single dose of digoxin, 5 micrograms/kg body weight, may be given.

Vitamin A deficiency: Children with vitamin A deficiency are likely to be photophobic and keep their eyes closed. It is important to examine the eyes very gently to prevent damage and rupture. If the child has night blindness or shows any eye signs of deficiency/xerophthalmia, give orally vitamin A on days 1, 2 and 14 (for age >12 months, give 200,000 IU; for age 6–12 months, give 100,000 IU; for age 0–5 months, give 50,000 IU). If there is corneal clouding or ulceration, give additional eye care to prevent extrusion of the lens:

- Instill 1% chloramphenicol eye drop or tetracycline eye ointment 2–3 hourly as for 7–10 days in the affected eye for 5–7 days
- Instill atropine eye drops (1%), 1 drop three times daily for 3-5 days
- Cover with eye pads soaked in saline solution and bandage for 5–7 days.

Dermatosis: Hypo or hyper with desquamation and/or weeping skin lesions (often ulceration) are commonly seen in and around the buttocks of children with SAM especially edematous malnutrition (kwashiorkor/marasmic kwashiorkor). Affected areas should be bathed in 1% potassium permanganate solution for 15 minutes daily. This dries the lesions, helps to prevent loss of serum, and inhibits infection.

Skin candidiasis and oral candidiasis/thrush: Fungal infection in skin, mouth and perianal region is not uncommon with SAM. Candidiasis should be treated with anti-fungal cream (e.g. clotrimazole) 2–3 times daily for 1–2 weeks. Oral candidiasis should be treated with oral nystatin (100,000 IU four times daily) for 5–7 days.

Continuing diarrhea and dysentery: Diarrhea is a common feature of malnutrition but it should subside within the first week of treatment. In the rehabilitation phase, loose, poorly formed stools are no cause for concern provided weight gain is satisfactory. **Mucosal damage** and **giardiasis** are common causes of continuing diarrhea. Treat giardiasis with metronidazole (7.5 mg/kg 8-hourly for 7 days). Treat invasive diarrhea/dysentery (e.g. shigellosis) with pivmecillinm 15 mg/kg/6 hourly for 5 days or ciprofloxacin 10 mg/kg/12 hourly for 3 days. Sometimes the diarrhea is due to lactose intolerance. Treatment with cereal containing F-75 (a low-lactose feed) usually cures the condition but may take time.

COMMUNITY-BASED MANAGEMENT OF SAM

A small proportion of cases usually can receive this facility-based treatment because active case finding in the community is rare or absent, many families cannot afford the economic and opportunity costs associated with facility-based inpatient care, and health facilities cannot reasonably handle such a high case load. If SAM is identified in the early stages when complications are absent, the technical aspects of treatment are very simple. Feeding therapeutic diets including F-75 and F-100 at home is not recommended because of the propensity of these liquid diets to become contaminated in the home environment. To overcome this problem, ready-to-use therapeutic food (RUTF) has been developed and used in field situations. It is now being used in emergency relief programs. If prepared as per prescription, RUTF has the nutrient composition of F-100 but is more energy dense and does not contain any water. Bacterial contamination, therefore, does not occur and the food is safe for use also in home conditions. The prototype RUTF is made of peanut paste, milk powder, vegetable oil, mineral and vitamin mix as per WHO recommendations. It is available, as a paste in a sachet, does not require any cooking and children can eat directly from the sachet. Local production of RUTF has commenced recently and several studies have concluded that local-RUTF is as good as the prototype RUTF. A supplementary feeding program providing food rations to children improved to moderate acute malnutrition (to prevent them from sloping back to SAM) and families of the affected child should be in place. So should be a stabilization centre for taking care of acutely ill severely malnourished children who need facility-based care based on WHO guidelines.

Therefore, to maximize coverage and access to management of SAM children, an approach with the following defined components is most appropriate:

- **Active case seeking in the community for SAM** practicing rapid screening technique such as mid-upper arm circumference (MUAC)
- **Management at the facility level** for SAM children who has illness/complication
- **Management at the community level** for SAM children having no illness or complication, and children discharged from facility-based inpatient care.

There are many advantages of a combined facility-based and community-based approach as follows:

- Active case-finding in the community helps to identify SAM children early, before medical complications occur. Thus , only 10–15 % of SAM children will require facility-based inpatient treatment. It also allow health facilities to focus resources on the specialized care of SAM children with complications. It benefit the uncomplicated SAM children by reducing exposure to hospital-acquired infections and also benefits families by reducing the time that caregivers spend away from home and other siblings, and by reducing opportunity costs. It also helps in maximum coverage and access for treatment and thus reduces default cases.

The development of the community-based approach for the management of severe acute malnutrition should provide a new impetus for putting this recommendation into practice. It is urgent, therefore, that this approach, along with preventive action, be added to the list of cost-effective interventions to reduce child mortality (Table 15.5).

MICRONUTRIENT DEFICIENCIES IN CHILDREN

Micronutrients are essential ingredients necessary for homeostasis and are affected by a variety of factors including maternal nutrition status, dietary intake, existing morbidity and body losses. Micronutrient (including vitamin and mineral) malnutrition remains common in developing countries. It affects any age group, but young children and women of reproductive age are the main victims. Not only severe, rather moderate deficiency

Table 15.5: A model for community-based management of severe acute malnutrition without complications, including locally produced ready-to-use therapeutic foods (RUTF). Until community-based care is in place, all children with SAM should be treated through facility-based care in a health facility

Independent additional criteria	• No appetite • Medical illness/complication	• Appetite present • Medical illness/complication
Intervention	Facility-based care • 24 hours medical care • Diet F-75 then gradually to • F-100 and/or similar • local diet	Community-based care • Child lives at home • Diet: RUTF • Weakly/fortnightly follow up at outpatient/ Community Clinic/ Primary Health and Nutrition Care Center
Transfer criteria from facility to community-based criteria	Reduced edema No complication Good appetite/appetite test passed (acceptable intake of RUTF)	Discharge when attaining ≥ – 2 WHZ or MUAC ≥125 mm in 6–59 months old children

Table 15.6: Prevalence of the three major micronutrient deficiencies by WHO region[14-16]

WHO region	Anaemia[a] (total population)		Insufficient iodine intake[b] (total population)		Vitamin A deficiency[c] (preschool children)	
	No. (millions)	% of total	N (millions)	% of total	N. millions	% of total
Africa	244	46	260	43	53	49
Americas	141	19	75	10	16	20
South-East Asia	779	57	624	40	127	69
Europe	84	10	436	57	No data available	
Eastern Mediterranean	184	45	229	54	16	22
Western Pacific	598	38	365	24	42	27
Total	2030	37	1989	35	254	42

[a]Based on the proportion of the population with hemoglobin concentrations below established cut-off levels.
[b]Based on the proportion of the population with urinary iodine <100 µg/L.
[c]Based on the proportion of the population with clinical eye signs and/or serum retinol ≤0.70 µmol/L.

can lead to serious adverse effects on various functions of the body. Globally, the four most common forms of micronutrient malnutrition are iron, vitamin A, iodine, and zinc deficiencies. According to the WHO World Health Report, almost one third of the world's population is affected by these four micronutrients deficiencies, and majority living in developing countries (Table 15.6). It is estimated that micronutrient deficiencies account for about 7.3% of the global burden of disease. Iron and vitamin A deficiency ranking among the 15 leading causes of the global disease burden.[13] Around 0.8 million deaths (1.5% of the total) can be attributed to iron deficiency each year as well as to vitamin A deficiency.

Of various micronutrient deficiencies of relevance to children, iron, vitamin A, zinc, and iodine deficiency represent the few for which there is considerable body of evidence for adverse outcomes and intervention strategies and mentioned here.

■ IRON DEFICIENCY

Iron is involved in various bodily functions, including the transport of oxygen in the blood, and brain development. Infants, toddlers, preschoolers and teenagers are at high risk of iron deficiency, mainly because their increased needs for iron. Iron deficiency is the most prevalent nutritional problem in the world. Out of 2 billion global anemia cases, 47% of under-5 children have anemia,[17] and iron deficiency alone accounts for 50%.[18] Among the two categories of iron present in food, heme iron present in meat, fish and poultry, and its absorption dose not hamper with others constituents of food. But the non-heme iron's absorption are reduced by bran, polyphenols), and phytate found in legumes and whole grains.

Main causes of iron deficiency in children: Prematurity and low birth weight, continuing exclusive breastfeeding beyond six months, low intake of meat or fish or poultry and high intake of cereals and legumes, gastrointestinal problem including celiac disease, persistent diarrhea, hookworm infestation.

Signs and symptoms of iron deficiency: Lethargy, loss of appetite, recurrent infections, educed cognitive performance, behavioral problems, breathlessness, and growth retardation.

Assessment of iron status: Anemia is the most common clinical condition with iron deficiency and can be detected by paleness in the palm, nail bed or palpebral conjunctiva. Hemoglobin, hematocrit, mean red cell volume, reticulocyte count are the common lab investigations to detect iron deficiency. Specific investigations are ferritin, transferrin saturation, soluble transferrin receptor, erythrocyte zinc protoporphyrin levels and bone marrow biopsy.[19-21]

Treatment in children: Oral elemental iron: 3 mg/kg/day for three months.

Prevention of iron deficiency: Following measures help in increasing iron level and prevent iron deficiency. Delaying cord clamping at birth, especially in preterm infants ensures adequate transplacental transfer of blood and iron supplies. In addition to exclusive breastfeeding for the first six months, supplementation of iron drop in preterm or low birth weight infants by 3–4 months of age is beneficial in maintaining iron level in the body. Before 12 months of age cow's milk should be avoided. Timely introduction of good quality complementary foods just after six months of age and promotion of iron and zinc containing foods (especially minced meat, liver, and poultry) are advised. Vitamin C helps the body to absorb more iron, so make sure the child has plenty of fruit and vegetables. In vegetarian populations, offer peas, broccoli, spinach, beans etc (these are good sources of non-heme iron). In populations at high risk of nutritional anemia use of sprinkles with microencapsulated iron also helps to prevent and treat anemia. Care must be taken when using iron supplements in malaria endemic areas because iron supplementation may increase morbidity and risk of hospitalization. Excessive intakes of tea and coffee often interferes iron absorption and should be avoided in children. Special attention should be given for prevention and treatment of infections, because infection is a frequent underlying cause of mild anemia in children. From more than one year of child's age 3–6 monthly administration of antihelminthic drug helps in prevention of iron and other nutrient deficiency.

VITAMIN A DEFICIENCY

Vitamin A is essential for immune system, light sensitive cells in the eye, integrity of epithelial tissues and mucous membrane, and the healthy growth and development of children. Vitamin A deficiency (VAD) is a public health problem in more than 50% of all countries, especially in low-income countries of Africa and South-East Asia, affecting young children and pregnant women. VAD is the leading cause of preventable blindness in children and increases the risk of disease and death from severe infections. An estimated 254 million preschool children are vitamin A deficient.[18] Low intake of dairy products, eggs, and fresh fruits and vegetables are the reasons for such deficiency. Xerophthalmia is the leading cause of preventable childhood blindness which is a consequence of long-term or severe vitamin A deficiency.[22]

Effect of vitamin A deficiency: Vitamin A deficiency leads to increased risk of blindness, and illness and death especially from measles and diarrhea. While severe ocular manifestations of vitamin A deficiency such as Bitot's spots, xerophthalmia and keratomalacia are fortunately decreasing, subclinical deficiency of vitamin A is relatively common in poor communities. The deficiency also causes squamous metaplasia of urinary tract and vaginal epithelium, and renal and vesical calculi. Its deficiency increases the severity of infection which, in turn, can reduce intake and accelerate body losses of vitamin A, thus it may result in needlessly high risk of death.

Treatment of vitamin a deficiency/xerophthalmia: Children with vitamin A deficiency are likely to be photophobic and keep their eyes closed. It is important to examine the eyes very gently to prevent damage and rupture. If the child has night blindness or shows any eye signs of deficiency/xerophthalmia, as mentioned before (in SAM management) give orally vitamin A on days 1, 2 and 14 (200,000 IU for age >12 months; 100,000 IU for age 6–12 months; and 50,000 IU for <6 month old children).

Management for subclinical deficient and prevention: Promoting breastfeeding is the best way to protect babies from VAD. Mangoes, pumpkin, carrot, sweet potatoes, and leafy vegetables are good sources of vitamin A. Food fortification is a cost effective measure for providing daily minimal needs for vitamin A. High-dose vitamin A supplementation within first seven days to the lactating mother helps in better supply of vitamin A to the baby through breast milk. Provision of vitamin A supplements every four to six months is an inexpensive, quick, and effective way to improve vitamin A status and save children's lives. It is estimated that this has the potential or reducing child mortality by 23% overall and by up to 50% for those with measles infection.

ZINC DEFICIENCY

Zinc is an essential micronutrient with a catalytic role in over a 100 specific metabolic enzymes, including perpetuation of genetic material, transcription of DNA, translation of RNA, and ultimately cellular division. Zinc is essential to perform functions, including healing of wounds, growth and repair of tissue, proper clotting of blood, correct thyroid function, metabolism of proteins, carbohydrates, fats and alcohol, fetal development, and sperm production. There are no conventional tissue reserves of zinc that can be released quickly in response to variations in dietary supply. Low intake of animal products, high phytate intake, malabsorption, persistent diarrhea and intestinal parasitic infestation the risk factors for zinc deficiency. Definitive data on prevalence of zinc deficiency are insufficient, but it is thought to be moderate to high in developing countries, especially in South Asia, most of sub-Saharan Africa, and the Western Pacific. About 20% of the world's population could be at risk of zinc deficiency.[23] Globally, zinc deficiency is responsible for approximately 16% of lower respiratory tract infections, 18% of malaria, 10% of diarrheal disease, and in total 1.4% (0.8 million) of deaths.[24]

Effect of zinc deficiency, management and dietary sources: Zinc deficiency in children results in increased risk of diarrhea, pneumonia, and malaria, as evidenced by many randomized placebo-controlled trials done in various populations in all regions of the world.[25] Severe deficiency results in anorexia, dermatitis, alopecia, retarded growth,

Annexure 1: Recipes for F-75 and F- 100

	Needs cooking	Does not need cooking	
	F-75	F-75	F-100
Whole milk powder* (g)	35	35	110
Rice powder (g)	35	–	–
Sugar (g)	70	100	50
Soya oil (g)	20	20	30
Mineral mix** (mL)	20	20	20
Water to make (mL)	1000	1000	1000
Energy (kcal/100 mL)	75	75	100

*Fresh cow's milk or dried skimmed milk may be used with altered proportion of ingredients
** CMV may be used (~3.2g or half of the supplied scoop). If not available, use separate micronutrients and vitamins

mental disturbance, delayed sexual maturation, and/or recurrent infections (impaired cell mediate immunity) and poor wound healing.[18] Plasma zinc <70 µg/dL generally reflects zinc deficiency in individual level. Treatment is oral elemental zinc 0.5 to 1 mg/kg/day. During each episode of diarrhea give 20 mg/day for 10–14 days (10 mg/day if age is <6 month). The major source of zinc intake is food e.g. meat, cheese, eggs, nuts, and legumes.

IODINE DEFICIENCY

Iodine is an essential component of thyroxine and triiodothyronine produced by the thyroid gland. These are required for normal neuronal migration and myelination of the brain during fetal and early postnatal life. Iodine deficiency has adverse effects on both pregnancy outcome and child development. Even deficiency in subclinical level during pregnancy impairs motor and mental development of the fetus and increases risk of miscarriage and fetal growth restriction.[5]It is the most wide spread, but easily avertable, cause of brain damage. Globally over 2.2 billion people are at risk for iodine deficiency, mostly in South Asia and sub-Saharan Africa. Current estimates suggest that 11 billion experience some degree of goiter.[26] Areas with a low level of iodine in soil and water and living in high-altitude regions far from the sea are the risk factors for iodine deficiency. Lack of iodine consumption results in increased risk of stillbirth, infant mortality, impaired cognitive function, hypothyroidism, goiter, etc.

Investigation: Low urinary iodine level, increased thyroid uptake of radioiodine (I^{131}), radionuclide thyroid scan, thyroid hormone assay, etc. help in diagnosing iodine deficiency disorder.

Treatment: Congenital hypothyroidism: oral thyroxine 10–15 µg/kg/day in neonate, 4 µg/kg/day in older children

Annexure 2: Composition and preparation of halwa

Ingredient	Amount	Energy (kcal)	Protein (g)
Rice or wheat flour (Atta)	200 g	682	24
Lentils (Mashur dal)	100 g	343	26
Oil (soya)	100 mL	900	–
Molasses (brown sugar or gur)	125 g	479	0.5
Water	600 mL (to make a thick paste)	–	–
Total weight of halwa	1,000 g	–	–
Total energy and protein per kg	–	2,404	50.5

100 g of cooked halwa contains 240 kcal and 5 g protein.
1 cup (130 g) of cooked halwa contains 312 kcal and 6.5 g protein.
The dal is soaked in water for 30 minutes and then crushed. Rice or wheat flour (atta) is fried on a hot pan for a few minutes. The atta, crushed dal and oil are mixed with water. Molasses (or sugar) is melted and added to the mixture to make a thick halwa

Annexure 3: Composition and preparation of *khichuri*

Ingredient	Amount	Energy (kcal)	Protein (g)
Rice	120 g	415	8
Lentils (mashur dal)	60 g	206	15.6
Oil (soya)	70 mL	630	-
Potato	100 g	97	1.6
Pumpkin	100 g	25	1.4
Leafy vegetable (shak)	80 g	22	2
Onion (2 medium size)	50 g	25	–
Spices*	50 g	22	1
Water	1,000 mL	–	–
Total weight of khichuri	1,000 g	–	–
Total energy and protein per kg	–	1,442	29.6

*Spices include ginger, garlic, turmeric and coriander powder.
100 g of cooked khichuri contains 145 kcal and 3 g protein.
1 cup (130 g) of cooked khichuri contains 190 kcal and 4 g protein.
Rice, dal, oil, spices and water are added to a pot and boiled. After about 20 minutes, the potatoes and pumpkin cut into pieces, and spices are added. Just 5 minutes before the rice is cooked, cleaned and chopped leafy vegetable is added. The pot is kept covered during cooking. Khichuri takes about 50 minutes to cook.

for endemic goiter of school age-children can be treated with Lugol's iodine 2 drops twice daily mixed with glass of water or milk, and thyroxine 950–100 µg/day.

Prevention and control: The most cost effective means to control iodine deficiency in populations is universal salt iodization. It has resulted in economic and social development in areas of iodine deficiency and declining iodine deficiency disorders globally.[27]

REFERENCES

1. WHO, 1995 (World Health Organization. Severe malnutrition: Report of a consultation to review current literature, 6-7 September 2004. Geneva, World Health Organization, 2005.

2. Black RE, Victora CG, Walker SP, and the Maternal and Child Nutrition Study Group. Maternal and child undernutrition and overweight in low-income and middle-income countries. Lancet 2013; published online June 6. http://dx.doi.org/10.1016/S0140-6736(13)60937-X.

3. Bhutta ZA, Das JK, Rizvi A, et al. The Lancet Nutrition Interventions Review Group, and the Maternal and Child Nutrition Study Group. Evidence-based interventions for improvement of maternal and child nutrition: what can be done and at what cost? Lancet2013; published online June 6. http://dx.doi.org/10.1016/S0140-6736(13)60996-4.

4. UNICEF. 2007 (web address: http://www.childinfo.org/areas/malnutrition/index.php

5. Uauy R, Desjeux J-F, Ahmed T, Hossain M, Brewster D, Forbes D, et al. Global Efforts to Address Severe Acute Malnutrition. Journal of Pediatric Gastroenterology and Nutrition. 2012;55(5):476-81.

6. Kapil U, Sachdev H. Management of Children with Severe Acute Malnutrition : A National Priority. Indian Pediatrics. 2010;47:651-3.

7. Black RE, Allen LH, Bhutta ZA, Caulfield LE, Onis Md, et al. Maternal and child undernutrition: global and regional exposures and health consequences. The Lancet. 2008;371(9608):243-60.

8. Millennium Development Goal. http://www.undp.org/content/undp/en/home/mdgoverview.html

9. Ahmed T, Ali M, Ullah M, Choudhury I, Haque E, Salam A, et al. Mortality in severely malnourished children with diarrhoea and use of a standardised management protocol. Lancet. 1999;353:1919-22.

10. WHO. Management of severe malnutrition: a Manual for physicians and other senior health workers. World Health Organization, Geneva; 1999.

11. WHO (2005). WHO, UNICEF and SCN Informal Consultation on Community-Based management of Severe Malnutrition in Children. Geneva, 21-23 November 2005. G World Health Organization, Geneva.

12. Alam NH, Hamandani JD, Dewan N, Fuchs GJ. Efficacy and safety of a modified oral rehydration solution (ReSoMaL) in the treatment of severely malnourished children with watery diarrhea Journal of Pediatrics. 2003;143:614-9.

13. World Health Organization: The World Health Report 2002 – Reducing Risks, Promoting Healthy Life. Geneva, World Health Organization, 2002.

14. World Health Organization: Iron Deficiency Anaemia: Assessment, Prevention and Control. A Guide for Programme Managers. Geneva, World Health Organization; 2001.

15. De Benoist B, Andersson M, Egli I, Takkouche B, Allen H. Iodine Status Worldwide. WHO Global Database on Iodine Deficiency. Geneva, World Health Organization; 2004.

16. World Health Organization, Nutrition Unit, UNICEF: Global Prevalence of Vitamin A Deficiency. Geneva, World Health Organization; 1995.

17. Black RE, Allen LH, Bhutta ZA, et al. Maternal and child under nutrition: global and regional exposures and health consequences. Lancet. 2008;371:243-60.

18. Allen L, Organization WH: Guidelines on Food Fortification with Micronutrients. World Health Organization; 2006.

19. Zimmermann MB, Hurrell RF. Nutritional iron deficiency. Lancet. 2007;370:511-20.

20. Zimmermann MB. Methods to assess iron and iodine status. Br J Nutr. 2008;99(suppl 3):S2-9.

21. Ramakrishnan U. Nutritional anemias. CRS Series in Modern Nutrition. Boca raton. CRC Press; 2001:260.

22. Sommer A: Vitamin A deficiency, child health, and survival. Nutrition. 1997;13:484-5.

23. Global Alliance for Improved Nutrition: Vitamin and Mineral Deficiencies. http://www.gainhealth.org/about-malnutrition/vit amin-and-minera l-def iciencies#footnoteref12_eIp9zl1 (accessed August 28, 2013).

24. World Health Organization: The World Health Report 2002 – Reducing Risks, Promoting Healthy Life. Geneva, World Health Organization; 2002.

25. Sazawal S, Black RE, Ramsan M, et al: Effect of zinc supplementation on mortality in children aged 1–48 months: a community-based randomised placebo-controlled trial. Lancet. 2007;369: 927-34.

26. Hetzel BS: The Prevention and Control of Iodine Deficiency Disorders. Nutrition Policy Discussion Paper No. 3. ACC/SCN, 1988.

27. World Health Organization, United Nations Children's Fund, International Council for the Control of Iodine Deficiency Disorders and Monitoring Their Elimination. A guide for Programme Managers. (WHO/NHD/01.1), 2nd edn. Geneva: World Health Organization; 2001.

Chapter

16

Pediatric Enteral Nutrition

INTRODUCTION

The purpose of this chapter is to educate the reader about the specific indications for providing enteral nutrition, the general principles governing selection of a specific enteral nutrition formulation, availability of devices and techniques to access the gastrointestinal tract, mode of administration of the enteral feed and potential complications. As this chapter is being written for a Textbook of Pediatric Gastroenterology, Hepatology and Nutrition, the focus will be on nutritional issues relevant to clinical settings involving the gastrointestinal, pancreatic and hepatobiliary system.

The American Society for Parenteral and Enteral Nutrition (ASPEN) has developed Enteral Nutrition Practice Recommendations which are intended to serve as a useful guide to practitioners of enteral nutrition all over the world.[1]

Definition: Enteral Nutrition (EN) is nutrition provided through the gastrointestinal tract via a tube, catheter or stoma that delivers nutrients distal to the oral cavity.[2]

AMERICAN SOCIETY OF PARENTERAL AND ENTERAL NUTRITION RECOMMENDATIONS

The strength of each Enteral Nutrition Practice Recommendation is based on the 2002 ASPEN (American Society of Parenteral and Enteral Nutrition) Guidelines for the use of parenteral and enteral nutrition in adult and pediatric patients, which are currently being applied for nutrition practices in most regions of the world.[3] The recommendations for the use of enteral nutrition, which are applicable to pediatric patients are as follows *(the letter in parenthesis at the end of each recommendation indicates the level of evidence).*

Practice Guidelines

Malnutrition and its Consequences

- Prevention and early detection of malnutrition in children throughout the developmental cycle should be integrated into all health care encounters. (B)
- Prevention and detection strategies should be adapted to the clinical setting and the needs of the pediatric patient. (C)
- A family centered approach should be used for prevention and early detection of malnutrition to address all the factors that may have an impact on the adequate delivery of nutrients to the child. (C)
- A nutrition screen, incorporating objective data such as height, weight, weight change, primary diagnosis and presence of comorbidities should be a component of the initial evaluation of all pediatric patients in ambulatory, hospital, home, or alternate site care settings. (C)
- The health care organization should determine the data elements to be included in the screening tool and who will perform the screen. (C)
- A procedure for periodic nutrition rescreening should be established. (C)
- A formal nutrition assessment should be carried out in any pediatric patient, independent of the care setting, who is identified by a nutrition screen as nutritionally at risk. (C)
- The nutrition assessment should be patient specific and include evaluation of the medical course, medication history, nutritional history, feeding skill level, analysis of typical and current diet, physical examination, anthropomorphic measurements, and laboratory data. (C)
- A written summary of the objective and subjective data collected for the nutrition assessment, of the explicit nutrition risk stratification, and of the specific recommendations to be incorporated into the

- nutrition care plan (protein, calorie, and micronutrient requirements, route of administration, and treatment goals and monitoring parameters) should be created and made available to the patient's care providers. (C)
- Nutrition goals should be developed as a part of the nutrition care plan. (C)
- The frequency of nutrition monitoring and re-assessment should be based on the patient's clinical course and upon an objective nutrition acuity rating. (C)
- Nutrition goals should include short-term and long-term objectives. (C)
- A plan for monitoring the effect of nutrition interventions should be stated in the nutrition care plan. (C)
- Specialized nutrition support (SNS) should be used in patients who cannot meet their nutrient requirements by oral intake. (B)
- When SNS is required, EN should generally be used in preference to PN. (B)
- When SNS is indicated, PN should be used when the gastrointestinal tract is not functional or cannot be accessed and in patients who cannot be adequately nourished by oral diets or EN. (B)
- Energy needs in infants and children should be estimated using standard formulas or nomograms and then adjusted according to the clinical course of the child. (B)
- Energy requirements should be adjusted depending on the route of SNS administration. (B)
- Energy needs for patients undergoing surgical procedures should be based on indirect calorimetry or adjusted down from standard formulas to avoid overfeeding. (B)
- Fluid needs vary with the age and weight of the child and should be adjusted accordingly. (B)
- Water and electrolyte requirements should be adjusted in pediatric patients undergoing surgical procedures or who have on-going losses from stomas or other sites. (B)
- Protein requirements should be adjusted according to the age of the child. (B)
- Histidine is a conditionally essential amino acid for neonates and infants up to 6 months of age and should be specifically supplemented. (B)
- Carbohydrates should comprise 40% to 50% of the caloric intake in infants and children. (C)
- Small amounts of carbohydrates should be used in infants and children who are not otherwise receiving nutrition support to suppress protein catabolism. (B)
- In infants who are lactose tolerant, lactose should be the predominate enteral carbohydrate administered in the first 3 years of life. (B)

- Preterm infants should receive a formula that has a 50/50 mixture of lactose and glucose polymers. (B)
- For the neonate, carbohydrate delivery in PN should begin at approximately 6 to 8 mg/kg per minute of dextrose and be advanced, as tolerated to a goal of 10 to 14 mg/kg per minute. (B)
- Carbohydrate administration should be closely monitored and adjusted in the postoperative period in neonates and children to avoid hyperglycemia. (B)
- Full term infants up to 1 year of age should be allowed an unrestricted fat intake. (A)
- Children between 1 and 2 years of age should have very limited or no restrictions on fat intake (B)
- Between age 2 and 5 to 6 years, children should transition from a high-fat diet to a fat-modified (moderate fat) diet (less than 30% of total energy from fats and less than 10% from saturated fats). (B)
- Vitamins and trace elements should be components of all PN solutions and enteral formulas. (A)
- Decisions regarding access for EN should be made considering the effectiveness of gastric emptying, gastrointestinal anatomy, and aspiration risk. (B)
- Nasoenteric tube placement should initially be attempted using a spontaneous or other bedside placement technique; if this is unsuccessful, fluoroscopic or endoscopic guidance should be used. (A)
- Radiographic confirmation of the feeding tube tip position should be obtained after placement of a nasogastric or nasoenteric access tube. (B)
- Gastric residuals should be checked frequently when feedings are initiated and feedings should be held if residual volumes exceed 200 mL on two successive assessments. (A)
- Feeding tubes should routinely be flushed with 20 to 30 mL of warm water every 4 hours during continuous feedings and before and after intermittent feedings and medication administration. (A)
- Standardized protocols for enteral nutrition ordering, administration, and monitoring should be utilized. (B)

GENERAL PRINCIPLES OF PEDIATRIC ENTERAL NUTRITION

Enteral nutrition (EN) has distinct advantages over parenteral nutrition (PN) from the standpoint of preservation of gut function, ease of administration, safety and overall cost.[4,5] Enteral nutrition mimics the normal gastrointestinal response following ingestion of a meal, with the exception of the oral phase. Intestinal structural and functional changes occur through interaction between nutrients and neuroendocrine peptides, cytokines and hormones.[6-8] The maintenance of gut mucosal mass,

Table 16.1: Indications for pediatric enteral nutrition

Inability to ingest adequate nutrition orally
- Disorders of sucking and swallowing
  - Permaturity
  - Neurological and neuromuscular disorders (e.g. cerebral palsy, dysphagia)
- Congenital abnormalities of the upper gastrointestinal tract of airways
  - Tracheoesophageal fistula
- Tumors
  - Oral cancer
  - Head and neck cancer
- Truma
- Critical illness
  - Mechanical ventilation
- Severe gastroesophageal reflux
- Drug related
  - Chenotheraphy
- Severe food aversion
- Severe depression

Disorders of digestion or absorption
- Cystic fibrosis
- Short-bowel syndrome
- Inflammatory bowel disease
- Congenital abnormalities of the gastrointestinal tract
  - Microvillus inclusion disease
  - Tufting enteropathy
- Enteritis
- Intractable diarrhea of infancy
- Autoimmune enteropathy
- Immunodeficiency
  - AIDS
  - Severe combind immunodeficiency
- Postgastrointestinal surgery
- Graft-versus-host disease
- Solid organ transplantation
- Interstinal fistulae
- Chronic liver disease
  - Biliary atresia
  - Alagille's syndrome

Disorders of gastrointestinal motility
- Chronic pseudo-obstruction
- Ileocolonic Hirschsprung's diseease

Increased nutritional requirements
- Cystic fibrosis
- Chronic renal disease
- Congenital heart disease
- Chronic pulmonary disease
  - Bronchopulomonary dysplasia
- Burn injury

Psychiatric and behavioral disorders that interfere with oral intake
- Anorexia nervosa
- Severe behavioral disorders
  - Autism

Contd...

Contd...

Metabolic diseases
- Inborn errors of metabolism
- Diabetes mellitus

Acute or acute/chronic pancreatitis

Administration of disease treatment
- Ketogenic diet in epilepsy
- Administration of pharmaceutical agents
- Bowel washouts in severe chronic constipation

which includes the gut-associated lymphoid tissue (GALT) is assisted by enteral nutrients. There is a reduction in gut mucosal mass and suppression of GALT function during periods of "bowel rest" as, for example, during prolonged starvation.[9] This, in turn, decreases the production of secretory IgA in the gut and increases gut permeability resulting in bacterial translocation.[10,11]

INDICATIONS FOR ENTERAL NUTRITION

Enteral nutrition must be considered in any child with a functioning gastrointestinal tract who is not able to meet his or her energy and nutrient requirements solely through the oral route. Enteral feeding may be necessary in children with growth failure, growth faltering or deficit in weight. This may be defined as weight for height less than the 5th percentile below the mean for sex and age or body mass index for age (BMI for age) less than minus 2 standard deviations (SD).[12] Table 16.1 broadly lists the indications for pediatric enteral nutrition.[13]

PEDIATRIC ENTERAL NUTRITION FORMULATIONS

At a stage when enteral nutrition support was still evolving, blenderized feeds were used as a source of enteral nutrition. Over the years, it was observed that this approach led to nutritional imbalance, feed intolerance and tube blockage, and was largely replaced with ready-to-use commercially available enteral formulations. Based on these observations, current recommendations support use of commercial enteral nutrition formulations all over the world, including developing nations in the South-East Asian region.[14] Currently, there is a wide range and availability of commercial ready-to-use enteral nutrition formulations for use in infants and children and most of these are isocaloric complete balanced nutritional formulations and provide complete macro- and micronutrient requirements as the only source of nutrient intake. Preterm infant, full term infant and pediatric enteral nutrition formulations have been specifically designed based on age and stage of development of the infant and child. A modular feed consists of a specialized combination of nutrients for providing a nutritional supplement or addressing a specific nutrient requirement.

In recent years, with the recognition that the approach to enteral nutritional intervention requires to be tailored to meet the energy and nutrient requirements in specific clinical settings, disease-specific enteral nutrition formulations have been designed and are now widely available, such as formulations for hepatic, renal and diabetic patients. Immune-enhancing formulations for use in the critically ill setting are available.[15-17]

Enteral nutrition formulations for delivery into the gastrointestinal tract may be polymeric, oligomeric or monomeric.

Polymeric formulations: Most patients with a normally functioning gastrointestinal tract will tolerate gastric administration of a polymeric formula containing intact protein derived from cow's milk or soybean. The non-nitrogen to nitrogen energy ratio in these formulations is approximately 150 to 1. The source of carbohydrate is starch. Maltodextrin, corn syrup and hydrolyzed corn starch are common ingredients. The lactose content in these formulations is variable. The fat source is polyunsaturated fatty acids (PUFA) derived from sunflower, safflower or soybean oil or from animal fat. In polymeric formulations used in patients with malabsorption, the fat source is predominantly medium-chained triglycerides (MCT). Some formulations contain soluble fiber as an additive—the main advantage being normalization of intestinal transit. But, addition of soluble fiber also has another important advantage—it is a source of energy. Approximately 20% of normal digestive activity occurs in the proximal colon and soluble fiber gets converted to short-chained fatty acids (SCFA) in the proximal colon, which provide an important and useful source of energy. Most polymeric formulations are isocaloric (provide 1 kcal/mL on reconstitution).

Oligomeric formulations: In patients with underlying gastrointestinal disease or significant malabsorption, oligomeric formulations are preferred. The protein in these formulations is available as hydrolyzed protein either in the form of peptides or a combination of peptides and aminoacids. Most oligomeric formulations are lactose-free.

Medium-chained triglycerides are the major source of fat in these formulations. An important clinical indications for administering oligomeric formulations is for nasojejunal feeding in patients with severe acute pancreatitis.

Monomeric (elemental) formulations: Elemental formulations contain completely digested macronutrients (the basic building blocks)—glucose is the source of carbohydrate; amino acids are the source of protein

and medium-chained triglycerides are the source of fat. Monomeric formulations are both lactose and gluten-free. Protein from these formulations has very high biological value—this is evident from the essential to non-essential amino acid ratio. Important clinical indications for using monomeric formulations are intestinal failure and short bowel syndrome.

Disease-specific enteral formulations: The most widely used formulations in this category are formulations for patients with hepatic disease, renal disease and diabetes mellitus. These formulations are designed to have a preponderance of a specific nutrient or nutrients which are indicated and have been documented to be of possible benefit in these specific clinical settings. Formulations for hepatic patients are enriched with branched-chained amino acids (BCAA) and medium-chained triglycerides (MCT). The advantage of using MCT as a source of fat in these patients is ready availability due to bypassing the carnitine pathway. BCAA stimulate hepatic protein synthesis and contribute to decreased ammonia production and there is clear evidence that they are useful in encephalopathy in chronic liver disease.[18] The BCAA content in these formulations is 40–45%. Enteral formulations for patients with renal disease are of two types—formulations for patients with chronic renal disease who are not being dialyzed (predialysis) and those for patients undergoing regular dialysis (post-dialysis). The major difference between these two types of formulations is the protein content—the later containing almost twice the protein content of the former, the rationale being that dialysis removes the toxic metabolites and in patients undergoing regular dialysis, the protein supplementation can be liberal (even up to 1.2 times the normal requirement). Enteral formulations for patients with diabetes mellitus are rich in monounsaturated fatty acids (MUFA). The sensitivity of the cells of the body to the effects of insulin is increased by MUFA.

Immune-enhancing enteral formulations: These formulations contain either one or a combination of three major immunonutrients—glutamine, arginine and n-3 fatty acids. Over the years, the important role and potential benefit of glutamine as an immunomodulator has been very well established, especially from the standpoint of its effect in critically ill children on reduction in time taken to wean the patient off the ventilator and in patients with multi-organ failure. Glutamine has also been demonstrated to prevent intestinal mucosal injury resulting from chemotherapy and radiation therapy in patients with cancer. In pediatric patients, however, unlike adults where the potential benefit of glutamine and other immunonutrients in immune-enhancing formulations has clearly been established, the evidence is not very convincing and the issue remains controversial.[19,20] The source of n-3 fatty acids in most immune-enhancing formulations is fish oil, but an algal source has also been recognized and is a contributor to some formulations.

Formulations for Infants and Young Children with Cow's Milk Protein Allergy

Cow's milk protein allergy (CMPA) is an entity characterized by allergy to both the fractions of protein present in cow's milk, namely, casein and whey protein. Any formulation that is designed specifically for this condition must be hypoallergenic and devoid of both casein and whey protein. The term CMPA is a misnomer and is also used to describe allergy to buffalo milk as well as all enteral formulations containing milk protein of animal origin. The ideal formulation for CMPA is an extensively hydrolyzed formulation which, unfortunately are not readily available in some regions of the world such as South Asia. Partially hydrolyzed peptide-based as well as soy milk-based formulations have also been used in CMPA but they are less hypoallergenic as compared to extensively hydrolyzed formulations. Furthermore, approximately 15–20% infants with CMPA receiving soy milk based formulations continue to be symptomatic. Flow chart 16.1 depicts a very practical approach to decide on the type of enteral feed to be administered.

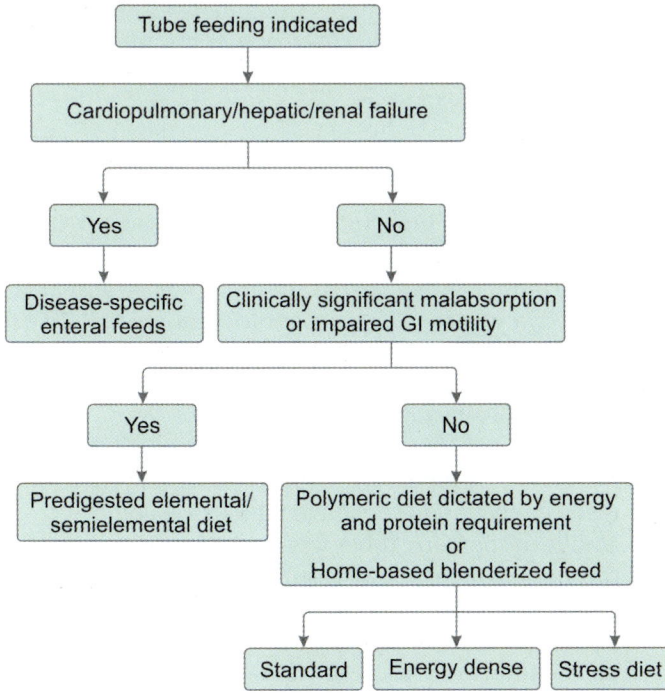

Flow chart 16.1: Practical approach to choice of diet in critically ill

Table 16.2: Protocol for continous tube feeding	
Term infants	1–20 mL/h
Children (1–10 years)	10–30 mL/h
Adolescents	25–30 mL/h

Table 16.3: Increase volume two hourly	
Lower limit in each category	
Term infants	1 mL/h
Children (1–10 years)	10 mL/h
Adolescents	25 mL/h

The administration of the enteral feed requires a practical approach, which is tailored to the needs of the pediatric patient in the specific clinical setting but as a general rule, the feed is advanced gradually, beginning with the lower limit in each category. The volume of the feed is increased first and then the concentration. Tables 16.2 and 16.3 depict the volume of feed with which feeding is initiated at different ages.

ENTERAL NUTRITION DELIVERY— ACCESS TECHNIQUES AND DEVICES

Patients with an intact and functional gastrointestinal tract who are unable to maintain adequate oral energy intake and require either short-term (less than 4 weeks) or long-term (more than 4 weeks) enteral feeding. The following are the indications for enteral feeding tube placement:[21]

- Impaired swallowing owing to neurological conditions or traumatic injury.
- Obstruction of the gut lumen caused by strictures or malignant lesions of the gastrointestinal tract.
- Clinical settings associated with increased energy and protein catabolism such as burns, inflammatory bowel disease and cystic fibrosis.
- Postpyloric feeding is practiced when obstruction or motility disorders prevent gastric feeding.
- For gastric decompression due to inoperable intestinal obstruction or gastroparesis.
- For ensuring hydration and timely administration of medication.

Enteral access techniques can be divided, from a practical standpoint, into two broad categories—invasive and non-invasive. The non-invasive techniques of enteral access consist of nasogastric, nasoduodenal (postpyloric) and nasojejunal feeding-nasogastric tubes can be placed directly, nasoduodenal and nasojejunal tubes can be placed either endoscopically or fluoroscopically. The invasive techniques of accessing the gastrointestinal tract

Flow chart 16.2: Enteral feeding tube decision tree

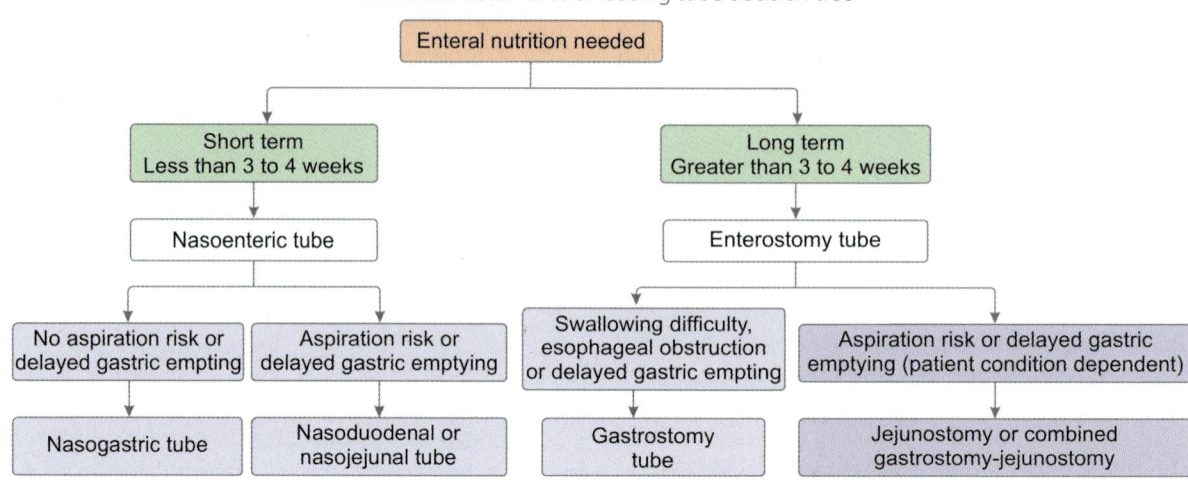

(*Source:* Guenter P, Silkroski M. Enteral Feeding Access Devices. Tube Feeding Practical Guidelines and Nursing Protocols; 2001)

consist of gastrostomy and jejunostomy, both of which may be placed either endoscopically (percutaneous endoscopic gastrostomy and jejunostomy) or surgically.

Flow chart 16.2 depicts a systematic and logical approach to decide the specific access technique for delivering an enteral feed.[22]

Noninvasive Techniques of Enteral Access

Nasogastric feeding: Nonsurgical or nonendoscopic placement of a feeding tube into the stomach is most commonly preferred and practiced universally owing to cost and ease of access. The nasal route is always preferred except in very premature infants or in those with congenital nasopharyngeal malformations. The nasogastric tube diameter for use in pediatric patients is small, ranging from size 5-12 Fr. Owing to the small diameter, there is an increased possibility of tube blockage as compared to those used in adult patients and it is recommended that the nasogastric tube be flushed with water or saline after every feed. Currently, tubes for nasogastric feeding are made of polyurethane, elastomer or flexible silicone and may require a guide wire (stylet) for assisted placement. Despite their increased flexibility, they have a longer life span and they may be adapted to incorporate some specialized features such as a double port proximally to enable both feeding and side injections (medication), a combination of distal end and side exit ports to prevent blockage , plastic coated stylets to prevent tube perforation, markings on the tube to facilitate appropriate tube selection and positioning and a rounded, bullet-shaped, non-weighted tip to facilitate easy insertion. Table 16.4 provides information about sizes of enteral feeding tubes to be used at different ages.

Table 16.4: Size of enteral tube		
	Tube french size	*Tubel length (cm)*
Premature to neonate	4–5	38–41
Infants to young children	5–8	41–91
Older children to aolesoents	8–14	91–114

Nasoduodenal and nasojejunal tube placement: Postpyloric placement of feeding tubes can be blind, endoscopically or fluoroscopically. The endoscopic technique has clear advantages and is preferred over the other methods of postpyloric tube placement. The tube is inserted under direct vision using a guidewire through the lumen of the tube by employing the drag and pull technique and radiation exposure is avoided.[23-25]

Invasive Techniques of Enteral Access

Gastrostomy and jejunostomy tubes are used for long-term enteral feeding (beyond 4 weeks). These tubes can be placed either surgically or endoscopically and offer distinct advantages over nasoenteric tubes in clinical situations that demand prolonged enteral feeding:

1. They are fixed to the anterior abdominal wall and this prevents displacement of the tube.
2. Unlike nasogastric tubes, they do not require repeated insertion—a practice which may result in psychological disturbances and aversion to food in the child.
3. Unlike nasoenteric tubes where repeated friction with the nasal mucosa may result in sinusitis or chronic nasal discharge and interference with breathing, these problems are not encountered with gastrostomy and jejunostomy feeding tubes. Figures 16.1 to 16.3

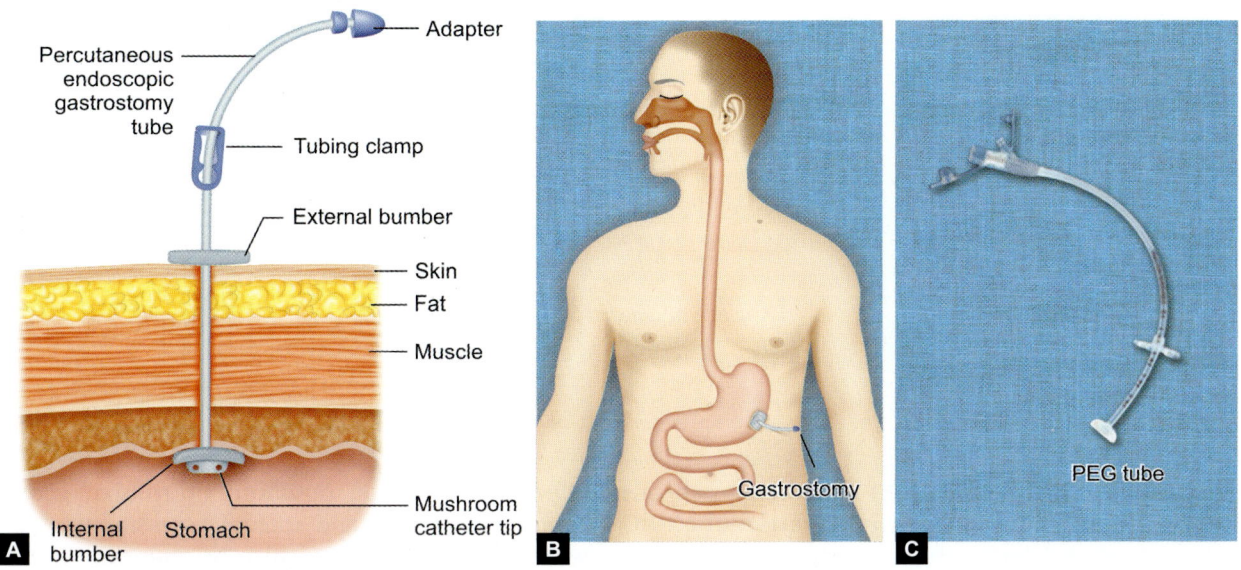

Figs 16.1A to C: Percutaneous endoscopic gastrostomy (PEG)

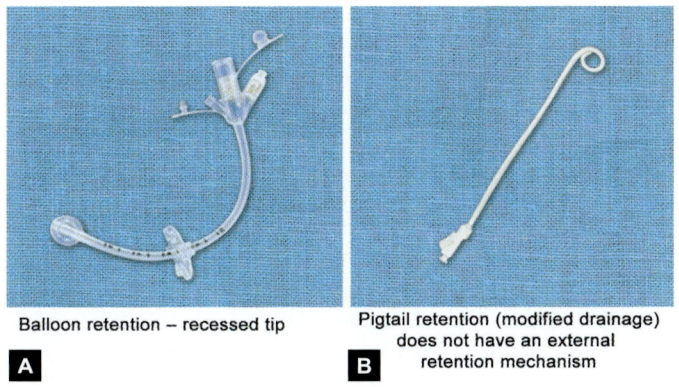

Figs 16.2A and B: Gastrostomy tubes; examples of balloon and pigtail retained gastrostomy tubes

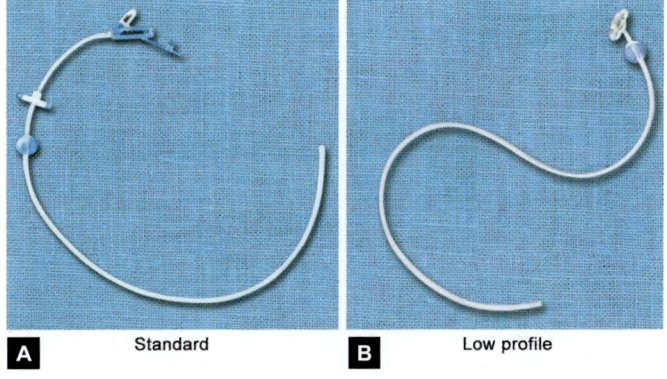

Figs 16.3A and B: Jejunostomy tubes

illustrate the basic components of a tube utilized for percutaneous endoscopic gastrostomy (PEG) and the types of gastrostomy and jejunostomy tubes.

Gastrostomy tubes (Figs 16.2A and B): These tubes have a large diameter (14-24 Fr) and are designed to deliver a large volume of feed with a minimal risk of occlusion. They are of the following types:

❑ Standard gastrostomy tube with a cupped internal bolster, sliding external bolster and a separate cap distally, with a large internal feeding port and a smaller side port for administering medication.
❑ Balloon type gastrostomy replacement tube with a balloon type internal bolster, a sliding external bolster and a one piece external tube with three openings—one each for feeding, medication and inflation.

❑ Gastrostomy device with a balloon type internal bolster and a shaft of fixed length to match the length of fistula.

Currently, the percutaneous endoscopic technique (PEG) is preferred and surgical placement of a gastrostomy tube is reserved for patients in whom PEG is contraindicated, have undergone a failed PEG placement or in patients who are to undergo a surgical procedure in conjunction with PEG placement. Surgical gastrostomy can be performed as an open surgical technique or laparoscopically and in skilled hands, the laparoscopic gastrostomy is not only faster but also safer, associated with reduced patient discomfort and duration of hospital stay.[26]

Jejunostomy tubes (Figs 16.3A and B): Percutaneous endoscopic jejunostomy feeding can be carried out either

Table 16.5: Complications associated with enteral feeding

Gastrointestinal	Pulmonary	Infectious	Mechanical	Metabolic
Intestinal discomfort	Aspiration pneumonia	Bacterial feed contamination	Tube occlusion	Fluid and electrolyte imbalance
Bloating	Incorrect tube placement	Chronic nasal discharge	Mechanical irritation causing inflammation, ulceration, perforation	Hyperglycemia
Diarrhea	Tube dislodgement into airway	Sinusitis	Gastrostomy tube migration and intestinal obstruction	Hypoglycemia
Nausea and Vomiting	Jejunal tube-dislodgement, ampullary obstruction, jaundice	Refeeding syndrome		
Exacerbation of GER		Dumping syndrome		

by direct placement of the tube (DPEJ—direct percutaneous endoscopic jejunostomy) or by the creation of a PEG and placement of a double-lumen tube (percutaneous endoscopic gastrostomy jejunostomy). The technique of DPEJ is similar to PEG, the difference being that the tube is placed in the jejunum. Transillumination of the bowel through the anterior abdominal wall and a sharp indentation easily visualized within the small bowel by the endoscopist is mandatory before the endoscopist punctures the jejunum.

The needle-catheter jejunostomy technique is the most commonly used technique for surgical placement of the jejunostomy tube. It involves the insertion of a large-bore needle into the seromuscular layers of jejunum distal to the ligament of Treitz. When there is a high risk of infection or bleeding, severe intestinal disease or adhesions, the insertion of a tube into the jejunum (Stamm technique) or a direct jejuna stoma (Maydl technique) is preferred.

Mode of enteral feeding: Enteral feeds may be administered as a continuous infusion using an infusion (feeding) pump and the mode of feeding is referred to as continuous tube feeding. Bolus feeding refers to a mode of feeding where a fixed volume of feed is delivered regularly into the gastrointestinal tract at a specified time interval and mimics physiological feeding. Intermittent feeding may be used during transition from continuous to bolus feeding and refers to feeding, which is administered as a continuous infusion interspersed with periods of a few hours of bowel rest when no feed is administered.

COMPLICATIONS ASSOCIATED WITH ENTERAL FEEDING

Complications associated with enteral nutrition therapy are recognized[27-31] and Table 16.5 summarizes these complications. They can have a significant detrimental effect on achieving optimum nutritional goals and a thorough physical and mental assessment of the child with a detailed dietary history and prior information regarding feed tolerance and any pre-existing metabolic or electrolyte abnormalities will go a long way in preventing these complications.

REFERENCES

1. Enteral nutrition practice recommendations. Bankhead et al. J Parenter Enteral Nutr. 2009;33(2):122-66.
2. American Society for Parenteral and Enteral Nutrition Board of Directors and Standards Committee: Teitelbaum D, Goenther P, Howell WH, Kochevar ME, Roth J, Seidner DL. Definition of terms, style and conventions used in ASPEN Guidelines and Standards. Nutr Clin Pract. 2005;20:281-85.
3. ASPEN Board of Directors and the Clinical Guidelines Task Force. Guidelines for the use of parenteral and enteral nutrition in adult and pediatric patients. J Parenter Enteral Nutr. 2002;26(Suppl): 1SA-138 SA. Errata 2002; 26:144.
4. Braunschweig CL, Levy P, Sheehan PM, et al. Enteral compared with parenteral nutrition: A meta-analysis. Am J Clin Nutr. 2001;74:534-42.
5. Heyman MB, Harmatz P, Acree M, et al. Economic and psychologic costs for maternal caregivers of gastrostomy-dependent children. J Pediatr. 2004;145:511-6.
6. Wong WM, Wright NA. Epidermal growth factor, epidermal growth factor receptors, intestinal growth and adaptation. J Parenter Enteral Nutr. 1999;23:S83-8.
7. Chen K, Nezu R, Wasa M, et al. Insulin-like growth factor – 1 modulation of the intestinal epithelial cell restitution. J Parenter Enteral Nutr. 1999;23:S89-92.
8. Ziegler TR, Estivariz CF, Jones CR, et al. Interactions between nutrients and peptide growth factors in intestinal growth repair and function. J Parenter Enteral Nutr. 1999;23:S174-83.
9. Li J, Kudsk KA, Gocinski B, et al. Effects of parenteral and enteral nutrition on gut-associated lymphoid tissue. J Trauma. 1995;39:44-51.
10. Alverdy JC, Aoys E, Moss GS. Total parenteral nutrition promotes bacterial translocation from the gut. Surgery. 1988;104:185-90.

11. Kudsk KA, Li J, Renegar KB. Loss of upper respiratory tract immunity with parenteral feeding. Ann Surg. 1996;223:629-38.

12. Ramachandran P, Gopalan HS. Assessment of nutritional status in Indian preschool children using WHO 2006 Growth Standards. Indian J Med Res. 2011;134:47-53.

13. Duggan C, et al. Nutrition in Pediatrics, 4th Edition, Hamilton, Ontario, Canada: BC Decker Inc; 2008.

14. Technical Consultation on Hospital Nutrition Practices in South-East Asia, New Delhi, India, 30 November-1 December, 2010. World Health Organization. 2012.

15. Heyland DK, Novak F, Drover JW, et al. Should immunonutrition become routine in critically ill patients? A systematic review of the evidence. JAMA. 2001;286:944-53.

16. Kenler AS, Swails WS, Driscoll DF, et al. Early enteral feeding in postsurgical cancer patients: Fish oil structured lipid-based polymeric formula versus a standard polymeric formula. Ann Surg. 1996;223:316-33.

17. Schloerb P. Immune-enhancing diets; Products, components and their rationales. J Parenter Enteral Nutr. 2001;25:S3-7.

18. Plauth M, Cabre E, Riggio O, Assis- Camilo M, Pirlich M, Kondrup J, Ferenci P, Holm E, von Dahl S, Mueller MJ, Nolte W. ESPEN Guidelines on Enteral Nutrition: Liver Diseas. Clin Nutr. 2006;25:285-94.

19. Brissoulis G, Filippou O, Hatzi E, et al. Early enteral administration of immunonutrition in critically ill children: Results of a blinded randomized controlled trial. Nutrition. 2005;21:799-807.

20. Lima AAM, Brito LFB, Ribiero HB, et al. Intestinal barrier function and weight gain in malnourished children taking glutamine supplemented enteral formula. J Ped Gastroent Nutr. 2005;40:28-35.

21. Technology Status Evaluation Report of the American Society of Gastrointestinal Endoscopy. In: Gastrointestinal Endoscopy. 2010;72(2):236-48.

22. Goenther P, Silkroski M. Enteral feeding access devices. Tube feeding practical guidelines and nursing protocols; 2006.

23. Chellis MJ, Sanders SV, Dean JM, et al. Bedside transpyloric tube placement in the pediatric intensive care unit. J Parenter Enteral Nutr. 1996; 20:88-90.

24. Guiterrez ED, Balfe DM. Fluoroscopically guided nasoenteric tube placement. Results of a 1- year study. Radiology. 1991;178:759-62.

25. Dranoff JA, Augood PJ, Topazian M, et al. Transnasal endoscopy for enteral tube feeding placement in critically ill patients. Am J Gastroenterol. 1999;94:2902-4.

26. Rosser JC, Rodas EB, Blancaflor J, et al. A simplified technique for laparoscopic jejunostomy and gastrostomy tube placement. Am J Surg. 1999;177:61-5.

27. Bott L, Husson MO, Guimber D, et al. Contamination of gastrostomy feeding systems in children in a home-based enteral nutrition program. J Pediatr Gastroenterol Nutr. 2001;33:266-70.

28. Ramage IJ, Harvey E, Geary DF, et al. Complications of gastrostomy feeding in children receiving peritoneal dialysis. Pediatr Nephrol. 1999;13:249-52.

29. Israel DM, Hassal E. Prolonged use of gastrostomy for enteral hyperalimentation in children with Crohn's Disease. Am J Gastroenterol. 1993;90:1084-8.

30. Weiss B, Fradkin A, Ben-Akun M, et al. Upper gastrointestinal bleeding due to gastric ulcers in children with gastrostomy tubes. J Clin Gastroenterol. 1999;29:48-50.

31. Bastow MD. Complications of enteral nutrition. Gut. 1986;27:51-5.

Chapter

17

Parenteral Nutrition

Mohammad Nurul Akhtar Hasan, Sandipan Sarkar, Garima Garg, Parvathi U Iyer

▮ INTRODUCTION

The prevalence of malnutrition among critically-ill patients has remained largely unchanged over the last two decades[1-3] especially in those with a protracted clinical course. The metabolic response to stress, injury, surgery, or inflammation is not easily predicted. These metabolic alterations are also likely to change during the course of illness in the pediatric intensive care unit (PICU). Metabolic alterations are more common in children, majority of which are hypometabolic; these children who have a pathologic pattern of metabolism are also at a greater risk of dying.[4] Both underfeeding and overfeeding are common in pediatric intensive care units (PICUs), resulting in major energy and other nutritional imbalances. There is paucity of published research on the various aspects of nutritional support in the PICU and compiling evidence-based best practice guidelines is challenging.

Thus the main goal of nutritional therapy (NT) in the PICU is not to "achieve growth" but to largely minimize protein catabolism, meet energy needs as well as to prevent deficiencies of essential nutrients.[3] Unfortunately, these goals are not always met and underfeeding continues to be common in many PICUs.[5] Hazards of underfeeding are multiple, including increased vulnerability to infections, occult and symptomatic hypoglycemia, need for prolonged ventilation as well as increased mortality.[3]

Parenteral nutrition (PN) came of age in 1964 with the demonstration that beagle puppies could be nourished successfully from 12 weeks of age to maturity by providing all nutrients intravenously. The first application of total parenteral nutrition in an infant with extreme short bowel syndrome was reported three years later in 1967. Since then there has been a plethora of literature not only on the benefits of TPN but also on complications related to its use. These complications have included both nutritional deficiencies and excesses, infections, complications related to both inadequate and excessive energy and protein intake, liver disease as well as toxicities from product contamination.[6]

In the critically-ill child, the optimal implementation of nutritional therapy includes accurate assessment of the nutritional requirements, early initiation of nutritional therapy, prevention of under and overfeeding and close monitoring for energy and protein imbalance. A clear understanding of energy needs is the first step in nutritional planning for the critically-ill child and calculating the required energy intake is a fundamental step in prescribing PN for a patient. It would be appropriate here to recapitulate some common terms and definitions.

Basal metabolic rate (BMR) is the energy expenditure of a recumbent child or adult in a thermo-neutral environment after a 12- to 18-hour fast just after awakening and prior to initiation of the daily routine. Basal metabolic rate is an indicator of the energy expenditure needed for performing the essential basic vital physiological functions of the body.

Resting energy expenditure (REE) is a term used to describe the energy expenditure of an individual at rest in a thermo-neutral environment. The difference between BMR and REE usually does not exceed 10%.[7]

Total energy expenditure (TEE) is the total of the energy requirement for maintaining basal metabolism, energy requirement for performing physical activity, thermoregulation and thermic effect of food ingested.

Energy needs can be either measured directly or estimated using the many available formulae (Tables 17.1 to 17.3). Indirect calorimetry is considered the gold standard for the measurement of metabolic rate and substrate utilization,[3,7,8] but the Harris-Benedict equation is a more practical means of estimating the basal energy expenditure (BEE) in adults.[7] Estimation of energy needs were conventionally based mainly on body size, i.e. weight, height and body surface area, however, it has been suggested that prediction of energy needs should be based on fat free mass or organ tissue mass, to take into account differences in body composition.[8]

Total daily energy requirements are usually estimated by adding to the REE or BMR of the healthy child, the

Table 17.1: Equations for calculating REE and BMR (kcal/day) in infants from 0–3 years*

Source	Gender	Equation
WHO	Male	REE = 60.9 x Wt – 54
	Female	REE = 61 x Wt – 51
Schofield	Male	BMR = 0.17 x Wt + 15.17 x Ht – 617.6
	Female	BMR = 16.25 x Wt + 10.232 x Ht – 413.5

*Wt—body weight in kilograms; Ht—length in meters.

Table 17.2: Equations for calculating REE and BMR (kcal/day) in children from 3–10 years*

Source	Gender	Equation
WHO	Male	REE = 22.7 x Wt + 495
	Female	REE = 22.5 x Wt + 499
Schofield	Male	BMR = 19.6 x Wt + 1.303 x Ht + 414.9
	Female	BMR = 16.97 x Wt + 1.618 x Ht + 371.2

*Wt—body weight in kilograms; Ht—length in meters.

Table 17.3: Equations for calculating REE and BMR (kcal/day) in children from 10–18 years and above

Source	Gender	Equation
WHO	Male	REE = 17.5 x Wt + 651
	Female	REE = 12.2 x Wt + 746
Schofield	Male	BMR = 16.25 x Wt + 1.372 x Ht + 515.5
	Female	BMR = 8.365 x Wt + 4.65 x Ht + 200
Harris-Benedict (>18 yr)	Male	REE = 66 + (13.7 x Wt) + (5 x Ht) – (6.8 x age)
	Female	REE = 655+ (9.6 x Wt) + (1.8 x Ht) – (4.68 x age)

Table 17.4: Energy requirement recommendations in various clinical situations

Stress factors	% BEE
Elective surgery	110
Medical illness of non-critical nature	120
Trauma	135–150
Burns	150–160
Sepsis	160–180

increased energy expenditure associated with activity, stress, disease state, injury and growth (Table 17.4). Stress factors have to be added to this BEE.[8-10]

PREFERRED ROUTE OF NUTRIENT DELIVERY

What is the preferred route of nutrient delivery in critically-ill children? In critically-ill children with a functioning gastrointestinal tract (GIT) the gut remains the preferred route of nutrient delivery (Grade C). Enteral nutrition has the added advantage of being more cost effective with no added risk of nosocomial infections.[3] Studies on current PICU practices of nutrient delivery have shown that ~ 20% of PICU admissions receive parenteral nutrition, 9% get parenteral and enteral nutrition but majority (55%) receive nutrient therapy by the enteral route.[11]

TOTAL PARENTERAL NUTRITION AND PARTIAL PARENTERAL NUTRITION

Parenteral nutrition (PN) is defined as delivery of nutrients intravenously, e.g. via the bloodstream. The components of PN are in elemental or predigested form: Protein as amino acids, carbohydrate (CHO) as dextrose, fat as lipid emulsion and electrolytes, vitamins and minerals.[12]

❑ Total parenteral nutrition (TPN) is when the required nutrition is administered totally parenterally and the patient does not receive any other form of nutrition. Partial parenteral nutrition (PPN) is when the patient receives part of the nutritional requirement from non-parenteral sources also.

❑ TPN has a higher concentration of constituents, i.e. is often hyperosmolar and needs to be administered through larger veins. PPN comes in a lesser concentration and can be delivered through a peripheral vein.

❑ TPN is not a preferred option for long-term nutritional supplementation.

ROUTE OF ADMINISTRATION

Central veins can handle higher macronutrient concentrations as compared to peripheral vessels, without the risk of thrombophlebitis or vessel damage.[12-15] True peripheral veins cannot tolerate concentrations of more than 900 mosm/L. Concentrations of calcium ≤5 mEq/L and potassium ≤40 mEq/L may be administered via the peripheral venous route. Ideally the peripheral veins are suitable for administration of isotonic fat emulsions and hypocaloric dextrose solutions (i.e. <10% dextrose), hence their use is limited to prevention of starvation and minimizing nitrogen loss.[16]

Peripherally inserted central catheter (PICC) is a short-term central access. The catheter is inserted through either the basilic vein or brachial vein of the arm. It enables use of concentrated, high osmolarity solutions since the tip of the catheter lies near the superior vena cava and mimics a central catheter.

The subclavian vein is the most suitable vein for parenteral nutrition as this is comfortable for the patient and carries less risk of dislodgement compared to an internal jugular vein cannula. It has less thrombophlebitis risk compared to the femoral vein. A dedicated lumen should be available for administration of PN. A central venous line should be placed with strict aseptic precautions and dressed with a sterile dressing every 48 hours.[17] The European Society for Clinical Nutrition and Metabolism (ESPEN) has issued specific guidelines on the use of central venous catheters with regard to access, care, diagnosis and treatment of complications.[18]

INDICATIONS FOR PARENTERAL NUTRITION

In general infants and children in the PICU need to be fed because lack of feeding is associated with increased morbidity and mortality.[3] PN should be initiated in all sick infants and children whose nutrient needs cannot be met by the enteral route within three days of admission to the PICU.[13-15]

Specific indications for PN in infants and children include medical and surgical indications are described in Table 17.5.

Potential cardiac indications for PN are conditions causing bowel ischemia:[19]

❑ Severe coarctation of aorta
❑ Interrupted aortic arch
❑ Large PDA
❑ Postcardiac surgery: Severe low cardiac output state (LCOS)
❑ Qp: Qs mismatch following aortopulmonary (Blalock-Taussig) shunt surgery

In summary, infants and children who cannot eat, who should not eat or who cannot eat enough are the candidates for PN in the PICU and pediatric ward.

Table 17.5: Specific indications for PN in infants and children include medical and surgical indications

Medical indications	Surgical indications
BW <1000 g	Necrotizing enterocolitis
Protracted diarrhea with severe malnutrition	Severe peritonitis
Patient who has failed EN	Small bowel obstruction
Extended period of starvation ??	Meconium ileus
Paralytic ileus	Intestinal atresia
Severe short bowel syndrome	Tracheoesophageal fistula
Mesenteric ischemia	Malrotation
Severe pancreatitis	Omphalocele, gastroschisis
Chronic diarrhea and vomiting in the extremely undernourished undergoing surgery, chemotherapy and so on	Anastomotic leaks in the early postoperative period following bowel resection

The **components** of PN are macronutrients [Dextrose, proteins (amino acids), fat] and micronutrients (electrolytes, vitamins, minerals, trace elements).

SOURCES OF ENERGY

Controversy surrounds the choice of nutrient as the main source of energy. However, a few basic principles can be agreed upon:

❑ There is a minimum amount of glucose that must be provided in order to prevent hypoglycemia and a maximum limit that results in excessive carbon-dioxide production and/or hepatic steatosis both of which need to be avoided.

❑ There is a minimum requirement (both dose and frequency) of intravenous fat emulsion to prevent essential fatty acid deficiency, and a maximum dose beyond which intravenous fat may have deleterious effects.

❑ Amino acids must be provided in adequate amounts to prevent hypoproteinemia but there are adverse consequences if given in excess.

During acute illness, the aim should be to provide energy as close as possible to the measured energy expenditure in order to minimize negative energy balance. In the absence of indirect calorimetry, ICU patients should receive at least 25 kcal/kg/day to start with, with escalation to the target requirement over the next 2–3 days.

The popular distribution of calories is 50–55% from carbohydrate, 10–15% from proteins and 30–40% from fats.[1,12,13] However, controversies exist regarding choice of nutrient as the source of energy—whether carbohydrate or lipid should be the principal source. The current distribution of non-protein calories is 60–75% from Carbohydrates (reduced from 80–85%) and 30–35% from fat due to the increasingly recognized superiority of lipids. Lipids are highly calorie dense as they provide 9 kcal/g as opposed to carbohydrates which give 3.4 kcal/g. In addition, lipids provide essential fatty acids, can be administered via peripheral lines and have no hyperglycemia related complications.[1,12,13,20]

Although protein is a potential energy substrate, it should be utilized only as a metabolic fuel to prevent negative catabolism, to maintain lean body mass and for tissue growth. Amino acid if used in excess, as an energy fuel may cause deleterious effects like azotemia and metabolic acidosis. Thus the currently recommended Nitrogen : Nonnitrogen calorie ratio is : 1 : 150–200. Glucose and lipids should provide sufficient calories to avoid protein catabolism. A healthy preterm neonate needs 100–150 kcal/kg/day, whereas a term neonate needs 100–120 kcal/kg/day.

CARBOHYDRATE REQUIREMENT

The minimal amount of carbohydrate required is about 2 g/kg of glucose per day. Hyperglycemia, glucose >10 mmol/L (180 mg/dL), contributes to infections and mortality in the critically-ill patient and should be avoided. However, variable mortality rates have been reported in PICU patients when blood glucose is maintained between 4.5 and 6.1 mmol/L (80–110 mg/dL)[20,21] and an unequivocal recommendation on this is, therefore, not possible at present. There is a higher incidence of severe hypoglycemia in patients treated with a tight glycemic control protocol.[13,21] Estimates of glucose utilization by the brain are shown in Table 17.6.[19] These estimates vary with age and, at first glance, reflect the minimum amount of glucose that must be provided to prevent hypoglycemic brain injury.[20] The surviving sepsis campaign has recommended tight glucose control in critically-ill adults based on results of a single trial that showed decreased mortality in critically-ill adults. Both hypoglycemia and glucose variability also are associated with increased length of stay and mortality and hence undesirable in the critically-ill child.[21] On the other hand, persistent hyperglycemia in the neonate receiving PN may warrant insulin therapy.[22] Insulin should be used only for those patients in whom other methods of glucose control, such as reduction of glucose infusion rates, elimination of medications predisposing patients to hyperglycemia, and correction of underlying causes of hyperglycemia (i.e. sepsis) have failed.[22]

Glucose infusion rate (GIR) = % dextrose/100 × volume in 24 hr ÷ wt (kg) ÷ 1.44 GIR is to be titrated as per random blood sugar level. The goals are to avoid hypoglycemia <50 mg/dL and avoid hyperglycemia >125 mg/dL.

The GIR rates are given in the Table 17.7.[12,13]

PROTEIN REQUIREMENT

The principal goal of protein/amino acid administration in critical·illness is to provide precursors for protein synthesis in tissues having a high turnover of protein and to protect skeletal muscle mass and function from disuse

Table 17.6: Estimates of glucose consumption by the brain

Age	Utilization (mg/kg/min)	Utilization (g/kg/d)
Newborn	8.0	11.5
1 year	7.0	10.1
5 years	4.7	6.8
Adolescent	1.9	2.7
Adult	1.0	1.4

Table 17.7: GIR infusion rates

Age	Initiate	Advance	Maximum
<1 yr	6–9 mg/kg/min	1–2 mg/kg/min	10–12 mg/kg/min
1–10 yr	1–2 mg/kg/min	1–2 mg/kg/min	8–10 mg/kg/min
>10 yr	1–2 mg/kg/min	1–2 mg/kg/min	5–6 mg/kg/min

Table 17.8: Parenteral amino acid supply considered adequate for most patients

Age	Initiate	Advance	Maximum
Preterm infants	0.5–1 g/kg/day	0.5–1 g/kg/day	1.5–4 g/kg/day
Term neonates	0.5–1 g/kg/day	0.5–1 g/kg/day	1.5–4 g/kg/day
< 1 yr	1–2 g/kg/day	1 g/kg/day	4 g/kg/day
1–10 yr	1–2 g/kg/day	1 g/kg/day	1.5–3 g/kg/day
>10 yr (Adolescent)	1 g/kg/day	1 g/kg/day	0.8–2.5 g/kg/day

atrophy. Amino acid requirements varyfrom 2.5 g/kg/d for preterm infants to 0.75 g/kg/d for adolescents[12,23,24] (Table 17.8). When PN is indicated, a balanced amino acid mixture should be infused at approximately 1.3–1.5 g/kgideal body wt/day in conjunction with an adequate energy supply. Amino acid solutions are the main source of protein. Available solutions contain nine essential amino acids; cysteine, tyrosine, taurine and arginine as the semiessential amino acids. Standard amino acid (AA) solutions are referred to as "balanced" when the composition of essential amino acids (EAA) is comparable to individual amino acid requirements in healthy subjects.[25] The objective is to achieve a blood urea nitrogen (BUN) value between 10 and 15 mg/dL which indicates an intake of amino acids that is adequate for protein anabolism (Laine and Shulman, unpublished data). In a normal healthy state, intravenous infusion of amino acids administration causes stimulation of whole body and muscle protein synthesis. In contrast, infusion of glucose and insulin preferentially inhibits proteolysis.[26,27] Administration of a combination of glucose, insulin and amino acids is associated with a greater anabolic effect than administration of insulin or amino acids alone.[26] In the setting of a pediatric intensive care unit (PICU), the amino acid component of the parenteral nutrition (PN) infusate should provide 0.2–0.4 g/kg/day of L-glutamine (equivalent to 0.3–0.6 g/kg/day alanyl-glutamine dipeptide).

Table 17.9 shows the differences between neonatal and pediatric amino acid solution.

Components of intralipid include triglycerides which are the source of calories and essential fatty acids (EFA),

Table 17.9: Differences between neonatal and pediatric amino acid solution	
Neonatal amino acid	Pediatric amino acid
• Contain low methionine, proline and phenylalanine • Contains taurine for brain development • Contains cysteine	Contains excess methionine, proline and phenylalanine

Table 17.10: Parenteral lipid infusion guidelines[12]***

Age	Initiate	Advance	Maximum
<1 yr	1 g/kg/day	1 g/kg/day	3 g/kg/day
1–10 yr	1 g/kg/day	1 g/kg/day	2–3 g/kg/day
>10 yr	1 g/kg/day	1 g/kg/day	1–2.5 g/kg/day

***goals dependent on total kcal goals
***do not exceed 60% of kcal via lipid (concern regarding ketosis)
***maximum lipid clearance 0.15 g/kg/H

Table 17.11: Current recommendations of intralipid use in sick children[12,13,14]

- Sepsis, thrombocytopenia: Can use judiciously
- Hyperlipidemia:
  - Neonates and infants: Stop when serum TG >250 mg/dL for 24–48 hr→ restart at slower infusion rate (@0.02–0.04 g/kg/hr)
  - In older children: Stop when serum TG > 400 mg/dL
- Liver failure: Reduce/stop lipid in cholestasis
- Renal failure: No problem
- ARDS: Lower dose lipid permitted
- Pancreatitis: Usually acceptable to give lipid, watch serum TG level

egg phospholipids which is an emulsifier and glycerine which makes the admixture approximately isotonic.

A key role of intravenous fat emulsion is the prevention of essential fatty acid deficiency. In the absence of intravenous fat emulsion, endogenous adipose tissue and the liver are probably the sources of essential fatty acids.[28] In order to prevent the mobilization of fatty acids for energy, essential fatty acids must be provided in amounts necessary to both replace deficits and supply ongoing needs for metabolism. Intravenous fat emulsions with high concentration of phospholipids (i.e. 10% emulsions) should be avoided as they carry a higher risk of producing high serum levels of triglycerides, cholesterol, and phospholipids than other emulsions (i.e. 20% and 30% emulsions).[29,30] Thus, 20% intralipid is preferred over 10% intralipid solutions and also has the added advantage of being more energy dense.

Several studies have shown specific clinical advantages of long chain triglycerides/medium chain triglycerides (LCT/MCT) mixtures over use of soybean LCT alone, but this requires confirmation by controlled prospective trials. In infants and children mixtures of mixed LCT/MCT lipid emulsions can be considered generally safe.[12,13,31] Olive oil-base for parenteral nutrition is also well-tolerated in critically-ill patients. Addition of *docosahexaenoic* acid *(DHA)* and *eicosapentaenoic acid (EPA)* to lipid emulsions has demonstrable positive effects on cell membranes and inflammatory processes. Fish oil-enriched lipid emulsions possibly decrease the length of stay in critically-ill patients particularly in those with lung injury.[32-34] However, current evidence does not consistently support the routine use of immune enhancement in children.[3]

Recognized adverse effects of intralipid therapy are egg allergy, hypertriglyceridemia, and immunosuppression. Thus contraindications to lipid therapy include severe egg allergy, pancreatitis associated with hyperlipidemia and high baseline triglycerides levels of >400 mg/dL. Hence, precautions should be taken in neonatal hyperbilirubinemia since lipids can displace bilirubin from albumin, leading to kernicterus or bilirubin encephalopathy; thus it is a good idea to limit lipids to 1 gm/kg/day in neonates on phototherapy.[12-14]

There has been concern that intravenous lipids induce thrombocytopenia. However, available data does not support this.[35,36] Early studies suggested that infusion of intravenous lipid emulsion impairs neutrophil function but recent data are not supportive and have demonstrated normal immune function.[36] There is a theoretical risk involved in administration of lipids to a neonate with severe respiratory distress owing to an imminent risk of developing pulmonary embolism and PGI_2 (Prostacyclin) formation, which may cause an alteration in the ventilation/perfusion ratio.[37] In contrast, lipids, when administered as a slow infusion over 24 hours, are not associated with worsening of respiratory distress. Embolism is mostly related with larger droplet of (>0.5 micro M). This can be avoided by following recommended guidelines and use of droplet filters.

Intravenous lipid emulsions (LCT, MCT or mixed emulsions) can be administered safely at a rate of 0.7 g/kg up to 1.5 g/kg over 12 to 24 hours[12-14] (Table 17.10). Table 17.11 shows the current recommendation of intralipid use in sick children.

What Happens if Lipid is not Given?

Essential fatty acid deficiency can occur within days particularly in preterm infants and neonates which can be prevented by providing at least 0.5 g/kg/day of lipid (2–4% of total kcal). Symptoms of fatty acid deficiency are shown in Table 17.12.[12-14,38]

Table 17.12: Symptoms of fatty acid deficiency

- Alopecia, scaly dermatitis
- Increased capillary fragility
- Poor wound healing
- Increased platelet aggregation
- Increased susceptibility to infection
- Fatty liver
- Growth retardation in infants and children

Table 17.13: Daily electrolyte and mineral requirements for pediatric patients*

Electrolytes	Preterm/ Neonates	Infants/Children	Adolescent/ Children >50 kg
Na	2–5 mEq/Kg	2–5 mEq/Kg	1–2 mEq/Kg
K	2–4 mEq/Kg	2–4 mEq/Kg	1–2 mEq/Kg
Ca	2–4 mEq/Kg	0.5–4 mEq/Kg	10–20 mEq/day
Phos	1–2 mmol/Kg	0.5–2 mmol/Kg	10–40 mmol/day
Mg	0.3–0.5 mEq/Kg	0.3–0.5 mEq/Kg	10–30 mEq/day
Acetate	As needed to maintain acid-base balance		
Chloride	As needed to maintain acid-base balance		

*Assumes normal age-related organ function and normal losses.

Table 17.14: Estimated needs of vitamins (dose/day)

Vitamins	Term infants (≥2.5 kg)	Preterm infants (≤2.5 kg)
Lipid Soluble		
A (µg)	700	280
D (IU)	400	160
E (mg)	7	2.8
K (mg)	200	80
Water Soluble		
Thiamine (mg)	1.2	0.48
Riboflavin (mg)	1.4	0.56
Niacin (mg)	17	6.8
Pantothenate (mg)	5	2
Pyridoxine (mg)	1	0.4
Biotin (µg)	20	8
Vitamin B_{12} (µg)	1	0.4
Ascorbic acid (mg)	80	32
Folic acid (µg)	140	56

Note: Requirements of vitamin should be tailored according to underlying disease conditions.

Electrolytes

Critically-ill infants and children are prone to fluid and sodium overload, and renal injury is frequent. Therefore, it is neither adequate nor appropriate to propose guidelines for the use of electrolytes on the basis of body weight or as a fixed element of parenteral nutrition. The highly variable requirements should instead be determined by plasma electrolyte monitoring. This is especially important in case of cardiac surgery patients who require strict maintenance of body electrolytes especially K^+, Ca^{++}, Mg^{++}, etc.[12-14]

Daily requirements of electrolyte and mineral for pediatric patients is shown in Table 17.13.

Are Micronutrients Required in PICU Patients?

Vitamins, Minerals and Trace Elements

The 1998 National Advisory Group on Standards and Practice Guidelines underlined the importance of establishing optimal trace element and vitamin formulations for both adult and pediatric patient populations.[39] In April 2000, the US Food and Drug Administration (FDA) amended the multivitamin formulation for adult patients to bring it into accordance with the 1988 recommendations of the American Medical Association-FDA Public Workshop Committee providing micronutrients to include the full range of trace elements and vitamins as an integral part of nutritional support.[39]

Administration of Multivitamins in Children[12]

All PN prescriptions should include a daily dose of multivitamins and trace elements (Grade C for adults).[12,13] Daily requirements of vitamins for infants and children is shown in Table 17.14.

The daily requirements for both water and fat-soluble vitamins can be easily provided in TPN. Water soluble vitamins should be administered regularly to parenterally fed patients preferably on a daily basis.

Features of vitamin deficiency is shown in Table 17.15.

Table 17.15: Features of vitamin deficiency

Micronutrient and vitamins	Clinical signs of deficiency
Thiamine	Congestive cardiac failure, lactic acidosis
Ascorbic acid	Scurvy
Copper	Arrhythmia, altered immunity
Selenium	Acute cardiomyopathy
Zinc	Delayed wound healing, infections

Practical Aspects of Multivitamin Administration in Children

There is an acute shortage of pediatric intravenous multivitamins worldwide so the following recommendations have been made:[40]

❑ Water-soluble vitamins should be administered regularly to parenterally fed patients, preferably on a daily basis. When feasible, vitamin preparations should be added to the lipid emulsion (Grade D)

❑ Switch to enteral multivitamins when enteral intake is greater than 50% of needs

❑ Supplement intravenous vitamin K daily (total daily dose = 200 μg). The vitamin K content of the adult multivitamin product should be noted when supplementing with additional vitamin K

❑ Children >2.5 kg or 36 weeks gestation: 5 mL of adult vitamins solution

❑ Infants <2.5 kg or <36 weeks gestation: 1 mL/kg up to a maximum of 2.5 mL/day adult MVI.

❑ Children >11 years: Full adult dose (10 mL)

Note: Adult intravenous multivitamin products contain propylene glycol and polysorbate which may be toxic to neonates.

Trace Elements

Trace elements are crucial with long-term parenteral nutrition >3 weeks in pediatrics (Grade D).[12,13]

Parenteral nutrition solutions usually contain some of the various trace minerals due to contamination of the components (e.g. amino acids, calcium gluconate, multivitamins) with trace metals.[41] In one report zinc, copper, manganese, and selenium were found in greatest concentration but contamination will vary depending on the commercial products used to prepare the PN.[41] Heat and storage time can modestly reduce the levels of some trace elements as well.[41]

Manganese (Mn)

The FDA-approved trace element formulation results in relatively high levels of copper and manganese, which may be associated with toxicity during prolonged home PN. Manganese toxicity has also been described during its acute administration in critically-ill patients where it has led to neurotoxicity. Manganese is an essential trace mineral that is normally excreted in bile and has a special affinity for the extrapyramidal system.[42,43] Manganese accumulation can be detected in the basal ganglia as symmetric, increased signal intensity on T-1 weighted magnetic resonance images.[44] These changes are reversible when Mn is removed from the PN.[44-47] Clinical symptoms are usually but not always reversible. Manganese and copper may be withheld in patients with hepatic dysfunction.

Chromium (Cr)

Chromium plays an important role in the metabolism of lipids and carbohydrates and is an essential micronutrient. Both chromium excess and deficiency have been reported in patients receiving PN for 3 weeks or more (long-term).[48,49] Effort should be made to identify PN components with low or no Cr contamination.[50] A high serum Cr competes with iron for binding to transferring and an intake of 0.2 mg/kg per day has been recommended for infants and children (maximum of 5 mg/day) receiving PN.

Iron

Patients receiving long-term PN (3 weeks or more) should receive iron supplementation. In children receiving long-term iron supplementation parenterally, the risk of iron overload requires periodic monitoring of iron status using serum ferritin. Parenteral iron must be supplemented to very low birth weight infants receiving PN. The dose of iron for infants and children (50–100 mg/kg per day) is based on calculations extrapolated from studies showing that lower doses may be inadequate to maintain iron balance and represents "expert opinion". The dose in premature infants may be as high as 200 mg/kg per day. During short-term PN (i.e. <3 weeks) iron supplementation is usually unnecessary. The preferred modality of iron administration is a regular daily dosing.[12,51,52]

Copper

The parenteral (intravenous) dose of copper for infants and children is 20 mg/kg per day. The concentrations of plasma copper and ceruloplasmin must be monitored in patients receiving long-term PN and also in parenterally fed patients with burns or with cholestasis, and the dose of copper administered requires appropriate modification.

Zinc

Zinc (Zn) is a very important mineral involved in the metabolism of energy, proteins, carbohydrates, lipids and nucleic acids and is required for tissue accretion. Standard trace element preparations do not provide this amount and further supplementation (zinc sulphate) by adding to the PN infusate may be necessary in the preterm infant or in patients with high loss of zinc from the body (diarrhea, stomal losses or severe skin disease).[12,51] An intravenous intake of 250 mg/kg/day and 100 mg/kg/day, respectively, for infants less than or more than 3 months of age and 50 mg/kg/day for children (maximum of 5.0 mg/day).[51] Zn is the only trace element that should be added to solutions of patients on short-term PN.[12,51,53]

Is Anything Else We Should Add to PN?

Carnitine

Carnitine is a quaternary ammonium compound biosynthesized from the amino acids lysine and methionine. It is required for the transport of fatty acids from the cytosol into the mitochondria during the breakdown of lipids for the generation of metabolic energy. It is currently added to neonatal PN and adult PN in selected cases only. American Society for Parenteral and Enteral Nutrition (ASPEN) recommends the routine addition of 2 to 5 mg/kg/d to the PN for neonates if no enteral source is provided. Carnitine synthesis and storage is suboptimal at birth and in the preterm on prolonged PN. In infants requiring prolonged PN (>2–3 weeks) a parenteral source of carnitine may be provided at 10–20 mL/kg/d until EN can be established.[12]

Cysteine

It is an essential amino acid. It lowers pH of parenteral nutrition solution and may need additional acetate to prevent acidosis. Low pH enhances solubility of calcium and phosphorus. Cysteine should be supplemented in PN @ 30–40 mg/g protein.

Selenium

Selenium (Se) acts as an antioxidant by being an essential component of active glutathione peroxidase (GSHPx), an enzyme that may protect against oxidative tissue damage. Current trace elements contain no selenium. An intravenous selenium supply of 2 to 3 µg/kg per day is recommended for parenterally fed LBW infants. Selenium deficiency causes cardiac and skeletal myopathy, increased risk of bronchopulmonary dysplasia, hypothyroidism and a weakened immune system.

Fluid Requirements

Fluids are a very essential part of parenteral nutrition. Fluid volume should be increased over the first 7 days depending on status of serum electrolytes, clinical assessment of hydration and underlying pathology (e.g. heart failure, renal failure) with the aim of delivering 100–150 mL/kg/day by the end of a week to 10 days if possible. Fluid requirement can be calculated by the Holiday-Segar formula (Table 17.16).

A number of complications of PN have been described. In fact the potential dangers of PN have been highlighted in the article "death by parenteral nutrition.[54] PN has been shown to be associated in ill adults with increases in infection rates, multiorgan failure, length of stay and greater chance of death.

Complications with the Use of PN

TPN related complications include:
- Catheter related:
  - Pneumothorax, hemothorax, hydrothorax (TPN solution)
  - Intravascular displacement, catheter embolism-sheared tip, infections
  - Air embolism, venous thrombosis, pulmonary embolism, extravasations
- Sepsis: Mostly due to carbohydrate or lipid, catheter related
- Metabolic:
  - Dextrose related: Hyperglycemia/hypoglycemia, dehydration/fluid overload
  - Protein related: Azotemia, hyperammonemia, metabolic acidosis
  - Lipid related: Hyperlipidemia, hyperbilirubinemia
  - Electrolyte imbalances, hyperammonemia, acid-base imbalance
  - Fatty liver, bone demineralization
  - Coagulopathy, thrombocytopenia
- Re-feeding syndromes, growth retardation, trace element deficiency
- PN associated cholestasis (PNAC).

The re-feeding syndrome is characterized by hypophospatemia, hypomagnesemia, hypokalaemia and hyperinsulinemia and may be observed in patients kept nil by mouth for greater than 7–10 days, chronic alcoholics, severe cachexia and those with severe systemic derangements on initiation of TPN.[55,56] Correction of electrolyte abnormalities, administration of thiamine in alcoholics and those with severe malnutrition and a regular check of electrolyte levels may help to prevent this re-feeding syndrome.

Most common contaminants of PN are aluminum and manganese.[12-14]

Aluminum toxicity is a real problem especially with renal compromise on long-term PN in infants and neonates. Safe intake of aluminum in PN is set at 5 µg/

Table 17.16: Holiday-Segar formula	
Body weight	Fluid requirement per day
1–10 kg	100 mL/kg
11–20 kg	1000 mL/kg + 50 mL/kg above 10
Above 20 kg	1500 mL/kg + 20 mL/kg above 20

kg/day. Manganese toxicity has also been reported in long-term PN patients. Manganese concentrations of 8 to 22 µg/day have been reported even in formulations with no added manganese. This may lead to neurological symptoms as discussed above.

Long-term adverse effects including all the above-mentioned short-term complications along with vitamin, mineral deficiency/toxicity, and aluminium toxicity in infants with impaired renal system.

Known Causes of Risk Factors of Parenteral Nutrition Associated Cholestatis (PNAC)[12-14]

PNAC is more often transient than progressive:
- ❑ Risk factors include: Prematurity, increased duration of PN, fasting, infections
- ❑ Suggested etiologies are: Amino acid imbalance, CHO: Fat ratio imbalance, nutrition deficiency, phytosterol, inflammation, lack of enteral feeding.

Prevention and Treatment of PNAC[12-14]

- ❑ Prevention: By early initiation of trophic enteral feed (Grade A), protection of PN from light
- ❑ Treatment: Limit carbohydrates, limit IV fat <1 g/kg/d eliminate hepatotoxic drugs, cyclical PN (Grade C)
- ❑ Possible medications include: Ursodeoxycholic acid, cholestyramine, phenobarbitone ??

There is also emerging evidence that omega-3 fatty acid emulsion may be beneficial in prevention and treatment of cholestasis.

Despite complications PN is a valuable tool in the presence of gastrointestinal feed intolerance or failure, especially in neonates, preterm infants and small infants.[3,12-14]

Practice Guidelines for Administration of PN[12-14,53]

- ❑ All patients receiving PN should receive a parenteral vitamin preparation on a daily basis.
- ❑ Health care providers should choose PN components with the lowest aluminum content when possible to minimize parenteral aluminum exposure.
- ❑ Trace elements are crucial with long-term parenteral nutrition >3 weeks in pediatrics (Grade D).[12,13] When the use of a commercially available multiple trace element combination product increases the risk of trace element toxicity or deficiency states, the use of individual trace element products is warranted.
- ❑ Parenteral iron should not be routinely supplemented in patients receiving PN therapy. It should be limited to conditions of iron deficiency when oral iron supplementation fails.

Table 17.17: Parenteral nutrition monitoring	
Measurement	Frequency of measurement
Blood	
Glucose	2–3 times a day while increasing GIR, then once a day while on stable GIR
BUN, Cr	Twice a week initially, then weekly
Serum electrolytes	Twice a week initially, then weekly
Serum albumin, PCV	Weekly
LFT, serum TG	Weekly
Anthropometry	
Weight	Daily at the same time
Length	Weekly
Head circumfernce	Weekly
Nutrient intake calculation	Daily Energy in Kcal/kg/d, protein g/Kg/d

Contraindications to PN include a functional and accessible GI tract, aprognosis which does not warrant aggressive nutrition support (terminally ill children) and when risk exceeds benefitie (Anticipated duration of therapy <3 days unless severe malnutrition or extreme prematurity is present).[12-14]

How Should We Monitor Infants Receiving PN?

PN monitoring: Refer Table 17.17.[12-14]

How Should We Wean PN ?

Generally PN should be tapered slowly as oral or enteral feedings are introduced and advanced. Usually, PN is continued until 75–80% of energy needs are met enterally.[12-14]

▌ TOTAL NUTRIENT ADMIXTURE (TNA)

Parenteral nutrition admixtures (also called total nutrient admixtures or TNA, three-in-one solutions, or all-in-one solutions-AIO) are recent complex systems that make use of the fact that under certain conditions the glucose/amino acid solution may be mixed with intravenous fat emulsion and administered to the patient in one bag.[57,58] There are a number of potential advantages to PN admixtures but also some disadvantages.

These admixtures have the advantage of decreased risk of contamination with ease of administration. The bag contains a glucose solution (13%, 16% or 19%), a pediatric amino acid solution (Primene®, Baxter®) with electrolytes and olive oil based lipid emulsion (ClinOleic®, Baxter®) in different compartments separated by a seal, which can be broken to mix the components just before administration. The preparation does not contain trace elements or vitamins, which are added into the final mixture separately as per the clinical needs of the patients.[57-60] However, due to concerns of complexity, special attention should be paid to physicochemical and microbiological stability of the mixture, because of potential interactions among components that can be very hard to analyze.[58]

Parenteral Nutrition Admixtures: Advantages and Drawbacks (Table 17.18)

Stability of the mixture is a major concern. The emulsion in the TNA is stable for 28 days with refrigeration, followed by 2 days at room temperature.[58] TPN admixture prepared in a hospital pharmacy can also be stored without loss of stability for at least 60 hours.[58-62] But considering degradation of retinol palmitate and tocopherols, admixtures with vitamins need to be infused within 24 hours of compounding.[58-62]

The stability and compatibility of total parenteral nutrition admixtures is paramount to their safety. This is related to the stability of lipid-injectable emulsions and the compatibility of calcium and phosphate salts as well as

Table 17.18: Advantages and drawbacks of parenteral nutrition admixtures	
Advantages	Disadvantages
Nursing time for administration of PN is decreased	Particulate matter is difficult to see prohibiting visual inspection of solution
Rate of extrinsic touch contamination potentially reduced	Filtration must be performed with a larger filter (1.2 micron vs 0.22 micron)
Pharmacy preparation time decreased	
Admixtures support microbial growth less than fat emulsion alone	Support the growth of microorganisms better than glucose amino acid solutions
A two pump system is eliminated	Computer interfaced automated compounder expensive
Increased compliance of administering fat emulsion in the home patient population	Emulsion instability can be disrupted with high concentrations of electrolytes or when base solution component amounts exceed compatibility limits
The cost of 'Y' site tubing and additional supplies is saved	

globule size.[61-63] The most significant cause of precipitation is excessive concentrations of calcium phosphate and the most important cause of chemical instability is the oxidation of specific vitamins.[62-64] The addition of vitamins and trace elements to PN solutions induces a significant increase in peroxidation products, which are reduced when admixtures are protected from light. Iron should not be included in these solutions, even if solutions are light-protected.[62-65]

To minimize lipid peroxidation, AIO admixtures should be stored light-protected and refrigerated without trace elements. The trace elements should be only added immediately before administration or should be given separately.[62-67] MCT/LCT based lipid emulsion provides more physical stability of TPN admixtures than MCT-based emulsion.[67] On the other hand SMOF-lipid (lipid emulsion based on soybean oil, medium chain triglycerides, olive oil and fish oil) is more stable than that of MCT/LCT. Lipids with olive-oil containing emulsion contain mainly MUFA, has a lot of beneficial properties, primarily stability against lipid-peroxidation. This has implications for storage; peroxidation of lipids is much more pronounced in plastic (EVA) bags used for storage of TPNs than in glass bottles.

Infection is yet another major concern with TNA. Although earlier studies showed increased incidence of growth of pathogenic bacteria in TNA in comparison with traditional TPN,[68] recent studies revealed a low incidence of contamination of TNA.[69-71] Studies also showed that the administration of low-dose heparin in TNA may decrease the incidences of catheter obstruction and catheter related infections.[71]

The most common recommendation for the size of lipid droplets is less than 5 microns.[72,73] Diameters higher than 5 µm are still allowed in parenteral lipid emulsions and in therapeutic admixtures but they must not exceed the proportion of 0.05%.[72] Recent evidence suggests that TNAs (Total nutrient admixtures) with LDs of 5 µm or more constituting >0.4% of the final fat concentration are unstable.[72] The recent Food and Drug Administration Safety Alert recommends in-line filtration for all total parenteral nutrition admixtures.[72,73] In olive oil containing emulsions the larger droplets appear in the surface layer whereas in soya containing emulsion at the bottom. From the therapeutic point the emulsions of the bigger droplets within the upper layer are safer because the potentially dangerous big droplets could remain in the infusion bag after the administration.

In summary the TNA system of nutritional support has become very popular especially in Europe and offers some unique advantages over the traditional method of administering TPN. The establishment of all-in-one admixtures has made parenteral nutrition easier, increased their effectiveness and reduced complications.[73]

CONCLUSION

Appropriate nutritional therapy (NT) is essential to improve outcomes in critically-ill small infants and children. The enteral route constitutes the mainstay of nutritional therapy in sick children. However, parenteral nutrition (PN) continues to be a valuable nutritional tool in the presence of gastrointestinal feed intolerance or failure and insurgical bowel pathology especially in neonates, preterm infants and small children. Several complications associated with PN have been described, but most can be averted or managed effectively. Total nutrient admixtures (TNA) have gained increasing popularity, have several advantages and have attained increasing acceptance in various parts of Europe even in children.

ACKNOWLEDGMENTS

The authors are indebted to the Residents Dr Yukti Choudhry and Dr Harsheen Kaur of the Pediatric Intensive Care Unit of the Fortis Escorts Heart Institute for their contributions in the literature search, reviews and bibliography. We would also like to acknowledge with grateful thanks their assistance in reading the manuscript carefully and for making appropriate revisions.

CONFLICTS OF INTEREST

The authors have no conflicts of interest or sources of finding to disclose.

REFERENCES

1. Hulst J, Joosten K, Zimmermann L, Hop W, van Buuren S, Büller H, et al. Malnutrition in critically ill children: From admission to 6 months after discharge. Clin Nutr. 2004;23(2):223-32. [PubMed]
2. Pollack MM, Wiley JS, Kanter R, Holbrook PR. Malnutrition in critically ill infants and children.JPEN J Parenter Enteral Nutr. 1982;6(1):20-4. [PubMed]
3. Mehta NM, Compher C. ASPEN Board of Directors. ASPEN Clinical guidelines: Nutrition support of the critically ill child. J Parenter Enteral Nutr. 2009;33(3):260-76. doi: 10. 1177/0148607109333114. [PubMed]
4. Are patients fed appropriately according to their caloric requirements? McClave SA, et al. JPEN J Parenter Enteral Nutr. 1998.[[PubMed]
5. Oosterveld MJ, et al. Energy expenditure and balance following pediatric intensive care unit admission: a longitudinal study of critically ill children. PediatrCrit Care Med. 2006. [PubMed]
6. Spencer Carolyn T, Charlene C. The development of TPN: an interview with pioneer surgical nutritionist Jonathan E Rhoads. J Am Diet Assoc. 2001;101(7):747-50.
7. Harris JA, Benedict FG. Washington, DC: Biometric Studies of Basal Metabolism in Man. Carnegie Institution of Washington; 1919. Publication No 279.
8. Forchelli ML, Gura KM, Shulman RJ. Metabolism estimation, recommended energy, protein and fluid needs by age in pediatric nutrition in your pocket. Corkins MR, Shulman RJ (Eds). American Society for Parenteral and Enteral Nutrition (in press).
9. Hunter DC, Jaksic T, Lewis D, Benotti P N, Blackburn GL, Bistrian BR. Resting energy expenditure in the critically ill: estimations versus measurement. Br J Surg. 1988;75(9):875-8. [PubMed]
10. Boulanger BR, Nayman R, McLean RF, Phillips E, Rizoli SB. What are the clinical determinants of early energy expenditure in critically injured adults? J Trauma. 1994;37(6):969-74. [PubMed]
11. Taylor RM1, Preedy VR, Baker AJ, Grimble G. Nutritional Support in Critically Ill Children. Clin Nutr. 2003;22(4):365-9. [PubMed]
12. American Society for Parenteral and Enteral Nutrition. The A.S.P.E.N. pediatric nutrition support core curriculum; 2010.
13. Bozzetti F, Forbes A. The ESPEN clinical practice guidelines on Parenteral Nutrition: Present status and perspectives for future research. Clin Nutr. 2009;28(4):359-64.doi: 10.1016/j.clnu.2009.05.010. Epub 2009 Jun 12.
14. Braegger C, Decsi T, Dias JA, Hartman C, Kolacek S, Koletzko B, et al. Practical Approach to Paediatric Enteral Nutrition: A Comment by the ESPGHAN Committee on Nutrition. JPGN. 2010;51(1):110-22.
15. Dickerson RN, Brown RO, White KG. Parenteral Nutrition solutions. In: Rombeau JL, Caldwell MD (Eds). Parenteral Nutrition. 2nd ed. Philadelphia: WB Saunders. 1993;pp. 310-33.
16. Isaacs JW, Millikan WJ, Stackhouse J, Hersh T, Rudman D. Parenteral nutrition of adults with a 900 milliosmolar solution via peripheral veins. Am J ClinNutr. 1977;30(4):552-9.
17. ConlyJM, Grieves K, Peters B. A prospective, randomized study comparing transparent and dry gauze dressings for central venous catheters. J Infect Dis. 1989;159(2):310-9. [PubMed]
18. Pittiruti M, Hamilton H, Biffi R, MacFie J, Pertkiewicz M. ESPEN. ESPEN Guidelines on Parenteral Nutrition: Central Venous Catheters (access, care, diagnosis and therapy of complications) Clin Nutr. 2009;28(4):365-77 doi: 10.1016/j.clnu.2009.03.015. Epub 2009 May 21. [PubMed]
19. Macrae Duncan J. Renal, Gastrointestinal, Hepatic and Neurologic Dysfunction. Carol L Lake, Peter D Booker (Eds). Pediatric cardiac anesthesia, 4th ed. Lippincott Williams and Wilkins. 2005;pp. 705-22.
20. Kalhan SC, Kilic I. Carbohydrate as nutrient in the infant and child: range of acceptable intake. Eur J Clin Nutr. 1999;53(Suppl 1):S94-100.
21. Wintergerst KA, Buckingham B, Gandrud L, Wong BJ, Kache S, Wilson DM. Association of hypoglycemia, hyperglycemia, and glucose variability with morbidity and death in the pediatric intensive care unit. Pediatrics. 2006;118(1):173-9. [PubMed]
22. Arsenault D, Brenn M, Kim S, Gura K, Compher C, Simpser E. ASPEN Clinical Guidelines : Hyperglycemia and Hypoglycemia in the Neonate Receiving Parenteral Nutrition. American Society for Parenteral and Enteral Nutrition (ASPEN) Board of Directors and Mark PuderJPEN J Parenter Enteral Nutr. 2012;36:81 originally published online 16 December 2011.

23. Brown MR, Thunberg BJ, Golub L, Maniscalco WM, Cox C, Shapiro DL. Decreased cholestasis with enteral instead of intravenous protein in the very low-birth-weight infant. J Pediatr Gastroenterol Nutr. 1989;9(1):21-7. [PubMed]

24. National Advisory Group on Standards and Practice Guidelines for Parenteral Nutrition. Safe practices for parenteral nutrition formulations. J Parent Ent Nutr. 1998;22:49-66.

25. Young VR, Borgonha S. Nitrogen and amino acid requirements: the Massachusetts Institute of Technology amino acid requirement pattern. J Nutr. 2000;130(7):1841S-9S.

26. Tessari P, Inchiostro S, Biolo G, et al. Differential effects of hyperinsulinemia and hyperaminoacidemia on leucine-carbon metabolism in vivo. Evidence for distinct mechanisms in regulation of net amino acid deposition. J Clin Invest. 1987;79(4):1062-9. [PubMed]

27. Biolo G, Tipton KD, Klein S, Wolfe RR. An abundant supply of amino acids enhances the metabolic effect of exercise on muscle protein. Am J Physiol. 1997;273(1 Pt 1):E122–9. [PubMed]

28. Foote KD, MacKinnon MJ, Innis SM. Effect of early introduction of formula vs fat-free parenteral nutrition on essential fatty acid status of preterm infants. Am J Clin Nutr. 1991;54(1):93-7. [PubMed]

29. Haumont D, Deckelbaum RJ, Richelle M, Dahlan W, Coussaert E, Bihain BE, et al. Plasma lipid and plasma lipoprotein concentrations in low birth weight infants given parenteral nutrition with twenty or ten percent lipid emulsion. J Pediatr. 1989;115(5 Pt 1):787-93. [PubMed]

30. Haumont D, Richelle M, Deckelbaum RJ, Coussaert E, Carpentier YA. Effect of liposomal content of lipid emulsions on plasma lipid concentrations in low birth weight infants receiving parenteral nutrition. J Pediatr. 1992;121(5 Pt 1):759-63. [PubMed]

31. Putet G. Lipid metabolism of the micropremie. Clin Perinatol. 2000;27:57-69.

32. Pluess TT, Hayoz D, Berger MM, et al. Intravenous fish oil blunts the physiological response to endotoxin in healthy subjects. Intensive Care Med. 2007;33(5):789-97. Epub 2007 Mar 22. [PubMed]

33. Wachtler P, Konig W, Senkal M, Kemen M, Koller M. Influence of a total parenteral nutrition enriched with omega-3 fatty acids on leukotriene synthesis of peripheral leukocytes and systemic cytokine levels in patients with major surgery. J Trauma. 1997;42(2):191-8. [PubMed]

34. Singer P, Shapiro H, Theilla M, Anbar R, Singer J, Cohen J. Anti inflammatory properties of omega-3 fatty acids in critical illness: novel mechanisms and an integrative perspective. Intensive Care Med. 2008;34(9):1580-92. doi: 10.1007/s00134-008-1142/4. Epub 2008 May 7. [PubMed]

35. Spear ML, Spear M, Cohen AR, Pereira GR. Effect of fat infusions on platelet concentration in premature infants. JPEN J Parenter Enteral Nutr. 1990;14(2):165-8. [PubMed]

36. Herson VC, Block C, Eisenfeld L, Maderazo EG, Krause PJ. Effects of intravenous fat infusion on neonatal neutrophil and platelet function. JPEN J Parenter Enteral Nutr. 1989;13(6): 620-2. [PubMed]

37. Hageman JR, McCulloch K, Gora P, Olsen E K, Pachman L, Hunt C E. Intralipid alteration in pulmonary prostaglandin metabolism and gas exchange. Crit Care Med. 1983;11(10):794-8. [PubMed]

38. Stegink LD, Freeman JB, Wispe J, Connor WE. Absence of the biochemical symptoms of essential fatty acid deficiency in surgical patients undergoing protein sparing therapy. Am J Clin Nutr. 1977;30(3):388-93. [PubMed]

39. Shenkin A. Trace elements and vitamins in enteral and parenteral nutrition. In: Sobotka L, Allison S, Furst P, Meier R, Soeters P, (Eds). Basics in clinical nutrition. 3rd ed. Prague: Galen. 2004;pp. 169-75.

40. Parenteral Nutrition Multivitamin Product Shortage Considerations The American Society for Parenteral and Enteral Nutrition (ASPEN); 2012.

41. Hardy G, Reilly C. Technical aspects of trace element supplementation. Curr Opin Clin Nutr Metab Care. 1999;2:277-85.

42. Van Gossum A, Neve J. Trace element deficiency and toxicity. Curr Opin Clin Nutr Metab Care. 1998;1(6):499-507. [PubMed]

43. Dickerson RN. Manganese intoxication and parenteral nutrition. Nutrition. 2001;17:689-93.

44. Quaghebeur G, Taylor WJ, Kingsley DP, Fell JM, Reynolds AP, Milla PJ. MRI in children receiving total parenteral nutrition. Neuroradiology. 1996;38(7):680-3. [PubMed]

45. Fell JME, Reynolds AP, Meadows N, et al. Manganese toxicity in children receiving long-term parenteral nutrition. Lancet. 1996;347:1218-21.

46. Bertinet DB, Tinivella M, Balzola FA, de Francesco A, Davini O, Rizzo L, et al. Brain manganese deposition and blood levels in patients undergoing home parenteral nutrition. JPEN J Parenter Enteral Nutr. 2000;24(4):223-7. [PubMed]

47. Masumoto K, Suita S, Taguchi T, Yamanouchi T, Nagano M, Ogita K, et al. Manganese intoxication during intermittent parenteral nutrition: report of two cases. JPEN J Parenter Enteral Nutr. 2001;25(2):95-9. [PubMed]

48. Pluhator-Murton MM, Fedorak RN, Audette RJ, Marriage BJ, Yatscoff RW, Gramlich LM. Trace element contamination of total parenteral nutrition. 1. Contribution of component solutions. JPEN. J Parenter Enteral Nutr. 1999;23(4):222-7. [PubMed]

49. Lovrincevic I, Leung FY, Alfieri MA, et al. Can elevated chromium induce somatopsychic responses? Biol Trace Elem Res. 1996;55(1-2):163-71. [PubMed]

50. Bougle D, Bureau F, Deschrevel G, et al. Chromium and parenteral nutrition in children. J Pediatr Gastroenterol Nutr. 1993;17(1):72-4. [PubMed]

51. Greene HL, Hambidge KM, Schanler R, Tsang RC. Guidelines for the use of vitamins, trace elements, calcium, magnesium, and phosphorus in infants and children receiving total parenteral nutrition: report of the Subcommittee on Pediatric Parenteral Nutrient Requirements from the Committee on Clinical Practice Issues of the American Society for Clin Nutr. Am J Clin Nutr. 1988;48(5):1324-42. [PubMed]

52. Leung FY. Trace elements in parenteral micronutrition. Clin Biochem. 1995;28(6):561-6. [PubMed]

53. National Advisory Group on Standards and Practice Guideline for Parenteral Nutrition. Safe practices for parenteral nutrition formulations. J Parent Ent Nutr. 1998;22:49-66.

54. Marik PE, Pinsky M. Death by parenteral nutrition. Intensive Care Med. 2003;29:867-9.

55. Solomon SM, Kirby DF. The refeeding syndrome: A review. JPEN J Parenter Enteral Nutr. 1990;14(1):90-7. [PubMed]

56. Brooks MJ, Melnik G. The refeeding syndrome: an approach to understanding its complications and preventing its occurrence. Pharmacotherapy. 1995;15(6):713-26. [PubMed]

57. Mirkovic D, Antunovic M, Putic V, Aleksic D. Stability inventigation of total parenteral nutrition admixture prepared in a hospital pharmacy. Vojnosanit Pregl. 2008;65(4):286-90. [PubMed]

58. Telessy IG, Balogh J, Szabo B, Csempesz F, Zelko R. Kinetic stability of all-in-one parenteral nutrition admixtures in the presence of high dose Ca^{2+} additive under clinical application circumstances. Nutrition Journal. 2012;11:32. [PubMed]

59. Simmer K, Rakshasbhuvankar A, Deshpande G. Standardised Parenteral Nutrition. Nutrients. 2013;5(4):1058-70. [PubMed]

60. Deitel M, Friedman KL, Cunnane S, Lea PJ, Chaiet A, Chong J, et al. Emulsion stability in a total nutrient admixture for total parenteral nutrition. J Am Coll Nutr. 1992;11(1):5-10. [PubMed]

61. Sforzini A, Bersani G, Stancari A, Grossi G, Bonoli A, Ceschel GC. Analysis of all-in-one parenteral nutrition admixtures by liquid chromatography and laser diffraction: study of stability. J Pharm Biomed Anal. 2001;24(5-6):1099-109. [PubMed]

62. Driscoll DF. Stability and compatibility assessment techniques for total parenteral nutrition admixtures: setting the bar according to pharmacopeial standards. Currn Opin Clin Nutr Metab Care. 2005;8(3):297-303. [PubMed]

63. Télessy IG, Balogh J, Turmezei J, Dredán J, Zelkó R. Stability assessment of o/w parenteral nutrition emulsions in the presence of high glucose and calcium concentrations. J Pharm Biomed Anal. 2011;56(2):159-64. [PubMed]

64. Allwood MC, Kearney MC. Compatibility and stability of additives in parenteral nutrition admixtures. Nutrition. 1998;14 (9):697-706. [PubMed]

65. Grand A, Jalabert A, Mercier G, Florent M, Hansel-Esteller S, Cambonie G, et al. Influence of Vitamins, Trace Elements, and Iron on Lipid Peroxidation Reactions in All-in-One Admixtures for Neonatal Parenteral Nutrition. JPEN J Parenter Enteral Nutr. 2011;35(4):505-10. [PubMed]

66. Steger PJ, Mühlebach SF. Lipid peroxidation of intravenous lipid emulsions and all-in-one admixtures in total parenteral nutrition bags: the influence of trace elements. JPEN J Parenter Enteral Nutr. 2000;24(1):37-41. [PubMed]

67. Télessy IG, Balogh J, Csempesz F, Szente V, Dredán J, Zelkó R: Comparison of the physicochemical properties of MCT-containing fat emulsion in total nutrient admixture. Colloids Surf B Biointerfaces 2009;72(1):75-9. [PubMed]

68. D'Angio R, Quercia RA, Treiber NK, McLaughlin JC, Klimek JJ. The Growth of Microorganisms in Total Parenteral Nutrition Admixtures. JPEN J Parenter Enteral Nutr. 1987;11(4):394-7. [PubMed]

69. Didier ME, Fischer S, Maki DG. Total Nutrient Admixtures appear safer than Lipid Emulsion alone as Regards Microbial Contamination: Growth Properties of Microbial Pathogens at Room Temperature. JPEN J Parenter Enteral Nutr. 1998;22(5):291-6. [PubMed]

70. Montejo O, Cardona D, Sánchez F, Rigueira AI, Coll P, Bonal J. Microbiological Quality Control Study of "All-In-One" Total Parenteral Nutrition Admixtures. JPEN J Parenter Enteral Nutr. 2000;24(3):183-6. [PubMed]

71. Tang J, Li XH, Wang H, Xiong Y, Mu DZ. Administration of low-dose heparin in total nutrient admixture prevents central venous catheter-related infections in neonates. Zhongguo Dang Dai ErKeZaZhi. 2009;11(12):983-5. [PubMed]

72. Driscoll DF, Bacon MN, Bistrian BR. Effects of In-Line Filtration on Lipid Particle Size Distribution in Total Nutrient Admixtures. JPEN J Parenter Enteral Nutr. 1996;20(4):296-301. [PubMed]

73. Eisner F, Xieker D, Adolph M, Konigstainer A, Glatzle J. Parenteral nutrition via all-in-one admixtures in clinical practice: an approach for handling parenteral nutrition in clinical practice. Nutritional Therapy Metabolism. 2012;30(4):185-96.

Chapter 18

Probiotics in Gastrointestinal Disorders

Juliet Sio Aguilar

INTRODUCTION

Much progress has elapsed since Élie Metchnikoff, a Russian biologist and Nobel Prize winner in Medicine in 1908, first introduced the concept of probiotics. Metchnikoff observed the longevity of Bulgarian peasants who consumed fermented milk foods and proposed that lactobacilli may reduce the putrefactive effects of intestinal metabolism.[1] Subsequently, German physiologist, microbiologist, and physician Professor Alfred Nissle established that one of the key physiologic functions of the human gut microbiota is to defend the gut against exogenous microbial colonization; i.e. colonization resistance.[2] During World War I in 1917, Nissle isolated a strain of *Escherichia coli* (now named *Escherichia coli* Nissle 1917) from human stools and inoculated it into healthy typhoid carriers, which resulted in the eradication of *Salmonella* among these hosts. Since then and more dramatically in recent years, numerous investigations evaluating the use of probiotics in health and disease have evolved.

DEFINITIONS

Originating from the Greek word "biotikos", or that which relates to life, the term **probiotics** refers to viable microorganisms that enhance the intestinal microflora and are touted to confer a wide range of health benefits to the host. As the gut is the largest source of microbial stimulation and that 60–80% of immune system components are present in the gut, focus has been placed on the significance of intestinal microflora in modulating the diseases in man.[3,4]

Prebiotics are non-digestible nutrients that stimulate the growth and activity of intestinal microflora, enhancing the well-being of the host. These include fructo-oligosaccharides (such as inulin and other soluble substrates found in beans and fruits) and galacto-oligosaccharides (produced during the acidic hydrolysis of lactose). As these substrates require the enzymes fructosidase and β-galactosidase for fermentation which are produced only by bifidobacteria and some lactobacilli, the activity of these microflora are indirectly stimulated, benefiting the host.

Postbiotics are non-viable byproducts of microorganisms that exert beneficial activity in the host such as butyrate, a short-chain fatty acid resulting from the catabolism of undigested carbohydrates in the intestine. Such by-products are purported to promote intestinal growth and differentiation and to suppress inflammation through the generation of reactive oxygen species.

Synbiotics are nutrients with synergistic combinations of probiotics and prebiotics.

MECHANISMS OF ACTION OF PROBIOTICS

Various mechanisms have been identified as the modes of action of probiotics on the human host. These actions can be directed toward the pathogens or the host. Those that are aimed at the pathogens include (1) inhibition of the growth and translocation of pathogens through the production of lactic acid and bacteriocin; (2) production of antimicrobial substances like butyric acid and cytokines; (3) competition for binding and receptor sites of enteric pathogens; and (4) reduction of gut pH through lactic acid production. Those that are host-directed are (1) improvement of immune function by stimulating immunomodulatory cells; (2) restoration of normal intestinal flora during antibiotic therapy; (3) regulation of gut motility; (4) production of the enzyme lactase; and (5) reduction in fecal concentrations of enzymes, mutagens, and secondary bile salts which may potentially inhibit colon carcinogenesis.[1]

Characteristics and Dose

Various microorganisms have been recognized to have probiotic properties and are classified under various

Table 18.1: Probiotic species	
Genus	Species
Lactobacillus	L. acidophillus
	L. bulgaricus
	L. casei
	L. fermentum
	L. gasseri
	L. lactis
	L. plantarum
	L. reuteri
	L. rhamnosus GG
	L. sporogenes
Bifidobacterium	B. animalis
	B. bifidum
	B. breve
	B. lactis
	B. longum
	B. infantis
Streptococcus	S. mitis
	S. oralis
	S. sanguinis
	S. subtilis
	S. thermophilus
Saccharomyces	S. boulardii
Bacillus	B. clausii
Enterococcus	E. faecium

genera and species. Table 18.1 lists these microbes that have been purported to exhibit beneficial effects on the host.

The observed effects of probiotics can be strain-specific; thus, different strains of organisms may not necessarily exert the effects uniformly. For instance, the results obtained from studies with one strain may not always be generalized for another species.[3] Moreover, the beneficial effects of probiotics are also dose-dependent; this is noted in acute infectious diarrhea where the impact is greater for doses 10^{10} to 10^{11} colony-forming units per day.[2]

▮ STRAINS WITH DOCUMENTED EFFICACY

The benefits of probiotics in human health lie in the potential to enhance treatment of diseases and minimize the occurrence of diseases through prevention. The clinical applications in gastrointestinal disorders where its efficacy has been investigated include acute and persistent diarrhea; antibiotic-associated diarrhea; necrotizing enterocolitis; *Helicobacter pylori* eradication; functional bowel disorders, such as infantile colic, functional constipation, and irritable bowel syndrome; and inflammatory bowel diseases.

Acute Diarrhea

The clinical setting with the most extensive studies on probiotics in human health is acute diarrhea. Because diarrhea remains to be a leading cause of morbidity and mortality in many developing countries, and recurrent episodes of diarrhea especially during the first two years of life impact negatively on physical growth and cognitive function,[5,6] strategies to improve treatment and prevent diarrhea have been a subject of extensive research investigations, including the use of probiotics. Table 18.2 summarizes the various systematic reviews on the use of probiotics in the treatment of acute diarrhea.

Various systematic reviews on the use of probiotics in acute diarrhea have shown a consistent reduction in the duration of diarrhea by an average of one day compared to placebo. *Lactobacillus* GG however has been demonstrated to have the most consistent results.[9] The relative risk for developing prolonged diarrhea of more than 7 days has also been observed to be 0.25.[10,11] The number of individuals needed to treat (NNT) to achieve this benefit is five. No effect has been demonstrated with regards stool volume and frequency.

Among Turkish children 5 months to 5 years old with rotavirus gastroenteritis, *Bifidobacterium lactis* has been demonstrated to significantly reduce the duration of diarrhea when compared with *Saccharomyces boulardii* or placebo.[12] The mean duration of diarrhea for the comparative groups were 4.1 ± 1.3 days for *B. lactis*, 6.6 ± 1.7 days for *S. boulardii*, and 7.0 ± 1.6 days for ORS alone. A head-to-head comparison of four different probiotic strains and placebo given to Italian children 3 to 36 months with non-hospitalized acute diarrhea substantiates that no two probiotics are exactly alike in their clinical impact.[13] The mean duration of diarrhea was significantly shorter for the children given *L. rhamnosus* (78.5 hrs) and mixed strains of *L. delbreuckii* var *bulgaricus*, *S. thermophilus*, *L. acidophilus*, and *B. bifidum* (70.0 hrs) in comparison to those who were on ORS alone (115 hrs); p<0.001. The number of stools passed per day was also significantly lower in children given *L. rhamnosus* and mixed strains compared with the plain ORS group; p<0.001. No differences in the primary outcomes were observed for those children who received *S. boulardii* and *B. clausii*. No effect on the duration of vomiting, fever, and hospitalization rate was noted for any of the probiotic strains.

Based on recent evidence globally, the current recommendations of international societies such as European Society of Pediatric Gastroenterology, Hepatology and Nutrition (ESPGHAN) and World Gastroenterology Organization (WGO) Global Recommendations state Level IA evidence for efficacy of two probiotic strains in the treatment of acute diarrhea— *Lactobacillus GG* and *Saccharomyces boulardii*.[14,15]

Table 18.2: Meta-analyses on the efficacy of probiotics in acute diarrhea

Authors	Participants	Type of probiotics	Outcome
Allen SJ, et al. (2010)[7]	63 RCT/quasi-RCT studies (56 trials in infants and young children); n=8,014	Varied	• Reduced duration • Mean diff: 25 hours; (16–34 hours) • Diarrhea lasting >4 days • Risk ratio 0.41 (0.32–0.53)
Huang JS, et al. (2002)[8]	18 studies (<5 years)	Varied	• Reduced duration • Random-effects pooled estimate: • 0.8 day (-1.1 to -0.6); p<0.001
Szajewska H, Mrukowicz JZ (2001)[9]	DBRCT in infants and children	Varied (LGG with consistent results)	• Reduced duration • Weighted mean diff (WMD): -24.8 (-31.8 to -17.9)] Diarrhea lasting >3 days • Pooled risk: Fixed-effect model: 0.43 (0.34–0.53) Random-effect model: 0.40 (0.28–0.57)
Szajewska H, et al. (2007)[10]	8 RCTs in children; n=988	*Lactobacillus GG* (for 2–5 days; one ad libitum)	• No effect on stool volume and frequency • Significant reduction in duration WMD all cases:-1.1day (-1.9 to -0.3) • RVGE:-2.1 days (-3.6 to -0.6) • Diarrhea >7 days • RR: 0.25 (0.09–0.75) • Duration of hospitalization, WMD: -0.58 day (-0.8 to -0.4)
Szajewska H, et al. (2007)[11]	5 RCTs in children; n=619	*Saccharomyces boulardii* (for 4–6 days)	• Reduced duration WMD: -1.1 day (-1.3 to -0.8)] • Diarrhea >7days • RR: 0.25 (0.08–0.83); NNT 5 (3–20)

Abbreviations: RR, relative risk; WMD, weighted mean difference; NNT, numbers needed to treat; RVGE, rotavirus gastroenteritis.

Table 18.3: Meta-analyses on the use of probiotics in the prevention of diarrhea

Authors	Participants	Type of probiotics	Outcome

Szajewska H, et al. (2011)[18]	3 RCTs in children (1-month to 18 years)	*Lactobacillus rhamnosus GG*	• Lower rates of diarrhea:
			  – RR:0.37 (0.23–0.59)
			  – Symptomatic RVGE
			  – RR:0.49 (0.28–0.86)

Sazawal S, et al. (2006)[19]	34 RCTs (all in developed countries; most in healthcare setting than community-based)	*Lactobacillus rhamnosus GG, L. acidophilus, L. bulgaricus, S. boulardii* used singly or in combination	• Reduction in incidence:
			• Acute diarrhea
			  – Children: 57% (35–71%)
			  – Adults: 26% (7–49%)
			  – Travellers'diarrhea
			  – 8% (-6 to 25%)
			  – Protective effect
			  – not strain-specific

A large community-based intervention study in Kolkata, India, using the probiotic strain *Lactobacillus casei Shirota* for prevention of diarrheal disease showed a beneficial effect.[16]

Persistent Diarrhea

The impact of probiotics on the treatment of persistent diarrhea has been reviewed in a meta-analysis of four randomized controlled trials of 464 subjects.[17] Using varied strains of probiotics, the mean duration was reduced by 4 days (3.43-4.61 days) with stool frequency observed to be reduced in two studies and hospitalization shorter in one study. No adverse effects were documented. Because of the limited number of subjects studied, these findings should be interpreted with caution until further studies are available.

Diarrhea Prevention

Prevention of diarrhea through the use of probiotics has also been the subject of numerous investigations.

Table 18.3 tabulates two meta-analyses summarizing the relevance of prophylactic probiotics use in diarrhea.

The use of probiotics has been associated with a reduction in the incidence of acute diarrhea in children by 57–63% and a reduction in the risk of symptomatic RVGE by 50%. The strains investigated were primarily from the genus *Lactobacillus*.

Extensive studies have also been conducted on the relevance of probiotics in the prevention of antibiotic-associated diarrhea (AAD). Table 18.4 summarizes the significant findings. Despite great heterogeneity in strains, dose, and duration of administration of probiotics, an overall protective effect has been established with the use. A reduction in the incidence of AAD has been demonstrated to be 35–65%. The NNT to effect the desired benefit is seven. High doses of probiotics of at least 5 billion CFU/day have been observed to be more efficacious. Strain-specific efficacy needs to be further investigated.

Necrotizing Enterocolitis

Necrotizing enterocolitis (NEC), a leading cause of neonatal morbidity and mortality worldwide, occurs in 2–22% of very low birth weight infants weighing 1,500 g and below and carries a high mortality rate of 20–30%.[23,24] Survivors are at risk for long-term sequelae such as impairment in physical growth and neurodevelopmental capacities, short bowel syndrome, among others. The predisposing factors for the development of NEC include immaturity of the gastrointestinal tract with decreased intestinal barrier function and gut motility and a predilection for inflammation; enteral feeding; and abnormal bacterial colonization due to prolonged antimicrobial treatment, decrease in commensal bacteria, and increase in pathogenic organisms such as *Escherichia coli*, *Klebsiella*, *Clostridium perfringens*, *Staphylococcus epidermidis*, and *Rotavirus*. It is hypothesized that probiotics can promote the acquisition of commensal microbiota in the host, with prebiotics enhancing the growth of probiotic microorganisms and postbiotics mimicking the function or activity of the probiotic microorganisms.[24]

The efficacy of probiotics in improving neonatal outcomes among preterms has been difficult to ascertain owing to the variability in study designs, which have involved single or combination of agents with doses ranging from 10^5 to 10^{10} colony-forming units per day. Moreover, varying periods of initiation and supplementation have been tried, with initiation typically within a week after birth to more than a month of age. Two recently published meta-analyses on the probiotics supplementation among preterm infants have demonstrated the beneficial effects with prophylactic use. A relative risk of 0.35 [95% confidence

Table 18.4: Meta-analyses on the use of probiotics in the prevention of antibiotic-associated diarrhea			
Authors	*Participants*	*Type of Probiotics*	*Outcome*
Johnson BC, et al. (2011)[20]	16 RCTs in children (0–18 years); n=3432	*Bacillus* spp, *Bifidobacterium* spp, *Lactobacillus* spp, *Lactococcus spp*, *Leuonostoc cremoris*, *Saccharomyces* spp, *Streptococcus* spp; singly or combined	Great heterogeneity in strain, dose and duration but with overall protective effect For high dose trials (>5B cfu/day): NNT=7 (6–10)
Sazawal S, et al. (2006)[19]	34 RCTs (all in developed countries; most in healthcare setting than community-based)	*Lactobacillus rhamnosus* GG, *L. acidophilus*, *L. bulgaricus*, *S. boulardii* *used singly* or in combination	Antibiotic-associated diarrhea 52% (95% CI: 35–65%)
Kale-Pradhan PB, et al. (2010)[21]	10 RCTs in children and adults; n=1862	• Lactobacillus • Dose: 2 x 109 to 4 x 1010 CFU/day while on antibiotics; follow-up period 2 days to 3 months	• Reduction in risk • RR: 0.35 (0.19–0.67) • Subgroup analysis in children not significant
D'Souza AL, et al. (2002)[22]	9 RCTs	*S. boulardii* *Lactobacillus spp*	• Reduction in risk • OR: 0.39 (0.25–0.62) • OR: 0.34 (0.19–0.61

Abbreviations: RCT, randomized controlled trials; OR, odds ratio.

interval (CI): 0.23–0.55] for the development of NEC has been documented when probiotics were administered within 10 days of life and for a period of at least 7 days.[25] Another published meta-analysis noted that the use of *Bifidobacteria sp.* is associated with a lower incidence of NEC with a pooled relative risk of 0.30 (95% CI: 0.16-0.58) compared with *Lactobacillus sp.* alone [pooled RR of 0.37 (95% CI: 0.19-0.73)] or in combination with *Bifidobacteria sp.* [pooled RR of 0.33 (95% CI: 0.19-0.58)].[26] The impact on other outcome variables such as sepsis and mortality has not been as dramatic as that seen in NEC. A reduction in mortality was observed only with the use of *Lactobacillus sp.*, used singly [pooled RR of 0.61 (95% CI: 0.38–0.97)] or in combination with *Bifidobacteria sp.* [pooled RR of 0.47 (95% CI: 0.26–0.87)]. No beneficial effect was seen for the reduction in sepsis.[26]

Clinical studies on the use of prebiotics (such as fructo-oligosaccharides and galacto-oligosaccharides) and postbiotics are forthcoming.

Helicobacter pylori Eradication

Helicobacter pylori, a major cause of chronic gastritis and peptic ulcer disease, has long been established as a definite carcinogen for stomach cancer. High eradication failure rates in children (more than 30%), primarily due poor drug compliance, antibiotic resistance, and occurrence of side effects during treatment, have prompted investigations on the use of probiotics as an adjunct in the treatment of *H. pylori* infection. Improved eradication treatment and reduction in gastrointestinal side effects have been identified as outcome variables in these studies.

In a meta-analysis of 5 randomized controlled trials of 1,307 patients (90 of whom were children) using *S. boulardii* in addition to standard triple therapy, increased eradication rate [RR=1.13 (95% CI: 1.05–1.21)],

albeit minimally, and reduced risk of treatment-related adverse effects [overall: 0.46 (95% CI: 0.3-0.7); diarrhea: 0.47 (95% CI: 0.32–0.69)] were observed when compared with placebo.[27] In another systematic review of 10 trials (963 patients) examining the effect of fermented milk-based probiotic products, a pooled odds ratio of 1.91 (95% CI: 0.32-0.69) was observed for eradication by intention-to-treat analysis in the treatment group compared with the control group, with a pooled risk difference of 0.10 (95% CI: 0.05-0.15; p<0.0001). The pooled odds ratio for adverse effects was 0.51 (95% CI: 0.10–2.57; p=0.41) with significant heterogeneity by Cochran's Q of 68.5 (p<0.0001).[28]

A comparison of two RCTs on the use of mixed probiotic strains (*Lactobacillus spp.*, *Streptococcus thermophilus*, *Bifidobacterium spp.*) for the eradication of *H. pylori* is depicted in Table 18.5. Lower rates of therapy-related side effects, but not of eradication rates, following its adjunctive administration have been consistently demonstrated.[29,30]

With the promising benefits of probiotics on the eradication of *H. pylori* infection, it is anticipated that the progression of the disease to chronic gastritis and gastric cancer would be less likely.

Infantile Colic

Infantile colic, a common problem affecting 10–30% of infants globally, usually poses grave distress to both the infants and their parents or caregivers.[31] Excessive paroxysmal crying that occurs more commonly in the evenings can also predispose babies to the risk for child abuse by tired and exasperated caregivers. Because its cause can be multifactorial, the underlying cause, particularly if organic, warrants prompt investigation.

One of the purported pathophysiologic mechanisms for infantile colic relates to gut hormones particularly motilin. Motilin is believed to trigger hyperperistalsis

Table 18.5: RCTs on the use of probiotics in children for *H. pylori* eradication

Authors	Participants	Type of Probiotics	Outcome
Khodadad A, et al. (2013)[29]	DBRPCT in children (3-14 yrs; mean = 9.09 years); n=66	*Lactobacillus acidophilus, L. rhamnosus, L. bulgaricus, L. casei, Streptococcus thermophilus, Bifidobacterium infantis* and *breve*	• Rate of eradication higher in probiotic group OR=4.37 (95% CI: 1.07–17.62; p=0.04) • Lower rate of nausea/vomiting (6.1% vs. 27.3%; p=0.02) and diarrhea (6.1% vs. 24.2%; p=0.039) in probiotic group during treatment
Tolone S, et al. (2012)[30]	RCT (mean age of 8.3 + 3.4 years); n=68 histopathologically proven *H. pylori* infection	*Lactobacillus plantarum, L. reuterii, L. casei* subsp rhamnosus, *B. infantis* and *longum; L. salivarius, L. acidophilus, Strep thermophilus, L. sporogenes* Strength: 19 x 10^9	Rate of eradication similar: • in probiotic (82.3%) vs. control (76.4%), p=0.1 • Lower rates of epigastric pain (17.6% vs. 5.8%), nausea (8.8% vs. 2.9%), vomiting (5.8% vs. 0) and diarrhea (23.5% vs. 0); all (p<0.05)

and consequently abdominal pain. Recent epidemiologic studies have implicated exposure to cigarette smoking as an underlying cause for infantile colic. Increased levels of plasma and intestinal motilin have been documented with smoking, and high levels of intestinal motilin have been associated with increased risk for infantile colic.[31]

Randomized, double-blind, placebo-controlled trials using *Lactobacillus reuteri*, administered orally at 5 drops 10^8 colony-forming units) once daily 30 minutes before feeding (in the morning for three weeks, have reported promising results for colicky breastfed infants.[32,33] Crying time at the end of a 3-week intervention was significantly reduced by 69% and sustained at 78% reduction a week after the probiotic was discontinued.[32] The response rate to treatment was significantly higher in the treatment group than the placebo group [RR 4.3 (95% CI: 2.3–8.7) at day 14; RR 2.7 (95% CI: 1.85–4.1) at day 21; and RR 2.5 (95% CI: 1.8–3.75) at day 28]. The number of responders (defined as 50% reduction in crying from baseline) was significantly higher in the *L. reuteri* group compared with the placebo group on day 7 (20 vs. 8; p=0.006), day 14 (24 vs. 13; p=0.007), and day 21 (24 vs. 15; p=0.036). A significant increase in fecal *Lactobacilli* (p=0.002) and a reduction in fecal *Escherichia coli* were noted in the *L. reuteri* group (p=0.001).[33]

As the experience on *L. reuteri* in infantile colic is limited with small study sizes (n=80 for Szajewska et al. and n=46 for Savino et al.), further studies are necessary to confirm these encouraging preliminary results.

Functional Constipation

Chronic constipation, a common condition in developed countries, is fast gaining grounds in the developing countries. Functional constipation, as defined in the Rome III classification, exists when two or more of the following features are present in a child with a developmental age of at least 4 years, with weekly symptoms for at least two months: two or fewer bowel movements per week; at least one episode of fecal incontinence per week; history of excessive volitional stool retention or stool withholding; history of painful or difficult bowel movements; history of large stools obstructing the toilet; and presence of large fecal mass in the rectum.[34] Because only 60% of children with constipation respond to conventional treatment, this drawback has opened the horizon to other treatment options.[35]

Growing interest in the use of probiotics in functional constipation has been premised on the fact that colonic microbiota impacts on the motility of the colon through enhancement of an acidic milieu.[36] Probiotics such as *Bifidobacteria spp.* and *Lactobacillus spp.* can effect lowering of the colonic pH through the production of lactic acid, acetic acid, and other similar acids, which then promotes colonic peristalsis and shortens transit time.

Current studies on its use among constipated children are few. In a systematic review of five RCTs, two of which involved children, findings have been dichotomous.[37]

Table 18.6: Outcome on the use of *L. casei rhamnosus* Lcr35 in 45 constipated children				
Parameter	L. casei rhamnosus Lcr35	Magnesium oxide (MgO)	Mean difference (95% CI)	p
Abdominal pain (times)	1.9 ± 1.6	6.7 ± 3.3	-4.8 (-6.6 to -3)	0.03*
Change in appetite	0.7 ± 0.8	0.7 ± 0.6	0 (-0.6 to 0.6)	0.81
Defecation frequency (times/day)	0.57 ± 0.17	0.37 ± 0.1	0.2 (0.1 to 0.3)	0.03*
Hard stools passed (%)	22.4 ± 14.7	75.5 ± 6.1	-53 (-63 to -43)	0.01*
Use of glycerin enema (times)	1.6 ± 1.9	4.0 ± 2.1	-2.4 (-4 to -0.8)	0.04*
Use of lactulose (times)	4.4 ± 3.6	6.2 ± 3.8	-1.8 (-4.7 to 1.1)	0.66
Fecal soiling (times)	2.1 ± 3.8	2.7 ± 1.4	-0.6 (-3.2 to 2)	0.95
Treatment success (>3 spontaneous BMs per week with no fecal soiling at end of 4 weeks)	14/18	1/9	RR = 7 (1.1 to 45)	0.01*

Abbreviations: (*) - significant findings
(*Source*: Bu LN, Chang MH, Ni YH, et al. Pediatr Int. 2007;35)

The trial using *L. casei rhamnosus* Lcr35 demonstrated a significant increase in defecation frequency, reduction in the proportion of patients passing hard stools, decrease in abdominal pain, and reduction in the use of glycerin enema as shown in Table 18.6.[38]

The other study using *Lactobacillus* GG as an adjunct to lactulose in the treatment of 84 children (2–16 years) with constipation did not show any significant findings.[39] On the other hand, a preliminary study using a probiotic mixture of *Bifidobacteria bifidum, B. infantis, B. longum, Lactobacillus casei, L. plantarum,* and *L. rhamnosus* among 20 constipated children (4–16 years) demonstrated favorable outcomes such as increased frequency of defecation, decreased episodes of fecal incontinence, and decrease in abdomen pain.[35] Further studies are needed to further elucidate on the use of probiotics in functional constipation.[40]

Irritable Bowel Syndrome

Irritable bowel syndrome (IBS) is defined as recurring abdominal discomfort or pain in the absence of an anatomic, inflammatory, metabolic, or neoplastic process, that is associated with two or more of the following, occurring at least 25% of the time at least once a week for a period of two months: (1) onset associated with a change in stool frequency; (2) onset associated with a change in stool appearance; and (3) improvement with defecation.[34] Current evidence suggests that the gut microbiome is altered in patients with IBS, thus affecting gut secretion and motility.[41] Because alterations in the immune cell profile have also been observed in these patients and that probiotic intake can change the blood cytokine levels and fecal microflora, studies have been undertaken to investigate the efficacy of probiotics in IBS.[42] The results of a meta-analysis of 10 studies that evaluated outcome variables such as pain, distension, stool frequency, stool consistency, flatulence, straining, and urgency, are summarized in Table 18.7. Notable are the findings that pain, distention, and flatulence are significantly reduced in IBS patients following treatment with probiotics.

No impact on stool frequency and consistency, straining, and urgency was observed. It appears that the

Table 18.7: Efficacy of probiotics in the treatment of irritable bowel syndrome			
Outcome variable and authors	*No. of participants*	*Type of probiotics*	*Overall estimates standardized mean differences (95% CI)*
Pain			
Kim et al, 2005; Kajander et al, 2005; Kim et al, 2003	154	*Bifidobacterium breve*	-0.34 (-0.66; -0.02)
Zeng et al, 2008; Drouault-Holowacz et al, 2008; Guyonnet et al, 2007; Kim et al, 2003	202	*Bifidobacterium longum*	-0.48 (-0.91; -0.06)
Simrén et al, 2010; Williams et al, 2009; Zeng et al, 2008; Drouault-Holowacz et al, 2008; Kim et al, 2005; Kim et al, 2005; Kim et al, 2003 Kim et al, 2003 Kim et al, 2003	328	*Lactobacillus acidophilus*	-0.31 (-0.61; -0.01)
Distension			
Kim et al, 2005; Kajander et al, 2005; Kim et al, 2003	154	*Bifidobacterium breve*	-0.45 (-0.77; -0.13)
Kim et al, 2005; Kim et al, 2003	73	*Bifidobacterium infantis; Lactobacillus casei; Lactobacillus plantarum*	-0.53 (-1.00; -0.06)
Flatulence			
Kim et al, 2005; Kajander et al, 2005; Kim et al, 2003	154	*Bifidobacterium breve*	-0.42 (-0.75; -0.10)
Kim et al, 2005; Kim et al, 2003	73	*Bifidobacterium infantis; Lactobacillus casei; Lactobacillus plantarum*	-0.60 (-1.07; -0.13)
Zeng et al, 2008; Kim et al, 2005; Kim et al, 2003	102	*Bifidobacterium longum; Lactobacillus acidophilus; Lactobacillus bulgarius; Streptococcus salivarius ssp. thermophilus*	-0.61 (-1.01; -0.21)

(*Source*: Ortiz-Lucas M, Tobias A, Saz P, Sebastian JJ. 2013;39)
All studies had heterogeneity index of 0.0, except for those involving *B. longum* (I2=49.5) and *L. acidophilus* (I2=42.3))

efficacy of probiotics in the treatment of IBS patients may be species-specific.

Inflammatory Bowel Diseases

The incidence of inflammatory bowel diseases (IBD) has been observed to be on the rise especially in developed countries in the recent years. While ulcerative colitis and Crohn's disease are immunologic disorders that have a genetic basis, not all individuals with the genetic defect develop the disease. It is purported that other causes such as environmental factors influence its occurrence. With a shift to a predominantly high-fat, high-carbohydrate diet, such dietary modification provokes a change in the gut microbiome of the genetically-susceptible host, and brings about a reduction in commensals and an increase in pathogenic organisms. The alteration in the gut flora leads to an increased exposure to harmful bacterial products (such as H_2S) and a decreased exposure to beneficial bacterial by-products (such as short-chain fatty acids), ultimately resulting in intestinal inflammation.[43] The use of probiotics has been hypothesized to be beneficial in IBD through restoration of protective commensal species such as *Faecalibacterium prausnitzii* and *Clostridium spp.*[41]

Clinical studies on the efficacy of probiotics in IBD have so far yielded conflicting results.[44] The reports for ulcerative colitis have been encouraging as beneficial effects in inducing and maintaining remission have been observed using a combination of *Lactobacillus*, *Bifidobacterium*, and *Streptococcus* probiotic species and *Escherichia coli* Nissle 1917.[41,45] However, no consistent effects have been documented for the treatment and prevention of relapses in Crohn's disease.[41,44]

REFERENCES

1. Ötles S, Çagındı Ö, Akçiçek E. Probiotics and health. Asian Pac J Cancer Prev. 2003;4:369-72.
2. Wolvers D, Antoine JM, Myllyluoma E, Schrezenmeir J, Szajewska H, Rijkers GT. Guidance for substantiating the evidence of beneficial effects of probiotics: prevention and management of infections by probiotics. J Nutr. 2010;140:698S-712S.
3. Minocha A. Probiotics for preventive health. Nutr Clin Pract. 2009;24:227-41.
4. Gill HS, Guarner F. Probiotics and human health: a clinical perspective. Postgrad Med J. 2004;80:516-26.
5. Niehaus MD, Moore SR, Patrick PD, Derr LL, Lorntz B, Lima AA, Guerrant RL. Early childhood diarrhea is associated with diminished cognitive function 4 to 7 years later in children in a Northeast Brazilian shantytown. Am J. Trop Med Hyg. 2002; 66:590-3.
6. Moore SR, Lima AAM, Conaway MR, Schorling JB, Soares AM, et al. Early childhood diarrhea and helminthiasis associate with long-term linear growth faltering. Int J Epidemiol. 2001;30:1457-64.
7. Allen SJ, Martinez EG, Gregorio GV, Dans LF. Probiotics for treating acute infectious diarrhea. Cochrane Database Syst Rev 2010 Nov 10;(11):CD003048.
8. Huang JS, Bousvaros A, Lee JW, Diaz A, Davidson EJ. Efficacy of probiotic use in acute diarrhea in children: a meta-analysis. Dig Dis Sci. 2002;47:2625-34.
9. Szajewska H, Mrukowicz JZ. Probiotics in the treatment and prevention of acute infectious diarrhea in infants and children: a systematic review of published randomized, double-blind, placebo-controlled trials. J Pediatr Gastroenterol Nutr. 2001;33 Suppl 2:S17-25.
10. Szajewska H, Skórka A, Ruszczyński M, Gieruszczak-Białek D. Meta-analysis: Lactobacillus GG for treating acute diarrhoea in children. Aliment Pharmacol Ther. 2007;25:871-81.
11. Szajewska H, Skórka A, Dylag M. Meta-analysis: Saccharomyces boulardii for treating acute diarrhoea in children. Aliment Pharmacol Ther. 2007;25:257-64.
12. Erdoğan O, Tanyeri B, Torun E, Gönüllü E, Arslan H, Erenberk U, Oktem F. The comparition of the efficacy of two different probiotics in rotavirus gastroenteritis in children. J Trop Med. 2012;2012:787240. doi: 10.1155/2012/787240. Epub 2012 Jun 19.
13. Canani RB, Cirillo P, Terrin G, Cesarano L, Spagnuolo MI, De Vincenzo A, et al. Probiotics for treatment of acute diarrhoea in children: randomised clinical trial of five different preparations. BMJ. 2007 Aug 18;335(7615):340.
14. Guarino A (Coordinator), Ashkenazi S, Gendrel D, Lo Vecchio A, Shamir R, Szajewska H. European Society for Pediatric Gastroenterology, Hepatology and Nutrition/European Society for Pediatric Infectious Diseases. Evidence-Based Guidelines for the Management of Acute Gastroenteritis in Children in Europe: Update 2014. JPGN. 2014;59:132-52.
15. World Gastroenterology Organisation Global Guidelines Probiotics and Prebiotics. World Gastroenterology Organization. 2011;1-28.
16. Sur D, Manna B, Niyogi SK, Ramamurthy T, Palit A, Nomoto K, et al. Role of probiotic in preventing acute diarrhoea in children: a community-based, randomized, double-blind, placebo-controlled field trial in an urban slum. Epidemiol Infect. 2011;139:919-26.
17. Bernaola AG, Bada Mancilla CA, Carreazo Pariasca NY, Rojas Galarza RA. Probiotics for treating persistent diarrhoea in children. Cochrane Database Syst Rev 2013 Aug 20;8:CD007401. doi: 10.1002/14651858.CD007401.pub3.
18. Szajewska H, Wanke M, Patro B. Meta-analysis: the effects of Lactobacillus rhamnosus GG supplementation for the prevention of healthcare-associated diarrhoea in children. Aliment Pharmacol Ther. 2011;34:1079-87.
19. Sazawal S, Hiremath G, Dhingra U, Malik P, Deb S, Black RE. Efficacy of probiotics in prevention of acute diarrhoea: a meta-analysis of masked, randomised, placebo-controlled trials. Lancet Infect Dis. 2006;6:374-82.
20. Johnston BC, Goldenberg JZ, Vandvik PO, Sun X, Guyatt GH. Probiotics for the prevention of pediatric antibiotic-associated diarrhea. Cochrane Database Syst Rev. 2011 Nov 9; 11:CD004827. doi: 10.1002/14651858. CD004827.pub3.

21. Kale-Pradhan PB, Jassal HK, Wilhelm SM. Role of Lactobacillus in the prevention of antibiotic-associated diarrhea: a meta-analysis. Pharmacotherapy. 2010;30:119-26.

22. D›Souza AL, Rajkumar C, Cooke J, Bulpitt CJ. Probiotics in prevention of antibiotic associated diarrhoea: meta-analysis. BMJ. 2002;324(7350):1361.

23. Bernardo WM, Aires FT, Carneiro RM, de Sá FP, Rullo VEV, Burns DA. Effectiveness of probiotics in the prophylaxis of necrotizing enterocolitis in preterm neonates: a systematic review and meta-analysis. J Pediatr (Rio J).2013;89:18-24.

24. Patel RM, Denning PW. Therapeutic use of prebiotics, probiotics and postbiotics to prevent necrotizing enterocolitis. What is the current evidence? Clin Perinatol. 2013;40:11-25.

25. Deshpande G, Rao S, Patole S, Bulsara M. Updated meta-analysis of probiotics for preventing necrotizing enterocolitis in preterm neonates. Pediatrics. 2010;125:921-30.

26. Wang Q, Dong J, Zhu Y. Probiotic supplement reduces risk of necrotizing enterocolitis and mortality in preterm very low-birth-weight infants: an updated meta-analysis of 20 randomized, controlled trials. J Pediatr Surg. 2012;47:241-8.

27. Szajewska H, Horvath A, Piwowarczyk A. Meta-analysis: the effects of *Saccharomyces boulardii* supplementation on Helicobacter pylori eradication rates and side effects during treatment. Aliment Pharmacol Ther. 2010;32:1069-79.

28. Sachdeva A, Nagpal J. Effect of fermented milk-based probiotic preparations on *Helicobacter pylori* eradication: a systematic review and meta-analysis of randomized-controlled trials. Eur J Gastroenterol Hepatol. 2009;21:45-53.

29. Khodadad A, Farahmand F, Najafi M, Shoaran M. Probiotics for the treatment of pediatric *Helicobacter pylori* infection: a randomized double blind clinical trial. Iran J Pediatr. 2013;23:79-84.

30. Tolone S, Pellino V, Vitaliti G, Lanzafame A, Tolone C. Evaluation of *Helicobacter pylori* eradication in pediatric patients by triple therapy plus lactoferrin and probiotics compared to triple therapy alone. Ital J Pediatr. 2012;38:63.

31. Kheir AEM. Infantile colic, facts and fiction. Ital J Pediatrics 2012; 38:34.

32. Szajewska H, Gyrczuk E, Horvath A. *L. reuteri* DSM 17938 for the management of infantile colic in breastfed infants: a randomized, double-blind, placebo-controlled trial. J Pediatr. 2013;162:257-62.

33. Savino F, Cordisco L, Tarasco V, Palumeri E, Calabrese R, Oggero R, Roos S, Matteuzzi D. *Lactobacillus reuteri* DSM 17938 in infantile colic: a randomized, double-blind, placebo-controlled trial. Pediatrics 2010; 126:e526-33.

34. Rasquin A, Di Lorenzo C, Forbes D, Guiraldes E, Hyams JS, Staiano A, Walker LS. Childhood functional gastrointestinal disorders: Child/adolescent. Gastroenterology. 2006;130:1527-37.

35. Bekkali N, Bongers MEJ, Van den Berg MM, Liem O, Benninga MA. The role of a probiotics mixture in the treatment of childhood constipation: a pilot study. Nutr J. 2007;6:17.

36. Picard C, Fioramonti J, Francois A, Robinson T, Neant F, Matuchansky C. Bifidobacteria as probiotic agents – physiological effects and clinical benefits. Aliment Pharmacol Ther. 2005;22: 495-512.

37. Chmielewska A, Szajewska H. Systematic review of randomised controlled trials: probiotics for functional constipation. World J Gastroenterol. 2010; 16: 69-75.

38. Bu LN, Chang MH, Ni YH, Chen HL, Cheng CC. *Lactobacillus casei rhamnosus* Lcr35 in children with chronic constipation. Pediatr Int. 2007;49:485-90.

39. Banaszkiewicz A, Szajewska H. Ineffectiveness of Lactobacillus GG as an adjunct to lactulose for the treatment of constipation in children: a double-blind, placebo-controlled randomized control trial. J Pediatr. 2005;146:364-69.

40. Tabbers MM, Boluyt N, Berger MY, Benninga MA. Nonpharmacologic treatments for childhood constipation: systematic review. Pediatrics. 2011;128:753-61.

41. Sanders MA, Guarner F, Guerrant R, Holt PR, Quigley EMM, Sartor RB, Sherman PM, Mayer EA. An update on the use and investigation of probiotics in health and disease. Gut 2013;62: 787-96.

42. Ortiz-Lucas M, Tobias A, Saz P, Sebastian JJ. Effect of probiotic species on irritable bowel syndrome symptoms: A bring up to date meta-analysis. Rev Esp Enferm Dig (Madrid). 2013;105:19-36.

43. Leone V, Chang EB, Devkota S. Diet, microbes, and host genetics: the perfect storm in inflammatory bowel diseases. J Gastroenterol. 2013;48:315-21.

44. Dylag K, Hubalewska-Mazgaj M, Surmiak M, Szmyd J, Brzozowski T. Probiotics in the mechanism of protection against gut inflammation and therapy of gastrointestinal disorders. Curr Pharm Des. 2013 Jun 10. [Epub ahead of print].

45. Schultz M, Butt G. E. coli Nissle 1917 in the treatment of Inflammatory Bowel Disease. Practical Gastroenterol. 2010;34:11-9.

Section 3

Hepatology

Anatomy, Development and Physiology of the Hepatobiliary System

Dhanasekhar Kesavelu

Anatomy, development and physiology of the hepatobiliary system are include:
- Functional anatomy: Sectors and segments
- Anatomy of the biliary tract and bile duct epithelial cells
- Development of the liver and bile ducts
- Liver physiology including hepatocellular function
- Hepatocyte death and regeneration.

INTRODUCTION

The liver is the largest gland in the body. The liver performs major actions such as bile secretion and various other metabolic functions. It is also called as 'hepar' from which the adjective 'hepatic' originates which names the structures that link the liver.

It is located in the right hypochondrium and the majority of it is widely covered by the ribs and diaphragm. An average adult male has a liver weighing 1600 grams and female adult around 1300 grams. It is reddish brown in color and is friable in live subjects.

The understanding of the developmental anatomy and physiology of the liver and biliary tree offers the clinician a good insight into the origin of their patient's diseases and disorders but gives a good understanding about future therapies.

FUNCTIONAL ANATOMY: SECTORS AND SEGMENTS

The liver is divided into the right and left functional lobes and these do not correspond or relate to the anatomical lobes and this is based on the intrahepatic distribution of hepatic artery, portal vein and the biliary ducts.[1]

The right lobe is further subdivided into anterior and posterior segments and the left lobe into medial and lateral segments. Hence the livers four segments are as follows:[2]
- Right anterior
- Right posterior
- Left lateral
- Left medial

Liver anatomy can be described using two different aspects: morphological anatomy and functional anatomy. The traditional morphological anatomy is based on the external appearance of the liver and does not show the internal features of vessels and biliary ducts branching, which are of obvious importance in hepatic surgery. In 1957, C Couinaud divided the liver into eight functionally independent segments.[3]

Couinaud Classification (Fig. 19.1)

The Couinaud classification of liver anatomy divides the liver into eight functionally independent segments. Each segment has its own vascular inflow, outflow and biliary drainage.[2] In the center of each segment there is a branch of the portal vein, hepatic artery and bile duct. In the periphery of each segment there is vascular outflow through the hepatic veins.

Right hepatic vein divides the right lobe into anterior and posterior segments.

Middle hepatic vein divides the liver into right and left lobes. This plane runs from the inferior vena cava to the gallbladder fossa.

Left hepatic vein divides the left lobe into a medial and lateral part.

Portal vein divides the liver into upper and lower segments. The left and right portal veins branch superiorly and inferiorly to project into the center of each segment.

Because of this division into self-contained units, each segment can be resected without damaging those remaining. For the liver to remain viable, resections must proceed along the vessels that define the peripheries of these segments. This means, that resection-lines parallel the hepatic veins. The centrally located portal veins, bile ducts, and hepatic arteries are preserved.

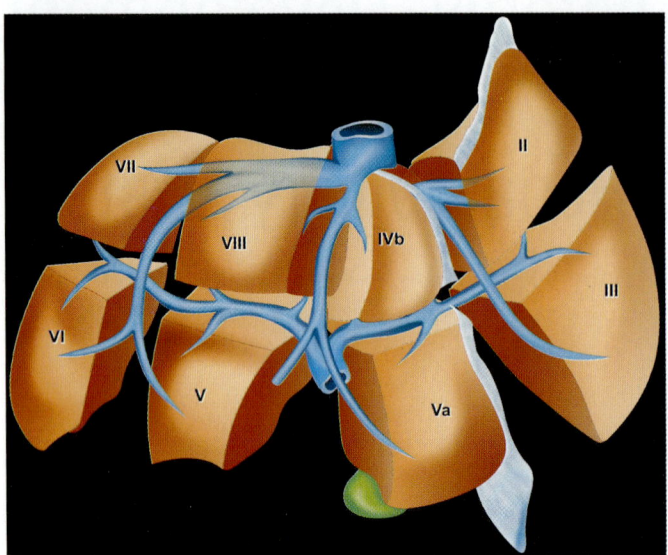

Fig. 19.1: Couinaud classification (*Source:* Reference from the University of Iowa College of Medicine, University of Iowa, College of Medicine: Couinaud classification http://dpi.radiology.uiowa.edu/nlm/app/livertoc/liver/8seg.html.)

The Numbering of Segments

There are eight liver segments. Segment 4 is sometimes divided into segment 4a and 4b according to Bismuth. The numbering of the segments is in a clockwise manner. Segment 1 (caudate lobe) is located posteriorly. It is not visible on a frontal view.

ANATOMY OF THE BILIARY TRACT AND BILE DUCT EPITHELIAL CELLS

The biliary system is a series of channels and ducts that conveys bile—a secretory and excretory product of hepatocytes—from the liver into the lumen of the small intestine.

The liver arises as a diverticulum in the 4th week from the ventral surface of duodenal foregut, close to its junction with the midgut. The septum tranversum arises from this diverticulum and grows ventrally and caudally, this is lined with endoderm. From this arise the hepatic buds which later form into the right and left lobes of liver. The buds develop into hepatic cylinders (epithelial trabeculae or sheets) these then branch and form a close meshwork. The space between them (meshwork) is filled with blood vessels and on cross section the organ looks like a vascular sponge. The continuous and rapid growth of these sheets leads to increase in the mass of liver. The mesenchymal cells of the septum transversum give rise to connective tissue and stroma.[3]

The diveticulum from the duodenum leads to formation of cystic duct and gallbladder and later gets canalized. During the embryonic period and gut rotation it then occupies the position in the medial border. The caudal surface of septum tranversum leads to projection of liver into the abdominal cavity. During this process the liver, falciform ligament, right and left triangular ligaments and lesser omentum.

By the age of three months the liver is almost filling the abdomen and both lobes are nearly equal in size. During the embryonic process the left lobe undergoes degeneration and shrinks in size and the right remains its original size. Until birth the liver remains large in size.

DEVELOPMENT OF HEPATIC VASCULATURE

The development of the hepatic vasculature is similar to the development of bile ducts. The endothelial cells are required for liver induction and migration form the lining of hepatic sinusoids. They then lead on to form the lobule by directing the migration of hepatoblasts into the cords.[5] Moreover during fetal development the placenta and maternal liver perform necessary functions. Liver enzymes are activated by loss of blood at birth.[6] It is a very complicated process by how the liver enzymes get activated and there is a huge interindividual variability. An abnormal liver function test at infancy due to systemic insults explains the immaturity of the liver before it achieves its full potential. The drastic transition for the fetus from parturition to extrauterine life is handled by the anatomic and physiologic development of liver.[3]

LIVER PHYSIOLOGY INCLUDING HEPATOCELLULAR FUNCTION

The liver function can be classified under multiple categories:
- The liver as metabolic organ, i.e. the liver as endocrine and exocrine liver
- The liver as a filtering system
- The liver as metabolic organ
- The liver as hematopoietic organ

The Liver as Metabolic Organ—the Liver as Endocrine and Exocrine Liver

The two functions are endocrine, i.e. excretion into sinusoidal system and exocrine indicating excretion into biliary system.

The endocrine function of the liver starts after birth when the fetus starts functioning independently and the liver starts synthesizing glycogen de novo. The main circulating and transport protein in fetus is α-fetoprotein. The levels fall by term as the synthesis of albumin starts then, which leads to fall in the levels of α-fetoprotein. The production of coagulation factors is vital function of liver which is dependent on vitamin K. The gut is devoid of bacteria which produce vitamin K and hence the reason for neonatal vitamin K administration. Fatty acids oxidation allows the utilization of fats in breast milk to be transported to the portal system and the process of fatty oxidation and ketogenesis is provided by the liver. The regulation half lives of hormones like insulin and estrogen is done by liver. The liver responds to insulin by initiating gluconeogenesis and storing carbohydrates as glucagon.

The exocrine functions are bile acid synthesis which at infancy acts as trophic factors for developing bile tree and the overall synthesis is less than the mature infant with recued efficiency when compared with adult. Overall the hepatocyte has reduced ability to excrete bile acids into the canalicus until first year of life. The liver acts a major route for excretion of metabolites and the immaturity will lead to increased risk of cholestasis in the first few months of life. The liver is the main site of cholesterol synthesis which is regulated by bile acid composition and from the enterohepatic circulation.

The Liver Filter

The kuppfer cells that line the sinusoids, in the liver play a major role in elimination of toxins, medications, bacteria (which are derived from gut), the liver along with the kidney are very vital in eliminating and excreting the xenobiotics. The principle defense is provided by the liver against bacteria entering the portal circulation through the intestines.

The Liver as Hematopoietic Organ

In the fetus starting from the 4th and 5th week of life the liver is the major site for hematopoiesis and peaks towards the early third trimester. The liver ceases to function as extra-hemopoietic site with due course of time. It is the marrow which guarantees a constant supply of Kuppfer cells to keep the line of defense against enteric organisms.

HEPATOCYTE DEATH AND REGENERATION

It is a well-known phenomenon that liver has a regenerative potential and it is very remarkable. Mice models have shown that the liver volume is restored two weeks after hepatectomy. Recent scientific advancements have shown

that the donor liver volume doubles in donors in 7 days and 14 days in recipients.[3] The structure does not get replaces but the volume does. The regeneration of liver happens because of the following cells hepatocytes, hepatocyte progenitors, endothelial cells, leukocytes and stellate cells. The hepatocytes start replicating after 24 hours post-injury and biliary endothelial cells and biliary cells in 72 hours. In situations where there is severe hepatocyte compartment injury, oval cells take over. The stem cells are unique that they have self-maintenance and multipotency.

The two major types of cells are hepatic stem cells and oval cells. Hepatic stem cells are pluripotent which are in the canals of hering.[5] These cells could be remnants of liver when it was a major hematopoietic organ.

Oval cells reside in portal tracts and are known as hepatocyte progenitor cells.[7,8] They are organ specific cells and conditional stem cells. They can differentiate into hepatocytes, cholangiocytes and abnormal ductular reactive cells.

Current evidence suggests that these cells respond to different permissive conditions and their developmental pathways are activated by a complex process that leads to hepatocyte regeneration in active and chronic liver diseases. As scientific advances progress we will have better knowledge about this complex process in the future.[9,10]

REFERENCES

1. BD Chaurasia's Human Anatomy, Volume 2, 4th Edition, CBS Publishers & Distributors; 2013.
2. Grays Anatomy.
3. Wyllie R, Hyams S (Eds). Textbook of Pediatric gastrointestinal and Liver Disease, 3rd Edition, Saunders Elsevier-ISBN 07216-3924-0.
4. Nelson Textbook of Pediatrics, 19th Edition, Elsevier, 2011.
5. McLin V, Balistreri W. Approach to neonatal cholestasis.In: Walker WA, Goulet O, Kleiman RE, Sherman PM, Shneidr B, Sanderson IR (Eds). Pediatric Gastrointetinal Disease, 4th Edition. Hamilton, ON:BC Decker. 2004; 1079-92.
6. Crosby HA, Nijar SS, de Goyet J de V, et al. Progenitor cells of the biliary epithelial cell lineage. Semin Cell Dev Biol. 2002; 13:397-403.
7. Desmet V. Organizational principles, In: Arias E, Boyer J, Chisari F. et al (Eds). The Liver: Biology and pathobiology, 4th edn. London: Lippincott, Wiliams & Wilkins;2001:3-16.
8. Desmet V.Congenital diseases of the intrahepatic bile ducts variations on the theme 'ductal plane malformations' Hepatology. 1992;16:1069-86.
9. Di Campli, Gasbarrini G, Gasbarrini A. A medicine based on cell transplantation—is there a future for treating liver disease? Aliment Pharmacol Ther. 2003;18:473-80.
10. Crosby HA, Nijjar SS, de Goyet J de V, et al. Progenitor cells of the biliary epithelial cell lineage. Semin Cell Dev Biol. 2002;13;397-403.

Approach to Common Liver: Symptoms and Signs

Siham Al Sinani

■ INTRODUCTION

Liver disease in children is not uncommon, considering its varied etiology. Manifestations of liver disease in the pediatric age group vary. This chapter will cover some common symptoms and signs of liver disease in children, their definition, pathophysiology, presentation and differential diagnosis. This chapter will include laboratory investigations, evaluation and management of some of the common manifestations of liver disease in children.

■ JAUNDICE

Definition[1]

❑ The term *jaundice* originated from the French *jaune*, which means "yellow" or icterus (Greek *ikteros*) refers to yellowish discoloration of skin, sclerae, and mucous membranes that results from deposition of bile pigment bilirubin.

❑ It is a sign of hyperbilirubinemia which is defined as total serum bilirubin concentration >1.4 mg/dL after 6 months of age.

Bilirubin Metabolism

❑ Bilirubin is the end product of heme-containing compounds degradation, hemoglobin (70–80%) and other hemoproteins (20–30%).

❑ The conversion from heme to bilirubin follows a 2-step process that occurs mainly in the reticuloendothelial system:
  • Heme is converted to biliverdin by heme oxygenase enzyme.
  • Biliverdin is converted to bilirubin by biliverdin reductase enzyme.

• Unconjugated bilirubin is a hydrophobic compound that is tightly bound to serum albumin and is transported to the liver for conjugation and clearance.

❑ Metabolism of bilirubin in the liver follows distinct steps:
  • Bilirubin is taken up across the sinusoidal membrane of the hepatocyte by a membrane receptor carrier.
  • Bilirubin then binds to ligandin, an intracellular binding protein and is conjugated with glucuronic acid in the endoplasmic reticulum by the enzyme bilirubin glucuronosyltransferase (BGT) to form bilirubin glucuronides (monoglucuronides—15% and diglucuronides—85%). Neonates have a higher concentration of bilirubin monoglucuronides in their bile because of lower BUGT enzyme activity.
  • Water-soluble bilirubin glucuronides are excreted into bile through the apical canalicular membrane (mediated by an adenosine triphosphate-dependent export pump).

❑ In the intestine, bilirubin glucuronides are deconjugated by bacteria:
  • The resulting bilirubin is converted to urobilinogen and then reabsorbed in the terminal ileum, a process known as enterohepatic circulation.
  • Some urobilinogen is oxidized by intestinal bacteria to brown stercobilin that is excreted in feces.
  • The reminder of urobilinogen is transported by blood to the kidneys, where it is converted to urobilin and excreted, givig the urine its color.
  • Newborns are more likely to absorb bilirubin from the intestine because they lack bacterial flora to form nonabsorbable urobilinoids.

Differential diagnosis: It is age specific.

Neonatal hyperbilirubinemia can be cause by a number of etiologies (Table 20.1). Table 20.2 summarizes neonatal

Table 20.1: Causes of neonatal hyperbilirubinemia

Increased bilirubin production:
- Feto-maternal blood group incompatibilities
- Extravascular blood
- Polycythemia
- Red blood cell abnormalities (hemoglobinopathies or membrane and enzyme defects)
- Induction of labor

Decreased bilirubin excretion:
- Increased enterohepatic circulation
- Breastfeeding
- Inborn errors of metabolism
- Drugs and hormones
- Prematurity
- Hepatic hypoperfusion
- Cholestatic syndromes
- Biliary tree obstruction/anomalies

Combined causes:
- Sepsis
- Intrauterine infection
- Congenital cirrhosis

Table 20.2: Causes of neonatal cholestasis (conjugated Hyperbilirubinemia)

Anatomic abnormalities/obstruction:
- Biliary Atresia
- Choledochal cyst
- Inspissated bile/mucous plug
- Cholelithiasis or biliary sludge
- Tumors/masses (intrinsic/extrinsic)
- Neonatal sclerosing cholangitis
- Spontaneous perforation of bile ducts

Infection:
- Viral: HIV, CMV, HSV, rubella, parvovirus B19, echovirus, adenovirus, HIV
- Bacterial: Sepsis, UTI, syphilis, listeriosis, tuberculosis
- Protozoal: Toxoplasma

Metabolic/genetic:
- Genetic
  - Alagille syndrome
  - Nonsyndromic paucity of interlobular bile ducts
  - Progressive familial intrahepatic cholestasis (types 1–3)
  - Benign recurrent intrahepatic cholestasis
  - Congenital hepatic fibrosis/Caroli's disease
  - Cystic fibrosis
- Disorders of carbohydrate metabolism
  - Galactosemia
  - Fructosemia
  - Type IV glycogenosis
- Disorders of amino acid metabolism
  - Tyrosinemia
  - Hypermethioninemia
- Disorders of lipid metabolism
  - Wolman, Niemann-Pick, Gaucher disease, cholesterol ester storage disease
- Disorders of bile acid synthesis
  - 3-beta-hydroxysteroid dehydrogenase/isomerase deficiency
  - 4-oxosteroid 5-beta-reductase deficiency
- Peroxisomal disorders: Zellweger syndrome
- Mitochondrial disorders
- Other metabolic defects:
  - Urea cycle defects
  - Citrin deficiency
  - Alpha-1-antitrypsin deficiency
  - Panhypopituitarism
  - Hypothyroidism

Toxic:
- Drugs
- Parenteral nutrition

Chromosomal disorders:
- Autosomal trisomies
- Turner syndrome

Miscellaneous:
- "Idiopathic" neonatal hepatitis
- Shock/hypoperfusion/vascular
- Intestinal obstruction

cholestasis etiologies. Causes of jaundice in infants and older children are summarized in Table 20.3.

Definition of Neonatal Cholestasis

Neonatal cholestasis (NC) is defined as prolonged conjugated hyperbilirubinemia that occurs in the newborn period. It results either from diminished bile flow and/or excretion, which can be caused by a number of disorders (Table 20.2). It affects approximately 1 in 2500 newborns (excluding infants with parenteral nutrition-associated cholestasis), but estimates vary depending on the definition.

Neonatal cholestasis is defined as a serum conjugated bilirubin concentration >1.0 mg/dL if the total serum bilirubin is <5.0 mg/dL or >20 % of the total serum bilirubin if the total serum bilirubin is >5.0 mg/dL.[1] It is defined histologically by evidence of bile stasis in hepatocytes and bile ducts.

Physiological jaundice (unconjugated hyperbilirubinemia) typically resolves by age of 2 weeks. Between 2–15 % of newborns are still jaundiced at 2 weeks of age.[2] Although most of these infants have benign breast milk jaundice, a few will have biliary atresia. NASPGHAN suggests that the evaluation for cholestasis may be delayed until 3 weeks of age in jaundiced infants who are most likely to have breast milk jaundice if they have a normal physical examination, no history of dark urine or light stools, and can be reliably monitored.[1]

Table 20.3: Causes of jaundice in infants and older children

Infections:
- Hepatitis A, B, C, D, E viruses
- Adenovirus
- EBV, CMV, herpes virus
- Influenza
- Sepsis, UTI

Anatomical/obstructive:
- Cholelithiasis
- Caroli's disease
- Autosomal recessive polycystic kidney disease (ARPKD)

Immunological:
- Autoimmune hepatitis
- Primary sclerosing cholangitis

Genetic:
- PFIC
- Gilbert's syndrome, Dubin-Johnson, Rotor syndrome, Crigler-Najjar syndrome
- CF
- A1AT deficiency
- Wilson disease

Metabolic:
- Storage disorders: Glycogen storage disorders (types 1, 4)
- Lipid storage disorders
- Urea cycle defects
- Mitochondrial disorders
- Peroxisomal disorders

Drug-induced liver injury

Vascular
- Hepatic outflow obstruction (Budd Chiari, infiltrative disorders)
- Portal vein thrombosis

Systemic disease:
- Malignancies
- Immunodeficiency syndromes

Non-alcoholic fatty liver disease (NAFLD)

Jaundice in Infants and Older Children

Jaundice in the older infant and child is always pathologic.[1] Causes of jaundice at this age group vary (Table 20.3).

Complications of Cholestasis

- ❑ Malabsorption and malnutrition:
  - Steatorrhea
  - Growth failure
  - Fat-soluble vitamin deficiencies
  - Mineral and trace element deficiencies
- ❑ Bile constituents (bile acids, cholesterol) retention:
  - Pruritus
  - Xanthomas
  - Jaundice

- ❑ Hepatic fibrosis/cirrhosis:
  - Portal hypertension, variceal bleeding
  - Ascites
- ❑ End stage liver disease

Evaluation

- ❑ **History:**
  - Age and gender of child/neonate.
  - Onset of jaundice (neonatal or later).
  - Duration of jaundice.
  - Part of body involved in discoloration.
  - Pallor.
  - Stool and urine color or recent changes.
  - Stool pattern: Delayed meconium may be seen in CF or hypothyroidism; diarrhea may suggest infectious cause, metabolic cause or PFIC.
  - Fever, anorexia.
  - Abdominal pain.
  - Vomiting, poor feeding (metabolic causes).
  - Skin rash, bruises, bleeding tendency (may indicate coagulopathy or vitamin K deficiency)
  - Pruritus, arthritis, conjunctivitis.
  - Lethargy (may indicate metabolic disease, sepsis, hypothyroidism, panhypopituitarism), confusion, abnormal behavior, sleep disturbance, irritability (irritability may indicate metabolic disease or sepsis).
  - Nutritional, growth and developmental history.
  - Hepatitis risk factors (neonatal history—congenital infections—prenatal US, neonatal infections, isoimmune hemolysis, travel, possible exposure, blood transfusion, IV drug use).
  - Consanguinity: It increases the risk of an autosomal recessive disorder.
  - Nutritional history: Breastfeeding, galactose containing formulas).
  - Family history of jaundice, hemolytic disorder, liver disease, neuropsychiatric disorders, or inherited disorders.
  - Exposure to medications, herbal remedies.
  - Chronic illnesses: Congenital heart disease, CF, hematologic disorders, autoimmune disorders.
  - Medical intervention (if any).
- ❑ **Physical examination:** Signs that might lead to etiology of jaundice, liver disease, liver dysfunction or its complications).
  - General appearance (lethargy, irritability, itching, poor growth, dysmorphic features, developmental delay).
  - Vital signs and lymph nodes examination.
  - General examination: Stigmata of chronic liver disease (clubbing, palmar erythema, spider nevi, muscle wasting).

- Skin examination: Jaundice, scratch marks, xanthomas, or signs of autoimmune disorders.
- Eye examination: Icterus and pallor. Additional signs such as cataract (in galactosemia), posterior emryotoxon (Alagille syndrome, requires slit lamp examination), retinal changes (metabolic or infectious etiology), Kayser-Fleischer rings (Wilson disease).
- Systemic examination: For both associated signs of possible etiology or consequences of chronic liver disease (such as cardiac murmur, hypoxia, cardiac failure, pericardial effusion, pneumonia, pleural effusion, palpable kidneys in case of polycystic kidney disease).
- Musculoskeletal examination: Arthritis (autoimmune disease).
- Abdominal examination: Distension, pigments, caput medusae, umbilical hernia, previous surgical scars, tenderness, ascites, hepatomegaly (span, edge), shrunken liver, liver consistency, signs of portal hypertension, splenomegaly, masses or tumors.
- Neurological examination: Encephalopathy.

❑ **Laboratory investigations:**
- Total and conjugated serum bilirubin levels.
- Liver enzymes (transaminases).
- Alkaline phosphatase: High ALP indicates either biliary obstruction or intrahepatic cholestasis.
- Gamma glutamyl transpeptidase (GGT): Elevated GGT is found in diseases of the liver, biliary tract, and pancreas, and reflects the same spectrum of hepatobiliary disease as alkaline phosphatase. In pediatrics age group, low GGT cholestasis indicates a set of disorders.
- Full blood count: To rule out hemolysis, total white blood count and its differential to rule out infections. High platelets' count might indicate infectious or inflammatory etiology whereas thrombocytopenia might indicate hypersplensim. Blood smear is important to rule out hemolysis, infectious, metabolic or malignant (infiltrative) causes.
- Electrolytes and renal function: These might be abnormal if cholestasis is associated with renal disease such as metabolic causes.
- Bone profile: If cholestasis is prolonged affecting vitamin D absorption or secondary to renal disorder.
- Synthetic liver function:
  - Coagulation profile: An elevated INR that corrects with vitamin K administration suggests impaired intestinal absorption of fat-soluble vitamins and is compatible with obstructive jaundice. On the other hand, an elevated INR that does not correct with vitamin K suggests impaired synthetic function.

- Glucose level: Hypoglycemia in liver failure.
- Albumin level: Hypoalbuminemia in liver failure (if other causes are ruled out).
- Cholesterol and ammonia levels.
- Creatine kinase: To rule out muscular pathology.
- Fat soluble vitamin levels: As part of nutritional assessment in chronic cholestasis.
- Investigations for specific underlying etiology of cholestasis (Table 20.4).

Management of Cholestatic Jaundice[3,4]

❑ Identify and treat potentially treatable disease.
❑ Recognize complications of cholestasis for which medical therapy may improve the quality of life and prognosis, such as:
- Malabsorption and malnutrition: Secondary to increased metabolism, decreased fat absorption. Treatment is by:
  - Provide adequate caloric and protein intake.

Table 20.4: Investigations for specific underlying etiology of cholestasis

Disease	Diagnostic workup
Biliary atresia	Abdominal US, liver biopsy, cholangiogram
Choledochal cyst	Abdominal US
Any other anatomical cause	Abdominal US, cholangiogram, abdominal CT, others as indicated
Inborn error of metabolism	• Newborn screening and urine reducing substances (Galactosemia) • Urine succinylacetone (Tyrosinemia) • Serum amino acids and urine organic acids (Others)
TORCH	Urine CMV, others as indicated
UTI, sepsis, viral hepatitis	Urine culture, other cultures or viral studies based on clinical picture
Alagille syndrome	Echocardiogram, spine X-ray, ophthalmologic examination, liver biopsy.
Endocrine causes	TFT, early am cortisol, glucose, brain MRI (pituitary gland)
Cystic fibrosis	Newborn screening (serum immunoreactive trypsinogen), sweat chloride test, CFTR gene mutation analysis
Progressive familial intrahepatic cholestasis (PFIC types 1–3)	LFT, GGT level, liver biopsy, genetic mutation
A1AT deficiency	A1AT level and phenotype
Bile acid synthesis defect	Total serum bile acids, urine bile acid FAB

- Supply MCT containing formula/supplement as fat source.
- Supplement fat-soluble and water-soluble vitamins
- Correct/prevent mineral and trace elements deficiencies
- Bile constituents (bile acids, cholesterol) retention:
  - Ursodeoxycholic acid 15–30 mg/kg/day in two doses
  - Phenobarbital
  - Rifampin 10 mg/kg/day in two doses
  - Cholestyramine 0.25–0.5 mg/kg/day in three doses
  - Opioid antagonists
  - Biliary diversion procedures
- Hepatic fibrosis/cirrhosis:
  - Portal hypertension, variceal bleeding:
    - Vasopressin infusion, octreotide
    - Variceal banding, sclerotherapy
    - Portosystemic shunts
    - Propranolol (prophylaxis or therapeutic)
  - Ascites:
    - Sodium intake limitation
    - Spironolactone
    - Loop diuretics
    - Albumin infusions
    - Paracentesis
- End stage liver disease
  - Liver transplantation.

PRURITUS

Definition

Pruritus, or itch, is an unpleasant sensation that provokes the desire to scratch. Generalized pruritus may have underlying causative disease: dermatologic pruritus, renal pruritus, cholestatic pruritus, hematologic pruritus, endocrine pruritus, pruritus related to malignancy, and idiopathic generalized pruritus.

Pruritus is a well-known feature of chronic cholestasis (intra- and extrahepatic) in both adults and children. It can be persistent or intermittent, generalized or localized to specific parts of the body, usually the palms and soles. It is often more troublesome at night; in the presence of tight, constrictive clothes; and in hot, humid weather.[5] Pruritus can interfere with sleep, daily activities, normal cognitive development and school performance. It can also lead to excoriation and secondary skin infections.

Pathogenesis

Penicillate interdermal nerve endings have been implicated as the sensors that mediate general pruritus; however, the mediators that stimulate these nerve endings in cholestasis are still unknown. Several hypotheses have been proposed.[6]

Bile Acids (BA)

Pruritus due to cholestasis was thought to be caused by the accumulation and deposition of BA in the skin.[6] There are observations that are not consistent with a primary role for BA as the cause of pruritus such as:
- Intermittent disappearance of pruritus despite persistence of elevated plasma BA levels.[7]
- Absence of pruritus in some patients with cholestasis and high plasma BA levels.[7]
- No correlation between presence or severity of pruritus and concentrations of BA in skin of patients with cholestasis (in a carefully done study).[8]
- BA resins used to treat pruritus of cholestasis also decrease pruritus in patients with uremia and polycythemia vera (not associated with BA retention).

Elevated plasma BA is also thought to cause direct hepatocyte toxicity by altering the hepatocyte membrane and allowing leakage of hepatocyte contents (some of which are pruritogens) into the bloodstream rather than their effect on nerve.[9]

Endogenous Opioids

Centrally-mediated mechanism for pruritus associated with increased opioid neurotransmission. Endogenous opioid levels are elevated (via an uncertain mechanism) in patients with chronic liver disease[10] and many reports have shown a reduction in cholestatic pruritus in patients treated with opioid antagonists.[11,12]

Histamine

Opioid peptides have been shown to increase histamine release from mast cells[13] leading to elevated venous histamine levels.

Serotonin

Connection between serotonin and endogenous opiate system in the hypothalamus suggests that serotonin may also contribute to the mechanism of cholestatic pruritus.[14]

Lysophosphatidic Acid and Autotaxin

Role for lysophosphatidic acid (LPA) in cholestatic pruritus.[15] Patients with cholestatic pruritus had significantly increased serum concentrations of LPA and autotaxin activity. These observations need confirmation, but suggest a potential role for inhibition of autotaxin as therapeutic strategy.

Evaluation

- ❑ **History:**
  - Primary dermatologic disorders can cause pruritus.
  - Pruritus onset, duration, severity, location, provoking factors, time relation, and relationship to activities such as bathing.
  - A review of systems to uncover a systemic disease.
  - Drug and medications history—that can cause itching.
- ❑ **Physical examination:**
  - Differentiate between systemic versus primary dermatologic conditions.
  - Signs of liver disease: Jaundice, palmar erythema, spider angiomata, clubbing, white nails, splenomegaly, and ascites.
- ❑ **Laboratory investigations:** Directed to the cause and complications of cholestasis.

Treatment

- ❑ Correction of the underlying hepatobiliary disease.
- ❑ General measures:
  - Cool baths.
  - Moisturizers.
  - Finger nails trimming.
  - Long-sleeve nightshirts.
- ❑ Intrahepatic cholestasis with moderate-severe pruritus (if definitive therapy is not possible), the following options are available.[16-21]

Rifampin

10 mg/kg/day PO divided into two doses (total 150–600 mg/ day). Effect can take place in up to 1–3 months.
- ❑ Mechanism of action: Unknown, but possible mechanisms:
  - Inhibit the uptake of toxic BA.
  - BA cause hepatocyte membrane injury, resulting in the release of pruritogenic substances and increased production of enkephalins. Rifampin is thought to induce the mixed function cytochrome P-450 isoenzyme system, thereby enhancing the degradation of enkephalins and toxic BA and preventing hepatocyte injury.[16,17]
  - Rifampin has been shown to activate the human glucocorticoid receptor, and pruritus severity has been found to decrease with prednisolone in adult patients with primary biliary cirrhosis.[16,17]
- ❑ Side effects:
  - Staining body secretions orange-red.
  - Idiosyncratic hypersensitivity reactions (hemolytic anemia, renal failure, and thrombocytopenic purpura).

- Long-term use of rifampin monotherapy can result in development of resistant organisms.

Phenobarbital

10 mg/kg/day PO divided into two doses. Effect can take place in few days.
- ❑ Mechanism of action is unknown, but the following could be possible mechanisms:[18]
  - Induces hepatic and microsomal enzymes to increase the conjugation and excretion of bilirubin.
  - Decreases the serum concentrations and half-lives of the primary bile salts through increased fecal excretion, resulting in decreased pruritus. These two mechanisms occur independently of each other.
- ❑ Side effects:
  - Somnolence is a dose-related. Start with low dose initially and increase gradually.
  - Can be associated with respiratory depression especially in patients with underlying respiratory disease.

Ursodeoxycholic Acid

15–20 mg/kg/day PO divided into two doses.
- ❑ Mechanism of action: A hydrophilic bile acid with potent choloretic properties. It protects the hepatocyte against the cytotoxic effects of hydrophobic BA by the following:[19]
  - Reducing endogenous bile acids toxicity by competitively inhibiting their absorption from the intestine, thereby reducing their concentration.
  - Increasing hydrophilic (nontoxic) bile acid concentrations.
- ❑ Side effects: Relatively safe drug. Diarrhea is common.

Opioid Antagonists

For example, oral naltrexone.[20,21] Significant side effects and withdrawal reactions may limit its general use.

Antihistamine

For example, oral hydroxyzine:
- ❑ Children <6 years: 50 mg/day in 4 divided doses as needed
- ❑ Children >6 years and adolescents: 50–100 mg/day in 4 divided doses as needed
- ❑ Alternate dosing:
  - Weight ≤40 kg: 2 mg/kg/day divided every 6–8 hours as needed (max single dose: 25 mg).
  - Weight >40 kg: 25–50 mg once daily at bedtime or twice daily.

Bile-binding Resins

Cholestyramine 0.25–0.50 g/kg/day (initial dose usually limited to ≈1 g daily) in 3 divided doses. Maximum dosage is 4 g daily in children ≤10 years and 8 g daily in children >10 years. Effect can take place in 1–2 weeks. Cholestyramine (and colestipol) should be diluted in juice or water and taken before breakfast (greatest amount of bile acids available for binding are thought to be in the gallbladder before breakfast). Patients with an intact gallbladder should take cholestyramine 30 minutes before and 30 minutes after breakfast. A third dose should be taken after lunch to maximize the effectiveness and minimize the adverse events.

- ❏ Mechanism of action: Cholestyramine is hydrophilic, water insoluble anion-exchange resin that binds BA, it therefore:
  - Prevents BA absorption through the enterohepatic circulation.
  - Increases fecal excretion of BA.
- ❏ Side effects:
  - Adverse gastrointestinal effects: Constipation, abdominal discomfort, and fat malabsorption (including fat soluble vitamin deficiency).
  - Can interfere with the absorption of many drugs, it should be given 2–4 hours before or after the administration of other drugs.
  - Unpleasant taste, but this can often be overcome by administering the bile-binding resin in a pill or capsule form (for older patients).

Other Medical Therapeutic Options

- ❏ Ondansetron: Serotonin antagonists and selective serotonin-reuptake inhibitors—evaluated for the treatment of cholestatic pruritus in adults, with varying reports of efficacy. Not evaluated for the treatment of cholestatic pruritus in children but may be potential options in the future.[14]
- ❏ Leukotriene antagonists approved for seasonal allergies because of their ability to inhibit the histamine and leukotriene cascade. Not evaluated for the treatment of cholestatic pruritus in adults or children, but they may be a promising option in the future.
- ❏ Extrahepatic biliary obstruction (if definitive therapy is not possible): Biliary diversion or ileal exclusion is usually effective.
- ❏ Liver transplantation: In severe unremitting pruritus.

■ HEPATOMEGALY

Hepatomegaly (increased liver size) can be seen in many disorders. Because of the variability in liver size

Table 20.5: Estimated mean liver span (cm) in infants, Children, and adolescents by percussion		
Age in years	Males	Females
0.5 (6 months)	2.4	2.8
1	2.8	3.1
2	3.5	3.6
3	4.0	4.0
4	4.4	4.3
5	4.8	4.5
6	5.1	4.8
8	5.6	5.1
10	6.1	5.4
12	6.5	5.6
14	6.8	5.8
16	7.1	6.0
18	7.4	6.1
20	7.7	6.3

(Bate's Guide to Physical Examination and History Taking)[22]

and shape, it is not a very reliable sign of liver disease. In order to determine if hepatomegaly is present, liver span should be measured. This can be done by percussing the upper margin and palpating the lower margin along the midclavicular line. In children younger than 2 years of age, the liver edge can extend to 3.5 cm below the right costal margin in the mid clavicular line. In older children, the liver edge rarely extends beyond 2 cm below the right costal margin. Liver span increases with body weight and age in both genders. It correlates more with the weight than the height (Table 20.5).[22] A liver span 2-3 cm smaller or larger than the mean is considered abnormal.[22]

Note: The liver can be displaced inferiorly by the diaphragm or thoracic organs giving the impression of hepatomegaly. Pneumothorax or pleural effusion may also displace it. A retroperitoneal mass, choledochal cyst, or perihepatic abscess can also be mistaken as hepatomegaly. Children with orthopedic disorders such as narrow chest wall or pectus excavatum may be mistakenly labeled to have hepatomegaly. A normal variant of the right lobe of the liver, called a Riedel lobe, may extend BCM and be confused as pathological live enlargement.[23]

Pathophysiology

Hepatomegaly can represent intrinsic liver disease or may be the presenting physical finding of a generalized disorder. Hepatomegaly mechanisms are summarized in Table 20.6.

Table 20.6: Hepatomegaly mechanisms

Inflammation:
- Infection
  - Viral (hepatitis A-E, CMV, EBV, coxsackievirus),
  - Bacterial (sepsis, abscess, cholangitis)
- Toxins, drugs, neonatal hepatitis, radiation,
- Autoimmune disease

Excessive storage:
- Glycogen: GSD, DM, PN
- Lipids: Wolman disease, Niemann-Pick disease, Gaucher disease
- Fat: Fatty acid oxidation defect, obesity, DM, PN, MPS type I-IV, mitochondrial disease, malnutrition, galactosemia
- Metals: Copper (Wilson disease), iron (hemochromatosis)
- Abnormal proteins: Alpha-1- antitrypsin, carbohydrate-glycoprotein deficiency
- Kupffer cell hyperplasia (Hypervitaminosis A)

Infiltration:
- Primary neoplastic tumors: Hepatoblastoma, hepatocelluar carcinoma
- Primary non-neoplastic tumors: Hemanigomas, hemangioendothelioma, teratoma, focal nodular hyperplasia
- Metastatic or disseminated tumors: Leukemia, lymphoma, neuroblastoma, histocytosis, Wilms tumor
- Cysts: Parasitic cysts, choledochal cysts, polycystic liver disease
- Hemophagocytic syndromes
- Extramedullary hematopoiesis

Vascular congestion:
- Suprahepatic obstruction (CHF, restrictive pericardial disease, hepatic vein thrombosis (Budd-Chiari), or suprahepatic vascular webs
- Intrahepatic: Veno-occlusive disease (post-BMT).

Biliary obstruction (congenital, acquired):
- Cholelithiasis, choledochal cysts, biliary atresia
- Tumors: Hepatic, biliary, pancreatic, duodenal

Abbreviations: GSD, glycogen storage disease; DM, diabetes mellitus; PN, parenteral nutrition; CHF, congestive cardiac failure; BMT, bone marrow transplantation.

Table 20.7: History of hepatomegaly and its implications

Information	Implication
Maternal infection	TORCH, HIV, viral hepatitis
Fetal US	Congenital anomaly
Consanguinity/similar condition in family	Autosomal recessive genetic disorder
Fever, rash, pharyngitis, cough, SOB, poor feeding, exposure, contaminated food, vomiting, diarrhea, etc	Infectious cause
Growth and development	Congenital infection, genetic/ metabolic or chronic disease.
History of trauma	Hematoma
Blood transfusion/organ transplant	Infectious cause
Sexually active/ drugs use	Infectious cause
Foreign travel	Infectious cause
Medications intake/ herbal remedies/toxins	Intoxication
Chronic illnesses	Cardiac, CF, DM, hematological disease, obesity, etc

Evaluation

- **History:** Hepatomegaly rarely presents alone. It usually accompanies other clinical signs and symptoms based on the underlying pathophysiology. Symptoms that might represent an underlying etiology should always be looked for (Table 20.7).
- **Physical examination:** Hepatomegaly should always be confirmed by a careful physical examination.
  - *General physical examination:*
    - Skin: Petechiae and purpura (chronic liver disease, malignancy); pruritus/jaundice (liver disease); rashes (infection).
    - Head and neck: Icterus, cherry red retinal spots or cloudy cornea (lipid storage disease), Kayser-Fleischer ring (Wilson's disease).
    - CNS: Altered level of consciousness, seizures (hypoglycemia due to storage disease, end stage liver disease).
    - CVS and respiratory: Murmur, abnormal heart sounds (S3, S4) (congenital heart diseases), abnormal breath sounds (alpha-1 antitrypsin deficiency).
    - Abdominal: Distension, tenderness, ascites, hepatomegaly (see specific liver examination below), splenomegaly (hemolytic anemia).
    - Musculoskeletal: Joint tenderness (autoimmune hepatitis), bone pain (malignancy).
  - *Liver examination:*[22-24]
    - Liver size and span (see normal values above). >3.5 cm below the right costal margin in a newborn is abnormal.
    - Liver consistency and edge: A firm, enlarged liver may indicate a storage disease, infiltrative process, veno-occlusive disease or neoplasia. Liver edge that is firm, irregular or nodular is suggestive of cirrhosis or malignancy. Rubbery liver can indicate hepatitis.
    - Liver tenderness: It may indicate acute hepatitis or inflammatory or congestive process.
- **Laboratory investigations:**[23, 25]
  - CBC with differential and peripheral blood smear.
  - AST, ALT, GGT, alkaline phosphatase, bilirubin (total and direct), total protein, albumin.
  - Liver synthetic function.

- Serum electrolytes and BUN and bone profile.
- Hepatitis serology.
- Additional investigations based on clinical suspicion: EKG, echocardiogram, lipid profile, serum ceruloplasmin level, alpha-1- antitrypsin, HIV, blood culture, autoantibodies, alpha fetoprotein, bone marrow aspiration and biopsy.
- ☐ **Imaging:**[23,25]
  - Abdominal ultrasound with Doppler.
  - Abdominal CT or MRI (hepatic masses, biliary tree, anatomical obstructions).
  - Echocardiogram (congenital heart defects).
  - MRCP and or ERCP (stones).
- ☐ **Liver biopsy**

SPLENOMEGALY

Definition

Splenomegaly is enlargement of the spleen resulting from abnormalities of the lymphoid, reticuloendothelial, or vascular components of the spleen.

The spleen is a hematopoietic organ supporting the megakaryotic, lymphoid, erythroid, myeloid, and reticuloendothelial systems.

Spleen's Functions

- ☐ Hematopoietic: A major hematopoietic organ during fetal life and children with bone marrow failure.
- ☐ Phagocytic.
- ☐ Immunologic
  - A major lymphoreticular organ: A filter for infectious organisms.
  - Removes senescent and abnormal erythrocytes.
  - Removes particulate material.
  - Acts as a site of IgM and properdin production.
- ☐ Reservoir for blood-borne elements.

Normal Spleen Size[26]

Spleen weighs 11 g at birth, 55 g at 6 years and 125 g (100–250 g) at puberty.

It is palpable below the left costal margin in about 30% of neonates, 10% of normal children, and more than 2% of normal 19-year-old people. When tip of spleen is felt beyond 2 cm below the left costal margin, it is abnormal.[22,26] Table 20.8 illustrates ultrasound measurements of normal spleen length in infants and children.

Prevalence

- ☐ A soft spleen is normally palpable in 15–30% of neonates.

Table 20.8: Ultrasound measurements of the normal spleen length (from the dome to the tip)[27]

Age	Upper limit of splenic length
3 months	6 cm
12 months	7 cm
6 years	9.5 cm
12 years	11.5 c m
>=15 years (girls)	12 cm
>=15 years (boys)	13 cm

- ☐ By 1 year of age, 10% of healthy infants have a palpable spleen.
- ☐ After 10 years of age, 1% of children have palpable spleens.

Signs of Abnormal Splenomegaly

- ☐ 2 cm below left costal margin
- ☐ Abnormally rough surface
- ☐ Tender
- ☐ Hard

Causes of Splenomegaly (Table 20.3): S-P-L-E-E-N[28]

- ☐ **S**equestration of red blood cells: Hereditary spherocytosis, congenital or acquired hemolytic anemias.
- ☐ **P**roliferation secondary to infection (viral, bacterial, fungal or parasitic infections, infective endocarditis), chronic inflammation (systemic lupus erythematosus, JIA).
- ☐ **L**ipid deposition disorders: Gaucher or Niemann-Pick disease.
- ☐ **E**ndowment: Congenital splenic hemangioma, hamartoma, or cysts.
- ☐ **E**ngorgement: Splenic trauma (intracapsular hematoma), sequestration crisis in sickle cell disease, chronic heart failure, or portal hypertension.
- ☐ i**N**vasion: Granulomatous, histiocytic, lymphoproliferative, or malignant hematologic disease.
- ☐ Common mechanisms and etiologies of splenomegaly are illustrated in Tables 20.9 and 20.10.

Table 20.9: Mechanisms of splenomegaly

Reactive: Infections, inflammatory, autoimmunity, or hemolysis
Congestive: Anatomical obstruction or backflow of blood.
Infiltrative: May be of a benign (storage disease) or a malignant origin

Table 20.10: Etiology of splenomegaly

Infection:
- Viral: Hepatitis, CMV, EBV, HIV
- Bacterial: Septicemia, *Salmonella*, brucella, tuberculosis, infective endocarditis
- Parasitic: Malaria, schistosomiasis, toxoplasmosis, leishmaniasis
- Fungal: Candidiasis, histoplasmosis, coccidioidomycosis

Hematologic:
- Acute and chronic hemolytic anemias: Congenital and acquired
- Acute splenic sequestrations: Sickle cell disease (children).
- Extramedullary hematopoiesis: Thalassemia major, osteopetrosis, myelofibrosis

Inflammation:
- Systemic lupus erythematosus
- Systemic onset JIA
- Serum sickness
- Sarcoidosis

Infiltrative:
- Nonmalignant:
  - Gaucher's disease
  - Niemann-Pick disease
  - Glycogen storage disease
- Malignant:
  - Leukemias
  - Lymphomas
  - Langerhans cell histiocytosis
  - Hemophagocytic lymphohistiocytosis
  - Primary splenic tumors
  - Metastatic solid tumors

Congestive:
- Congestive heart failure
- Cirrhosis/portal hypertension
- Thrombosis of portal, hepatic, or splenic veins

Primary splenic disorders:
- Splenoptosis: Normal size spleen that moves freely within the peritoneal cavity
- Cysts
- Hemangiomas and lymphangiomas
- Subcapsular hemorrhage
- Accessory spleen

Table 20.11: History and its implications in splenomegaly

Information	Implication
Family history: Anemia, jaundice, splenomegaly, splenectomy, autoimmune disease	Hereditary hematological, storage, inflammatory causes
Neonatal history: Omphalitis or umbilical vein catheterization	Portal vein thrombosis
Postnatal history: Persistent jaundice	Hemolytic anemias
Fever, pharyngitis, malaise, poor feeding, cough	Viral (EBV, CMV), bacterial infection
Fever, night sweats, malaise, weight loss, rash, arthralgia, bone pain, abnormal bruising	Inflammatory, infectious, or malignant cause
Travel	Infectious cause
Trauma	Subcapsular hemorrhage
Known history: Congenital heart disease, storage disease, liver disease, blood transfusions or surgeries	Congestive, infiltrative causes

Evaluation

In most cases, the cause of splenomegaly can be determined by history and physical examination.[22,28]

❑ **History:** History and its implications in children with splenomegaly is summarized in Table 20.11.

❑ **Physical examination:**
- *General physical examination:*
  - Skin: Petechiae and purpura (thrombocytopenia, autoimmune disorder, malignancy); jaundice (hemolytic anemia or liver disease); rashes (infection, lupus, JIA, infective endocarditis).
  - Head and neck: Icterus, cherry-red retinal spots or cloudy cornea (lipid storage disease), lymph nodes (infection, inflammation, malignancy), mouth ulceration (autoimmune disorder).
  - Cardiac and respiratory: Murmur, shortness of breath, fatigue (anemia, heart failure, infective endocarditis)
  - Abdomen: Distension, tenderness, ascites, hepatomegaly (liver disease, gallstones, trauma, and hemolytic anemia).
  - Muskeloskeletal: Arthritis (JIA, lupus, hepatitis), bone pain (malignancy).
  - Neurologic: Poor vision (osteopetrosis), uveitis, iritis (sarcoidosis or JIA), loss of developmental milestones (storage diseases, chronic infection, or immunodeficiency).
- *Splenic examination:*
  Note:
  - Spleen moves downward with inspiration and enlarges diagonally across the midline toward the right ileac fossa.
  - An enlarged spleen may extend down into the pelvis.
  - Palpation and percussion are important techniques in the physical examination of the child with suspected splenomegaly.

Palpation (Bimanual):

- Patient should be supine and relaxed.
- Relaxation is improved if legs and neck are slightly flexed.
- Begin in the right lower quadrant.
- Move across the abdomen toward the left upper quadrant.
- Normal palpable spleen: Soft, smooth, nontender and is < 1–2 cm below the left costal margin.
- Pathologically enlarged spleen: Usually firm with abnormal surface and is often associated with signs and symptoms of an underlying disease.
- Spleen may be tender if it has enlarged quickly, for example, in splenic sequestration, or splenic trauma with subcapsular hemorrhage.
- When portal hypertension causes splenomegaly, dilatation of the superficial abdominal veins can be seen.
- Although a palpable spleen could be normal, concomitant finding of hepatomegaly is usually pathologic.

Percussion:

- Percussion cannot confirm splenic enlargement but can raise suspicion.
- Castell's method: Percuss the lowest intercostal space in the left anterior axillary line. Dullness to percussion indicates splenomegaly.
- Traube's space: Bound superiorly by the 6th rib, laterally by the mid-axillary line and inferiorly by the costal margin. Dullness to percussion indicates splenomegaly.
- Enlarged spleen replaces the tympani of stomach and colon with dullness of a solid organ.
- If tympani is prominent, especially laterally, then splenomegaly is not likely.
- A change from tympani to dullness on inspiration at the lower intercostal spaces in the left anterior axillary line suggests splenic enlargement.

- ❑ **Laboratory investigations**
  - The initial laboratory testing of a child with splenomegaly should include:
    - Complete blood count
    - Leukocyte differential
    - Reticulocyte count
    - Peripheral blood smear
  - Further laboratory investigations should be directed at the suspected diagnosis:
    - AST, ALT, GGT, alkaline phosphatase, bilirubin, prothrombin time, total protein and albumin.
    - Viral serology (EBV, CMV, parvovirus B19, HIV etc.), acid beta-glucosidase (Gaucher disease),

autoimmune work-up, bone marrow aspirate and biopsy.
    - Tissue biopsy depending upon the clinical suspicion (lymph node, liver, etc).

- ❑ **Splenic imaging:**
  - Ultrasound (to quantify splenic enlargement, cysts or abscess).
  - CT scan or MRI (trauma, focal splenic pathology, malignancy, identify parenchymal disease).
  - Radioactive (Tc-99m) sulfur colloid scintigraphy (assesses splenic function).

Complications of Splenomegaly

- ❑ Rupture of the enlarged and friable spleen is possible if the child participates in contact sports.
- ❑ Hypersplenism can cause cytopenias and severe anemia.

Management

- ❑ Treatment of splenomegaly should be aimed at the underlying disease entity.
- ❑ Splenectomy: It may be indicated to help control or stage some diseases that cause splenomegaly:
  - Hereditary spherocytosis
  - Autoimmune thrombocytopenia or hemolysis
  - Lymphoma, Hodgkin's disease
  - Chronic, severe hypersplenism.
- ❑ Postsplenectomy (auto- or post-procedure), all children:
  - Are at risk for fulminant bacteremia, particularly from *Streptococcus pneumoniae*, *Haemophilus influenzae*, *Neisseria meningitides*.
  - Should receive appropriate immunizations.
  - Daily antimicrobial prophylaxis against pneumococcal infections (in addition to immunization) is recommended:
    - In children <5 years of age
    - For ≥1 year after splenectomy.

When to Refer to Specialist

- ❑ Splenomegaly with concomitant hepatomegaly.
- ❑ Palpation of a hard spleen.
- ❑ Suspicion of malignancy or other infiltrative disorders.
- ❑ Evidence of hemolytic anemia.

ASCITES

Definition

Ascites is the accumulation or retention of free fluid within the peritoneal cavity.[29]

Pathogenesis

Ascites represents a disturbance of the intravascular volume homeostasis.[30] It occurs when hydrostatic and osmotic pressures of the hepatic and mesenteric capillaries produce a net transfer of fluid from blood vessels to lymphatic vessels at a rate that exceeds the drainage capacity of the lymphatics. This could be associated with factors such as:[30,31]

- Decreased plasma colloid osmotic pressure.
- Increased capillary pressure.
- Increased colloid osmotic pressure of the ascitic fluid.
- Decreased ascitic fluid hydrostatic pressure.

Etiology

It varies with age (Tables 20.12 to 20.14).[32]

Table 20.12: Causes of fetal ascites[32]

Hepatic causes:
- CMV infection
- Neimann-Pick disease type C
- Biliary atresia
- Neonatal hemochromatosis

Nonhepatic causes:
- Gastrointestinal disorders:
  - Meconium peritonitis
  - Intestinal malrotation
  - Intussusception
  - Jejunal atresia
  - Cystic fibrosis
- Infection:
  - Parvovirus
  - Syphilis
  - CMV
  - Toxoplasmosis
- Genitourinary tract disorders:
  - Hydronephrosis
  - Polycystic kidney disease
  - Urinary tract obstruction
  - Ovarian cyst
- Chylous ascites
- Cardiac causes:
  - Arrhythmias
  - Cardiac failure
- Chromosomal abnormalities:
  - Trisomies
  - Turner syndrome
  - Others
- Other causes:
  - Inborn error of metabolism
  - Hemolytic anemia
  - Hydrops fetalis
  - Idiopathic

Evaluation[29,31,32]

- **History:**
  - Abdominal distension
  - Recent weight gain
  - Associated abdominal pain
  - Symptoms of infections: Fever, travel, rash, etc.
  - Symptoms of possible cause:
    - Chronic liver disease
    - Gastrointestinal
    - Cardiac
    - Renal
    - Neoplastic
    - Inflammatory
    - Allergic
    - Trauma/surgeries
  - Chemicals/drugs
- **Physical examination:**
  - *General examination:*
    - Weight/growth parameters
    - Jaundice
    - Clubbing
    - Spider angiomas
    - Palmar erythema

Table 20.13: Cause of neonatal ascites

Hepatobiliary causes:
- Cirrhosis
- A1AT deficiency
- Congenital hepatic fibrosis
- Hepatitis
- Budd-Chiari syndrome
- Perforated bile duct
- Ruptured cystic mesenchymal hamartoma

Nonhepatic causes:
- Gastrointestinal:
  - Intestinal malrotation
  - Intussusception
  - Jejunal atresia
- Pancreatitis
- Chylous ascites
- TPN
- Metabolic storage disorder:
  - Lysosomal storage disease
  - Wolman's disease
- Renal:
  - Obstructive uropathy
  - Spontaneous or traumatic bladder rupture
  - Nephrotic syndrome
- Cardiac:
  - Arrhythmias
  - Cardiac failure
- Others

Table 20.14: Causes of ascites in infants and children

Hepatic causes:
- Portal hypertension:
  - Presinusoidal causes: Portal vein thrombosis
  - Sinusoidal causes: Cirrhosis, vitamin A toxicity
  - Postsinusoidal causes: Veno-occlusive disease, Budd-Chiari syndrome, congestive cardiac failure, constrictive pericarditis
- Biliary: Perforated bile duct
- Liver transplantation

Nonhepatic causes:
- Chylous ascites: Traumatic and nontraumatic
- Renal:
  - Nephrotic syndrome
  - Dialysis- associated.
- Cardiac:
  - Hear failure
- Ventriculoperitoneal shunts
- Neoplasma:
  - Neurofibromatosis
  - Mesenteric fibromatosis
  - Malignant mesothelioma
- Inflammatory/serositis:
  - Infectious causes: Spontaneous bacterial peritonitis, tuberculosis
  - Allergic: Eosinophilic gastroenteritis
  - Immunologic causes: SLE, vasculitis, HSP
  - Pancreatic causes: Pancreatitis
  - Chemical cause: Talc peritonitis
- Others:
  - Chronic granulomatous disease
  - Thoracic duct obstruction.
  - Abdominal trauma.
  - Congenital diaphragmatic hernia
  - Pseudo-ascites: Celiac disease, omental cysts

Table 20.15: High and low gradient SAAG

High gradient (>1.1 g/dL) ascites	Low gradient (<1.1 g/dL) ascites
- Portal hypertension (cirrhosis) Alcoholic ascites - Cardiac failure - Massive liver metastases - Fulminant hepatic failure - Budd-Chiari syndrome - Portal vein thrombosis - Veno-occlusive disease - Myxedema	- Peritoneal carcinomatosis - Tuberculosis peritonitis - Pancreatic ascites - Biliary ascites - Nephrotic syndrome - Serositis (connective tissue disease)

- ❑ **Diagnostic paracentesis: to diagnose etiology.**[29,31,32]
  - Serum-ascitic albumin concentration gradient (SAAG) (Table 20.15).
  - Ascitic fluid white blood cells (WBC): High in bacterial peritonitis (>250 neutrophils/mm³), low in cirrhosis (<250 cells/mm³).
  - Ascitic fluid culture: Polymicrobial infection indicates intestinal perforation.
  - Ascitic fluid protein: <2.0 g/dL in cirrhosis, >2.0 g/dL is seen in infection, Budd-Chiari and pancreatic ascites.
  - Ascitic fluid amylase: High in pancreatitis or intestinal perforation.
  - Ascitic urea and creatinine: High in uro-ascites (higher than serum).
  - Ascitic fluid bilirubin: High in biliary tree or upper GI perforation.
  - Chylous ascites: Milky appearance, high ascitic fluid triglycerides (higher than serum).

Paracentesis Location

Left lower abdominal quadrant, 2 finger breadths above and 2 finger breadth medial to anterior superior iliac crest is the best location (thinner abdominal wall and larger pool of fluid).

Treatment[30,32]

- ❑ Sodium restriction:
  - Limit it to 1–2 mEq/kg/day (max 1000 mg/day).
  - Should not interfere with nutrient ingestion.
- ❑ Diuretics:
  - To promote sodium excretion. Through diuresis.
  - Spironolactone (2–3 mg/kg/day divided into 2–4 doses in infants, 100–200 mg/day in 2 divided doses in children and adolescents—maximum dose is 400 mg/day).
  - Furosemide: Indicated when spironolactone fails (1–4 mg/kg/day in infants, 40–160 mg/day in older children—maximum dose is 160 mg/day).
  - Watch for electrolytes and fluid disturbances associated with diuretics.

  - Signs of possible underlying etiology (see history above)
- Abdominal examination:
  - Distension
  - Bulging flanks
  - Umbilical collateral veins
  - Dullness to percussion: Dull ascites filled flanks, tympanitic mid abdomen (gas filled center), shifting dullness (minimum fluid required to illicit shifting dullness is 1.5–3.0 L).
  - Fluid thrill (wave) test: Requires 4 hands (2 examiners) and a cooperative patient.
- ❑ **Imaging:**
  - Plain abdominal X-rays: It can detect ascites indirectly, by changes in hepatic angle or flank stripe sign.
  - Abdominal US: Most sensitive. 10–20 mL required for ascites to be detected in an infant (100 mL in adults).
  - Computed tomography (CT)/MRI: For ascites and underlying etiology detection.[30]

- Can combine spironolactone and furosemide (monitor for hypovolemia and electrolyte imbalance).
❏ Large volume paracentesis in refractory ascites or if restricting respiratory efforts.
❏ TIPSS and peritoneovenous shunting: In disabling intractable ascites. Complications could fatal.
❏ Liver transplantation.

TRANSAMINITIS

Definition

Transaminitis is elevated serum amniotransferases' (AST and ALT) levels. AST (aspartate aminotransferase) and ALT (alanine aminotransferase) are normally present in serum in low concentrations in the healthy people. These enzymes are present in several different tissues.

Note

❏ AST and ALT are used to identify released from damaged hepatocytes.
❏ AST is found in high concentrations in liver, skeletal muscle, heart muscle, kidney, brain, pancreas, lung, leukocytes, and red blood cells.
❏ ALT is more specific for liver disease, because it is present in low concentrations in other tissues.
❏ A disproportionately isolated increase in AST suggests: Hemolysis, acute rhabdomyolysis, myopathy, myocardial disease, or a recent vigorous physical activity.
❏ A high ratio of AST : ALT > 4 in the appropriate clinical setting might indicate Wilson disease.
❏ Transaminitis may be the only manifestation of celiac disease.
❏ There is a poor correlation between degree of transaminitis and extent of liver cell damage. Rapidly declining transaminases with increasing cholestasis and worsening of coagulopathy reflects massive liver damage and poor prognosis in a child with acute liver failure.

The pattern of LFT abnormalities may suggest the underlying cause of the patient's liver disease to be of hepatocyte injury (elevated aminotransferases) or cholestasis type (elevated alkaline phosphatase, GGT and or direct bilirubin). The magnitude of the LFT abnormalities and the ratio of AST to ALT may make certain diagnoses more or less likely. In this chapter, hepatocellular pattern only will be discussed. Cholestasis was discussed at a different stage of this chapter. Hepatocellular pattern occurs when disproportionate elevation in the serum aminotransferases compared with the alkaline phosphatase, serum bilirubin may or may not be elevated and tests of synthetic function may or may not be normal.

Differential Diagnosis

Differential diagnosis for transaminitis is broad but can be categorized according to its duration and severity into (Tables 20.16 to 20.19).[32,33]

Table 20.16: Chronic, mild elevation: ALT >AST (<150 u/L or < 5× normal)

Hepatic cause:
- Chronic viral hepatitis
- Bacterial infections (brucellosis, tuberculosis, etc.)
- Medications and toxins
- Autoimmune hepatitis
- Steatohepatitis
- Alpha 1 antitrypsin deficiency
- Wilson disease

Nonhepatic cause:
- Celiac disease
- Hyperthyroidism

Table 20.17: Chronic mild elevation: AST >ALT (<150 u/L or <5 × normal)

Hepatic cause:
- Cirrhosis
- Alcohol related liver disease

Nonhepatic cause:
- Myopathy
- Hypothyroidism
- Strenuous exercise
- Macro-AST

Table 20.18: Acute, severe elevation: ALT > AST (> 1000 u/L, or >20–25 × normal)

Hepatic cause:
- Acute viral hepatitis
- Bacterial infections (sepsis, abscess, brucellosis, tuberculosis, etc.)
- Autoimmune hepatitis
- Ischemic hepatitis
- Medications/toxins
- Wilson disease
- Acute Budd-Chiari syndrome
- Hepatic artery ligation
- Acute bile ducts obstruction

Table 20.19: Acute, severe elevation: AST > ALT (> 1000 u/L, or > 20–25 × normal)

Hepatic cause:
- Cirrhosis
- Alcohol related liver disease

Nonhepatic cause:
- Acute rhabdomyolysis
- Myopathy

Evaluation

- ❑ **History:**
  - Age, gender of patient.
  - Duration of transaminitis.
  - Prenatal, natal and postnatal history.
  - History of:
    - Symptoms related to the liver disease or etiology (fever, fatigue, malaise, anorexia, nausea, jaundice, abdominal pain, etc.)
    - Symptoms of extrahepatic manifestations (skin rash, arthritis).
    - Exposure to hepatotoxins (medications and herbal remedies).
    - Risk for viral hepatitis (blood transfusion, IV drugs use, travel to endemic area, exposure to patient with jaundice).
    - Symptoms of disorders that are associated with liver disease (Diabetes mellitus, obesity, gallstones, inflammatory bowel disease, celiac disease, thyroid disease, etc.)
    - Family history of hepatitis, inherited or acquired liver disease or predisposing factors.
- ❑ **Physical examination:**
  - Complete physical examination (growth, extrahepatic manifestations).
  - Jaundice.
  - Signs of chronic liver disease (Mental status changes, edema, ascites, clubbing, petechiae, ecchymosis, spider angiomas).
  - Hepatosplenomegaly, abdominal tenderness or masses.
  - Signs of cardiac, respiratory, dermatological or joint disease.
- ❑ **Investigations:**
  - Liver enzymes (might require repeating to determine if chronic or acute).
  - Synthetic liver function.
  - Electrolytes, renal function and bone profile: Especially if chronic liver disease, metabolic or causes are suspected.
  - Underlying etiology (see tables above).
- ❑ **Serological testing and imaging:**
  - For etiologies listed in the above tables
  - Ultrasound with Doppler.
- ❑ **Histopathologic examination:**
  - Important adjunct in evaluation of children with hepatitis.

Management

- ❑ Identify and treat potentially treatable disease.
- ❑ Recognize complications of acute and chronic hepatitis (portal hypertension, ascites, liver dysfunction).

▌UPPER GASTROINTESTINAL BLEEDING

Definition

Upper gastrointestinal bleeding (UGIB) is bleeding from a site proximal to the ligament of Treitz.[34,35] In this section, the emphasis is mainly on liver-related causes of UGIB.

Epidemiology[34,35]

- ❑ 5% of all indications of upper endoscopies in pediatric age group.
- ❑ Incidence is higher in critically sick children (6–25%).
- ❑ Only 0.4% is life-threatening.

Presentation[34,35]

- ❑ Hematemesis: Vomiting of bright red blood (usually indicates a large volume or rapidly bleeding lesion.
- ❑ Coffee-ground emesis: Appearance of dark denatured blood (by contact with gastric acid).
- ❑ Melena: Black tarry stools caused by oxidation of blood from GI tract proximal to colon by intestinal bacteria (as little as 50–100 mL can cause melena).

Causes of UGIB

See Table 20.20.[34,35]

Portal Hypertension Related UGIB

Variceal Bleeding

- ❑ Accounts for 5–11% of GI bleeding in children.
- ❑ Esophageal varices grading:
  - Grade I: Disappear with air insufflation.
  - Grade II: Nonconfluent varices remain unchanged with insufflation.
  - Grade III: Large, tense protruding into esophageal lumen.
  - Grade IV: Near complete luminal obstruction by varices, cherry-red spot with impending hemorrhage.

Portal Hypertensive Gastropathy

- ❑ Seen in portal hypertension regardless of etiology (>90% is seen with cirrhosis).
- ❑ Endoscopic features vary with severity of portal hypertension:
  - Mosaic pattern of erythematous patches separated by white lattice.
  - Cherry red spots
  - Diffuse hemorrhage.

Table 20.20: Common etiologies of UGIB in children

Neonates:
- Swallowed maternal blood
- Hemorrhagic disease of the newborn
- Stress gastritis
- Peptic ulcer disease
- Vascular anomalies
- Coagulopathy
- Cow milk protein intolerance

Infants:
- Stress gastritis
- Peptic ulcer disease
- Mallory-Weiss tear
- Vascular anomaly
- Gastrointestinal duplication
- Esophageal/gastric varices
- Foreign body (FB)
- Hereditary telangiectasia

Children/adolescents:
- Mallory-Weiss tear
- Esophagitis/gastritis
- Peptic ulcer disease
- Variceal bleeding
- Caustic ingestion
- Vasculitis (HSP)
- Crohn's disease
- Hemobilia
- Foreign body (FB)
- Tumors
- Telangiectasia

Evaluation

- **History:**
  - Prenatal, natal and postnatal history.
  - Vitamin K injection after delivery.
  - Birth asphyxia, umbilical catheterization.
  - Maternal conditions (e.g. cracked nipples).
  - Bleeding tendency and other sites of bleeding.
  - Onset of vomiting (e.g. extensive retching, hematemesis or food content at the beginning of vomiting).
  - Description of vomitus (hematemesis, coffee ground).
  - Nose or gum bleeds.
  - Presence of melena.
  - Abdominal pain or distension.
  - Retrosternal pain.
  - Caustic or foreign body ingestion.
  - Symptoms of chronic liver disease.
  - Extraintestinal manifestation: Skin rash, petechiae, purpura, arthritis, mouth ulcers, etc.

- Medications intake (aspirin, NSAIDs, steroids, anticoagulants/thrombotics, etc.)
- Family history of UGIB, liver disease, telangiectasia, bleeding tendencies.

- **Physical examination:**
  - Vital signs, cardiovascular stability, orthostatic changes, level of consciousness.
  - Pallor, restlessness.
  - Signs of chronic liver disease.
  - Skin rash: Purpura, petechiae, hemangioma, and telangiectasia.
  - Epistaxis or blood in hypopharynx.
  - Abdominal tenderness, hepatosplenomegaly, ascites, masses.
  - Rectal examination for melena.

- **Laboratory investigations:**
  - Complete blood count, platelet count, differential, reticulocyte count.
  - Coagulation profile (PT, INR, PTT).
  - Liver function tests.
  - Blood group, cross match.
  - Inflammatory markers when indicated.

- **Imaging (usually after consideration of differential diagnosis):**
  - Plain X-ray film of neck/chest or abdomen: May show FB or free air (suggestive of perforation).
  - Upper GI contrast study: Radiolucent FB, duplication cysts, etc.
  - Abdominal ultrasound: When portal hypertension is suspected.
  - Radilabeled RBC scan: For bleeding lesions with flow of 0.1 mL/min.
  - Angiography: For bleeding lesions of 0.5 mL/min or higher (therapeutic intervention can be done at the same time).

- **Endoscopy:**
  - Not indicated in hemodynamically stable child without anemia.
  - Is contraindicated if child is unstable or has severe anemia.
  - Both diagnostic and therapeutic.

Management[34,35]

- Stabilization of patient.
- Nasogastric tube insertion: To identify source of bleeding location and for irrigation.
- Resuscitation with fluids, blood and blood products.
- Correction of anemia, coagulopathy, electrolytes imbalance or fluid loss.

❑ Pharmacologic intervention:
- Acid suppression: Proton pump inhibitor (0.1 mg/kg bolus followed by 0.1 mg/kg/hour infusion).
- Sucralfate (40–80 mg/kg/day in 2–4 doses/day): facilitates ulcers healing by binding to base.
- Octreotide: May be used in both variceal and non-variceal bleeding.
  - Reduces splanchnic, decreases gastric acid secretion and portal blood flow.
  - Dose: 1 μg/kg bolus followed by 1–3 μg/kg/hour infusion.
  - Reduce dose over a 12-hour period when bleeding is controlled.
  - Discontinue when dose is 25% of initial dose.
  - Can cause peripheral vasoconstriction: May worsen renal function.

Endoscopic Intervention[36,37]

❑ **Esophageal/gastric variceal bleeding management:**
- Injection sclerotherapy.
- Band ligation.
- Intraesophageal balloon tamponade.

❑ **Nonvariceal bleeding management:**
- Epinephrine injection (1:10,000) (9 mL normal saline to 1 mL epinephrine): Effect through tamponade and vasoconstriction.
- Other sclerosing agents' injections: Normal saline, hypertonic saline, 50% dextrose, ethanol, polidocanol, sodium tetradecyl sulfate.
- Thermocoagulation: Using heater probe and mono/bipolar coagulators. Argon plasma coagulation is useful for vascular ectasia, bleeding ulcer, postpolypectomy bleeding, Mallor-Weiss tear and Dieulafoy lesion.
- Hemostatic clip/ligation devices

❑ **Interventional radiology in UGIB:**
- Useful in massive acute arterial bleeding, portal hypertension and vascular anomalies, after failed endoscopic therapy.
- Imaging used: CT, CT angiography, tagged RBC radionuclide study, and angiography.
- Examples of techniques: Provocation angiography, embolization (coils, particles, gelfoam, NBCA), vasoconstrictor infusion, TIPSS, portal varix embolization, partial splenic embolization, portal vein recanalization, and others.

REFERENCES

1. Moyer V, Freese DK, Whitington PF, Olson AD, Brewer F, Colletti RB, et al. North American Society for Pediatric Gastroenterology, Hepatology and Nutrition. Guideline for the evaluation of cholestatic jaundice in infants: recommendations of the North American Society for Pediatric Gastroenterology, Hepatology and Nutrition. J Pediatr Gastroenterol Nutr. 2004;39(2):115.
2. Kelly DA, Stanton A. Jaundice in babies: implications for community screening for biliary atresia. BMJ. 1995;310(6988):1172.
3. Boyer JL. New perspectives for the treatment of cholestasis: lessons from basic science applied clinically. J Hepatol. 2007;46(3):365-71.
4. Emerick KM, Whitington PF. Neonatal liver disease. Pediatr Ann. 2006;35(4):280-6.
5. Mela M, Mancuso A, Burroughs AK. Review article: pruritus in cholestatic and other liver diseases. Aliment Pharmacol Ther. 2003;17:857-70.
6. Jones EA, Bergasa NV. The pruritus of cholestasis. Hepatology. 1999;29:1003-6.
7. Murphy GM, Ross A, Billing BH. Serum bile acids in primary biliary cirrhosis. Gut. 1972;13(3):201.
8. Ghent CN, Bloomer JR, Klatskin G. Elevations in skin tissue levels of bile acids in human cholestasis: relation to serum levels and pruritus. Gastroenterology. 1977;73(5):1125.
9. Ghent CN. Pruritus of cholestasis is related to effects of bile salts on the liver, not the skin. Am J Gastroenterol. 1987;82(2):117.
10. Thornton JR, Losowsky MS. Plasma leucine enkephalin is increased in liver disease. Gut. 1989;30(10):1392.
11. Summerfield JA. Naloxone modulates the perception of itch in man. Br J Clin Pharmacol. 1980;10(2):180.
12. Casale TB, Bowman S, Kaliner M. Induction of human cutaneous mast cell degranulation by opiates and endogenous opioid peptides: evidence for opiate and nonopiate receptor participation. J Allergy Clin Immunol. 1984;73:775-81.
13. Bergasa NV, Jones EA. The pruritus of cholestasis. Semin Liver Dis. 1993;13:319-27.
14. Kiefel JM, Cooper ML, Bodnar RJ. Serotonin receptor subtype antagonists in the medial ventral medulla inhibit mesencephalic opiate analgesia. Brain Res. 1992;597:331-8.
15. Kremer, AE, Martens, JJ, Kulik, W, et al. Increased serum autotaxin activity in cholestatic pruritus (abstract). Hepatology. 209; 50:376A.
16. Tandon P, Rowe BH, Vandermeer B, Bain VG. The efficacy and safety of bile acid binding agents, opioid antagonists, or rifampin in the treatment of cholestasis-associated pruritus. Am J Gastroenterol. 2007;102(7):1528.
17. Podesta A, Lopez P, Terg R, Villamil F, Flores D, Mastai R, et al. JP. Treatment of pruritus of primary biliary cirrhosis with rifampin. Dig Dis Sci. 1991;36(2):216.

18. Bloomer JR, Boyer JL. Phenobarbital effects in cholestatic liver diseases. Ann Intern Med. 1975;82(3):310.

19. Batta AK, Salen G, Mirchandani R, Tint GS, Shefer S, Batta M, et al. Effect of long-term treatment with ursodiol on clinical and biochemical features and biliary bile acid metabolism in patients with primary biliary cirrhosis. Am J Gastroenterol. 1993;88(5):691.

20. Wolfhagen FH, Sternieri E, Hop WC, Vitale G, Bertolotti M, Van Buuren HR. Oral naltrexone treatment for cholestatic pruritus: a double-blind, placebo-controlled study. Gastroenterology. 1997;113(4):1264.

21. Terg R, Coronel E, Sorda J, Munoz AE, Findor J. Efficacy and safety of oral naltrexone treatment for pruritus of cholestasis, a crossover, double blind, placebo-controlled study. J Hepatol. 2002;37(6):717-22.

22. Bickley L, Szilagyi P, Bates B. Bate's Guide to Physical Examination and History Taking, 10th ed. Philadelphia: Wolters Kluwer Health/Lippincott Williams and Wilkins; 2009.

23. Kliegman R, Behrman, Jenson H, Stanton B. Nelson Textbook of Pediatrics, 18th ed. Philadelphia: Saunders; 2007.

24. Lawson EE, et al. Clinical Estimation of liver span in infants and children. Am J Dis Child. 1978;132(5):474-6.

25. Novak D, Suchy FJ, Balistreri WF. Disorders of the liver and biliary system. Oski's Pediatrics: Principles and Practice of pediatrics. 4th ed. Philadelphia, PA: Lippincott Williams and Wilkins; 2006: Chapter 367.

26. Krumbhaar EB, Lippincott SW. The postmortem weight of the "normal" spleen at different ages. Am J Med Sci. 1939;197:344.

27. Rosenberg HK, Markowitz RI, Kolberg H, Park C, Hubbard A, Bellah RD. Normal splenic size in infants and children: sonographic measurements. AJR Am J Roentgenol. 1991;157(1):119.

28. McMillan J, Nieburg P, Oski FA. The whole pediatrician catalogue. WB Saunders, Philadelphia. 1977;p.21.

29. Hou W, Sanyal AJ. Ascites: diagnosis and management. Med Clin North Am. 2009;93(4):801-17.

30. McDiarmid SV. End-stage liver disease. In: Kleinman R, Sanderson IR, Goulet O, Sherman PM, Mieli-Vergani G, Shneider BL(Eds). Walker Pediatric Gastrointestinal Disease. Hamilton, Ontario: BC Decker Inc. 2008;1138-41.

31. Hardy S, Kleinman RE, Cirrhosis and chronic liver failure. In: Suchy FJ, Sokol RJ, Balistreri WF (Ed.) Liver Disease in Children. New York, NY: Cambridge University Press. 2007;108-14.

32. Colleti RB, Krawitt EL. Ascites. In: Wyllie R, Hyams JS (Eds). Pediatric Gastrointestinal Disease: Pathophysiology, Diagnosis and Management. Philadelphia, Pennsylvania: WB Saunders Company. 1999;04-12.

33. Suchy FJ, Sokol RJ, Balistreri WF. Liver Diseases in Children. 3rd ed. New York, NY: Cambridge University Press; 2007.

34. Boyle JT. Gastrointestinal bleeding in infants and children. Pediatr Rev. 2008;29:39-52.

35. Gigler MA, Whitfield KL. Upper gastrointestinal bleeding. In: Kleinman RE, Sanderson IR, Goulet O, Sherman PM, Mieli-Vergani F, Shneider BL (Eds). Walker's Pediatric Gastrointestinal Disease. 5th ed. Hamilton, Ontario: BC Decker Inc. 2008;1286-90.

36. Cardenas A. Management of acute variceal bleeding: emphasis on endoscopic therapy. Clin Liver Dis. 2010;251-62.

37. Kay MH, Wyllie R. Therapeutic endoscopy for nonvariceal gastrointestinal bleeding. J Pediatr Gastroenterol Nutr. 2007;157-71.

Chapter

21

Interpretation of Liver Function Tests

BR Thapa, Ravinder Goyal, Srikanth KP

INTRODUCTION

Liver has to perform different kinds of biochemical, synthetic and excretory functions, so no single biochemical test can detect the global functions of liver.[1, 2] All laboratories usually employ a battery of tests for initial detection and management of liver diseases and these tests are frequently termed "liver function tests", although they are of little value in assessing the liver function per se. In spite of receiving lot of criticism for this terminology, the phrase 'liver function tests' is firmly entrenched in the medical lexicon and used widely. It might be argued that 'liver injury tests' would be a more appropriate terminology.[3] Moreover, the clinical history and physical examination play important role to interpret the functions. The role of specific disease markers, radiological imaging and liver biopsy cannot be underestimated.

USES

The various uses of liver function tests (LFT) include[4]
- *Screening:* They are a non-invasive yet sensitive screening modality for liver dysfunction
- *Pattern of disease:* They are helpful to recognize the pattern of liver disease. Like being helpful in differentiating between acute hepatitis and various cholestatic disorders and chronic liver disease. (CLD)
- *Assess severity:* They are helpful to assess the severity and predict the outcome of certain diseases like neonatal hepatitis, hepatitis B and hepatitis C.
- *Follow-up:* They are helpful in the follow up of certain liver diseases and also helpful in evaluating response to therapy like autoimmune hepatitis and Wilson disease.

LIMITATIONS[5]

- *Lack sensitivity:* The LFT may be normal in certain liver diseases like compensated cirrhosis, non-cirrhotic portal fibrosis (NCPF), congenital hepatic fibrosis (CHF), etc.
- *Lack specificity:* They lack specificity and are not specific for any particular disease. Serum albumin may be decreased in CLD and also in nephrotic syndrome. Aminotransferases may be raised in both cardiac and hepatic diseases.

Except for serum bile acids and alanine aminotransferase (ALT), the LFT are not specific for liver diseases, which may be affected by pathological processes outside the liver.

CLASSIFICATION OF LFT

Liver function can be studied under following headings
- Organic anion metabolism: Bilirubin, urobilinogen, bile salts
- Indicators of cell necrosis: Alanine aminotransferase (ALT), aspartate aminotransferase(AST)
- Indicators of cholestasis: Alkaline phosphatase (ALP), gamma glutamyl transpeptidase (γGT), 5' nucleotidase
- Protein synthesis: Albumin, prealbumin, prothrombin time (PT), international normalized ratio(INR), procollagen III peptide
- Markers of specific diseases: Ceruloplasmin (Cp), α1 antitrypsin(α1AT) , α fetoprotein (αFP).

TESTS OF THE LIVER'S CAPACITY TO TRANSPORT ORGANIC ANIONS

Serum Bilirubin

Most of the bilirubin is formed by the breakdown of hemoglobin, and other pyrole ring containing molecules like myoglobin and cytochromes in the body tissues. The bilirubin is bound to albumin in the circulation and dissociates in the liver, and free bilirubin enters liver cells, where it is bound to cytoplasmic proteins. Subsequently, it is taken by the smooth endoplasmic reticulum (SER) and it is conjugated by the enzyme **glucuronyl transferase**. However, small amount of bilirubin remains unconjugated (free bilirubin) and remains bound to albumin hence, not excreted in the urine, whereas each bilirubin molecule in SER reacts with two uridine diphosphoglucuronic acid (UDPGA) molecules to form bilirubin diglucuronide. This glucuronide, which is more water-soluble than the free bilirubin, is then transported against a concentration gradient by active process into the bile canaliculi. A small amount of the conjugated bilirubin escapes into the blood, where it is bound less tightly to albumin than is free bilirubin, and is excreted in the urine. Thus, the total plasma bilirubin normally includes free bilirubin plus a small amount of conjugated bilirubin. Most of the conjugated bilirubin passes via the bile ducts to the intestine.

In the intestine the conjugated bilirubin is acted upon by bacteria and gets converted into unconjugated bilirubin and stercobilinogen. The conjugated bilirubin is impermeable in the intestinal mucosa, whereas unconjugated bilirubin is permeable and goes into the enterohepatic circulation. Some of the stercobilinogen gets absorbed into circulation and is excreted in urine as urobilinogen.

The diazo method involved in bilirubin estimation is not very accurate, especially in detecting low levels of bilirubin. Direct bilirubin over estimates bilirubin esters at low bilirubin levels and under estimates them at high concentration. Thus, slight elevation of unconjugated bilirubin not detected, which is of value in detecting conditions like Gilbert syndrome. A newer highly accurate method of estimation involves alkaline methanolysis of bilirubin followed by chloroform extraction of bilirubin methyl esters and later separation of these esters by chromatography and spectrophotometric determination at 430 nm.

Diagnostic Value of Bilirubin Levels

Bilirubin in body is a careful balance between production and removal of the pigment. Hyperbilirubinemia seen in acute hepatitis is directly related to the degree of injury to the hepatocytes.

Hyperbilirubinemia: It results from overproduction and impaired uptake, conjugation, excretion and regurgitation of unconjugated or conjugated bilirubin from hepatocytes to bile ducts. Approach to jaundice in neonatal period is given in Flow chart 21.1.

Increased unconjugated bilirubin: This results from overproduction and impaired uptake and conjugation.

Flow chart 21.1: Algorithmic approach to hyperbilirubinemia in neonatal period

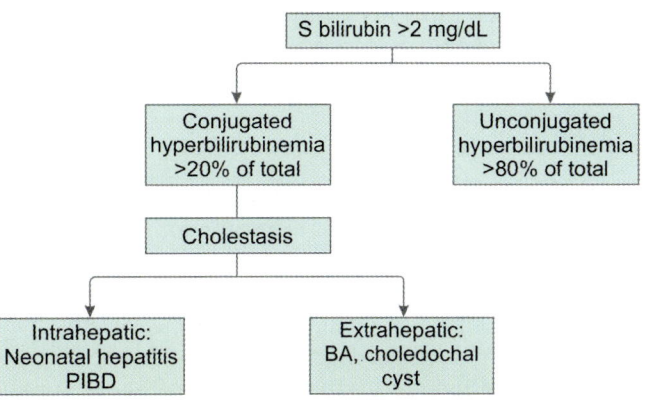

Hyperbilirubinemia Due to Hemolysis

Unconjugated bilirubin itself is not soluble in water and is bound to albumin and thus does not appear in urine. Hemolysis with overproduction of bilirubin and concomitant reduced GFR cause decreased excretion and can lead to high bilirubin levels. Bilirubin levels in excess of 25 mg/dL may be seen in hemolysis in association with liver disease due to underlying G_6PD deficiency.

Drugs

Serum bilirubin level can increase by intake of drugs like salicylates, sulfonamides, free fatty acids which displace bilirubin from its attachment to plasma albumin. Bilirubin may shift from tissue sites to circulation leading to increased levels.

Increased conjugated bilirubin: Conjugated bilirubin is increased when there is hepatocellular necrosis, impaired intrahepatic excretion and regurgitation of conjugated bilirubin from hepatocytes or bile ducts.

Prognostic Value of Bilirubin Levels

Bilirubin may be of prognostic value in conditions like fulminant hepatic failure where deep jaundice is associated with increased mortality. Other causes of extreme hyperbilirubinemia include severe parenchymal disease, septicemia and renal failure.

Urine Bilirubin

The presence of urine bilirubin indicates hepatobiliary disease. Because the renal threshold for conjugated bilirubin is low and the laboratory methods can detect low levels of bilirubin in urine. Conjugated bilirubin may be found in urine when the serum bilirubin levels are normal, e.g. early acute viral hepatitis. Tests strips impregnated with diazo reagent are easy to use and detect as little as 1–2 μmol bilirubin/L.

Urobilinogen

An increase in the urobilinogen in urine is a sensitive indicator of hepatocellular dysfunction. It can be detected in urine in the early phase of viral hepatitis, drug-induced hepatitis, alcoholic liver damage, well compensated cirrhosis or malignant disease of the liver. It is markedly increased in hemolysis. In obstructive jaundice urobilinogen disappears from urine. It may be intermittently present in case of gallstone. Urobilinogen gives a purple reaction to Ehrlich's aldehyde reagent. A dipstick containing this reagent allows rough and ready quantification. Freshly voided urine should be used.

Bile Salts

The bile acids are group of compounds that belong to acidic sterols, and are synthesized from cholesterol in the liver. Two principal bile acids synthesized by the liver are cholic acid and chenodeoxycholic acid. The bile salts are sodium and potassium salts of bile acids, and all those secreted into the bile are conjugated to glycine or taurine. In common with vitamin D, cholesterol, a variety of steroid hormones, and the digitalis glycosides, bile acids also contain the cyclopentanoperhydrophenanthrene (CPPA) nucleus. In the colon, bacteria convert cholic acid to deoxycholic acid and chenodeoxycholic acid to lithocholic acid. Since they are formed by bacterial action, deoxycholic acid and lithocholic acid are called secondary bile acids.

The bile acids perform several important functions, e.g. elimination of cholesterol from body, promotion and secretion of bile, elimination of endogenous and exogenous toxic substances including bilirubin, xenobiotics, and drug metabolites.

Functions of Bile Salts

The bile salts in the intestine reduce the surface tension and, in conjunction with phospholipids and monoglycerides, are responsible for the emulsification of dietary fat during digestion and absorption. They are amphipathic, i.e. they have both hydrophilic and hydrophobic domains, one surface of the molecule is hydrophilic because the polar peptide bond and the carboxyl and hydroxyl groups are on that surface, whereas the other surface is hydrophobic. Therefore, the bile salts tend to form cylindrical disks called micelles. The micelles play an important role in keeping lipids in solution and transporting them to the brush border of the intestinal epithelial cells, where they are absorbed. This detergent action of the bile salts help in absorption of the fats and the important fat-soluble vitamins (A, D, E and K) in the body.

Ninety to ninety-five percent of the bile salts are absorbed from the small intestine. Some are absorbed by nonionic diffusion, but most are absorbed from the terminal ileum by an extremely efficient Na^+–bile salt cotransport system powered by basolateral Na^+–K^+ ATPase. The remaining 5–10% of the bile salt enters the colon and deconjugated by the colonic bacteria and converted to the salts of deoxycholic acid and lithocholic acid. Lithocholate is relatively insoluble and is mostly excreted in the stools (only 1% is absorbed) whereas deoxycholate is completely absorbed and in the liver they get reconjugated.

The absorbed bile salts are transported back to the liver in the portal vein and re-excreted in the bile (enterohepatic circulation). Those lost in the stool are replaced by synthesis in the liver; the normal rate of bile salt synthesis is 0.2–0.4 g/day. The total bile salt pool of 2.0–4.0 g recycles repeatedly via the enterohepatic circulation (10–12 times/day), stimulated by postprandial contraction of gallbladder. Each day less than 5% is lost in the stool. This bile acid loss is compensated by hepatic synthesis of newly formed bile acids in the liver. When bile is excluded from the intestine, up to 50% of ingested fat appears in the feces. A severe malabsorption of fat and fat-soluble vitamins occurs when there is resection of terminal ileum.

In the preterm and term neonates there is a relatively reduced bile acid pool but rapid expansion of pool occurs during first few months of life, which ensures adequate absorption of fat and fat soluble vitamins and also leads to promotion of bile flow. Normal values of primary and total bile acids at different ages are given in Table 21.1.[6]

Inborn Error of Bile Acid Synthesis

Synthesis of bile acids in the liver involves a complex series of reactions at least 14 enzymatic steps. A failure to perform any of these enzymatic reactions will block bile acid production with failing to produce "normal bile acids"[7]. This results in the accumulation of unusual bile acids and intermediary metabolites. This will reduce the bile flow, leading to decreased intraluminal solubilization of fat and fat-soluble vitamins. Some of the intermediate metabolites produced because of blockade in the bile acid biosynthetic pathway may be toxic to hepatocytes. Nine inborn errors of bile acid metabolism have been identified that lead to enzyme deficiencies and impaired bile acid synthesis in infants, children, and adults. The clinical presentation occurs in the form of neonatal cholestasis,

Table 21.1: Normal values of primary and total bile acids at different ages[6]

Age	Primary bile acid (µM/L)	Total bile acid (µM/L)
Day 1	11.7	17.6
Day 2	14.5	18.9
Day 3	16.6	19.9
Day 4	21.4	24.0
Day 5	21.9	23.9
Day 6	24.3	27.1
1 month	24.7	27.1
2 months	22.8	25.2
3 months	20.2	22.6
5 months	15.0	17.0
1 year	10.8	15.3
2 years	8.1	12.0
3 years	8.7	13.5
4–6 years	4.1	6.3
7–9 years	3.2	4.8
10–15 years	2.9	4.4

neurologic disease, or fat and fat-soluble vitamin malabsorption. Untreated patients develop progressive liver disease leading to serious morbidity or mortality due to intestinal malabsorption.

Unexplained prolonged cholestasis in neonatal period, infancy, childhood or even during adulthood, a high index of suspicion of inborn errors of metabolism in bile acid synthesis should be considered. Among the diagnostic tools gas chromatography–mass spectrometry (GC-MS) continues to be the principal confirmatory analytical tool. The most significant advances in mass spectrometry in recent years have been the introduction of fast atom bombardment–mass spectrometry (FABMS) and electrospray mass spectrometry, both of which are referred to by the generic term liquid secondary ionization mass spectrometry (LSIMS). Although these molecular diagnostics are best to identify inborn errors of bile acid metabolism, the turnaround time for the assay is sometimes slow. As a screening test, in assessing infants with conjugated hyperbilirubinemia, it may be practical to measure serum bile acids by a standard laboratory technique that will identify primary and secondary bile acids and guide for further evaluation by GCMS or LSIMS.

The early diagnosis of in born errors of bile acids is important because, if untreated these conditions or invariably fatal. The replacement therapy with specific bile acids is helpful. Ultimately the defect can only be corrected by liver transplantation.

TESTS FOR HEPATOCYTIC NECROSIS

The liver contains thousands of enzymes however, majority of these do not have clinical significance.

Enzymes that Detect Hepatocellular Dysfunction

Aminotransferases

The aminotransferases (transaminase) are the most frequently utilized and specific indicators of hepatocellular necrosis. These enzymes are AST also known as glutamate oxaloacetate transaminase (SGOT) and ALT also known as glutamic pyruvate transaminase (SGPT) catalyze the transfer of the α amino acids of aspartate and alanine respectively to the α keto group of ketoglutaric acid. ALT is primarily localized to the liver whereas the AST is present in a wide variety of tissues like the liver, heart, skeletal muscle, kidney and brain.

AST: aspartate + α ketoglutarate = oxaloacetate + glutamate

ALT: alanine + α ketoglutarate = pyruvate + glutamate

AST is present in both the mitochondria and cytosol of hepatocytes, whereas ALT is localized to the cytosol. The cytosolic and mitochondrial forms of AST are true isoenzymes and immunologically distinct.[8]

About 80% of AST activity in human liver is contributed by the mitochondrial isoenzyme, whereas most of the circulating AST activity in normal people is derived from the cytosolic isoenzyme. Normal AST/ALT ratio is 0.8 if it is more than one it indicates CLD. Normal values AST, ALT and GGT are given in Table 21.2. Algorithm to approach mild and sustained rise of aminotransferases is given in Flow chart 21.2.

Significant elevation of mitochondrial AST occurs after extensive tissue necrosis.[8] Because of this, assay of mitochondrial AST has been advocated in myocardial infarction. Mitochondrial AST is also increased in CLD. Their activity in serum at any moment reflects the relative rate at which they enter and leave circulation. Virtually no aminotransferases are present in the urine or bile and hepatic sinusoids are the primary site for their clearance.

Table 21.2: Normal values of ALT, AST, and GGT (U/L) at different ages

	ALT(U/L)	AST(U/L)	GGT (U/L)
Neonate	0–40	<120	<200
Infant	10–80	<80	<120
Children	10–40	10–50	<35

Flow chart 21.2: Algorithmic approach to mild and sustained rise of aminotransferases

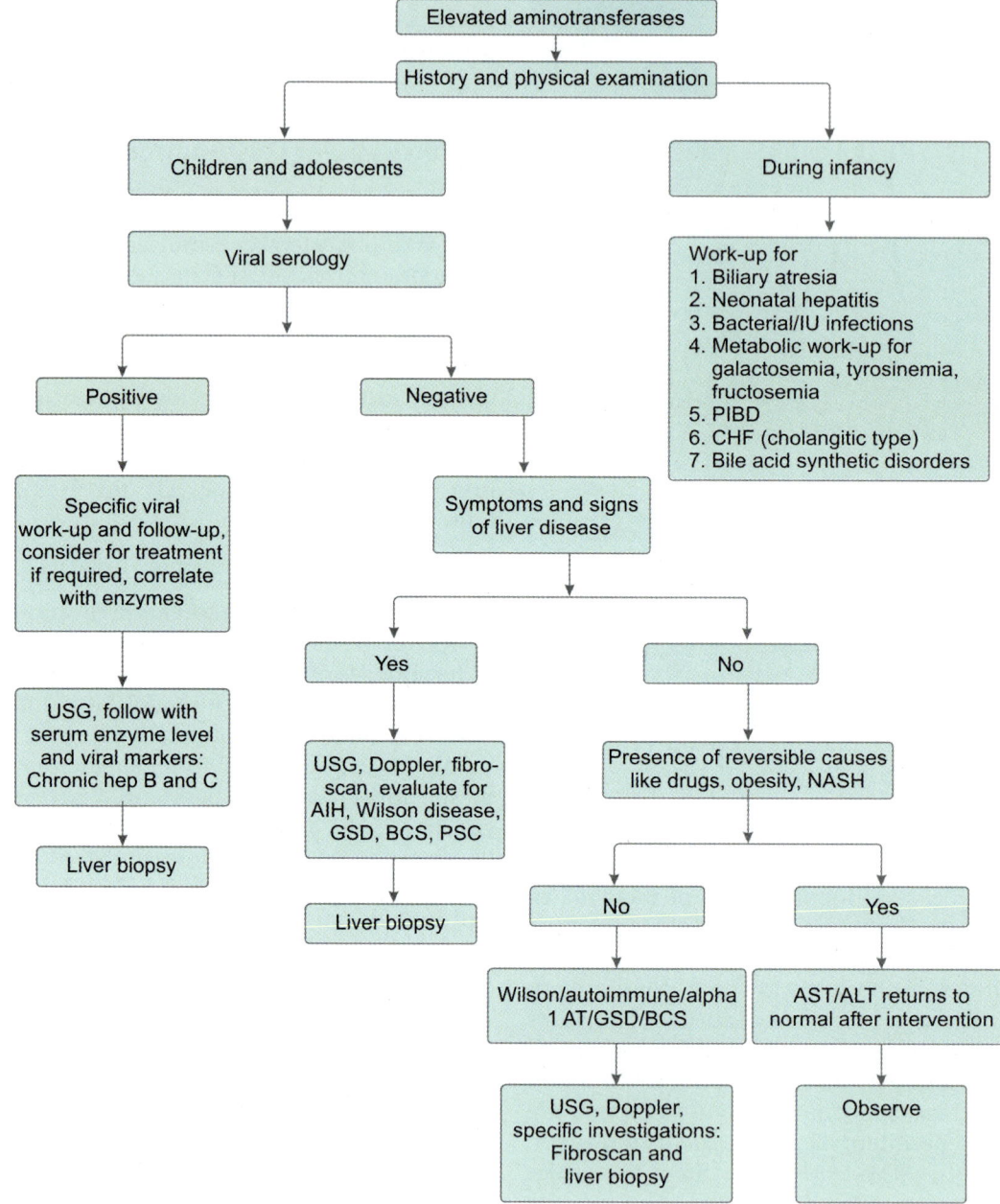

Mild, Moderate, and Severe Elevations of Aminotransferases

Severe (>20 times, 1000 U/L): The AST and ALT levels are increased to some extent in almost all liver diseases. The highest elevations occur in severe viral hepatitis; drug or toxin induced hepatic necrosis and circulatory shock. Although enzyme levels may reflect the extent of hepatocellular necrosis they do not correlate with eventual outcome. In fact declining AST and ALT may indicate either recovery or poor prognosis in fulminant hepatic failure.[9]

Moderate (3–20 times): The AST and ALT are moderately elevated in acute hepatitis, neonatal hepatitis, chronic hepatitis, autoimmune hepatitis, drug induced hepatitis, alcoholic hepatitis, and acute biliary tract obstructions.[10] The ALT is usually more frequently increased as compared to AST except in chronic liver disease.

Mild (1–3 times): These elevations are usually seen in sepsis induced neonatal hepatitis, biliary atresia (BA), fatty liver, cirrhosis, non alcoholic steatohepatitis (NASH), drug toxicity, myositis and even after vigorous exercise. One third to one half of healthy individuals with an isolated elevation of ALT on repeated testing have been found to be normal.

AST : ALT Ratio

The ratio of AST to ALT is of use in Wilson disease, CLD and alcoholic liver disease and a ratio of more than 2 is usually observed. The lack of ALT rise is probably due to pyridoxine deficiency. In NASH the ratio is less than one in the absence of fibrosis on liver biopsy. In viral hepatitis the ratio is usually less than one. The ratio invariably rises to more than one as cirrhosis develops possibly because of reduced plasma clearance of AST secondary to impaired function of sinusoidal cells. ALT exceeds AST in toxic hepatitis, viral hepatitis, chronic active hepatitis and cholestatic hepatitis. Falsely low aminotransferase levels have been seen in patients on long term hemodialysis probably secondary to either dialysate or pyridoxine deficiency.[11] Low levels have also been seen in uremia.[12]

Mitochondrial AST : Total AST Ratio

This ratio is characteristically elevated in alcoholic liver disease.[8] Abstinence from alcohol improves this ratio. It is also seen to be high in Wilson's disease.

Other Enzymes of Hepatocellular Necrosis

These include glutamate dehydrogenase, isocitrate dehydrogenase, lactate dehydrogenase, and sorbitol dehydrogenase. None of these tests have proved to be useful in practice than the aminotransferases

Lactate Dehydrogenase (LDH)

LDH is widely distributed in the body and has to be notes to be raised in ischemic hepatitis, acute and CLD, malignant liver infiltration, in skeletal and cardiac muscle injury, hemolysis, stroke and renal infarction. In liver disease it lacks specificity. Normal values in children are given in Table 21.3.

Enzymes that Detect Cholestasis

Alkaline Phosphatase (ALP)

ALP is a family of zinc metalloenzymes, with a serine at the active center; they release inorganic phosphate from various organic orthophosphates and are present in nearly all tissues. In liver, ALP is found histochemically in the microvilli of bile canaliculi and on the sinusoidal surface of hepatocytes. ALP from the liver, bone and kidney are thought to be from the same gene but that from intestine and placenta are derived from different genes.[13]

In liver two distinct forms of ALP are also found but their precise roles are unknown. In healthy people most circulating ALP originates from liver or bone.

The internationally recommended reference method uses p-nitrophenol phosphate as substrate, in alkaline buffer. Fresh unhemolysed serum is the specimen of choice for the estimation. Heparinized plasma may also be used. The test should not be done on plasma if citrate, oxalate or EDTA were used as anticoagulants; they form a complex with zinc and the alkaline phosphatase, causing irreversible enzyme inactivation.

Average values of ALP vary with age and are relatively high in childhood and puberty and lower in middle age and higher again in old age. Males usually have higher values as compared to females. The levels correlate with person's weight and inversely with the height of person. Normal values are given in Table 21.4.[14] Not uncommonly isolated elevated levels of ALP in otherwise healthy persons return to normal on follow-up.

Elevated ALP

Highest levels of ALP occur in cholestatic disorders. Elevations occur as a result of both intrahepatic and extrahepatic obstruction to bile flow and the degree of elevation does not help distinguish between the two. ALP levels are likely to be very high in BA but not diagnostic.

Table 21.3: Normal values of lactate dehydrogenase at different ages		
Age	U/L	
0–5 days	730–1650	
1–3 years	400–720	
4–6 years	375–700	
7–9 years	335–590	
	Male	Female
10–11 years	345–550	305–605
12–13 years	375–590	305–505
14–15 years	290–570	315–460
16–19 years	275–525	275–525

Table 21.4: Normal values of ALP at different ages[14]		
Age	U/L	
Preterm	Up to 1500	
Term neonate	Up to 700	
Infant	250–1000	
2–5 years	250–850	
6–7 years	250–1000	
8–9 years	250–750	
	Male	Female
10–11 years	250–730	250–950
12–13 years	275–875	200–730
14–15 years	170–970	170–460
16–18 years	125–720	75–270

The mechanism by which ALP reaches the circulation is uncertain; leakage from the bile canaliculi into hepatic sinusoids may result from leaky tight junctions. and the other hypothesis is that the damaged liver cell fail to excrete ALP made in bone, intestine and liver. In acute viral hepatitis, ALP is usually either normal or moderately increased. Hepatitis A may present with marked and prolonged cholestasis and elevated of alkaline phosphatase. Tumors may secrete ALP into plasma and there are tumor specific isoenzymes, such as Regan, Nagao and Kasahara isoenzymes.[15] Elevated serum levels of intestinal ALP have been found in patients with cirrhosis, particularly those with blood group type O, and may be associated specifically with intrahepatic disease as opposed to extrahepatic obstruction.[16]

Hepatic and bony metastasis can also cause elevated levels of ALP. Other diseases like infiltrative liver diseases,

abscesses, granulomatous liver disease and amyloidosis may also cause a rise in ALP. Mildly elevated levels of ALP may be seen in cirrhosis and congestive cardiac failure. Drugs like cimetidine, frusemide, phenobarbitone and phenytoin may increase levels of ALP. Approach to elevated ALP is given in Flow chart 21.3.[17]

Low ALP

Low levels of ALP occur in hypothyroidism, pernicious anemia, zinc deficiency and congenital hypophosphatasia. Wilson's disease complicated by hemolysis and FHF may also have very low levels of alkaline phosphatase. Ratio of ALP and bilirubin is low in fulminant Wilson disease. This might be the result of replacement of cofactor zinc by copper and subsequent inactivation of alkaline phosphatase.[18]

Flow chart 21.3: Algorithmic approach to marked rise of alkaline phosphatase

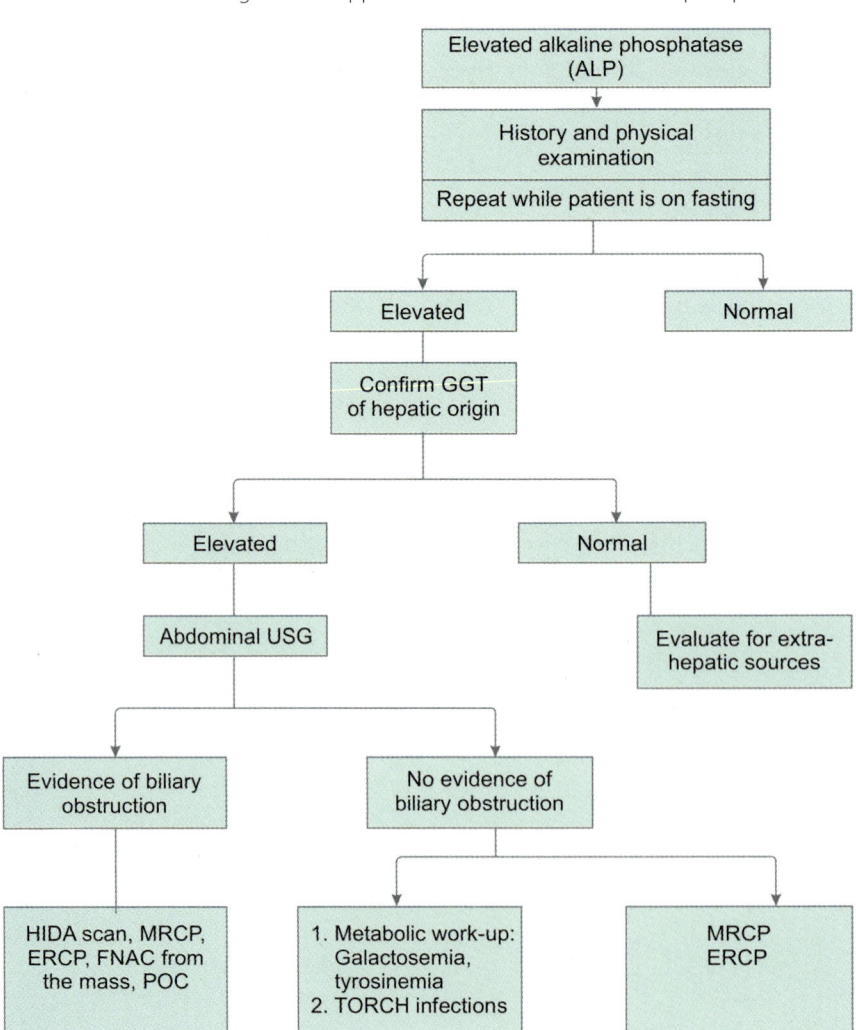

Regardless of the cause of acute hepatic failure a low ratio of ALP to bilirubin is associated with a poor prognosis.[19,20]

γ Glutamyl transpeptidase

GGT is a membrane bound glycoprotein which catalyses the transfer of γ glutamyl group to other peptides, amino acids and water. Large amounts are found in the kidneys, pancreas, liver, intestine and prostate. The gene for GGT is on chromosome 22. The levels of GGT are high in neonates and infants up to 1 year and also increase after 60 years of life. Men have higher values. Children more than 4 years old have serum values of normal adults. The normal range is 0–35 IU/L.

In acute viral hepatitis the levels of GGT may reach its peak in the second or third week of illness and in some patients they remain elevated for 6 weeks. Normal values of GGT are given in Table 21.2. Often clinicians are faced with a dilemma when they see elevated ALP levels and are unable to differentiate between liver diseases and bony disorders and in such situations measurement of GGT helps as it is raised only in cholestatic disorders and not in bone diseases. In liver disease GGT activity correlates well with ALP levels but rarely the GGT levels may be normal in intra hepatic cholestasis like in some familial intrahepatic cholestasis.[21] But, it is raised in cases of PFIC type III and BA, where ALP may be normal other conditions causing elevated levels of GGT include uncomplicated diabetes mellitus, acute pancreatitis and myocardial infarction. Drugs like phenobarbitone, phenytoin, paracetamol, tricyclic antidepressants may also increase the levels of GGT. Nonhepatic causes of increased levels of the enzyme include anorexia nervosa, Gullian–Barre syndrome, hyperthyroidism, obesity, and dystrophica myotonica.

As a diagnostic test the primary usefulness of GGT is limited to the exclusion of bone disease, as GGT is not found in bone.

Other Enzymes that Detect Cholestasis

These are the other enzymes that are not routinely estimated to detect cholestasis, e.g. 5'nucleotidase, leucine aminopeptidase. 5' nucleotidase behaves like ALP in the body during deceased state.

TESTS OF THE LIVER'S BIOSYNTHETIC CAPACITY

Serum Proteins

The liver is the major source of most the serum proteins. The parenchymal cells are responsible for synthesis of albumin, fibrinogen and other coagulation factors and

Table 21.5: Normal values of serum protein and albumin at different ages			
Total protein (g/dL)		Albumin (g/dL)	
Neonate	5.5–7.0	Newborn	2.5–5.0
1–3 years	6.0–7.0	1 years	3.5–5.0
>3 years	6.0–8.0	4 years and older	3.7–5.0

most of the α and β globulins.[22, 23] Normal values of serum proteins and albumin are given in Table 21.5.

Albumin

Albumin is quantitatively the most important protein in plasma synthesized by the liver and is a useful indicator of hepatic function. Because the half-life of albumin in serum is as long as 20 days, the serum albumin level is not a reliable indicator of hepatic protein synthesis in acute liver disease. Albumin synthesis is affected not only in liver disease but also by nutritional status, hormonal imbalance and capillary leak.[24] Liver is the only site of synthesis of albumin.

The serum levels are typically depressed in patients with cirrhosis and ascites.[25] In patients with or without ascites, the serum albumin level correlates with prognosis. In addition the rate of albumin synthesis has been shown to correlate with the Child-Pugh score.

Normal serum values range from 3.5 g/dL to 5.0 g/dL. The average adult has approximately 300–500 g of albumin. The serum levels at any time reflect its rate of synthesis, degradation, and volume of distribution. Normal values are given in Table 21.5. Corticosteroids and thyroid hormone stimulate albumin synthesis by increasing the concentration of albumin mRNA and tRNA in hepatocytes.

The serum albumin levels tend to be normal in diseases like acute hepatitis, drug-related hepatotoxicity and obstructive jaundice. Albumin levels below 3 g/dL in hepatitis should raise the suspicion of CLD like cirrhosis, which usually reflects, decreased albumin synthesis. In ascites there may be normal synthesis but the levels may appear reduced because of increased volume of distribution. Hypoalbuminemia is not specific for liver disease and may occur in protein malnutrition, nephrotic syndrome and chronic protein losing enteropathies.

Prealbumin

The serum prealbumin level is 0.2–0.3 g/L. these levels fall in liver disease presumably due to reduced synthesis. Because of its short half-life, changes may precede alteration in serum albumin. Determination of prealbumin has been considered particularly useful in drug-induced hepatotoxicity.

Serum Ceruloplasmin

Normal plasma level is 20–40 mg/dL. It is synthesized in the liver and is an acute phase protein. Plasma concentration rise in infections, rheumatoid arthritis, pregnancy, non-Wilson liver disease and obstructive jaundice. This is an important diagnostic marker in Wilson disease, in which the plasma level is usually low in 80–90% of the patients. Low levels may also be seen in neonates, Menke's disease, kwashiorkor, and marasmus, protein losing enteropathy, copper deficiency, nephrotic syndrome, and aceruloplasminemia.

Procollagen III Peptide

The serum concentration of this peptide appears to increase not only with hepatic fibrosis but also with inflammation and necrosis. Serial measurement of procollagen III may be helpful in the follow up of chronic liver disease.

α1 Antitrypsin

α1 antitrypsin is a glycoprotein synthesized by the liver and is an inhibitor of serine proteinases, especially elastase. Its normal concentration is 1–1.6 g/L. it is an acute phase protein, serum levels increase with inflammatory disorders, pregnancy and after oral contraceptive pills (OCP). The various alleles coded are M, F, S, Z and null forms. PiZZ homozygotes are associated with neonatal hepatitis. Cirrhosis in adults has been found with ZZ, MZ, SZ and FZ phenotypes. Liver disease is usually seen with deficiency of α1 antitrypsin, an inherited disorder. Deficiency should be confirmed by quantitative measurement and genetic studies.

α Fetoprotein

This protein is the principal one in fetal plasma in early gestation and is subsequently present at very low levels. It is increased in hepatocellular carcinoma (HCC) and more than 90% of such patients have raised levels. Raised values are also found in other liver diseases like chronic hepatitis, in regeneration phase of acute hepatitis and in hepatic metastasis. This is also raised in adenomas associated with tyrosinemia.

αFP elevation is less frequent when HCC arises in non-cirrhotic liver. Serial determination is of value in cirrhotic patients and rise in the values should raise the suspicion of HCC. Normal values are given in Table 21.6.[26]

Prothrombin Time (PT)

Clotting is the end result of a complex series of enzymatic reactions that involve at least 13 factors. The liver is the major site of synthesis of 11 blood coagulation proteins: Fibrinogen, prothrombin, labile factor, stable factor, christmas factor, stuart prower factor, prekallikrein and high molecular weight kininogen. Most of these are present in excess and abnormalities of coagulation only result when there is substantial impairment in the ability of the liver to synthesize these factors. The standard method to assess is the one stage prothrombin time of quick, which evaluates the extrinsic coagulation pathway. The results of this test may be expressed in seconds or as a ratio of the plasma prothrombin time to control plasma time. Normal control usually is in the range of 9–11 seconds. A prolongation of more than 3 seconds is considered abnormal. Normal values are shown in Table 21.7. The prolonged PT is not specific for liver diseases and is seen in various deficiencies of coagulation factors, DIC, and ingestion of certain drugs.

In acute and chronic hepatocellular disease the PT may serve as a prognostic indicator. In acute hepatocellular

Table 21.6: Normal values of α fetoprotein at different ages[26]

Age	Mean α fetoprotein level (ng/mL)
Premature	134,734
Newborn	48,408
Newborn to 2 weeks	33,113
2 weeks to 1 month	9,452
1 month	2,654
2 months	323
3 months	88
4 months	74
5 months	46.5
6 months	12.5
7 months	9.7
8 months	8.5

Table 21.7: Normal values of coagulation profile at different ages

	Age			
	1–5 years	6–10 years	11–16 years	Adult
PT	11	11.1	11.2	12
INR	1	1.07	1.02	1.10
aPTT	30	31	32	33
Fibrinogen	2.76	2.79	3.0	2.78

disease worsening of PT suggests an increased likelihood of acute hepatic failure. The PT is a predictor of outcome in cases of acetaminophen over dosage and acute alcoholic hepatitis. Prolongation of PT is also suggestive of poor long-term outcome in CLD.

If the PT returns to normal or improves by at least 30%within 24 hours of a single parenteral injection of vitamin K1 (5–10 mg), it may be surmised that parenchymal function is good and that hypovitaminosis K was responsible for the original prolongation of PT. Patients with parenchymal disease by contrast will show only minimal improvement. Most patients with extrahepatic obstruction like BA would respond promptly to a single injection of vitamin K1. The PT is particularly important in the management of patients with liver disease. It is important to perform before procedures like liver biopsy and kidney biopsy and it permits an assessment of the tendency to bleed. In many centers the International normalized ratio (INR) is done in place of PT.

To assess the severity of liver disease the Child-Pugh scoring was in use and proved very good to predict the outcome of the disease. Now with the upsurge of liver transplantation the model for end stage liver disease (MELD) and pediatric end stage liver disease (PELD) scoring system is being followed to prioritize the transplant surgery. Because of the shortcomings of the biochemical liver function tests, the quantitative function tests are used and are shown to be very sensitive but their utility in pediatric age group is limited.

Liver Biopsy

Liver biopsy is routinely practiced in pediatric gastroenterology and hepatology centers. It is an essential investigation to make the exact diagnosis of liver disease in infants and children. Histological confirmation of the CLD has great bearing on the treatment and the outcome of the disease. The liver function test (LFT), noninvasive biomarkers and imaging has limitations in the infants and children. Thus, liver biopsy remains an important tool in evaluation, to make diagnosis, disease staging and therapeutic decisions during post-transplant period.[27, 28]

Prerequisites for Liver Biopsy

Detailed history and clinical examination of the patient are very important to make the decision whether the disease is acute or chronic. LFT are also helpful in this regard. Before attempting, it is imperative to obtain hemogram, prothrombin time, INR and blood grouping and cross matching of the patient. These should be done within 24 hours of the procedure. PT should be with 3 sec of the upper limit and INR should be less than 1.5 and platelet count should be above 80000/µL, for hemoglobin less than 6 g/dL, blood transfusion should be given and a unit of blood should be readily available if necessitated to transfuse after the procedure. In case of border line lab parameters FFP and PC should be available during the procedure. Prophylactic antibiotics are indicated in case of valvular heart disease, prosthesis in the body and previous documented bacteremia.

Before the liver biopsy US abdomen is mandatory to assess the size, echo texture of the liver, intrahepatic bile ducts cysts, hemangiomas, tumors, Chilaiditi syndrome (small bowel loops between the shrunken liver and anterior abdominal wall) and position of lungs and gallbladder. USG is also helpful to make exact site for introduction of biopsy needle. Various types of needles used are Vim Silverman needle, Mehgni needle and true cut needles. Now liver biopsy guns of varying sizes are available for all the age groups.

Indications of Liver Biopsy

In case of asymptomatic liver disease with raised enzymes (1.5–2 times), for several months or more than 3 months and in case of hepatitis B and C for more than 6 months, becomes an indication for liver biopsy. Overall symptomatic liver disease and indications for liver biopsy are given in Table 21.8.

Contraindications

Absolute contraindications are liver disease with severe coagulopathy (PT > 4 sec, INR > 1.5 or platelets <80000/cm3, vascular lesions, hemangioma, cystic lesions, dilated intrahepatic bile ducts, bacterial cholangitis, uncooperative patients and impossibility of blood transfusion. But relative contraindications are ascites, obesity, amyloidosis and hemophilia.

Methods of Liver Biopsy

❑ Percutaneous
❑ Transvenous
❑ Surgical
❑ Fine needle aspiration (FNA).

Percutaneous Liver Biopsy

Percutaneous liver biopsy is possible through transthoarcic intercostals and subcostal routes depending upon the span and palpable liver below the left costal margin. By palpation and percussion blindly, it can be performed by an experienced resident doctor. To be on safer side it is performed under US/CT guidance . People have done liver biopsy from bare area of liver with gross ascites and

Table 21.8: Indications for liver biopsy in children	
Neonatal cholestasis • Biliary atresia • Paucity of intrahepatic bile ducts (PIBD) • Neonatal hepatitis • Neonatal sclerosing cholangitis (NSC) • Congenital hepatic fibrosis (CHF)	Infections • Chronic hepatitis B • Chronic hepatitis C
Metabolic liver diseases • α1 antitrypsin deficiency • Wilson disease • Indian childhood cirrhosis • Glycogen storage disease • Galactosemia • Fructosemia • Tyrosinemia	Autoimmune hepatitis • AIH • Primary sclerosing cholangitis (PSC) • Overlap syndrome
Biliary • Secondary biliary cirrhosis • Biliary atresia	Vascular • Budd-Chairi syndrome • Venoocclusive disease

Drug/toxin induced liver injury
Systemic diseases
• Sarcoidosis
• Tuberculosis
• Lymphoma
• Amyloidosis
• AIDS
	Miscellaneous
	• NASH
	• Tumors—benign and malignant
	• Post-transplant
	  – Acute rejection
	  – Chronic rejection
	  – Infection
	  – Drug toxicity
	  – Hepatic fibrosis

coagulopathy. Track can plugged with gel foam to avoid bleeding. Biopsies can be obtained from both the lobes of the liver. Transvenous routes like transjugular and transfemoral have been tried when there is coagulopathy. The limitation is that biopsy sample is usually very small. Laparoscopic liver biopsy has been done from both the lobes the liver selectively. Surgical biopsies include preoperative wedge and core needle biopsy and fine needle aspiration (FNA). Percutaneous FNA is also well known procedure to aspirate material from tumor, granulomatous and cystic lesions.

Liver Biopsy Procedure

Patient should be hospitalized for liver biopsy. The procedure and its associated complications should be explained to the parents. Written consent should be obtained at the same time. Patient should be fasting for 4–6 hours with intravenous (IV) fluids at normal maintenance. Liver biopsy should be done in a dedicated area where monitoring facilities with resuscitation kit, emergency drug tray and portable USG facilities are available.[29] Sedation is required in young infants and children as they are apprehensive before the procedure. IV ketamine (1 mg/kg) or propofol (2 mg/kg) are used. Monitor pulse rate, respiratory rate and saturation during the procedure. Mark the area by USG, intercostal or sub-costal in the mid axillary line, sterilize the area and inject lignocaine locally before insertion of needle. Give 5 mm cut in the dermis, ask the patient to hold the breath, if possible and insert the cutting needle to take the liver biopsy. One or two passes are allowed but not more than 3 passes in any case. After biopsy, pressure over the local site is applied followed by proper bandage. Patient is kept in right lateral position for atleast one hour. Post-procedure, observe the patient for any complications atleast for 24 hours. In case of respiratory distress, chest radiograph is required to rule out pneumothorax. If local pain with abdominal distension, request for abdominal USG to rule out peritoneal collection due to bleeding and bile leak. Adequate liver biopsy sample should be 1–3 cm long and 1.5–2 mm in diameter. Fragmented and small biopsy sample less 1 cm are not adequate for histopathological interpretation. In ideal situation biopsy sample should be sent for histopathology, microbiology, electron microscopy, immunohistochemistry, copper estimation and keep a part of it frozen for enzymatic and metabolic investigations.

Risks and Complications

Significant complications in percutaneous biopsy are 1:1000 with mortality of 1:10000. Nearly 30% of the patients' complaint of substantial pain at biopsy site after the procedure. Overall serious complications vary from 0 to 6.83%. The major complications include intraperitoneal injury/slicing of liver, bile leak and biliary peritonitis, injury to the duodenum, lung, GB and big vessels. The rate of complications in first 2 hours is 61%, within 10 hours is 82% and at 24 hours 96 % where as late complications occur in 4%.[30] Late complications are bleeding from the biopsy tract, arteriovenous fistula, hemobilia and seedling of the tumor in the tract.[31]

Limitations of Needle Biopsy

Percutaneous liver biopsy represents a small part of liver (1: 50000) and at the same time disease can be patchy and may not be representing the actually affected area, biopsy sample can be small and fragmented. The hepatic pathology particularly the fibrosis may not be uniformly distributed especially in case of hepatitis B, C and fatty liver disease. In a study of laparoscopically guided biopsy of right and hepatic lobes in a series of 124 patients of chronic hepatitis C, the biopsy samples from right and left lobes differed in the intensity of inflammation in 24.2% of the cases, and in the intensity of fibrosis in 31.1% of patient.[32] The diagnosis of cirrhosis was made in one lobe in 14.5%, but not in the other. In a similar study liver biopsies done in NASH were highly discordant.[33] This clearly indicates liver biopsy is for from an ideal test in this situation.

Antithrombotic Drugs

Patients on low molecular weight (LMW) heparin should stop medication one day before and can start one day after the liver biopsy, whereas on warfarin stop 5 days before and start one day after the liver biopsy. Antiplatelet medications like acetylsalicylic acid, aspirin, clopidogrel, stop 7–10 days before and start 2–3 days after the biopsy.

Safety of Liver Biopsy

It is quite safe in experienced hand; however, one has to be alert to face any complications subsequently. It is also reported to be safe below the age of 3 months.

Transvenous Liver Biopsy

Transvenous (transjugular or transfemoral biopsy) indicated during coagulopathy, gross ascites, small hard liver, morbid obesity, when free and wedge HVP needed, during TIPS and failure of percutaneous liver biopsy.[34]

Laparoscopic and Surgical Biopsies

These are usually targeted to the affected areas of the liver; the biopsy sample can be in the form of wedge biopsy or core biopsy or fine needle aspiration. Bleeding can be controlled under vision.

Fine Needle Aspiration (FNA)

Percutaneous FNA is indicated in case of diffuse lesions of the liver, granulomatous lesions, tumors and cystic lesions and is quite safe.

Limitations and Complications

Usually liver biopsy sample is very small and interpretations become difficult. In young infants and children this is not always feasible. The cost of the liver biopsy procedure is expensive. Complications range from 1.5 to 20% with mortality of 0.5%. Complications include neck hematoma, puncture of neck and intrathoracic arteries, transient Horner's syndrome, transient dysphonia, pneumothorax and arrhythmias, fever, infection, perforation of liver capsule and fistula between hepatic artery and portal vein and biliary leak.

Noninvasive Tests of Liver Disease

Liver biopsy is having certain limitations to diagnose liver disease. There is increasing evidence to suggest that laboratory tests and noninvasive tests and imaging studies are quite helpful to assess the liver in diseased state.

Specific Tests

Apart from LFT the other blood tests include like specific viral markers, to make diagnosis of viral hepatitis A, B, C, E and D and, markers of AIH, Wilson disease, hemochromatosis, α 1 AT deficiency, procoagulant state etc. However to assess the chronicity of liver disease in form of inflammation and fibrosis some noninvasive tests and imaging studies are very helpful.

Noninvasive Tests

Fibrosis and cirrhosis of liver are very important and dynamic changes occurring in the liver associated with some underlying known causes. Biopsy is not possible in every case and its own limitations due to patchy nature of the disease. There is need of noninvasive tests to assess fibrosis and cirrhosis affecting whole of liver. It is very important to pick up early and late stage of liver disease, especially in chronic hepatitis B and C infections. Clinical picture of advanced cirrhosis is quite evident from features of CLD like hard and irregular liver, splenomegaly, ascites, coagulopathy and encephalopathy, whereas in early stage of fibrosis and early cirrhosis all the clinical features may not be evident. Abnormalities in LFTs also suggest late cirrhosis, but these are not helpful in early stages of disease. Newer markers can detect lying down of the matrix resulting fibrosis in the liver. These can be divided into direct and indirect serological markers of fibrosis.[35]

Direct Serological Markers of Fibrosis

Direct serological markers of fibrosis due to deposition of matrix are procollagen type III amino terminal peptide (P3NP), type I and III collagens, laminin, hyaluronic acid and chondrex. P3NP is mostly widely studied marker of hepatic fibrosis and is evaluated in both acute and chronic liver injury. It reflects the histological stages of fibrosis in chronic liver diseases. Successful treatment of AIH leads to reduction P3NP.

Other markers of fibrosis are associated with matrix degradation, e.g. matrix metalloproteinase 2 and 3 (MMP 2 and 3), tissue inhibitor of metalloproteinase's 1 and 2 (TIMI-1 and TIM1-2), they are increased in liver fibrosis but not commercially available.

Indirect Serological Markers of Fibrosis

Various indirect serological markers of fibrosis have been used to detect extent of fibrosis and cirrhosis; however, findings are inconsistent. Some tests are quite sensitive and specific to avoid liver biopsy. Various tests are AST: ALT ratio (normal 0.8) more than 1 suggests of CLD but not specific. Other tests include AST: platelet ratio index (APRI), combination of prothrombin, GGT, apolipoprotein A1 level (CPGA) index, fibroindex, FIB 4 index, fibrometer, fibrotest and fibrosure, actitest and sequential algorithmic fibrosis evaluation (SAFE).[36] A meta-analysis have shown that fibrotest and actitest are reliable alternative to liver biopsy in chronic hepatitis C. SAFE is also has very good correlation to METAVIR scoring system with accuracy of 90.1%; thus, SAFE is having potential to avoid liver biopsy. All these tests need validation in infants and children.[37-40]

Imaging

Conventional Imaging Studies

Various conventional imaging studies recommended to use in liver diseases are USG, US Doppler, CT scan, MRI and ERCP. US of the liver are important to estimate size, echotexture and surface of the liver, intrahepatic bile ducts and biliary tree. US is very sensitive to visualize certain diseases like cysts, liver abscesses, hemangioma, tumors, secondaries, Caroli's disease, choledochal cyst, choledocholithiasis, assessment of portal vein (PV), hepatic veins and IVC. USG Doppler is very important to diagnose vascular diseases of the liver. CT is also very helpful in the same way as US of the liver. MRI is quite helpful in diagnosis of vascular diseases of the liver, e.g. BCS, EHPVO, etc. But these modalities are complimentary to each other. ERCP is minimally invasive modality which can diagnose hepatobiliary disorders and has great therapeutic value. However, these techniques are not good to detect extent of fibrosis.

Elastography

This is a noninvasive measurement to detect the stiffness of liver. Elastography is now widely used to detect hepatic fibrosis and can avoid liver biopsy. Elastography of liver can be performed by US or MRI.

Ultrasound Elastography

US elastography, also known as fibroscan or transient elastography is widely used to define fibrosis of liver. This has been applied even in young infants and children effectively. Fibroscan uses mild amplitude, low frequency (50 Hz) vibration transmitting through the liver. It induces elastic shear wave that propagates through the organ. The velocity of wave correlates with stiffness of the tissue, the wave travel faster through denser fibrotic tissue of the liver. This can detect fibrosis in whole liver as compared to liver biopsy. And can be repeated without any problem. Meta-analysis of 50 studies on the performance of fibroscan diagnosing liver fibrosis showed the area under curve (AUC) for significant fibrosis: 0.84 (95% CI 0.82–0.86), for severe fibrosis: 0.89 (95% CI 0.88–0.91), for cirrhosis: 0.94 (95% CI 0.93–0.95). Ultrasound elastography is having excellent accuracy to diagnose cirrhosis, irrespective of the underlying etiology. In other meta-analysis of 9 studies it diagnosed stage II to IV fibrosis with 70% sensitivity (95% CI 67%–73%) and 84% specificity (95% CI 80%–88%). This is a promising and reliable test to detect the extent of fibrosis in the liver even in children. Ultrasound elastography is less effective in obese patients, acute viral hepatitis, body mass index more than 30 and metabolic syndrome.[41-44]

Magnetic Resonance Elastography (MRE)

MRE appears to be more promising than ultrasound elastography. Technique is similar to US elastography. The vibration device is used to induce a shear wave in the liver. In this case the wave is detected by modified MR imaging machine and color coded images generated that depicts the wave velocity and stiffness throughout the liver. Studies have shown that CTP grade A cirrhosis the sensitivity is 93% and 82% specific. The direct comparison of varying degree of fibrosis was poor with APRI, fair with fibroscan and very good with MR elastography.[45]

Limitation

Very good and effective but cost is prohibitive and some patient with claustrophobia may not tolerate. This technique has great scope to eliminate the need of liver biopsy. The importance of liver biopsy diminishes with the accurate blood tests and noninvasive tests. However liver biopsy has a role in certain situations like diagnosis of infiltrative diseases, like granulomatous hepatitis, amyloidosis, sarcoidosis and fatty liver, NASH and evaluation of liver parenchyma after liver transplantation. The overwhelming liver disease symptomatology and signs also lessen the need of liver biopsy. In future elastography will be the largely replacing the need of liver biopsy in cases of chronic liver disease.

■ CONCLUSION

To conclude a single liver function test is of little value in screening for liver disease as many serious liver diseases may be associated with normal levels and abnormal levels might be found in asymptomatic healthy individuals. The use of battery of LFT, however, constitutes a highly sensitive tool to assess the liver disease. The number of false-negatives must be reduced by this. The use of battery of liver tests is also associated with high specificity especially when more than one test is abnormal.

The pattern of enzyme abnormality, interpreted in the context of the patient's characteristics, can aid in directing the subsequent diagnostic work-up. Awareness of the prevalence of known liver disease in specific population and of possible hepatic involvement during systemic illnesses or drug therapies may help the clinician identify the cause of alterations efficiently.

It is important to mention that in addition to LFT the role of liver biopsy, fibro scan and other imaging techniques cannot be underestimated in case of chronic liver disease in children. Liver biopsy is considered as gold standard in children; however, the recent advances in the noninvasive techniques like fibroscan and transient MR elastography may obviate the need of liver biopsy. The role of liver biopsy in certain liver disorders as discussed in the text cannot be ignored, e.g. post-transplantation assessment of liver. To make accurate diagnosis of liver disease it is essential to have detailed history and clinical examination of the patient, whether the disease is acute or chronic. The combination of various tests like LFT, specific disease markers, imaging studies and liver histology are more useful in reaching to a definitive diagnosis of the underlying liver disease rather than a single test.

REFERENCES

1. Thapa BR, Walia A. Liver function tests and their interpretation. Indian J Pediatr. 2007;74:663-71.
2. Schiff ER, Sorrell MF, Maddrey WC. Schiff's diseases of the liver. 10th ed. [edited by] Eugene R. Schiff, Michael F. Sorrell, Willis C. Maddrey. ed. Philadelphia ; London: Lippincott Williams & Wilkins; 2007.
3. Bacon BR, Di Bisceglie AM. Liver disease: diagnosis and management. New York ; Edinburgh: Churchill Livingstone; 2000.
4. Bircher J. Oxford textbook of clinical hepatology. 2nd ed. / edited by Johannes Bircher ... [et al.] ed. Oxford: Oxford University Press; 1999.
5. Green RM, Flamm S. AGA technical review on the evaluation of liver chemistry tests. Gastroenterology. 2002;123:1367-84.
6. Kawasaki H, Yamanishi Y, Miyake M, et al. Age- and sex-related profiles of serum primary and total bile acids in infants, children and adults. Tohoku J Exp Med. 1986;150:353-7.
7. Heubi J, Setchell K, Bove K. Inborn Errors of Bile Acid Metabolism. Semin Liver Dis. 2007;27:282-94.
8. Nalpas B, Vassault A, Charpin S, et al. Serum mitochondrial aspartate aminotransferase as a marker of chronic alcoholism: diagnostic value and interpretation in a liver unit. Hepatology. 1986;6:608-14.
9. Dunn M, Martins J, Reissmann KR. The disappearance rate of glutamic oxalacetic transaminase from the circulation and its distribution in the body's fluid compartments and secretions. J Lab Clin Med. 1958;51:259-65.
10. Katkov WN, Friedman LS, Cody H, et al. Elevated serum alanine aminotransferase levels in blood donors: the contribution of hepatitis C virus. Ann Intern Med. 1991;115:882-4.
11. Yasuda K, Okuda K, Endo N, et al. Hypoaminotransferasemia in patients undergoing long-term hemodialysis: clinical and biochemical appraisal. Gastroenterology. 1995;109:1295-300.
12. Cohen GA, Goffinet JA, Donabedian RK, et al. Observations on decreased serum glutamic oxalacetic transaminase (SGOT) activity in azotemic patients. Ann Intern Med. 1976;84:275-80.
13. Simko V. Alkaline phosphatases in biology and medicine. Dig Dis. 1991;9:189-209.
14. Hagerstrand I. Distribution of alkaline phosphatase activity in healthy and diseased human liver tissue. Acta Pathol Microbiol Scand A. 1975;83:519-26.
15. Gordon T. Factors associated with serum alkaline phosphatase level. Arch Pathol Lab Med. 1993;117:187-90.
16. Warnes TW, Hine P, Kay G. Intestinal alkaline phosphatase in the diagnosis of liver disease. Gut. 1977;18:274-8.
17. Kaplan MM. Serum alkaline phosphatase--another piece is added to the puzzle. Hepatology. 1986;6:526-8.
18. Shaver WA, Bhatt H, Combes B. Low serum alkaline phosphatase activity in Wilson's disease. Hepatology. 1986;6:859-63.
19. Reichling JJ, Kaplan MM. Clinical use of serum enzymes in liver disease. Dig Dis Sci. 1988;33:1601-14.
20. Sallie R, Katsiyiannakis L, Baldwin D, et al. Failure of simple biochemical indexes to reliably differentiate fulminant Wilson's disease from other causes of fulminant liver failure. Hepatology. 1992;16:1206-11.
21. Jansen PL, Muller M. The molecular genetics of familial intrahepatic cholestasis. Gut. 2000;47:1-5.
22. Forman WB, Barnhart MI. Cellular Site for Fibrinogen Synthesis. JAMA : the journal of the American Medical Association. 1964;187:128-32.
23. Anderson GF, Barnhart MI. Intracellular Localization of Prothrombin. Proceedings of the Society for Experimental Biology and Medicine Society for Experimental Biology and Medicine. 1964;116:1-6.
24. Jefferson DM, Reid LM, Giambrone MA, et al. Effects of dexamethasone on albumin and collagen gene expression in primary cultures of adult rat hepatocytes. Hepatology. 1985;5: 14-20.
25. Rothschild MA, Oratz M, Zimmon D, et al. Albumin synthesis in cirrhotic subjects with ascites studied with carbonate-14C. J Clin Invest. 1969;48:344-50.
26. Wu JT, Book L, Sudar K. Serum alpha fetoprotein (AFP) levels in normal infants. Pediatr Res. 1981;15:50-2.
27. Azzam RK, Alonso EM, Emerick KM, et al. Safety of percutaneous liver biopsy in infants less than three months old. J Pediatr Gastroenterol Nutr. 2005;41:639-43.

28. Rockey DC, Caldwell SH, Goodman ZD, et al. Liver biopsy. Hepatology. 2009;49:1017-44.

29. Amaral JG, Schwartz J, Chait P, et al. Sonographically guided percutaneous liver biopsy in infants: a retrospective review. AJR Am J Roentgenol. 2006;187:644-9.

30. Westheim BH, Ostensen AB, Aagenaes I, et al. Evaluation of risk factors for bleeding after liver biopsy in children. J Pediatr Gastroenterol Nutr. 2012;55:82-7.

31. Bravo AA, Sheth SG, Chopra S. Liver biopsy. N Engl J Med. 2001;344:495-500.

32. Regev A, Berho M, Jeffers LJ, et al. Sampling error and intraobserver variation in liver biopsy in patients with chronic HCV infection. Am J Gastroenterol. 2002;97:2614-8.

33. Ratziu V, Charlotte F, Heurtier A, et al. Sampling variability of liver biopsy in nonalcoholic fatty liver disease. Gastroenterology. 2005;128:1898-906.

34. Keshava SN, Mammen T, Surendrababu N, et al. Transjugular liver biopsy: What to do and what not to do. The Indian journal of radiology & imaging. 2008;18:245-8.

35. Carey E, Carey WD. Noninvasive tests for liver disease, fibrosis, and cirrhosis: Is liver biopsy obsolete? Cleve Clin J Med. 2010;77:519-27.

36. Sebastiani G, Halfon P, Castera L, et al. SAFE biopsy: a validated method for large-scale staging of liver fibrosis in chronic hepatitis C. Hepatology. 2009;49:1821-7.

37. Cales P, Oberti F, Michalak S, et al. A novel panel of blood markers to assess the degree of liver fibrosis. Hepatology. 2005;42:1373-81.

38. Oberti F, Valsesia E, Pilette C, et al. Noninvasive diagnosis of hepatic fibrosis or cirrhosis. Gastroenterology. 1997;113:1609-16.

39. Rossi E, Adams L, Prins A, et al. Validation of the FibroTest biochemical markers score in assessing liver fibrosis in hepatitis C patients. Clin Chem. 2003;49:450-4.

40. Poynard T, Imbert-Bismut F, Munteanu M, et al. Overview of the diagnostic value of biochemical markers of liver fibrosis (FibroTest, HCV FibroSure) and necrosis (ActiTest) in patients with chronic hepatitis C. Comp Hepatol. 2004;3:8-.

41. Fitzpatrick E, Quaglia A, Vimalesvaran S, et al. Transient elastography is a useful noninvasive tool for the evaluation of fibrosis in paediatric chronic liver disease. J Pediatr Gastroenterol Nutr. 2013;56:72-6.

42. Sandrin L, Fourquet B, Hasquenoph J-M, et al. Transient elastography: a new noninvasive method for assessment of hepatic fibrosis. Ultrasound Med Biol. 2003;29:1705-13.

43. Friedrich-Rust M, Ong M-F, Martens S, et al. Performance of transient elastography for the staging of liver fibrosis: a meta-analysis. Gastroenterology. 2008;134:960-74.

44. Talwalkar JA, Kurtz DM, Schoenleber SJ, et al. Ultrasound-based transient elastography for the detection of hepatic fibrosis: systematic review and meta-analysis. Clinical gastroenterology and hepatology : the official clinical practice journal of the American Gastroenterological Association. 2007;5:1214-20.

45. Huwart L, Sempoux C, Vicaut E, et al. Magnetic resonance elastography for the noninvasive staging of liver fibrosis. Gastroenterology. 2008;135:32-40.

Chapter 22

Neonatal Cholestasis

James Huang, Marion M Aw

INTRODUCTION

Neonatal cholestasis is the accumulation of bile components in the blood within the neonatal period. These components include bile acids, conjugated bilirubin and cholesterol. It most commonly presents to the physician as prolonged neonatal jaundice. Cholestasis is confirmed when the conjugated bilirubin fraction is greater than 20% of the total bilirubin level. In most cases of neonatal cholestasis serum bile acids are also elevated although they are seldom tested for.

Recent developments in molecular science and genetic profiling have allowed us to define distinct clinico-pathological entities in neonatal cholestasis, and may reveal potential molecular targets for therapy.

This chapter aims to provide a practical approach to an infant with cholestasis, as well as an outline of the management of such a child.

ETIOPATHOGENESIS OF NEONATAL CHOLESTASIS

Physiology of Bile Acid Synthesis and Transport

Bile acid synthesis occurs in the hepatocyte from sequential oxidation of cholesterol to form two primary bile acids, cholic acid and chenodeoxycholic acid. These two bile acids are secreted into the bile duct and subsequently into the intestinal lumen, whereby they undergo dehydroxylation to form secondary bile acids deoxycholic acid and lithocholic acid respectively. These bile acids are reabsorbed by intestinal enterocytes into the portal circulation, and are taken up by hepatocytes. Both primary and secondary bile acids can undergo conjugation in the hepatocyte with amino acids to form bile salts. The process of intestinal reabsorption and hepatic reuptake of bile acids is the enterohepatic circulation, as illustrated in Figure 22.1.

Bile acids and organic anions are taken up from the portal circulation into the hepatocyte via NTCP (sodium taurocholate cotransporting polypeptide) and OATP (organic anion-transporting polypeptide) transporters. They are secreted into the bile canaliculus via a variety of transporters including BSEP (bile salt export pump) and MRP2 (multidrug resistance-related protein). Bile salts can be absorbed at the level of cholangiocyte, enterocyte or renal tubular cell via the ASBT (apical sodium dependent bile acid transporter) transporter. Bile salts can also be excreted in the urine via MRP transporters in the renal tubular cell.

FXR (Farnesoid X receptor) is a nuclear receptor expressed in the hepatocytes and intestinal cells. It regulates homestasis of bile salt uptake by down-regulating the expression of ASBT. Knowledge of these nuclear receptors gives rise to the possibility of targeted novel molecular therapy in cholestatic diseases.[1]

Differential Diagnoses of Neonatal Cholestasis

Cholestasis can occur as a consequence of defects at any point in the process of bile acid synthesis, transport and secretion, and can result from structural or enzymatic defects.

The differential diagnoses of neonatal cholestasis are myriad as shown in Table 22.1 according to their pathophysiological mechanism .Of these diagnoses, a subgroup could potentially present as acute liver failure in the newborn period.

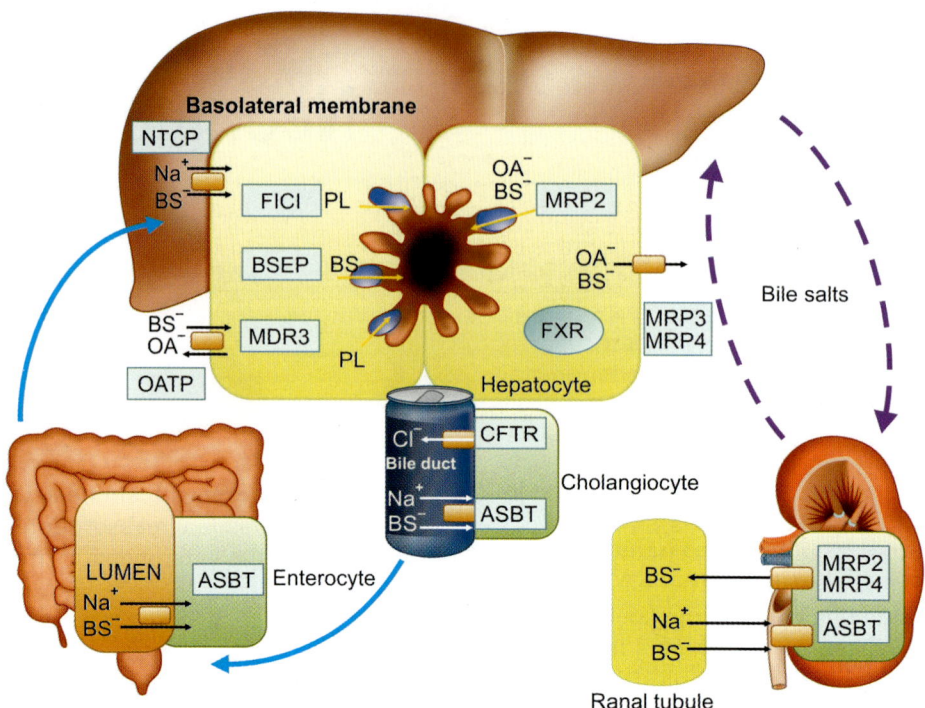

Fig. 22.1: Enterohepatic circulation and the key bile salt transporters

Abbreviations: NTCP, Na+-taurocholate cotransporting polypeptide; OATP, organic anion-transporting polypeptide; OA, organic anions; BS, bile salts; FIC1, familial intrahepatic cholestasis-1; BSEP, bile salt export pump; MDR3, multidrug resistance protein 3; MRP2/MRP3/MRP4, multidrug resistance-related protein; ASBT, apical sodium-dependent bile acid transporter; FXR, Farnesoid X receptor; CFTR, cystic fibrosis transport receptor.

Table 22.1: Differential diagnoses of neonatal cholestasis (adapted from Balistreri 2006)[2]		
Category	*Causes of neonatal cholestasis*	*May presents as acute liver failure*
Extrahepatic causes *intrahepatic form of choledochal cyst	Biliary atresia Choledochal cyst Caroli's disease * Inspissated bile syndrome Spontaneous perforation of bile duct Neonatal sclerosing cholangitis	No
Intrahepatic causes		
Familial (inherited) causes of intrahepatic cholestasis Disorders of embryogenesis	Alagille syndrome Ductal plate malformation (Caroli's disease)	No
Disorders of membrane transport and secretion	**Disorders of canalicular secretion** Bile salt export pump (BSEP) deficiency • PFIC type 2 (progressive) • BRIC type 2 (benign, recurrent) **Phospholipid transport- MDR3 deficiency** • PFIC Type 3 **Ion transport** Cystic fibrosis Complex, multiorgan disorders **FIC1 deficiency** • PFIC type 1, Byler's disease (progressive) • Recurrent, benign (BRIC type 1) • Alpha-1 antitrypsin deficiency • Neonatal ichthyosis-sclerosing cholangitis syndrome • Arthrogryposis-renal dysfunction-cholestasis syndrome (ARC) • Lymphedema-cholestasis (Aagenaes) syndrome	No No No No

Contd...

Contd...

Disorders of bile acid biosynthesis and conjugation	Bile acid synthetic enzyme deficiencies	Yes
Metabolic disorders	Cystic fibrosis	No
	Alpha-1 anti-trypsin deficiency	Yes
	Carbohydrate metabolism	Yes
	Galactosemia	Yes
	Amino acid metabolism	Yes
	Tyrosinemia type 1	
	Citrin deficiency (type 2 citrullinemia)	
	Arginase deficiency	
	Lipid metabolism	
	Niemann-Pick disease type C	
	Wolman's disease	
	Metal metabolism	
	Neonatal haemochromatosis	
	Mitochondrial disorders	
Sporadic causes of intrahepatic cholestasis		
Infections	*Bacterial*	
	Sepsis (in particular gram-negative sepsis) , listeria	Yes
	monocytogenes, syphilis	Yes
	Viral	
	TORCH intrauterine infections	
	Cytomegalovirus infections	
	Herpes simplex virus, including HHV-6	
	Echoviruses, adenoviruses, parvoviruses	
Endocrinopathies	Congenital hypothyroidism	No
	Congenital hypopituitarism	
Toxin effect	Drug-induced	Yes
	Parenteral nutrition induced	
Miscellaneous	Neonatal hemophagocytic lymphohistiocytosis	Yes
	Neonatal lupus	

APPROACH TO AN INFANT WITH CHOLESTASIS

In an infant with prolonged jaundice, a targeted history and physical examination should be conducted to identify:

CASE SCENARIO 1

R is a 2-month-old infant who has been referred from a general practitioner (GP) for persistent neonatal jaundice. His total bilirubin level done by the GP was 300 µmol/L. R was well at birth following a normal vaginal delivery at term. He was noted to be increasingly jaundiced over the past two weeks. On examination, he appears well-thrived but deeply jaundiced with no pallor. He is vigorous. He has a firm hepatomegaly measuring 5 cm from the right costal margin and a palpable splenic tip. He does not have ascites. The cardiac and respiratory examination is unremarkable.

His stools look cream-colored and his mother said the stools have changed from green/black to this paler color over the past three weeks.

- Signs and symptoms that would suggest the presence of cholestasis
- The ill infant who would need urgent medical evaluation
  - The septic infant
  - The infant with a metabolic decompensation
  - The infant in acute liver failure
- Physical signs that suggest early decompensated liver disease from liver cirrhosis
- Extrahepatic systemic features which could implicate the primary diagnosis.

HISTORY

A good history and physical examination (including stool inspection) is paramount in defining the need and urgency for further investigations. The symptoms of cholestasis—the presence of jaundice with high-colored urine and pale stools would alert one of its possibility.

A review of the child's birth history (specifically birth weight) and the mother's antenatal progress is a good starting point for evaluation. Points in the history suggestive of an infectious etiology include maternal fever and/ or localizing symptoms of an infection (e.g. rash, upper respiratory tract symptoms), especially at or around the time of delivery. Occasionally, the presence of cholestasis in pregnancy can suggest a diagnosis of progressive familial intrahepatic cholestasis (PFIC) type 3 in the infant. Perinatal risk factors for neonatal sepsis should also be evaluated. Early trimester maternal infections may result in distinctive clinical findings of in the newborn (microcephaly, cataracts, hepatosplenomegaly, and jaundice, rash). Systemic maternal illness (e.g. maternal lupus) can rarely manifest as transient cholestasis in the newborn.[3]

A review of the general health of the infant in the post-natal course is important. This includes a review of the child's feeding history and an assessment of the child's hydration (adequate weight gain, urine output, number of nappy changes, and weight of nappies). Worrisome symptoms such as lethargy, poor feeding and poor suck/latch, suggest neonatal sepsis or a possible metabolic decompensation and warrants urgent evaluation.

A detailed family history should be obtained, in particular the presence of consanguinity which should bring to mind the possibility of autosomal recessive cholestatic disorders (such as inborn errors of metabolism and the PFICs). In particular, a family history of cystic fibrosis or alpha-1 antitrypsin deficiency in siblings would be relevant.

If the history is suggestive of cholestasis, a review of possible complications should be obtained, in particular bleeding tendencies from vitamin K deficiency. This has implications on therapy, as infants have presented with life-threatening intracerebral haemorrhage after a missed diagnosis of biliary atresia.[4]

▮ PHYSICAL EXAMINATION

The child's anthropometric percentiles should be plotted. A low birth weight may be associated with an intrauterine infection or alpha-1 antitrypsin deficiency. Infants with biliary atresia usually thrive well early in the illness. A falsely high weight could be contributed by the presence of ascites.

An assessment on the general well-being of the infant, in terms of the child's tone, vigor of movements and irritability, would determine the need for urgent evaluation for sepsis and/or metabolic crises. Subtle signs of hepatic encephalopathy, initially manifested by irritability and subsequently drowsiness, can be missed.

The presence of pallor and jaundice should be verified. The presence of dysmorphic facial features could suggest certain specific pathologic entities (intrauterine infections, Alagille's, septo-optic dysplasia with congenital hypopituitarism). An ophthalmic examination should

be done, looking for cytomegalovirus retinitis, posterior embryotoxon and other ocular abnormalities associated with Alagille's syndrome.

An examination of the abdomen is vital, including the size and consistency of organomegaly and the presence of ascites. The presence of a hard, craggy liver with ascites is an ominous sign that cirrhosis has already occurred. The presence of ambiguous genitalia could suggest underlying hypopituitarism. The stool must be obtained for inspection to look for acholic stools.

The cardiorespiratory examination is important to look for associated cardiac malformations. It is important to look for dextrocardia and situs inversus, which can be associated with biliary atresia. The presence of cardiac malformations in a jaundiced infant may suggest Alagille's syndrome.

An assessment of the tone and reflexes of the infant should be done—brisk reflexes and clonus could suggest cerebral irritation in hepatic encephalopathy.

A review of any other systemic manifestations reported by the parents or other medical professionals can provide a clue to rarer etiologies. Lymphedema of the lower extremities is associated with lymphedema-cholestasis syndrome (Aagenaes syndrome).[5] Multiple joint contractures (arthogryposis multiplex congenita) are implicated in arthrogryposis-renal dysfunction-cholestasis (ARC) syndrome.

CASE SCENARIO 1 (CONT....)

Investigations reveal conjugated hyperbilirubinemia with a raised gamma-GT level. There is no hypoprothrombinemia. The albumin level is 39 g/dL. The plasma amino acid profile is unremarkable. The CMV IgM is positive. There is no evidence of CMV retinitis.

The ultrasound scan of the hepatobiliary system showed no intrahepatic duct dilatation but the gallbladder could not be visualized.

The HIDA scan done subsequently demonstrated absent biliary-enteric drainage.

▮ A DIAGNOSTIC APPROACH

The following basic laboratory investigations should be conducted for all patients with cholestasis.

Liver Function Test, Including Gamma Glutamyltranspeptidase (GGT) Level

Conjugated hyperbilirubinemia is defined as conjugated hyperbilirubin level >20% of total bilirubin level. NASPHGAN guidelines recommend that all children having jaundice beyond 2 weeks' age should have a conjugated bilirubin level measured.[6] Elevation of alanine aminotransferase levels (ALT) and aspartate aminotransferase levels (AST) can occur, but are non-specific findings in cholestatic disorders.

Gamma-glutamyltranspeptidase (Gamma-GT)

Gamma GT (GGT) is an enzyme bound to the canalicular membrane of cholangiocytes. The detergent effect of bile acids elutes GGT from the canalicular membrane into the bile. In cholestasis, GGT accumulates in bile and enters the bloodstream, causing a raised plasma GGT level. As this rise in plasma GGT level is dependent on the elution effect of bile acids, a *normal* plasma GGT level is seen in disorders which affect bile acid synthesis and secretion into the bile canaliculus, e.g. bile acid biosynthetic errors or progressive familial intrahepatic cholestasis.

In normal full-term neonates, the level of plasma GGT level can be up to seven times the upper limit of normal in an adult. [7]

Albumin Level, Coagulation Profile

Derangements would indicate decreased hepatic synthetic function. Prolonged PT could be also be secondary to vitamin K deficiency.

Full Blood Count/Complete Blood Count

Thrombocytopenia can result from (i) increasing spleen size from early portal hypertension and (ii) intrauterine infections. Leukopenia may be associated with neonatal sepsis.

Second-line Investigations

The indication for investigations in this list is guided by the index of clinical suspicion, after a thorough history taking and physical examination, together with initial blood investigations (Table 22.2).

Additional investigations may be considered if the initial diagnostic evaluation does not identify a specific etiology. In addition, a chip-based (Jaundice chip) genetic sequencing assay is available to detect mutations in genes associated with inheritable intrahepatic cholestasis;[8] JAG1 gene (Alagille syndrome), ATP8B1 (PFIC1/Byler's), ABCB11 (PFIC2), ABCB4 (PFIC3/MDR), and SERPINA1 (Alpha-1 antitrypsin deficiency).

Radiological Investigations

Ultrasound Scan of the Hepatobiliary System

All infants with features of cholestasis should undergo an ultrasound of the abdomen. Adequate fasting is essential to

Table 22.2: A summary of second-line investigations in an infant with cholestasis

Serology for TORCH infections Viral PCR for HHV-6, adenovirus, enterovirus Blood culture/urine culture	Infections
Plasma amino acids and urine organic acids	Organic acidemia Citrin deficiency (type 2 citrullinemia)
Urine for reducing substances and galactose-1-phosphate uridyl transferase (GAL-1-PUT) assay	Galactosemia
Urine for succinylacetone	Tyrosinemia type 1
Arterial ammonia and lactate	Organic acidemia Mitochondrial disorders Citrin deficiency
Thyroid hormone profile, insulin-growth factor-1, cortisol levels	Congenital hypopituitarism Congenital hypothyroidism
Immunoreactive trypsin Sweat test Genetic testing	Cystic fibrosis
Alpha-1 antitrypsin level and isoelectrofocusing	Alpha-1 antitrypsin deficiency
Ferritin level Lip or salivary gland biopsy	Neonatal hemochromatosis

visualize the gallbladder, and gives an option of observing the contraction of the gallbladder during a milk feed.

Ultrasonography can detect the presence of a choledochal cyst, including Caroli's disease. Biliary sludge in the biliary tree can be seen in inspissated bile syndrome. The presence of an atretic gallbladder and/or the constellation of the following findings: a gallbladder length less than 1.9 cm, a thin gallbladder wall and irregular wall contour (gallbladder ghost triad) is highly specific for biliary atresia.[9] The triangular cord sign (fibrosis of the porta hepatic region) seen on the ultrasound scan is also a highly specific sign for biliary atresia. However, a normal gallbladder, while making biliary atresia a less likely diagnosis, does not exclude biliary atresia. Note that as biliary atresia is a progressive obliterative cholangiopathy, biliary duct dilatation is typically not a feature.

The echo-texture of the liver can appear coarse and hyperechoic in a variety of cholestatic disorders. In addition, it is possible to detect congenital anomalies such as polysplenia/accessory spleen and situs inversus, associated with biliary atresiasplenic malformation (BASM) syndrome.

Hepatobiliary Iminodiacetic Acid Scan (HIDA) Scan

Hepatospecific imino-diacetic-acid (HIDA) is a lidocaine analog and competes with bilirubin for excretion in the hepatocyte.

The HIDA scan measures hepatic uptake of a radiotracer isotope and a delayed scan done by 24 hours demonstrates biliary-enteric drainage of the isotope. All patients are primed with biliary secretagogues such as phenobarbitone (5 mg/kg/day) or ursodeoxycholic acid for 3–5 days prior to the scan, to enhance biliary drainage.

A normal HIDA scan demonstrating good biliary-enteric drainage virtually excludes biliary atresia. However, absent biliary-enteric drainage on the HIDA scan has poor specificity for biliary atresia as false-positive results are common. As such, imaging modalities must be further employed to evaluate the patency of the biliary system.

Cholangiography in Defining Biliary Anatomy

The diagnosis and management of surgically amenable conditions in infant cholestasis invariably involve imaging the biliary system.

Modalities available include:

❏ Intraoperative cholangiogram
❏ Endoscopic retrograde cholangiopancreatography (ERCP)
❏ Magnetic resonance cholangiopancreatography (MRCP).

The gold standard in confirming the diagnosis of biliary atresia remains an intraoperative cholangiogram, which would demonstrate obstruction of flow within part of or through the entire extrahepatic bile duct. Rarely, up to one-third of patients with bile duct paucity can have similar findings on the intraoperative cholangiogram. The intraoperative cholangiogram is usually done concurrently with a liver biopsy.

Endoscopic retrograde cholangiopancreatography (ERCP) could also be an option in defining the patency of the biliary system in suspected cases of biliary atresia, before subjecting an infant to laparotomy.[10] However, it is technically challenging and few centres offer it as an option currently.

Newer modalities of imaging the biliary system, such as magnetic resonance cholangiopancreatography (MRCP) have been introduced as a noninvasive mode of visualizing structural anomalies of the biliary system e.g. choledochal cyst, Caroli's disease. The role of MRCP has also been discussed in the diagnosis of biliary atresia, but has not been universally adopted.

Histopathological Investigations

The liver biopsy can be conducted percutaneously as a means to avoid the morbidity and costs of a negative laparotomy (Figs 22.2 to 22.5). The key groups of histopathological features are shown in Table 22.3.

Table 22.3: Key groups of histopathological features	
Disorder	*Histopathological features*
Biliary atresia Alpha-1 antitrypsin deficiency Cystic fibrosis	Bile ductular proliferation Bile plugs Periportal fibrosis
Alagille syndrome Nonsyndromic bile duct paucity	Bile duct hypoplasia/paucity
Neonatal hepatitis (metabolic, infectious, intrahepatic cholestatic syndromes)	Giant cell transformation Lobular disarray

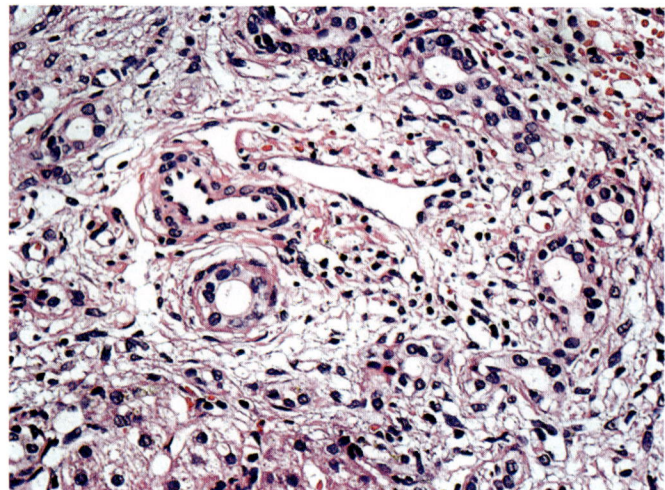

Fig. 22.2: Extrahepatic bile duct obstruction. The portal tract is expanded by stromal edema. There is increase in bile duct profiles (H & E, x200). (*Courtesy:* Professor Aileen Wee, Department of Pathology, National University of Singapore)

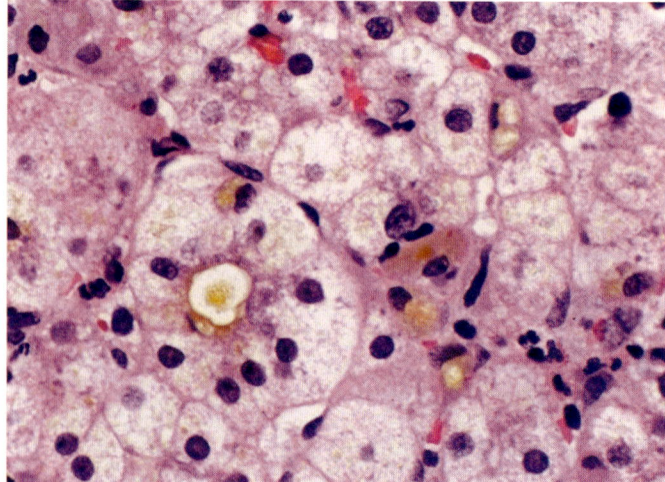

Fig. 22.3: Cholestasis. The hepatocytes are pale and swollen and show intracanalicular bile plugs (H & E x400) (*Courtesy:* Professor Aileen Wee, Department of Pathology, National University of Singapore)

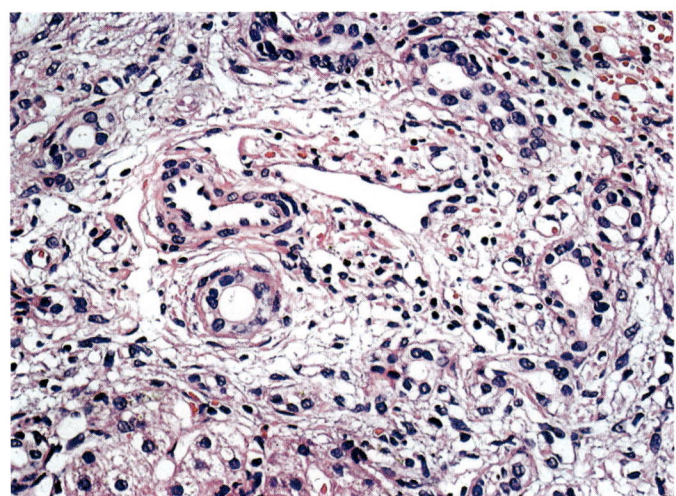

Fig. 22.4A: Extrahepatic biliary atresia with ductal plate malformation The portal tracts are expanded by stromal edema and fibrosis. The interlobular bile ducts are misshapen (H&E, x20). (*Courtesy:* Professor Aileen Wee, Department of Pathology, National University of Singapore)

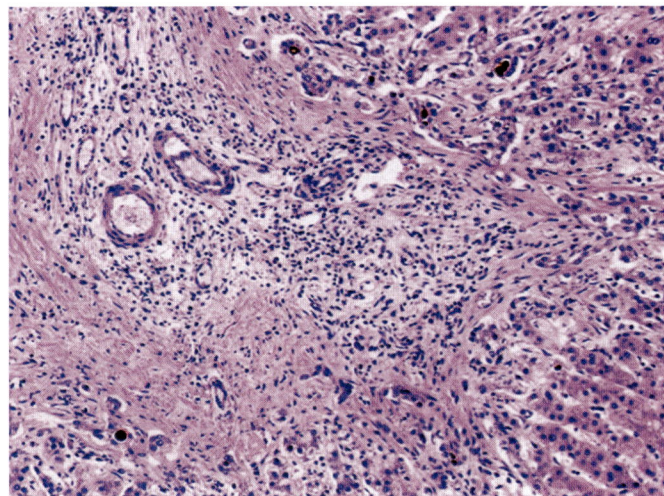

Fig. 22.5: Paucity of intrahepatic small bile ducts. The enlarged portal tract shows arterial and venous structures but absence of interlobular bile duct (H & E, x200) (*Courtesy:* Professor Aileen Wee, Department of Pathology, National University of Singapore)

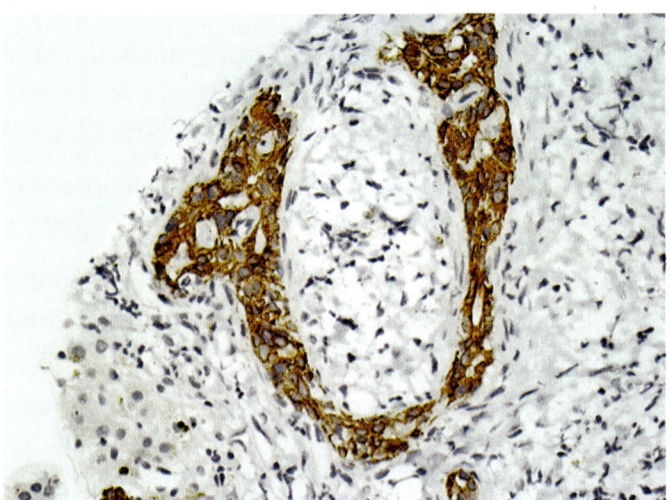

Fig. 22.4B: Ductal plate malformation. CK19 immunostain highlights misshapen ductal plate remnants encircling nubbin of loose fibrous stroma (x400) (*Courtesy:* Professor Aileen Wee, Department of Pathology, National University of Singapore)

Adjunctive techniques such as immunohistochemical staining can differentiate disorders; PAS-positive globules, diastase-resistant globules within hepatocytes is a feature of alpha-1 antitrypsin deficiency.

Electron microscopy can demonstrate coarse, granular bile (Byler's bile) in progressive familial intrahepatic cholestasis Type 1.

The liver biopsy can have equivocal histological features in up to 10% of cases, and may warrant further definitive investigations, such as cholangiography. Moreover, the histopathological features of cholestatic disorders can evolve through the course of the illness; the liver biopsy findings in biliary atresia early in the illness may be similar to that seen in neonatal hepatitis. Occasionally a repeat biopsy may be required.

Certain histopathological features on the liver biopsy such as micro- and macrovesicular fat with cholestasis can suggest metabolic disorders, such as citrin deficiency.

A percutaneous liver biopsy can potentially pick up infants with nonsyndromic bile duct paucity/mild cases of Alagille's syndrome thereby avoiding a laparotomy.

CASE SCENARIO 1 (CONTD....)

The presence of absent biliary-enteric drainage was suspicious for a diagnosis of biliary atresia. R underwent an exploratory laparotomy with an intraoperative cholangiogram and open trucut liver biopsy.

Intraoperatively, the gallbladder and extrahepatic bile ducts were found to be atretic. The cholangiogram demonstrated absence of flow of contrast through the extrahepatic bile ducts. A Kasai procedure was performed for the child in the same operative setting.

The liver biopsy was reviewed and demonstrated the presence of bile ductular proliferation and bile plugs, confirming the presence of biliary atresia.

Post-Kasai, the child resumed breastfeeding and was started on ursodeoxycholic acid and fat-soluble vitamin supplements until the jaundice cleared. He was also started on cotrimoxazole antibiotic prophylaxis.

The positive CMV IgM antibody could be a coincidental finding or could implicate cytomegalovirus infection as a possible aetiological factor in biliary atresia.

GENERAL PRINCIPLES OF MANAGEMENT

Surgical intervention is the first line of treatment in certain extrahepatic cholestatic disorders, e.g. biliary atresia, choledochal cyst. Medical management is the mainstay of therapy for most intrahepatic disorders of cholestasis until decompensated liver disease occurs with liver transplantation being inevitable.

Medical management of an infant with prolonged cholestasis is done in conjunction with nutritional management.[11]

❑ **Identify a treatable cause of intrahepatic cholestasis**
Metabolic disorders and endocrinopathies should be appropriately treated upon recognition.

❑ **Choleretic therapy and management of itch**
The use of choleretics such as ursodeoxycholic acid, phenobarbitone and rifampicin promote bile flow. This has multiple beneficial effects:

- Reducing toxic bile acid build-up within the hepatocyte and bile canaliculus
- Reducing the build-up of bile acids in skin and alleviating pruritus
- Enhancing absorption of fat-soluble nutrients and vitamins.

In particular, ursodeoxycholic acid has a reported action of protecting damaged cholangiocytes against the toxic detergent effect of bile acids and inhibition of apoptosis of hepatocytes.[12] Rifampicin, an established potent hepatic enzyme inducer, may have the effect of inducing hydroxylation of hydrophobic bile acids and thus reducing their toxic effect.[13]

Partial external or internal biliary diversion in infants with progressive familial intrahepatic cholestasis or Alagille syndrome[14] may slow down the progression of liver disease and provide symptomatic relief of intractable pruritus. There are potentially complications from a stoma. Further studies are needed to see if this postpones the need for liver transplantation in the above conditions.

Antihistamines are typically ineffective as monotherapy for cholestatic pruritus, but can be used as adjunctive therapy to choleretic agents listed above. Other potential agents include opioid antagonists such as naltrexone. Naltrexone can block the opioid-mediated neural pathways of afferent nerves which produce the sensation of itching.[15,16]

❑ **Nutritional management**
Infants with prolonged cholestasis may have failure to thrive, contributed by fat malabsorption, fat-soluble vitamin deficiency and increased metabolic demands from chronic liver disease.

Anthropometric measurements should be done at baseline and periodically during follow-up visits. Measurements of midarm circumference and triceps skinfold thickness are more definite indices of nutrition compared to weight (which may be affected by disproportionate organomegaly and ascites).

A diet high in medium-chain triglycerides with adequate supplementation of essential fatty acids is vital. Essential fatty acids such linoleic acid is vital for normal neurodevelopment. Suitable formulas include Alfare, Pregestimil and Neosure. Nasogastric feeding may be indicated for cachetic, malnourished infants. The caloric requirements of infants with cholestasis may be beyond 150 kcal/kg/day. There should not be any protein restriction unless the child is in decompensated liver disease with hepatic encephalopathy.

Fat-soluble vitamins (Vitamin A, D, E, K) should be prescribed either as individual vitamin supplements, or as a combination (AquaDEKs syrup) for ease of administration. The advantages of prescribing individual fat-soluble vitamins allow for titration of each vitamin, based on blood vitamin levels. There is to be caution in prescribing vitamin A, due to its risk of further hepatotoxicity.

Regular monitoring of the prothrombin time can assess the degree of vitamin K deficiency. Regular parenteral vitamin K therapy (intramuscular) can be administered, and the interval of injections to be decided based on the severity of hypoprothrombinemia.

An assessment of fat malabsorption, either through history from parents (asking specifically for oily, shiny stools) or by faecal fat analysis, should be conducted.

❑ **Psychosocial support**
Family care support is appropriate for families in view of the prolonged course of therapy required, and the inevitable need for liver transplant in subgroups of infants regardless of maximal medical therapy.

APPROACH TO THE PREMATURE INFANT WITH CHOLESTASIS

Much of the urgency of investigations in a full term infant is driven by the need to exclude biliary atresia promptly.

The approach of a premature infant with cholestasis is different, as the risk of biliary atresia is much lower. Several factors can contribute to cholestasis in a premature infant:

❑ Immaturity of biliary excretion
❑ Use of total parenteral nutrition
❑ Hemolysis
❑ Sepsis.

The basic laboratory investigations listed above, including newborn screening for metabolic disorders, could be performed according to index of suspicion. An ultrasound scan of the hepatobiliary system would be useful to detect the presence of dilated bile ducts and/or the biliary sludge. Further investigations such as hepatobiliary isotope scans and liver biopsy should be deferred until the corrected age is past term. Conservative management includes the use of choleretics and fat-soluble vitamins while cholestasis is present. Parenteral nutrition should be discontinued as far as enteral feeding can be escalated.

EXTRAHEPATIC CAUSES OF CHOLESTASIS

The first-line of treatment for extrahepatic cholestatic disorders is primarily surgical.

Biliary Atresia

Pathophysiology

Biliary atresia is the most commonest cause for children receiving liver transplantation, and prompt recognition of the diagnosis is paramount in order for early therapy to be instituted. Much of the diagnostic approach has been alluded to, earlier in the chapter.

The pathologic mechanism behind biliary atresia is a progressive fibrosing cholangiopathy that extends through all if not, part of the extrahepatic biliary tree. An inflammatory response occurs within the biliary ductules, with the peribiliary fibroblasts being activated and consequent proliferation of the biliary ductules. This chronic state of inflammation and progressive fibrosis eventually leads to cirrhosis, and current interventions in biliary-enteric bypass only serve as palliation prior to the inevitable need for liver transplantation.

The underlying aetiology for biliary atresia has been speculated to be an immune response to a viral infection, in particular echoviruses, rhinoviruses and cytomegaloviruses. It is rare in premature infants, and displays no form of inheritance.

There are two distinct clinical forms of biliary atresia:
- Post-natal form (80%)
- Embryonic form—associated with congenital malformations (situs inversus), cardiac malformations with three broad anatomical classifications of biliary atresia based on the Japanese classification system:
  - Type 1: Atresia restricted to the common bile duct
  - Type 2: Atresia of the common hepatic duct
  - Type 3: Atresia of the right and left hepatic duct (commonest anatomical subtype).

Early in the illness, the key clinical features are that of a well-thrived infant presenting with prolonged jaundice and acholic stools. Hepatomegaly is invariably present. Infants presenting late may have clinical features of cirrhosis with the onset of ascites and coagulopathy. Laboratory investigations reveal conjugated hyperbilirubinemia with raised transaminases and GGT level.

Diagnostic Approach to Biliary Atresia

There is still controversy on the best diagnostic approach for biliary atresia. Ultrasonographic features of the 'triangular cord sign' and 'gallbladder ghost triad' are highly specific but poorly sensitive for the condition. A hepatobiliary isotope scan has almost 100% sensitivity for biliary atresia but has false-positive results.

A percutaneous liver biopsy can have equivocal histopathological findings in up to 10% of cases, and may not detect bile ductular proliferation early in its course. The histopathological features of bile ductular proliferation, bile plugs and portal fibrosis were the best indicators of biliary atresia, versus giant cell transformation with lobular disarray in neonatal hepatitis[17] (see Figs 22.4A and B).

The gold standard remains as intraoperative cholangiography, which demonstrates absence of flow through part of or the entire extrahepatic biliary tree. Other modalities such as endoscopic retrograde cholangiography and magnetic resonance imaging are promising in diagnostic accuracy, but are not universally adopted.

Mimics of Biliary Atresia

There are certain disease entities which closely mimic the clinical presentation of biliary atresia. They should be considered preoperatively prior to subjecting an infant to a laparotomy.
- Alpha-1 antitrypsin deficiency
  This condition has almost identical histopathological features to biliary atresia. It is to be suspected in all infants born to consanguineous parents with or without a family history of pulmonary/hepatic disease.
- Cystic fibrosis
- Alagille's syndrome
  The characteristic syndromic facies may not be apparent. Recognition of the diagnosis warrants a percutaneous liver biopsy to look for characteristic bile duct paucity and avoids a laparotomy.
- Nonsyndromic bile duct paucity
- Inspissated bile syndrome.

Surgical Management

Surgical management for biliary atresia involves two main modalities:
- Kasai hepatic portoenterostomy
- Liver transplant—which may be offered as first-line curative treatment.

The Kasai hepatoportoenterostomy involves excision of the atretic biliary segments and forming a Roux-en-Y jejunal loop from the hepatic hilum to the small intestine. The success of the Kasai portoenterostomy in the early period is defined by the clearance of jaundice, rather than by improvement of transaminases or GGT levels. Long-term success of the Kasai procedure is however defined by survival rates of patients with their native livers.

It is critical that any infant with clinical features of cholestasis be expeditiously evaluated for biliary atresia prior to 60 days of life. The success of the Kasai hepatoportoenterostomy is greatly dependent on the timing of surgery. The likelihood of success of the Kasai hepatoportoenterostomy falls with time after 60 days of life.

Postoperative Complications

The immediate postoperative complications are similar to those experienced after abdominal surgery. These complications are usually rare after a Kasai procedure and include anastomotic leak, wound dehiscence and localised bleeding.

Ascending Cholangitis

Infants post-Kasai procedure are at risk of ascending cholangitis, and over 90% of infants would experience an episode of cholangitis after surgery before 1 year of age. Prompt institution of appropriate antibiotic therapy in established cholangitis helps the restoration of hepatic function. A child presenting with fever on a background of biliary atresia post-Kasai procedure, should be managed as ascending cholangitis unless proven otherwise.

Empirical antibiotic therapy with adequate gram-negative and anaerobic coverage for enteric organisms should be instituted after appropriate microbiological cultures are obtained.

Children with recurrent episodes of cholangitis may require a longer duration of antibiotic therapy (4–6 weeks). Options, such as home parenteral antibiotic therapy or outpatient parenteral antibiotic therapy should be explored for children requiring prolonged courses of antibiotics.

Antibiotic prophylaxis such as cotrimoxazole or neomycin can be used in an attempt to reduce the rates of recurrent cholangitis [18] but there is no conclusive evidence to support routine antibiotic prophylaxis.

Progressive Liver Disease

With improved quality of medical care, the overall survival rate for more than 20 years on native liver has increased but the morbidity rates of progressive liver disease remain high and has impact on the quality of life and development of the child.[19] It is inevitable in the course of biliary atresia that liver cirrhosis occurs, with the onset of sequelae of portal hypertension from decompensated liver disease. Patients suffer from complications, such as gastrointestinal variceal bleeding, growth failure and hepatopulmonary syndrome. These features are indications for liver transplantation.

Medical Management

Promoting Biliary Drainage

Unlike the aims of reducing bile acid accumulation and hepatocyte injury in intrahepatic cholestasis, the aim of chloretic use, such as ursodeoxycholic acid (UDCA) post-Kasai procedure is targeted towards the prevention of ascending cholangitis: the use of a choleretic may improve biliary flow and potentially expedite the clearance of jaundice after a Kasai procedure.[20]

The use of steroids perioperatively may enhance biliary flow post-Kasai procedure but has no proven benefit in reducing the incidence of cholangitis or long-term survival.[21]

Nutritional Support

While awaiting clearance of jaundice post-Kasai procedure, the general principles of management of a child with cholestasis apply. Once adequate bile drainage is achieved, no special formula or medium-chain triglyceride supplementation is required. Breastfed infants should continue breastfeeding and be weaned at the appropriate age.

Choledochal Cyst

Choledochal cysts are congenital cystic dilatations of the biliary tree and can occur in either the extrahepatic, intrahepatic biliary ducts or both. This presents in the neonatal period with clinical evidence of cholestasis—jaundice and acholic stools and a mass may be palpable in the right hypochondrial region. They can also present with acute cholangitis. The diagnosis can be confirmed on ultrasonography.

There are 5 different types of choledochal cysts. Type V or Caroli's disease involves cystic dilatations of the intrahepatic tree. If the disease is limited to one hepatic lobe, this is amenable to hepatic lobectomy. Bilobar involvement may warrant liver transplantation once biliary cirrhosis and portal hypertensive features set in.

The treatment of choice is excision of the choledochal cyst and a Roux-en-Y hepaticojejunostomy performed to restore biliary-enteric drainage after an intraoperative cholangiogram. Magnetic resonance imaging has allowed for better visualization of the biliary anatomy and enhanced presurgical planning.

Inspissated Bile Syndrome

Inspissated bile syndrome or the accumulation of biliary sludge in the biliary tree can be contributed by haemolysis, cystic fibrosis, dehydration, use of cephalosporins or sepsis.

A typical clinical scenario would be a premature infant who has had sepsis, is receiving intravenous parenteral nutrition and noted to have worsening cholestasis on serial liver tests. An ultrasound scan would be diagnostic in revealing the presence of biliary sludge and mild biliary duct dilatation.

Biliary sludge is predominantly composed of calcium bilirubinate. The use of cephalosporins, in particular ceftriaxone, is associated with ceftriaxone pseudolithiasis. This syndrome closely mimics biliary atresia, but as previous highlighted biliary duct dilatation is characteristically not a feature of biliary atresia.

Conservative management includes increasing hydration and use of chloretics, medium chain triglyceride formula and fat-soluble vitamins. If conservative management does not work to improve biliary flow, percutaneous or intraoperative flushing of the biliary tree with saline may be required.

Spontaneous Perforation of the Bile Duct

This is an extremely rare diagnosis, with less than 150 cases reported worldwide.[22] Infants present with symptoms of cholestasis and abdominal distension with bilous ascites. Bile-staining of the scrotum may be noted (biliscrotum) in male infants. Surgical management is the treatment of choice.

Intrahepatic Causes of Cholestasis

Advances in molecular science and genetic sequencing have allowed the entity of 'idiopathic neonatal hepatitis' to be further elucidated into different pathophysiologic categories of cholestasis syndromes. Idiopathic neonatal hepatitis was previously a diagnostic orphan group with a defined histopathological appearance of giant cell transformation, but with no identifiable cause of cholestasis. We now have better clarity on the etio-pathogenesis of inherited cholestatic disorders such as progressive familial intrahepatic cholestasis and primary bile acid deficiencies (Table 22.4). Knowledge of specific molecular targets (Fig. 22.6) also allows for genetic testing and targeted therapy in the future.

Infectious Causes

Bacteria, such as gram-negative bacilli produce endotoxin which has an inhibitory effect on hepatic secretion of bile. Organisms under the TORCHES complex—toxoplasmosis, rubella, cytomegalovirus, herpes viruses, and syphilis all can cause intrauterine infections of the infant associated with neonatal cholestasis.

In addition, hepatotrophic viruses, such as cytomegalo-virus and other viruses in the herpes family including HHV-6; enterovirus, adenovirus and parvovirus can all cause infectious neonatal hepatitis which can either resolve spontaneously, evolve into acute fulminant hepatitis with acute liver failure.

Neonatal cytomegalovirus (CMV) infection is the most common identified infectious cause of neonatal cholestasis. It can be transmitted via CMV infected cervicovaginal secretions or breastmilk. The diagnosis of cytomegalovirus neonatal hepatitis is made in conjunction with positive CMV IgM serology, rising CMV DNA PCR titres and CMV antigen assay. The histopathological features on liver biopsy show the characteristic viral inclusion

Table 22.4: A comparison of the three main groups of progressive familial intrahepatic cholestasis				
Type	*Pathophysiology*	*Clinical features*	*Investigations*	*Genes implicated*
PFIC type 1	FIC-1 defect Influences BSEP/FXR function and increases bile salt uptake but decreases bile salt secretion	Jaundice, itch Failure to thrive Extrahepatic features: Diarrhea Pancreatitis Hearing loss	Normal gamma-GT	ATP8B1
PFIC type 2	Failure of BSEP expression	Jaundice, itch (more severe) No extrahepatic features	Normal gamma-GT	ABCB11
PFIC type 3	MDR-3 Failure of secretion of phosphatidylcholine in bile	More progressive disease and more severe hepatitis	High gamma-GT	ABCB4

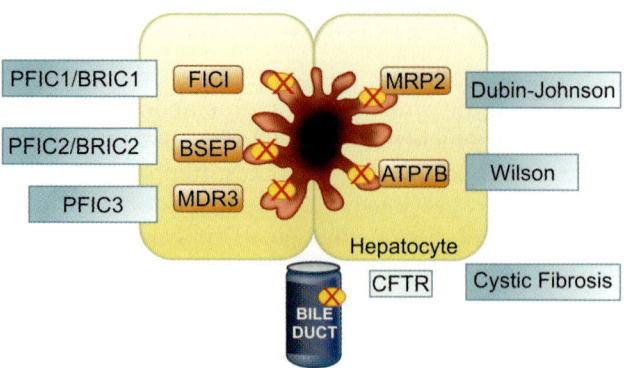

Fig. 22.6: Molecular defects in disorders of intrahepatic cholestasis *Abbreviations*: PFIC, progressive familial intrahepatic cholestasis; BRIC, benign recurrent intrahepatic cholestasis

bodies of cytomegalovirus infection. The presence of systemic disease, such as CMV retinitis, pneumonitis or encephalitis is an absolute indication for antiviral therapy. The decision to start antiviral therapy for isolated CMV neonatal hepatitis is controversial—there is little data on the efficacy of antiviral therapy in preventing progressive liver disease in CMV neonatal hepatitis. The degree of neonatal viraemia could increase the risk of long-term sequelae and may influence the decision to commence treatment.[23]

Endocrinopathies

Thyroid hormone, growth hormone and cortisol all have effects on bile transport and secretion. Congenital hypopituitarism and congenital hypothyroidism can result in cholestasis with a normal gamma-GT level. Hormone replacement can reverse the cholestasis.

Drug Effect/Toxic Effect

The cholestatic effects of total parenteral nutrition are well documented. Prenatal exposure to certain drugs, e.g. methamphetamine has rarely resulted in neonatal cholestasis.[24]

FAMILIAL (INHERITED) CAUSES OF INTRAHEPATIC CHOLESTASIS

Alagille Syndrome (AS) (Arteriohepatic Dysplasia)

Clinical Presentation

There is a spectrum of phenotypic severity: The presenting features include (i) bile duct paucity with chronic cholestasis, (ii) cardiovascular malformations, typically peripheral pulmonary stenosis or cyanotic heart disease, (iii) vertebral arch defects, (iv) posterior embryotoxon and other ocular defects such as Axenfeld anomaly/pupillary abnormalities, and anomalies of the optic disk, (v) renovascular abnormalities (renal artery stenosis) and cerebrovascular abnormalities (vascular aneurysms, Moyamoya disease), and (vi) dysmorphic facies.

Other associated features include poor growth and development.

Classic diagnosis criteria combine the presence of bile duct paucity on liver biopsy (see Fig. 22.5) with three of five systems involvement as listed above.

The clinical presentation is variable, and a single system involvement may predominate over the other.

Pathogenesis

This syndrome is associated with an autosomal dominant mutation in the JAGGED 1 gene on chromosome 20, and has variable penetrance. In over 50% of cases, this mutation occurs de novo. The JAGGED 1 gene is one of the key genes involved in the notch signaling pathway in embryogenesis, and the latter is vital in normal development.[25,26]

Diagnosis

The diagnosis of Alagille syndrome is clinical, and is made on recognizing the typical facies and the constellation of multisystem abnormalities. Occasionally, the typical facies is not recognised and the diagnosis is considered on the finding of bile duct paucity on liver biopsy.

The child should undergo vertebral X-rays, echocardiography and ophthalmological assessment.

The advent of genetic testing has proven useful in cases of atypical or mild cases of Alagille syndrome. JAG1 mutations can be found in approximately one third of patients presenting with only one or two clinical features of Alagille syndrome.[27]

Management

The general management of a child with Alagille's follows the management of a child with chronic cholestasis, including the use of chloretics, fat-soluble vitamins, and management of itch. Lipid-lowering therapy may be required for hypercholesterolemia, in view of possible long-term risks of atherosclerosis and cardiac morbidity.

Renovascular abnormalities may result in proteinuria or chronic hypertension, which warrants specific therapy. Monitoring for cerebrovascular aneurysms may be necessary in view of an increasingly recognised incidence of intracranial hemorrhage.

CASE SCENARIO 2

H is a 3-year-old boy who had presented with pallor and epistaxis. He was noted to have clubbing of his digits with firm hepatosplenomegaly and mild ascites. He had presented since infancy with mild jaundiced, but was not worked up till he became unwell at age 3 years. His liver function test showed mild conjugated hyperbilirubinemia, transaminitis with an elevated gamma-GT level. The parents have a consanguineous relationship (1st cousins).

The ultrasound scan showed hepatosplenomegaly with a normal gallbladder and no biliary duct dilatation. A liver biopsy done showed the presence of extensive cirrhotic changes in the absence of PAS+ve globules. Plasma/urine aminogram and urine organic acid profile was unremarkable. Autoimmune markers were negative; tests for alpha-1 antitrypsin deficiency were likewise negative.

Severe pruritus, poor hepatic synthetic function and portal hypertension are amongst the indications for liver transplantation. Partial biliary diversion may be considered as a bridge to transplant.

Progressive Familial Intrahepatic Cholestasis (PFIC)

There are three main types of PFICs:
- PFIC Type 1 (Byler's disease)
- PFIC Type 2
- PFIC Type 3/MDR-associated disease.

The main mode of pathogenesis in progressive familiar intrahepatic cholestasis is the inability to transport bile acids into the bile canalicus, leading to a build-up of toxic bile acids within the hepatocyte and liver injury. Genetic defects associated with each of the main subtypes of PFIC correspond to the defective expression of bile acid transporters (see Fig. 22.6).

PFIC Type 1

Etiopathogenesis

The underlying genetic defect lies within the FIC (familial intrahepatic cholestasis type-1 gene) gene, which has an official designation as ATP8B1. FIC gene is expressed not only in the liver, but also in high levels in the small intestine, pancreas and kidney.

The FIC1 gene regulates elements in bile salt transport:
- ASBT (Apical sodium dependent bile acid transporter) within the small intestine)
- FXR (Farnesoid X receptor)
- Bile salt export pump (BSEP) on biliary canalicular membranes

The loss of FIC1 gene in PFIC type 1 results in down regulation of the FXR receptor. The down regulation of FXR results in increased expression of ASBT transporters and increased uptake of bile acid from the gut.[28] Concurrently, the loss of FIC1 gene leads to diminished expression of BSEP on biliary canalicular membranes. The increased intestinal uptake of bile acids and decreased secretion of bile acids into the bile canaliculus eventually results in cholestasis.

Clinical Features

Affected infants present with features of cholestasis associated with failure to thrive and diarrhea (possibly related to the expression of FIC1 gene in the intestine). The accumulation of bile acids results in severe pruritus. Occasionally, pancreatitis and hearing loss has been associated. PFIC1 is a progressive disease which eventually results in cirrhosis and liver failure within the first decade of life.

Laboratory investigations show the presence of conjugated hyperbilirubinemia with a normal gamma-GT level. The latter is explained as the mechanism of cholestasis does not involve obstruction within the biliary canaliculus.

The histopathological features on liver biopsy show a bland appearance with biliary plugs and lobular disarray. Bile is noted to be coarse and granular on electron microscopy, commonly referred as 'Byler's bile'.

Management

Medical therapy is primarily supportive until the need for transplant. Surgical therapy can involve biliary diversion to an external stoma, and halting the reabsorption of bile acids. Liver transplant is the most effective form of treatment in those with progressive liver disease or cirrhosis. Due to the multiorgan expression of FIC1, extra-hepatic manifestations such as diarrhoea will continue to manifest post-transplant.

PFIC Type 2

Etiopathogenesis

The gene mutated in PFIC-2 is ABCB11 gene, which codes for the bile salt export pump (BSEP) transporter on the biliary canalicular membrane. The defective expression of BSEP transporters leads to reduced bile acid transport into the canaliculus and accumulation of bile salts.

Clinical Features

The symptoms are similar to that of PFIC-1 but with less extrahepatic manifestations. There are more severe symptoms of jaundice, itch and failure to thrive. Similarly, there is presence o f cholestasis with normal gamma-GT levels.

Management

Similar to PFIC-1, choleretics and biliary diversion can be attempted. Ursodeoxycholic acid is observed to be less effective as part of its efficacy is from the modification of activity of the BSEP transporter itself. Liver transplant is the key management for progressive liver disease and cirrhosis

Benign Recurrent Intrahepatic Cholestasis (BRIC) Type 1 and Type 2

These represent milder disease entities to their corresponding PFIC counterparts, and similarly arise from mutations in FIC1 and BSEP. These disorders present with recurrent episodes of jaundice and pruritus, associated with symptoms of fatigue, anorexia, pale stools and steatorrhoea. Recovery is spontaneous although each episode can last from weeks to months.

Progressive Familial Intrahepatic Cholestasis Type 3

Etiopathogenesis

The gene involved is ABCB4, which encodes for MDR3 (multidrug resistance protein-3), another type of transporter protein on the biliary canalicus. Unlike BSEP, the MDR3 mediates the secretion of phosphatidylcholine into bile. Phosphatidylcholine forms micelles with bile salts, and negates the toxic detergent effect on the cholangiocytes. Hence, in MDR-3 associated disease, a cholangiopathy occurs from the 'toxic bile' effect and explains a characteristic biochemical difference from PFIC-1/PFIC-2: the gamma-GT levels are elevated in PFIC-3.

Clinical Features

The onset of the disease is rarely in neonates. The typical features of cholestasis are present in patients. There may

---

CASE SCENARIO 2 (CONTD....)

The JaundiceChip gene sequencing assay was performed for H to identify genetic mutations in suspected PFIC Type 3. The assay revealed that H was homozygous for the ABCB4 gene mutation, confirming the diagnosis of PFIC type 3/MDR-associated disease. Genetic testing has been arranged to determine the carrier status of his parents.

As H has features of early decompensated liver disease, including faltering growth, he has been placed on a liver transplant waiting list.

---

be a positive family history in siblings and mothers of affected patients may report having suffered intrahepatic cholestasis of pregnancy. The gamma-GT level is characteristically elevated in PFIC-3.

Management

Ursodeoxycholic acid is used as a less toxic and more hydrophilic bile acid supplement to shift the biliary bile salt composition to one that is more hydrophilic. Patients who do not respond to ursodeoxycholic acid therapy should be considered for liver transplantation.

A comparison of the three main groups of PFIC is summarised in Table 22.4.

Disorders of Bile Acid Biosynthesis

These are responsible for up to 1–2% of cases of neonatal cholestasis.[29]

Etiopathogenesis

The primary bile acids cholic acid and chenodeoxycholic acid are synthesised from cholesterol through a pathway of multiple enzymatic reactions. Inborn errors of bile acid synthesis can be divided into primary and secondary disorders. Primary enzymatic disorders involve deficiencies in the enzymes catalysing the formation of cholic acid and chenodeoxycholic acids. These are listed as below:

❑ Cholesterol 7α-hydroxylase (CYP7A1) deficiency
❑ Oxysterol 7α-hydroxylase deficiency,
❑ Δ (4)-3-oxosteroid-5β-reductase deficiency
❑ 3-β-hydroxy-Δ(5)-C(27)-steroid dehydrogenase deficiency
❑ Cerebrotendinous xanthomatosis (sterol 27-hydroxylase deficiency)
❑ 2-methylacyl-CoA racemase deficiency
❑ Trihydroxycholestanoic acid CoA oxidase deficiency
❑ Amidation defects involving bile acid-CoA ligase deficiency and bile acid-CoA aminoacid N-acyltransferase (BAAT) deficiency.

Secondary disorders of bile acid biosynthesis include peroxisomal disorders such as Zellweger's (cerebrohepatorenal syndrome), in which the deficiency of hepatic peroxisomes lead to the decreased conversion of cholic acid precursors into cholic acid.[30]

The enzymatic deficiencies result in accumulation of toxic intermediate bile acid metabolites in the hepatocyte and subsequent progressive liver injury. Δ(4)-3-oxosteroid-5α-reductase deficiency is associated with rapid progression to liver failure if not promptly recognised.

Clinical Features

Affected infants present with features of cholestasis. However there is a characteristic absence of pruritus unlike most other cholestatic disorders.

Diagnosis

The laboratory investigations show the presence of conjugated hyperbilirubinemia with a normal gamma-GT level. The liver biopsy shows a non-specific histopathological appearance of giant cell hepatitis. Serum bile acids may be normal or low. The diagnosis is established through mass spectrometry of urinary bile acids, and each enzymatic deficiency has a characteristic urinary bile acid profile.

Management

Treatment of primary bile acid deficiency is via oral replacement of primary bile acid cholic acid. Early recognition of these rare disorders is vital, as prompt therapy can reverse cholestasis and hepatic injury.

Metabolic Disorders

These will be covered in brevity as a detailed discussion is available under Metabolic Disorders in the Infant.

Alpha-1 Antitrypsin Deficiency

This diagnosis stems from an abnormal genotype of protease inhibitor (PiZZ genotype), resulting in abnormal accumulation of alpha-1-antitrypsin polymers in the endoplasmic reticulum of hepatocytes and intrahepatic cholestasis.

The diagnosis is supported by low serum antitrypsin levels and protease inhibitor genotyping. Histopathological findings of bile ductular proliferation and bile plugs can be similar to biliary atresia, and PAS-staining of the abnormal polymers should be demonstrated on biopsy specimens. The progression to cirrhosis is typically slow and liver transplantation is curative.

Cystic Fibrosis

Neonatal cholestasis can rarely be the presenting feature of cystic fibrosis,[31] as the cystic fibrosis gene product (CFTR) is expressed in the biliary canaliculus and is responsible for chloride secretion into bile. Like in alpha-1 antitrypsin deficiency, the histopathological findings can closely mimic that of biliary atresia.

Galactosemia/Tyrosinemia

Galactosemia and tyrosinemia type 1 all can present as neonatal cholestasis with or without progression to acute liver failure. Prompt therapy potentially reverses cholestasis.

Citrin Deficiency

Citrin deficiency (type 2 citrullinemia) is increasingly recognized as a cause of neonatal cholestasis. The etiopathogenesis stems from a deficiency in citrin, a mitochondrial aspartate-glutamate carrier. This results in an inability to transfer high energy electrons in the form of NADH from cytosolic glycolysis into the mitochondria and a build-up of NADH in the cytosol. The high NADH levels result in suppression of glycolysis and galactose metabolism.

This results in a breakdown in mitochondrial aerobic metabolism and hepatocyte injury. A partial urea cycle defect occurs from a decrease in cytosolic levels of aspartate (citrulline reacts with aspartate to form arginosuccinate in the urea cycle).

Affected infants of citrin deficiency can present with jaundice, hypoglycemia and failure to thrive. There is also an associated hyperammonemia, and galactosemia.

The plasma aminogram is characteristic, and features multiple aminoacidemia including citrulline, methionine, threonine and tyrosine. Genetic testing for the involved gene SLC25A13 confirms the diagnosis. Percutaneous liver biopsy findings would classically reveal micro- or macro-vesicular steatosis.

The prognosis generally remains good with infants responding to a high fat, lactose-free diet alone by one year of age.[32]

Neonatal Hematochromatosis

This disorder carries an extremely poor prognosis, with affected infants progressing rapidly into acute liver failure.[33] There is increased iron deposition in the liver, heart and endocrine organs, resulting in multiorgan failure.

The clinical features are that of cholestasis with markedly decreased hepatic synthetic function (hypoalbuminemia, hypoglycemia, and marked coagulopathy).

The diagnosis should be suspected in any infant who manifests with signs of liver disease in utero or shortly after birth. Diagnosis is confirmed on buccal glandular biopsy.

Etiopathogenesis

The alloimmune hypothesis states that fetal liver injury occurs from maternofetal alloimmunity. Transplacental passage of maternal antibodies results in antifetal liver antigen antibodies and immune injury to the fetal liver. It is postulated that fetal liver injury causes reduced synthesis of hepcidin, which in turn, is responsible for the regulation of maternal–fetal iron flux.

There is a 60–80% probability that each subsequent child born would be affected, after an index case of neonatal haemochromatosis.[34] This observation is consistent with the patterns observed in other alloimmune gestational diseases (e.g. rhesus alloimmunisation).

Management

Liver transplantation is potentially curative although it is with extremely high risks given the small size of the infant and coexisting multiorgan failure. Medical therapy using a cocktail of antioxidants and iron chelators may be curative in the milder phenotypes.[35]

The use of high dose intravenous immunoglobulin in mothers with a previously affected child with neonatal hematochromatosis has promising results to date.[34]

■ SUMMARY

Neonatal cholestasis encompasses a heterogeneous group of disorders, broadly classified into extrahepatic and intrahepatic cholestatic pathologies. Much of the initial investigations of an infant with cholestasis is directed towards excluding biliary atresia, as the timing of surgical intervention greatly influences the eventual outcome. Advances in the knowledge of molecular genetics have allowed us to define distinct disease entities within the category of intrahepatic cholestatic disorders, and give rise to the possibility of targeted novel therapy.

REFERENCES

1. Cai SY, Boyer JL. FXR: a target for cholestatic syndromes? Expert Opin Ther Targets. 2006;10(3):409-21.
2. Balistreri WF, Bezerra JA. Whatever happened to "neonatal hepatitis"? Clin Liver Dis. 2006;10(1):27-53.
3. Brucato A, Cimaz R, Stramba-Badiale M. Neonatal lupus. Clin Rev Allergy Immunol. 2002;23(3):279-99.
4. Okada T, Sasaki F, Itoh T, Ota S, Todo S. Bleeding disorder as the first symptom of biliary atresia. Eur J Pediatr Surg. 2005;15(04):295-9.
5. Aagenaes O. Hereditary cholestasis with lymphoedema (Aagenaes syndrome, cholestasis-lymphoedema syndrome). New cases and follow-up from infancy to adult age. Scand J Gastroenterol. 1998;33(4):335-45.
6. Moyer V, Freese DK, Whitington PF, Olson AD, Brewer F, Colletti RB, et al. Guideline for the evaluation of cholestatic jaundice in infants: recommendations of the North American Society for Pediatric Gastroenterology, Hepatology and Nutrition. J Pediatr Gastroenterol Nutr. 2004;39(2):115-28.
7. Cabrera-Abreu JC, Green A. Gamma-glutamyltransferase: value of its measurement in paediatrics. Ann Clin Biochem. 2002; 39(Pt 1):22-5.
8. Liu C, Aronow BJ, Jegga AG, Wang N, Miethke A, Mourya R, et al. Novel resequencing chip customized to diagnose mutations in patients with inherited syndromes of intrahepatic cholestasis. Gastroenterology. 2007;132(1):119-26.
9. Tan Kendrick AP, Phua KB, Ooi BC, Tan CE. Biliary atresia: making the diagnosis by the gallbladder ghost triad. Pediatr Radiol. 2003;33(5):311-5.
10. Petersen C, Meier PN, Schneider A, Turowski C, Pfister ED, Manns MP, et al. Endoscopic retrograde cholangiopancreaticography prior to explorative laparotomy avoids unnecessary surgery in patients suspected for biliary atresia. J Hepatol. 2009; 51(6):1055-60.
11. Ng VL, Balistreri WF. Treatment options for chronic cholestasis in infancy and childhood. Curr Treat Options Gastroenterol. 2005; 8(5):419-30.
12. Paumgartner G, Beuers U. Mechanisms of action and therapeutic efficacy of ursodeoxycholic acid in cholestatic liver disease. Clin Liver Dis. 2004;8(1):67-81.
13. Marschall HU, Wagner M, Zollner G, Fickert P, Diczfalusy U, Gumhold J, et al. Complementary stimulation of hepatobiliary transport and detoxification systems by rifampicin and ursodeoxycholic acid in humans. Gastroenterology. 2005; 129(2):476-85.
14. Yang H, Porte RJ, Verkade HJ, De Langen ZJ, Hulscher JB. Partial external biliary diversion in children with progressive familial intrahepatic cholestasis and Alagille disease. J Pediatr Gastroenterol Nutr. 2009;49(2):216-21.
15. Wolfhagen FH, Sternieri E, Hop WC, Vitale G, Bertolotti M, Van Buuren HR. Oral naltrexone treatment for cholestatic pruritus: a double-blind, placebo-controlled study. Gastroenterology. 1997;113(4):1264-9.
16. Chang Y, Golkar L. The use of naltrexone in the management of severe generalized pruritus in biliary atresia: report of a case. Pediatr Dermatol. 2008;25(3):403-4.
17. Rastogi A, Krishnani N, Yachha SK, Khanna V, Poddar U, Lal R. Histopathological features and accuracy for diagnosing biliary atresia by prelaparotomy liver biopsy in developing countries. J Gastroenterol Hepatol. 2009;24(1):97-102.
18. Bu LN, Chen HL, Chang CJ, Ni YH, Hsu HY, Lai HS, et al. Prophylactic oral antibiotics in prevention of recurrent cholangitis after the Kasai portoenterostomy. J Pediatr Surg. 2003;38(4):590-3.
19. Bijl EJ, Bharwani KD, Houwen RH, de Man RA. The long-term outcome of the Kasai operation in patients with biliary atresia: a systematic review. Neth J Med. 2013;71(4):170-3.
20. Willot S, Uhlen S, Michaud L, Briand G, Bonnevalle M, Sfeir R, et al. Effect of ursodeoxycholic acid on liver function in children after successful surgery for biliary atresia. Pediatrics. 2008; 122(6):e1236-41.
21. Escobar MA, Jay CL, Brooks RM, West KW, Rescorla FJ, Molleston JP, et al. Effect of corticosteroid therapy on outcomes in biliary atresia after Kasai portoenterostomy. J Pediatr Surg. 2006; 41(1):99-103; discussion. 99-103.
22. Pereira ECMV, Yan J, Asaid M, Ferguson P, Clarnette T. Conservative management of spontaneous bile duct perforation in infancy: case report and literature review. J Pediatr Surg. 2012;47(9):1757-9.

23. Lanari M, Lazzarotto T, Venturi V, Papa I, Gabrielli L, Guerra B, et al. Neonatal cytomegalovirus blood load and risk of sequelae in symptomatic and asymptomatic congenitally infected newborns. Pediatrics. 2006;117(1):e76-83.

24. Dahshan A. Prenatal exposure to methamphetamine presenting as neonatal cholestasis. J Clin Gastroenterol. 2009;43(1):88-90.

25. Li L, Krantz ID, Deng Y, Genin A, Banta AB, Collins CC, et al. Alagille syndrome is caused by mutations in human Jagged1, which encodes a ligand for Notch1. Nat Genet. 1997;16(3):243-51.

26. Oda T, Elkahloun AG, Pike BL, Okajima K, Krantz ID, Genin A, et al. Mutations in the human Jagged1 gene are responsible for Alagille syndrome. Nat Genet. 1997;16(3):235-42.

27. Guegan K, Stals K, Day M, Turnpenny P, Ellard S. JAG1 mutations are found in approximately one third of patients presenting with only one or two clinical features of Alagille syndrome. Clin Genet. 2012;82(1):33-40.

28. Chen F, Ananthanarayanan M, Emre S, Neimark E, Bull LN, Knisely AS, et al. Progressive familial intrahepatic cholestasis, type 1, is associated with decreased farnesoid X receptor activity. Gastroenterology. 2004;126(3):756-64.

29. Heubi JE, Setchell KD, Bove KE. Inborn errors of bile acid metabolism. Semin Liver Dis. 2007;27(3):282-94.

30. Kase BF, Pedersen JI, Strandvik B, Bjorkhem I. In vivo and vitro studies on formation of bile acids in patients with Zellweger syndrome. Evidence that peroxisomes are of importance in the normal biosynthesis of both cholic and chenodeoxycholic acid. J Clin Invest. 1985;76(6):2393-402.

31. Lykavieris P, Bernard O, Hadchouel M. Neonatal cholestasis as the presenting feature in cystic fibrosis. Arch Dis Child. 1996; 75(1):67-70.

32. Hayasaka K, Numakura C, Toyota K, Kimura T. Treatment with lactose (galactose)-restricted and medium-chain triglyceride-supplemented formula for neonatal intrahepatic cholestasis caused by citrin deficiency. JIMD Rep. 2012;2:37-44.

33. Whitington PF. Neonatal hemochromatosis: a congenital alloimmune hepatitis. Semin Liver Dis. 2007;27(3):243-50.

34. Whitington PF, Hibbard JU. High-dose immunoglobulin during pregnancy for recurrent neonatal haemochromatosis. Lancet. 2004;364(9446):1690-8.

35. Flynn DM, Mohan N, McKiernan P, Beath S, Buckels J, Mayer D, et al. Progress in treatment and outcome for children with neonatal haemochromatosis. Arch Dis Child Fetal Neonatal Ed. 2003; 88(2):F124-7.

Chapter 23

Acute Hepatitis

Ramaswamy Ganesh, Malathi Sathiyasekaran

INTRODUCTION

Acute hepatitis is an abrupt onset of diffuse inflammation of the hepatocytes associated with hepatocellular necrosis and a characteristic constellation of clinical (jaundice, nausea, vomiting, right hypochondrial pain), biochemical (elevated serum bilirubin and transaminases) and pathological (hepatocellular inflammation and necrosis) features. The hallmark of acute hepatitis is the demonstration of increased transaminases (ALT) more than twice the upper limit of normal.

ETIOLOGY

Acute hepatitis may occur due to an infective or a non infective cause. In India infective causes are more common than noninfective with viruses constituting an important subset amongst the infections. The common causes of acute hepatitis are tabulated in Table 23.1. In this chapter acute viral hepatitis is discussed in detail.

Acute viral hepatitis (AVH) is a self-limiting disease with diffuse inflammation and/or necrosis of the hepatocytes caused by viruses and is characterized by an abrupt onset of symptoms with spontaneous resolution of illness usually within 4 weeks. Necroinflammation may progress to acute liver failure or continue beyond 6 months resulting in chronic hepatitis.[1]

The term "viral hepatitis" usually refers to hepatitis caused by the hepatotropic viruses, namely hepatitis A, B, C, D and E (HAV, HBV, HCV, HDV, HEV) though several other viruses including the less common hepatotropic viruses, such as hepatitis G virus (HGV)/GB virus-C (GBV-C)], Torque Teno virus (TTV), SEN and non-hepatotropic viruses, such as coxsackie, Epstein-Barr, HIV, cytomegalovirus (CMV) can present as acute hepatitis. Infections due to bacteria, spirochaete, protozoa and non infective causes, such as medications, metabolic, autoimmune and malignancy can present with acute hepatitis and must be differentiated from the common acute viral hepatitis for definitive management.

EPIDEMIOLOGY

The four common viruses that cause AVH are hepatitis A virus (HAV), hepatitis E virus (HEV), hepatitis B virus (HBV) and hepatitis C virus (HCV). In this "hepatitis alphabet" the two enterally transmitted viruses HAV and HEV have some similarity whereas the two parenterally

Table 23.1: Etiology of acute hepatitis	
Infective	*Noninfective*
Viruses—Hepatotropic; hepatitis A, B, C, D, E Nonhepatotropic: Dengue, TORCH, coxsackie, EB virus, HIV, Parvovirus B19	Drugs: Antituberculous drugs, anticonvulsants, dapsone
Bacteria—Typhoid Tuberculosis, Scrub typhus	Autoimmune: Autoimmune hepatitis, SLE
Spirochaete—Leptospirosis	Metabolic—Wilson's disease
Protozoa—Malaria, *Amoeba*	Vascular
Fungal	Miscellaneous: Malignancy, hemophagocytic lymphohistiocytosis (HLH)

transmitted viruses HBV and HCV share some common features.

Hepatitis A

Hepatitis A is still an important cause of acute viral hepatitis in India. According to WHO about 10–50 persons per 1,00,000 are infected annually and in India, 50–75% of acute sporadic hepatitis in children is due to HAV.[2] About two decades ago, it was not uncommon to isolate anti-HAV IgG antibodies, a marker of natural protection in more than 80–90% of children.[3] Improvement in socioeconomic status has resulted in a shift in epidemiology of HAV with children not acquiring protective antibodies naturally and, therefore, being more susceptible to the infection later in life. The recent introduction of vaccines has also changed the etiological profile of viral hepatitis. The relative incidence of HAV is probably less than before, although it is still prevalent in some parts of the country.

Hepatitis E

Hepatitis E virus is more common in North India, especially in areas situated around the river Ganges. HEV has been isolated in all the major epidemics of hepatitis in India and is the causative agent in 15–20% of sporadic acute hepatitis.

Hepatitis B

The prevalence of hepatitis B surface antigen (HBsAg) positivity in India is approximately 2–7%. In India sporadic acute hepatitis due to hepatitis B virus ranges from 10 to 15%. The incidence is decreasing following the universal immunization program. HBV has been classified into A–H genotypes. A genotype is pandemic, B and C are prevalent in Asia, D is seen in southern Europe, E in Africa, F in USA, UK and France A and D in India and H in Central America.[4]

Hepatitis C

The prevalence of hepatitis C virus in India is 1–2.5%. HCV as the causative agent for sporadic acute hepatitis is less than 1%.

ETIOPATHOGENESIS

Infections due to HAV and HEV are self-limiting and do not progress to chronicity. HBV and HCV infections can present as acute hepatitis and resolve but may also progress to chronic hepatitis, cirrhosis and hepatocellular carcinoma (HCC). HBV is more infectious than HCV and is spread by blood, blood products and body fluids. Perinatal transmission is also more common in HBV. The

several genotypes identified in HBV and HCV may modify the course of illness and response to therapy. All the major hepatotropic viruses are classified as RNA viruses except HBV which is a DNA virus.

Hepatitis A virus is a 27 nm spherical, non-enveloped entero virus of Picornaviridea family (Fig. 23.1). HAV is highly contagious and transmission occurs by orofecal route due to consumption of contaminated food or water. The virus is inactivated by boiling for 5 minutes, autoclaving or UV radiation. The incubation period for HAV is 2–7 weeks and fecal shedding occurs for 2–3 weeks before and 1 week after the onset of jaundice. Parenteral transmission has been reported. Transmission occurs during the preicteric stage of the disease. Antenatal HAV infection does not result in increased complications or clinical disease in the fetus or newborn. The virus can be isolated from the liver, bile, stools and blood during the late incubation period and preicteric phase of the illness. Natural infection confers life-long immunity. There is no evidence for chronic carrier state. Although HAV has a cytopathic effect in tissue culture, the hepatocyte injury is secondary to a host immune response. HAV infection causes periportal inflammation and pericentral cholestasis without significant cellular inflammation.[5]

Hepatitis E virus is a 30 nm RNA virus which has recently been assigned as a herpes virus and similar to HAV it is also transmitted by the orofecal route with an incubation period of 15–40 days. There are eight different genotypes identified till date. HEV infection during pregnancy is associated with a high maternal mortality and fetal deaths. The mechanism of hepatocyte injury due to HEV is still unknown but is most probably due to an immune mediated reaction.[5]

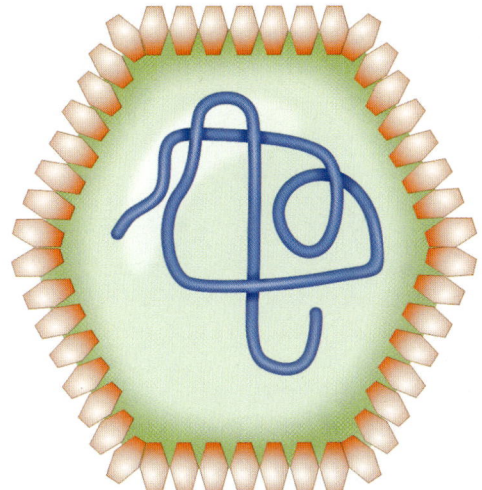

Fig. 23.1: Structure of hepatitis A virus

Hepatitis B virus is a complex hepadnavirus which causes an immune mediated injury. The intact HBV is the "Dane particle" or virion, which is double shelled and 42 nm in size (Fig. 23.2). Serologically, HBV is recognized by its three antigens namely surface (HBsAg), core antigen (HBcAg), and nucleocapsid (HBeAg) antigens and their corresponding antibodies, namely anti-HBs, anti-HBc and anti-HBe. HBV DNA can be detected quantitatively and is a sensitive marker of active replication. The severity of the illness depends on the degree of immune response by the host. HBV is a very infectious virus and contact with 0.00002 mL of infected blood is sufficient to acquire the infection. The incubation period of HBV infection is 60–180 days, and HBV is transmitted by blood, blood products and body fluids, including cervicovaginal secretions, semen, breast milk, saliva, sweat, pharyngeal secretions and tears. Perinatal transmission of HBV is a unique problem seen in children and is more common in areas of high endemicity. During the last decade numerous mutations have been described in the HBV genome. Mutation is defined as any change in the nucleic acid sequence of a genome. The various mutations that have been identified are precore or core, vaccine escape and envelope mutants. The problems with these mutant strains are evasion of vaccine, drug resistance, change in trophism and change in pathogenesis. The lysis of hepatocytes seen in acute HBV infection occurs as a result of polyclonal and multispecific immune response. The elimination of virus infected hepatocyte is dependent on the recognition of viral determinant protein on infected cell by cytotoxic "T" lymphocytes.[6]

Hepatitis C virus is a 30–80 nm RNA virus similar to a flavivirus and results in a complex immune response (Fig. 23.3). Recently nonimmunologic genes have also been recognized to influence its clearance. HCV is less infective but more sinister than HBV and is spread by blood and blood products. Apart from infection following perinatal transmission HCV is prevalent in those requiring multiple blood/blood product transfusions, IV drug users, hemodialysis and post organ transplant.

Hepatitis D virus is a defective virus with a small RNA molecule with HBsAg as envelope (Fig. 23.4). This virus can infect only those who are HBsAg positive.

Clinical Manifestations of AVH

In the majority of young children with AVH the illness is subclinical or anicteric whereas in the older age group the three classical stages of AVH namely the prodrome, icteric and convalescence may be more apparent. The clinical presentation is common to all the etiological types of viral hepatitis with a prodrome which usually lasts for 2–7 days characterized by nausea, vomiting, high colored urine, fever and right hypochondrial pain followed by jaundice, pale stools and tender hepatomegaly. The icteric stage lasts for 7–14 days, but may persist longer even for 12 weeks in older children. The child may present with pruritus which may be disturbing. The resolution of the illness is heralded by the disappearance of the constitutional symptoms, improvement in appetite and decrease in size of the liver. Certain features, such as presence of ascites, firm liver may

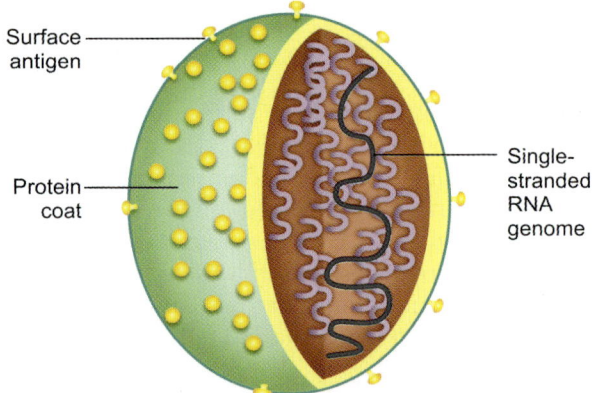

Fig. 23.3: Structure of hepatitis C virus

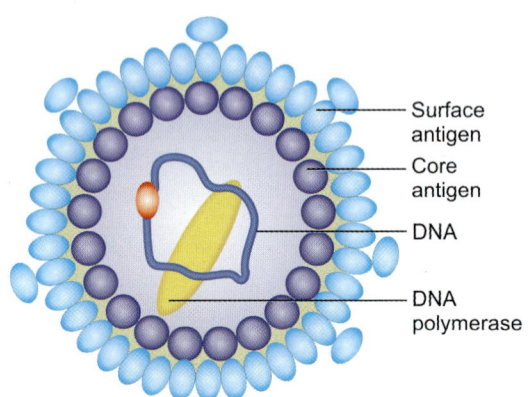

Fig. 23.2: Structure of hepatitis B virus

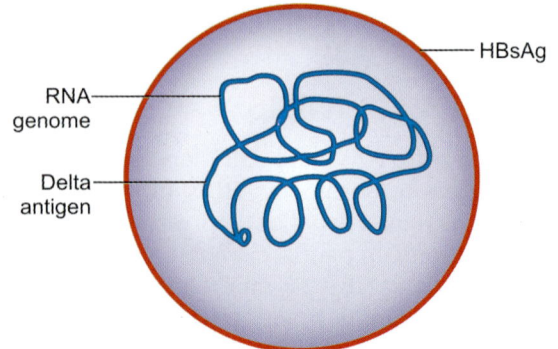

Fig. 23.4: Structure of hepatitis D virus

point to the existence of an underlying liver disease and a possibility of an acute on chronic liver disease should be considered. Prolonged fever, rash, arthralgia, arthritis, pallor, lymphadenopathy in a child with features of acute hepatitis may be pointers to a diagnosis of non-viral hepatitis.

Some characteristic clinical features in the illness caused by the different hepatotropic viruses have been described and help in understanding the natural history.

Hepatitis A

The characteristic features include an age dependent expression of clinical illness, low rate of fulminant disease and absence of chronicity. The clinical presentation varies with age of the child. In young children less than 6 years of age, the majority present as anicteric hepatitis and only 10% develop typical icteric illness. Whereas 40–60% of older children and 70–80% of adults will manifest with icteric hepatitis. In those presenting with jaundice the illness is heralded by a mild prodrome and recovery occurs within a period of 5–7 days. Older children with HAV infection may present with atypical manifestations, such as ascites, pleural effusion, firm hepatomegaly and disturbing pruritus. Cholestatic hepatitis is a distressing symptom of HAV infection more common in older children and may last for 12 weeks. Extrahepatic manifestations due to circulating immune complexes are uncommon and include evanescent skin rash, transient arthralgia, pancreatitis, vascultis, thrombocytopenia, triggering of autoimmune hepatitis, red cell aplasia, myocarditis, nephritis, cryoglobulinemia, and Guillian Barre syndrome. The incidence of acute liver failure occurs in less than 1% of acute infection with high fatality if liver transplant is not offered. Relapsing hepatitis has been reported however chronic hepatitis is not a feature of HAV infection. Co-infection with HEV or HBV may increase the morbidity. HAV infection in individuals with chronic liver disease is associated with increased mortality.

Hepatitis E

Infection due to HEV is similar to HAV; however, it is more commonly reported in young adults than in children.[7] The majority of clinical cases are icteric and extrahepatic manifestations are rare. Chronicity is not a feature of HEV but has been recently reported in immunosuppressed liver transplant individuals and in HIV infected patient. During HEV epidemics children usually have a milder or subclinical infection while pregnant women are more susceptible and present with acute liver failure with a high mortality of 1–20% and also increased still births.[8] The reason for the severity during pregnancy is probably related to suppressed cellular immunity and hormonal factors. The immunological changes include down regulation of the p65 component of nuclear factor (NF-κB) with a predominant T-helper type 2 (Th2) bias in the T-cell response along with host susceptibility factors, mediated by human leucocyte antigen expression. Recent reports from Chennai, South India, have demonstrated a lower incidence of mortality in pregnancy probably due to difference in genotypes.

Hepatitis B

The majority of children with acute HBV infection are anicteric. Those with icteric hepatitis may be symptomatic for 1–2 months and present with nausea, jaundice and hepatomegaly. A spectrum of immune mediated extrahepatic manifestations, such as aplastic anemia, rash, leukoclastocytic vasculitis, glomerulonephritis, Guillain-Barré syndrome, myocarditis, pancreatitis, urticaria, polyarteritis nodosa, migratory polyarthritis, cryoglobulinemia and popular acrodermatitis of childhood or Gianotti Crosti syndrome may be seen in HBV infection. Most of the older children clear the virus by 6 months and have natural seroconversion. The risk of chronicity in HBV infection is inversely proportional to the age of acquisition of the illness.[9]

Hepatitis C

In children this virus is an uncommon cause of acute hepatitis and has a benign and mild course with progression to acute liver failure in less than 1%. The symptoms of malaise, fatigue and jaundice are mild but the transaminases are elevated for a prolonged period. The incidence of chronicity is much more (40–50%) than seen in HBV infection. Chronic hepatitis can progress to cirrhosis and HCC. Sporadic hepatitis in children due to type C hepatitis is rare and is reported in children receiving multiple blood transfusions.

Hepatitis D

The clinical presentation of HDV depends on the status of the underlying HBV infection since Hepatitis D virus infects only those children who are HBsAg positive. Acute HDV infection can occur either as a coinfection with acute HBV infection or as a superinfection in an asymptomatic or symptomatic chronic HBsAg positive child.

Coinfection follows simultaneous exposure to an inoculum containing both HBV and HDV. The incubation period is same as that for HBV infection. A biphasic illness occurs which is uncommon in other forms of hepatitis. The incidence of acute liver failure is as high as 10%.

Superinfection can occur in an asymptomatic HBsAg positive child or in those with symptomatic HBV related to chronic liver disease. It results in deterioration of the pre-existing liver disease with the appearance or deepening of jaundice and worsening of ascites. Acute liver failure is as high as 20%.

ATYPICAL MANIFESTATIONS AND COMPLICATIONS OF ACUTE VIRAL HEPATITIS

Acute viral hepatitis in children is usually a self-limiting illness. However, atypical manifestations can occur in all the types of viral hepatitis. The common presentation is either the anicteric or classical icteric hepatitis. In HAV infection some atypical manifestations are seen in older children. The jaundice may be prolonged and associated with cholestatic features. Relapsing hepatitis has also been described in 1–15% of individuals. The relapse may be mild presenting with elevation of transaminases. Other atypical features seen in children with AVH are prolonged fever, hyperbilirubinemia and triggering of autoimmune hepatitis in susceptible individuals. Ascites has been reported in 8.7% of children with HAV infection in a study done in Chennai.[10] In a report from Lucknow, (UP) India ascitic form of sporadic AVH has been recognized as a separate entity which resolves spontaneously within 8 weeks.[11] The two major complications of AVH are acute liver failure and chronic hepatitis which increases the morbidity and mortality of the illness. Any child presenting with acute hepatitis who has deepening jaundice, vomiting, fever, significant anorexia, mucosal bleeds and change in sleep pattern should be very carefully observed for progression to acute liver failure and may warrant hospitalization. A decreasing liver size in addition to persistently prolonged prothrombin time uncorrected after injection vitamin K is diagnostic of Acute liver failure. Coinfections with HAV and HEV may not always worsen the natural history of the disease.

Diagnosis

Biochemical Investigations

The characteristic biochemical feature of acute hepatitis is the detection of elevated transaminases more than twice the upper limit of normal. In viral hepatitis alanine aminotransferase (ALT) is higher than aspartate aminotransferase (AST) indicating cytoplasmic rather than mitochondrial injury. The elevation is usually very marked more than 20 times upper of normal when the infection is due to the common hepatotropic viruses.

Such high elevation is usually seen only in hypoxic or toxic injury.[12] The level of transaminases however does not correlate with severity of the illness. In the icteric hepatitis the total serum bilirubin is increased with the direct component showing variable rise depending on the phase of illness. Apart from these two tests children with AVH do not require any other investigation unless hospitalized. Prothrombin time (PT) is the test of liver synthetic function. Elevated prothrombin time and international normalized ratio (INR) more than two are not good prognostic indices and indicate acute liver failure even in the absence of encephalopathy. A fall in serum albumin is uncommon in uncomplicated HAV infection. Persistent hypoglycemia and hyponatremia are also poor prognostic indices. Serum alkaline phosphatase may be normal or mildly elevated. The basic investigations in AVH, including complete blood counts, urine for bile salts and pigments should be done as a routine. Lymphopenia and neutropenia may occur during the course of illness.

Serological Tests

Except HBsAg as a screening test other biomarkers to confirm the viral etiology are usually not done unless there are atypical features.

Acute HAV infection is confirmed by the presence of immunoglobulin M (IgM) antibodies to HAV which appears at the onset of illness and remains positive for 4–6 months. Anti-HAV immunoglobulin G (IgG) is detected in the sera within 8 weeks of onset of symptoms and remains positive indefinitely. Polymerase chain reaction (PCR) for detection of viral particles in stool or blood is done only for research.

Acute HBV infection is diagnosed by the presence of the two markers, namely HBsAg and anti-HBcIgM. HBsAg is an early seromarker and is present 6 weeks following infection and is normally positive only for 6 months .Anti HBcIgM is detected soon after the appearance of HBsAg and decreases in titer by 3 months and indicates recent infection. The detection of HBsAg for more than 6 months following an acute infection is considered as chronic HBV infection. Anti-HBs a protective antibody appears once HBsAg clears. HBeAg is detected in the sera soon after the appearance of HBsAg and is a marker of infectivity and active viral replication. It usually disappears by 6 weeks; persistence of this antigen for more than 6 weeks indicates progression to chronicity. HBV DNA is a marker of viremia and infectivity. It is seen 2–3 weeks before the appearance of HBsAg in those with acute HBV infection and remains detectable even after HBsAg seroconversion. It is therefore of value only for monitoring chronic HBV infection.[13]

Acute HCV Infection Acute hepatitis (AHC) is usually asymptomatic and not perceived clinically. High transaminases >20 UL/N and presence of HCV RNA with anti HCV appearing later are characteristic of AHC. HCV RNA becomes positive within 2 weeks of exposure and anti HCV within 8–10 weeks of exposure.

Acute HDV Infection

Coinfection with HBV is diagnosed by the presence of HBsAg, anti-HBcIgM and low titres of anti-HDV IgM whereas in super -infection, high titres of anti-HDV IgM and HBsAg are present but anti-HBcIgM is absent.[14]

When atypical manifestations such as firm liver, ascites, abdominal veins or rash are present in children with acute hepatitis it is necessary to exclude other causes of acute hepatitis. Laboratory tests, such as IgM leptospirosis, IgM scrub typhus, blood Widal, blood culture, autoantibodies and ceruloplasmin are included in the work up. Ultrasound examination is done to exclude liver abscess or gallstones. Liver biopsy is not done in children with acute hepatitis, but is essential in those with suspected acute on chronic liver disease or chronic hepatitis.[15]

DIFFERENTIAL DIAGNOSIS

The differential diagnosis includes any condition presenting with elevated transaminases with or without jaundice. There are two main groups which have to be differentiated from viral hepatitis (i) hepatitis caused by the less common nonhepatotropic viruses and (ii) non-viral hepatitis. It is important that they are recognized since specific therapy is available for the non viral hepatitis unlike in the viral marker positive hepatitis where only supportive therapy is recommended.

Nonhepatotropic Viruses

Several nonhepatotropic viruses can cause acute hepatitis and, although they are less common in older children, they form an important group in neonates and young infants. Children with this form of hepatitis usually present with additional features of the underlying illness, such as the exanthem in measles or varicella apart from jaundice, hepatomegaly and elevated serum transaminases. The diagnosis is usually made clinically and if necessary confirmed serologically.[16]

Epstein Barr Virus

The Epstein Barr virus (EBV) infects more than 90% of the world's population and thus is the most prevalent human viral infection. It belongs to the Gammaherpesvirinae family and causes infectious mononucleosis. The common clinical presentation is prolonged fever, sore throat, evanescent rash, lymphadenopathy, hepatosplenomegaly and transient self-limited elevation of transaminases. The liver damage is characterized by lack of expression of EBV antigens in hepatocytes instead the EBV latency proteins are seen in the lymphocytes. The cytotoxic T lymphocytes target EBV-infected B lymphocytes causing collateral liver damage. Chronic hepatitis and cirrhosis are not sequelae. The diagnosis is confirmed by the detection of IgM antibody to the viral capsid antigen.

Measles Virus

Measles presenting with anicteric hepatitis is an atypical manifestation of the illness and usually results in spontaneous recovery. Measles virus can trigger autoimmune hepatitis type I within 3 months of the infection in susceptible individuals.

Cytomegalovirus

Cytomegalovirus is a ubiquitous herpes virus that infects majority of humans. CMV hepatitis in neonates presents as prolonged cholestasis and later may progress to cirrhosis. In older children it may occur in recipients of renal or liver transplant. The disease resembles EBV related mononucleosis without pharyngitis and posterior cervical lymphadenopathy. CMV hepatitis is a major problem in liver transplant patients. The infection is usually primary although reactivation can also occur. The diagnosis is made by isolation of the virus from urine or saliva using PCR. A fourfold rise in the antibody titre is also helpful in diagnosis. Liver biopsy demonstrates the characteristic nuclear and cytoplasmic inclusion bodies. Quantification of CMV DNA by PCR is also helpful for monitoring therapy.

Parvovirus B$_{19}$

Human parvovirus B$_{19}$ can present with hepatic dysfunction, elevated transaminases and acute liver failure with or without aplastic anemia.

Herpes Simplex 1 and 2

Herpes simplex virus (HSV) hepatitis is usually rare beyond the neonatal period unless the child is immune-compromised. It may present as part of a generalized herpetic disease in infants. In older children it is rare and the mucocutaneous lesions may be absent. The diagnosis is made by the presence of IgM antibodies and the isolation of virus from the vesicles or other tissue. Liver biopsy shows the characteristic inclusion bodies.

Dengue Virus

Dengue fever presents with the characteristic features of fever, hepatomegaly, rash, pleural effusion and features of capillary leak. In addition, there is a moderate elevation of transaminases especially AST more than ALT. In the presence of dengue shock syndrome, the transaminases may be very high in several thousands due to ischemic or hypoxic hepatitis. This elevation of transaminases unlike in viral hepatitis is associated with a significant rise in LDH which drops sharply once the child is resuscitated. The diagnosis is confirmed by the high hematocrit, low platelet, NS1 antigen and the presence of IgM dengue antibodies.

Human Herpes Virus-6

Liver dysfunction in association with human herpes virus (HHV)-6 virus infection may present as infectious mononucleosis like syndrome, hepatitis or acute liver failure. HHV-6 could enhance allograft rejection and increase severity of other infections, including CMV and HCV. Ganciclovir and valganciclovir are active against HHV-6 infection.

Varicella Zoster

Varicella zoster virus causing liver disease is unusual except in immunosuppressed children with HIV infection or post-transplant recipients.

Human Immunodeficiency Virus

Infants with HIV may present with acute cholestatic hepatitis and later progress to chronic hepatitis. Liver involvement in HIV infected individuals is indicative of a poor prognosis.

Echo, coxsackie and adenovirus may present in neonates and infants with acute liver failure.

Severe Acute Respiratory Syndrome-Coronavirus

Severe acute respiratory syndrome is a potentially lethal disease caused by SARS/coronavirus (CoV) which primarily affects the lung and intestine. Virus or viral products are also detected in the liver. Elevated ALT has been reported during the 1st week of illness and peaks by 2nd week. The liver disease due to SARS/CoV is of lesser significance compared to the lung involvement.

Exotic Viruses

Marburg, Ebola and Lassa are dangerous viruses which primarily target the liver. Lassa fever is caused by an arena virus and transmitted from rodents to man or from man to man. It causes acute liver failure with high mortality. Marburg virus disease is caused by an RNA virus transmitted by monkeys. The illness is characterized by features of hemorrhage, encephalopathy and hepatitis. Ebola resembles Marburg illness.

Infective Nonviral Causes: Bacterial Hepatitis

Salmonella

Typhoid hepatitis can mimic AVH and is differentiated clinically by the presence of toxemia, high fever and hepatosplenomegaly. Some children may also have mild ascites and pleural effusion similar to primary liver disease. The transaminases are moderately elevated (3–20 times the upper limit of normal) with an ALT/LDH ratio less than four whereas in AVH it is more than four. The diagnosis is confirmed by a positive blood culture for Salmonella typhi.

Bacterial Sepsis

Bacterial sepsis should be considered in children presenting with fever, jaundice, hepatosplenomegaly and mild elevation of transaminases. Liver involvement is secondary to parenchymal or biliary invasion as a part of a systemic manifestation of sepsis. The prolonged prothrombin time and mortality is due to disseminated intravascular coagulation (DIC) and sepsis rather than liver failure.

Tuberculosis

Tuberculous hepatitis should be considered in those children presenting with fever of unknown origin, hepatomegaly, mild to moderate elevation of transaminases and high alkaline phosphatase. Liver biopsy shows the characteristic caseating granuloma.

Brucellosis

This infection can occur in children who consume unpasteurized milk. It presents with fever, lymphadenopathy and elevated transaminases. The diagnosis is confirmed by a high initial titer for Brucella antibody more than 1:160 or a rising titer done 2 weeks apart.

Leptospirosis

The clinical presentation may range from inapparent infection to features of acute hepatitis or fatal disease. Jaundice, hepatosplenomegaly, fever, myalgia, congested conjunctiva, bleeding manifestations, hematuria, anuria, minimal ascites and pleural effusion are the common clinical features. Apart from rise in serum bilirubin and transaminases the C-reactive protein (CRP) and creatinine phosphokinase (CPK) may be elevated which helps differentiate it from viral hepatitis. The presence of IgM lepto confirms diagnosis.

Scrub Typhus

Scrub typhus or tsutsugamushi disease is a febrile illness caused by bacteria of the family Rickettsiaceae and named Orientiatsutsugamushi. Scrub typhus is endemic to a geographically distinct region, the so-called tsutsugamushi triangle, which includes Japan, Taiwan, China and South Korea. It has also been reported in India and recently there have been several reports from South India. The clinical feature resembles dengue fever with thrombocytopenia and elevated transaminases. The eschar may be identified in less than 50% of patients. Diagnosis is confirmed by the presence of IgM antibody. In an unpublished report from KKCTH Chennai during January-December 2012, scrub typhus constituted 155 cases out of 15229 inpatients (1%) and all had elevated transaminases.

Infective Nonviral Causes: Protozoal Hepatitis

Malaria

Malarial hepatitis or malarial hepatopathy (the term hepatopathy is preferable since inflammatory cells are not a characteristic feature on histology) is diagnosed when there is a threefold rise in ALT with or without rise in conjugated bilirubin, in the absence of clinical and serological evidence of viral and drug induced hepatitis and with a clinical response to antimalarials. It is usually seen with *Plasmodium falciparum* but may occur in *Plasmodium vivax* infection. The exact pathogenesis is unknown but could be due to impaired bilirubin transport caused by blockage of reticuloendithelial cells, microvilli damage or cytoadherence of parasites to the vascular endothelium leading to stagnant anoxemia.

Noninfective Causes

Drug Induced Liver Injury

The common drugs causing hepatitis are anticonvulsants, antituberculous drugs, antimetabolites, nonsteroidal anti-inflammatory drugs (NSAIDS), paracetamol, herbals and indigenous medications. It may be very difficult to differentiate drug induced liver injury (DILD) from viral hepatitis. The child presents with elevated transaminases with or without jaundice, rash and hepatomegaly. The absence of prodrome and the history of drug intake is a clue to diagnosis. The challenge is the onset of symptoms which occurs within 5–90 days of introducing the drug. On dechallenge, 50% drop in transaminases occurs within 8 days of stopping the drug.[17]

Autoimmune Hepatitis (AIH)

This is a progressive inflammatory liver disease of unknown etiology presenting with elevated transaminases, hypergammaglobulinemia, interface hepatitis, non-organ and liver specific antibodies and good response to immunosuppressive treatment. Children may present with type I or type II hepatitis. In type I hepatitis, antinuclear antibody (ANA) and anti-smooth muscle antibody (ASMA) are present whereas in the latter LKM1 antibody is detected.[18]

Obstructive Jaundice

Obstructive jaundice due to choledocholithiasis or biliary ascariasis can rarely mimic acute hepatitis. Abdominal pain and features of cholangitis are important clues to diagnosis. The direct bilirubin, alkaline phosphatase and ALT are elevated. Ultrasound helps in identifying the site and cause of obstruction.

Glycogen Storage Disease

In types I and III glycogen storage disease (GSD), the elevated transaminases may suggest anicteric hepatitis but the presence of massive hepatomegaly and other features such as short stature, doll-like faces, voracious appetite and early morning seizures will give a clue to a diagnosis of storage disorder. Jaundice is not a presentation. The liver biopsy shows swollen hepatocytes with glycogen [periodic-acid Schiff (PAS) positive and diastase sensitive] and steatosis in type I and PAS positive cells without steatosis in type III.

Wilson's Disease

Wilson's disease (WD) should be suspected in any child more than 3 years who presents with jaundice, elevated transaminases and a firm liver. Early appearance of free fluid, hemolysis, family history and a set back in school performance are pointers to suspect WD. The diagnosis is made by the presence of KF ring, decreased serum ceruloplasmin and elevated 24-hour copper and confirmed by liver biopsy, copper estimation in dry weight of liver and mutational studies.

Hemophagocytic Lymphohistiocytosis (HLH)

This is a condition characterised by multiorgan involvement secondary to hypercytokinemia. Clinically, it is characterized by fever, elevated transaminases, coagulopathy, central nervous system involvement and cytopenia. Hemophagocytosis in the bone marrow is a hallmark feature of this condition.

MANAGEMENT OF ACUTE VIRAL HEPATITIS

Supportive Therapy

Since the illness resolves spontaneously in the majority of children with AVH supportive therapy is all that is required. There is no necessity to restrict diet instead the child should get adequate calories. This will prevent endogenous breakdown of fat and protein. During the acute phase of illness strenuous physical exercise and hepatotoxic drugs should be avoided. Lactulose is given to children with constipation to prevent increase in levels of serum ammonia which may precipitate encephalopathy. Hospitalization is reserved only for those children with red flag signs, such as gastrointestinal bleed, altered sensorium, persistent fever or vomiting. Itching is a common but disturbing symptom observed during the cholestatic phase of AVH which responds to ursodeoxycholic acid at a dose of 15–20 mg/kg/day. Ascites if significant can be managed with spironolactone given over a short period. There is no role for NSAIDs in AVH which is strictly contraindicated because of its hepatotoxicity. Children who are already on anticonvulsants may require change in their medication. Sodium valproate and phenytoin can be replaced with phenobarbitone. Similarly, those who are on antitubercular therpy should be given ethambutol, streptomycin and fluoroquinolones instead of rifampicin, isoniazid and pyrazinamide.

Specific Therapy

Acute Hepatitis A and E

There is no specific antiviral therapy recommended for children with acute hepatitis A or E.

Acute Hepatitis B

Several antivirals are available for management of chronic hepatitis B in adults but at present there is no role for antivirals in treating either children or adults with type B acute viral hepatitis. These children with acute hepatitis B should be followed up for a period of 6 months to monitor spontaneous clearance of the virus.

Acute Hepatitis C

Children and adolescents who acquire acute HCV infection either following multiple blood transfusions or IV drug abuse should be monitored closely for 12 weeks for natural seroconversion. If HCV RNA persists after 12 weeks interferon should be initiated after checking the genotype. In asymptomatic adults with HCV genotype 1 infection a 12-week course of PEG–IFN initiated as early as possible is recommended whereas in icteric patients, HCV genotypes 2 and 3 treatment may be delayed as this group since there is better chance of clearing the virus and responding to chronic HCV therapy.

Acute Hepatitis D

The underlying Hepatitis B infection is treated and liver transplant is the option in those who ddo not respond to therapy.

TREATMENT FOR ACUTE HEPATITIS DUE TO OTHER NONHEPATOTROPIC VIRUSES

The treatment of acute hepatitis due to other non-hepatotropic viruses is also usually supportive. Some specific antiviral agents, such as acyclovir for herpes simplex, ganciclovir for CMV and highly active antiretroviral therapy (HAART) for HIV are available and may be used judiciously.

Treatment of acute hepatitis due to bacterial cause is with appropriate antibacterial agent depending upon the etiology identified.

Prevention

The most important aspect of therapy in AVH is prevention. The common viruses, such as HAV and HEV, can be prevented by improving personal, food and environmental hygiene. Effective immunization is available for HAV and HBV.[19]

Hepatitis A

❑ *Passive immunization*: HAV specific immunoglobulin is not available in India, and therefore, the available intramuscular preparation of immunoglobulin can be used. The dose is 0.02 mL/kg of immune globulin which should be administered within two weeks after exposure to HAV. There are however very few indications, such as newborns of HAV infected mothers and children with chronic liver disease who are exposed to HAV. Though the protection is immediate and effective it is transient. Immunoglobulin prophylaxis is not indicated for healthy household contacts.

❑ *Active immunization*: In India the shift in the epidemiology of hepatitis A virus has resulted in older children and adolescents from higher socioeconomic conditions presenting with HAV infection since they do not acquire natural antibodies. Effective and safe vaccine for HAV is available in India The vaccine is recommended on a one to one "named child" basis for children especially from higher socioeconomic group, adolescents and adults who are leaving homes for education or employment without past history of viral hepatitis or are antibody negative, all children and adults with underlying chronic liver disease and family contacts, all immuno compromised individuals, household contacts of acute HAV infection (within 10 days), children attending day care centers and creches, travellers from abroad (e.g. NRI's) visiting India or other endemic areas. Hepatitis A vaccine is a formalin inactivated suspension containing HM175 strain of the virus with aluminum hydroxide as the adjuvant. The vaccine is approved for use in children above two years of age, and is administered intramuscularly. The pediatric formulation contains not less than 720 ELISA units in 0.5 mL and can be used till 18 years of age. Two dose schedule is recommended, a prime boost schedule on an elected date (0) followed by a booster dose after 6 months. The same vaccine is given as a two dose schedule with 1 mL of vaccine containing 1440 Elisa units for individuals more than 18 years of age. Seroconversion occurs in up to 90% of children after the first dose and close to 100% after the second dose. IAP recommends two doses of HAV vaccine any time after 18 months of age.

A live attenuated human diploid cell vaccine from H_2 strain in China is also available. A single subcutaneous dose of 1 mL in children more than 2 years has been recommended. A novel inactivated vaccine using virosome with the added advantage of faster seroconversion and lesser side effects given at a dose is 0.5 mL intramuscularly has been reported.

Hepatitis B

- Active immunization: Hepatitis B vaccine is recommended for children and adults. The current IAP recommendation is to administer the recombinant genetically engineered subunit HBV vaccine intramuscularly in 3 doses of 10 µg for children less than 12 years and 20 µg for those more than 12 years. The three schedules endorsed by IAP are 0, 1 and 6 months or birth, 6 and 14 weeks or combination with triple antigen at 6,10, and 14 weeks. The genetically engineered recombinant DNA vaccine is safe and immunogenic. Immunogenicity is over 95 % after 3 dose schedule. An adequate response is defined as an anti HBs Ab level greater than 10 mIU/mL. Routine postimmunization testing for antibody levels is not necessary.
- Passive immunization: Hepatitis B immunoglobulin (HBIG) provides immediate passive immunity. It should be administered intramuscularly and not intravenously. In children, 32–48 IU/kg body weight and in neonates 100–200 IU is recommended. HBIG

does not interfere with antibody response to Hepatitis vaccine.Babies born to mothers who are HBsAg positive should receive the first dose of vaccine within 6 hours of birth and the HBIG should be given at a separate site. Subsequent doses of the vaccine should be given at 1, 2 and 12 months. Even without concurrent HBIG, the vaccine alone offers 90–95% protective efficacy in preventing vertical transmission. Risk factors for failure of immunization in newborns includes high level of maternal HBV DNA and low levels of maternal anti-HBc Abs.[19] Early administration of the vaccine is a cost effective method of prevention of disease in newborns. HBIG has also been recommended for those with history of acute exposure to HBsAg infected material (e.g. needle stick injury).

Hepatitis C and D

They can be prevented by avoiding unnecessary needle pricks, using disposable syringes and screened blood for transfusion.

SUMMARY

Acute hepatitis is a diffuse inflammation of the hepatocytes resulting in hepatocellular necrosis. Infections caused by hepatototropic viruses Hepatitis A, E, and B are the most common etiology followed by the nonhepatotropic viruses, bacteria, and drugs. Irrespective of the cause, acute hepatitis in children tends to be anicteric in most children and, therefore, may be missed. Elevated ALT is the characteristic biochemical feature of acuter hepatitis. Prolonged uncorrected prothrombin time is a useful prognostic index. Complications, such as acute liver failure, relapsing hepatitis and chronic hepatitis may occur. Underlying liver disease, malnutrition and hepatotoxic drugs increases the risk of complications.

REFERENCES

1. Craxi A, Stefano RD. Hepatitis due to non A-E viruses. In: Dooley JS, Lok Anna SF, Burroughs AK, Heathcote EJ (Eds). Sherlock's Diseases of the Liver and Biliary System. 12th edition. Wiley Blackwell Publication; 2011. pp. 427-37.
2. Malathi S,MohanavalliB,Menon T, et al. Clinical and viral marker pattern of acute sporadic hepatitis in Chennai,South India. J Tropical Pediatr. 1998;44:275-8.
3. Panda SK,DattaR,Gupta A, et al. Etiological spectrum of acute sporadic viral hepatitis in children in India.Tropical Gastroenterology. 1989;106-10.
4. Fung Sk, Lok AS. Hepatis B virus genotypes:do they play a role in the outcome of HBV infection? Hepatology. 2004;40:790-2.
5. Karayiannis P, Thomas HC. Enterically transmitted viral Hepatitis: Hepatitis A and Hepatitis E. In: Dooley Js, Lok As, Burroughs AK,

Heathcote JE (Eds). Sherlock's Diseases of the Liver and Biliary System 12th edition. Wiley Blackwell West Sussex; UK. 2011. pp.353-66.

6. Ganem D, Prince AM. Hepatitis B virus infection- natural history and clinical consequences. N. Engl J Med. 2004;350:1118-29.

7. Khuroo MS, Rustogi VK, Dawson GJ, et al. Spectrum of hepatitis E virus infection in India. J Med Virol. 1994;43:2810.

8. Jilani N, Das BC, Hussain SA, et al. Hepatitis E virus infection and fulminant liver failure during pregnancy. Gastroenterol Hepatol 2007;22:675-82.

9. Hochman JA, Balistreri WF. Acute and chronic viral hepatitis In: Suchy FJ, Sokol RJ, Balistreri WF (Eds): Liver disease in Children. 3rd edn. Cambridge University Press, NY USA. 2007:369-446.

10. Kamath SR, Sathiyasekaran M, Raja TE. Profile of viral hepatitis A in Chennai. Indian Pediatr. 2009;46:642-3.

11. Yachha SK, Goel A, Khanna V, et al. Ascitic form of sporadic acute viral hepatitis in children: a distinct entity for recognition. J Pediatr Gastroenterol Nutr. 2010;50(2):184-7.

12. Mohan Prasad VG, Nathan V. Hepatitis A virus. In: Mahtab MA, Rahman S (Eds). Liver-A Complete Book on Hepato-Pancreatico-Biliary Diseases. Elseiver India Pvt Ltd; 2009.pp.201-5.

13. Schiff ER. Viral hepatitis section V. In: Schiff ER, Sorrell ME, Maddrey WC (Eds). Schiff 's Diseases of the Liver, 10th edition. Philadelphia: Lippincot Williams & Wilkins; 2007.pp709-835.

14. Tagle M, Medina de Marioa, Schiff ER. Hepatitis A and E. In: Bacon BR, O'Grady JG, Di Bisceglie AM, Lake JR (Eds): Comprehensive Clinical Hepatology. 2nd edition. Mosby Elseiver; 2010.pp205-12.

15. Sathiyasekaran M, Ganesh R. Viral Hepatitis. IAP text book of Pediatrics, 4th edition, Jaypee publishers; New Delhi. 2009,pp655-67.

16. Sathiyasekaran Malathi. Acute Viral hepatitis. Common Viral infections. In: A Parthasarathy (Eds). Textbook of Pediatric Infectious Diseases Indian Academy of Pediatrics. Infectious Diseases Chapter. Jaypee Brothers; New Delhi. 2013;pp278-85.

17. Roberts EA. Drug induced Liver Disease. In: Suchy FJ, Sokol RJ, Balistreri WF (Eds). Liver disease in children. 3rd Edn. Cambridge University Press, NY USA. 2007:478-512.

18. Vergagni Gm,vergagni Diego.Autoimmune Hepatitis. In Suchy FJ, Sokol RJ, Balistreri WF (Eds). Liver disease in children 3rd Edn. Cambridge University Press, NY USA; 2007:447-58.

19. Agrawal R. Vaccines and Immunisation. In: A Parthasarathy (Ed): Textbook of Pediatric Infectious Diseases. Indian Academy of Pediatrics. Infectious Diseases Chapter. Jaypee Brothers. India; 2013:432-57.

Chapter 24

Chronic Viral Hepatitis

Neelam Mohan, Deepak Goyal

INTRODUCTION

Hepatitis is inflammation of the liver and is characterized by the presence of inflammatory cells in the tissue of the organ. Hepatitis is acute when it lasts less than six months and chronic when it persists longer than six months. This chapter includes chronic hepatitis due to hepatitis B and C viruses.

CLINICAL FEATURES OF CHRONIC VIRAL HEPATITIS

The clinical presentation of chronic viral hepatitis depends on the pace of progression of hepatocellular failure and fibrosis. Many children presents with findings discovered incidentally during routine physical examination, or as a result of an investigation of unrelated conditions. In such patients, it is referred to as latent or compensated. The child is apparently healthy, and there are no signs or symptoms of liver disease and a detailed history provides no evidence of antecedent illness. There may or may not be a large liver or palpable spleen. Biochemical tests may or may not show mild increases in hepatic transaminase.

As disease advances, eventually the clinical picture evolves to that of decompensated cirrhosis. There can be failure to thrive, muscle weakness, fatigue, jaundice, edema, ascites, and symptoms of fat soluble vitamin deficiency such as steatorrhea. Patient presents with symptoms due to complications, such as hematemesis, encephalopathy, ascites or infection, known as decompensated. This is mostly seen in adulthood. The complications of cirrhosis typically are related to impaired hepatic function or actual physical disruption of the liver parenchyma. Laboratory investigations may reveal elevated alkaline phosphatase, bilirubin, hepatic transaminase, and ammonia levels. The distinction between compensated and decompensated cirrhosis often is based on the severity of clinical and laboratory findings.

HEPATITIS B

Epidemiology

Worldwide the population has been divided into three zones based on the prevalence:[1] (1) High prevalence (> 8%)—includes most of the African countries, China, Canada, and part of South America. Early childhood infections are common in these region. (2) Intermediate (2%–7%)—includes India, Afghanistan, Russia. Infections occur in all age groupsin these regions. (3) Low (<2%)—includes North America, Southern countries of South America and Australia. Most infections occur in adults.

Mother to child transmission accounts for >50% of chronic infections in highly endemic areas. After exposure, the risk of chronicity is highest for newborns (90%), followed by infants and children <5 years of age (25–30%) than adolescents or adults (<5%).[2,3]

Virus Characteristics

The hepatitis B virus (HBV) belongs to a family of viruses, Hepadnaviridae. The virus contains both double stranded and single-stranded DNA. The intact virion, also known as Dane particle, is spherical and double-shelled particle with an outer lipoprotein envelope that contains three related envelope glycoproteins (or surface antigens) and is approximately 42 nm in diameter (Fig. 24.1).[4] Within the envelope is the viral nucleocapsid or core, which contains the partially double-stranded DNA; a DNA polymerase; and hepatitis B-e antigen (HBeAg). HBsAg is a 24-kDa protein, 20-nm in size and is the most abundant protein. It is produced in excess by the infected hepatocytes.[5]

Hepatitis B Virus Genotypes

There are eight genotypes of HBV, designated from A to H. Genotype A and D are predominant in India. Genotype A

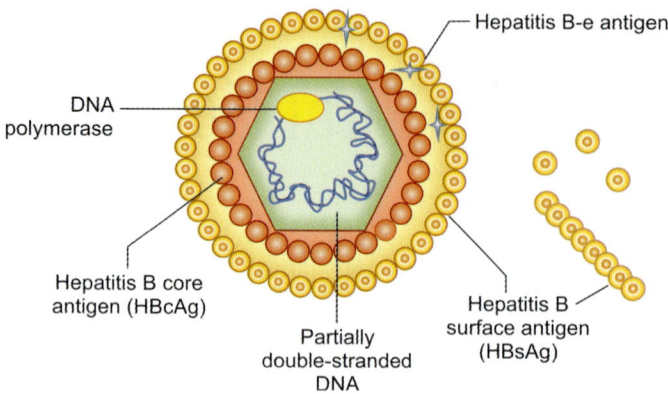

Fig. 24.1: Hepatitis B virus

is the predominant genotype in northern Europe and the United States. Genotypes B and C are the most prevalent genotypes and are confined to populations in eastern Asia and the Far East.[6]

Genotype is an important determinant in the development of hepatocellular carcinoma (HCC) and also is important in predicting response to therapy. Genotype B is more prevalent in the development of HCC in patients younger than 50 years.[7] In a multicenter study (N = 307) of chronic hep B patients, response rates to pegylated interferon was best with genotype A (47%), followed by B (44%); C and then D (25%).[8] HBeAg seroconversion occurs earlier in patients with genotype B than with genotype C.

Mutations of the Hepatitis B Virus Genome

HBV has a high mutation rate, around ten times that of similar viruses. Like most other polymerases, the reverse transcriptase lacks a proofreading capacity. This predisposes HBV to mutations either naturally or as the result of exposure to antiviral therapy. Mutations have been detected in almost all regions of the viral genome in patients with chronic HBV infection although the significance of many of these mutations is still not clear. The vast majority of mutations in the HBV genome are silent but some mutations can have potentially important implications:

Hepatitis B Surface Antigen Mutants

The typical mutation results in the substitution of glycine for arginine at amino acid position. This substitution prevents binding of neutralizing antibodies (anti-HBs). Patients harboring these "escape mutants" develop hepatitis despite adequate levels of anti-HBs and so these mutations can pose a potential threat to the success of vaccination programs.[9] Escape mutants have commonly been seen in post-liver transplant patients with HBV infection.

Mutations in the Pre-core, Basal Core Promoter and Core Genes

In cases of severe or fulminant hepatitis, mutations are seen in the pre-core and basal core promoter regions of genome of HBV. Cyotoxic T lymphocytes, a key mode of viral clearance are affected by these core gene mutations and thus may interfere with the response to interferon too. Risk of HCC is increased in the presence of these mutations. These patients do not have HBeAg positivity, but paradoxically have higher levels of HBV DNA along with elevated aminotransferase levels.[10]

Hepatitis B Virus DNA Polymerase Mutants

Drug resistance to nucleoside analogs may be secondary to the mutations in HBV polymerase. YMDD mutants (Y = tyrosine, M = methionine, D = aspartate), the most common mutation resulting in lamivudine resistance are seen in the C domain of the virus DNA. Similarly resistance to telbivudine and entecavir results from other nucleotide substitutes.

20% patients on lamivudine therapy develop resistance after one year of therapy and almost 70% develop in five years. Rates of resistance to adefovir, a nucleotide analog, are 0% at one year and 29% after five years.[4]

Pathogenesis

The virion attaches to host cell membranes. This is followed by fusion of the viral and host membranes and then nucleocapsid is released into the cytoplasm. The first step in viral replication involves conversion of the circular form of HBV DNA into a double-stranded, covalently closed circular form (cccDNA). CccDNA serves as a template for viral messenger RNA (mRNA) transcription and for future viral transcription.[11] After generation of mRNA, it is transported to the cytoplasm of hepatocytes, where the translation of viral mRNA produces various viral proteins—HBsAg, HBcAg, HBeAg and HBV DNA polymerase. This allows for assembly of progeny viral capsids. This RNA then undergoes reverse transcription into viral DNA. After this, some cores bud into the endoplasmic reticulum to get enveloped and are exported from the infected hepatocyte to infect other hepatocytes (Fig. 24.2).

The immune response to HBV is incompletely known yet. HBV is not directly cytopathic; instead, an immune response to infected hepatocytes is responsible for hepatic injury or for recovery. Eradication of the virus occurs via lysis by cytotoxic T cells (CTL). This is substantiated by the fact that HBV-infected individuals with immune defects often have mild acute liver injury but high rates of chronic carriage due to this fact.

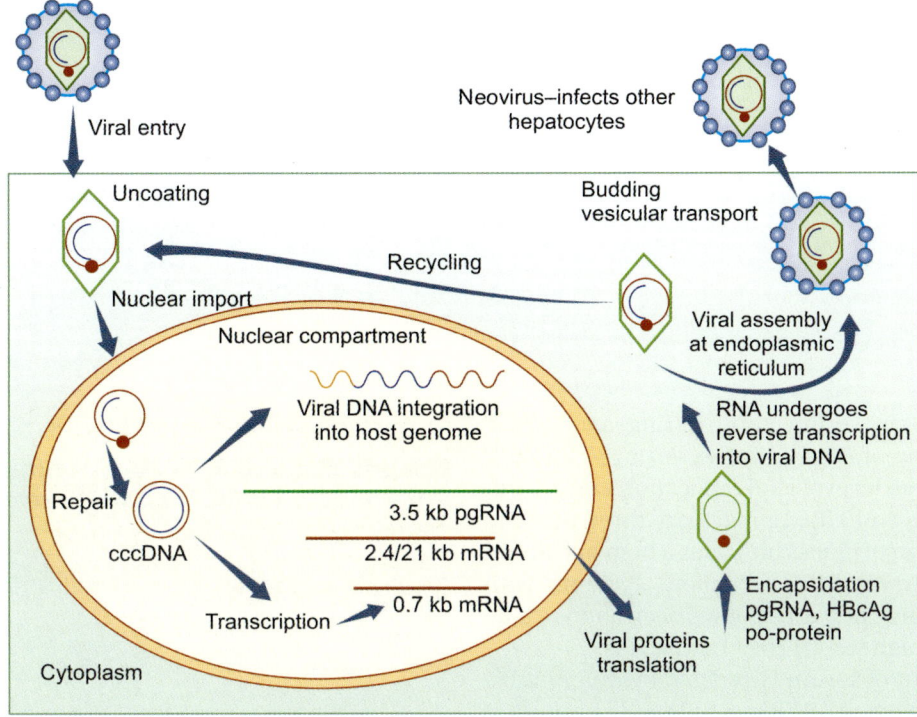

Fig. 24.2: Propagation of Hep-B virus

During acute HBV infection, most HBV DNA molecules are cleared rapidly from the liver via noncytopathic mechanisms mediated by cytokines released initially by cells of the innate immune system and later by HBV-specific CD8+ cells.

In persons with chronic HBV infection there is weak HBV-specific T-cell responses. CD8+ CTLs are thought to contribute to the disease process and result in apoptosis of infected hepatocytes. Direct killing of the infected cells and release of potent antiviral cytokines results from the binding of the cytotoxic T lymphocytes receptor to peptide—MHC complex on hepatocyte surface. Secondary to the presentation of viral peptides to class II MHC molecules CD4 helper T cells are activated and produce antiviral cytokines which neutralize antibody production. This results in limiting the intrahepatic spread of virus both in primary infection and re-infection.[11]

Perinatal Transmission

Perinatal transmission accounts for more than 50% of chronic infections in highly endemic areas. The risk of chronicity is very high in perinatal transmission, up to 90%. Most perinatal transmission occurs at or near the time of birth.[2,3] Around 90% of infants born to HBeAg-positive mothers develop chronic hepatitis B in contrast to infants of HBeAg-negative carrier mothers who have around 20% risk.

Specific risk factors for perinatal transmission are: (1) high maternal HBsAg titer; (2) Maternal HBeAg positivity (3) High viral load in maternal serum, and (4) If women acquires Hep-B in 3rd trimester.[12]

Risk of intrauterine infection with HBV have been correlated to polymorphism in the cytokine gene encoding the tumor necrosis factor-α and interferon-α. Perinatal transmission is responsible for a significant global burden of Hep B.

Mode of delivery has also a possible implication on HBV transmission and cesarean section has been assumed to have less transmission rate as compared to vaginal delivery. At this point, most obstetrical algorithms do not include change in the mode of delivery for HBsAg-positive women regardless of HBeAg status or level of viremia.

Diagnosis

In self-limited acute hepatitis, HBsAg usually becomes undetectable within 4–6 months. Persistence of HBsAg for more than six months implies chronic HBV infection. Anti-HBc subclass is the most important marker to differentiate acute and chronic Hep-B. During acute infection, anti-HBc is predominantly of the IgM class while it is IgG subtype in chronic states. It takes around 6 months before the disappearance of HBc-IgM in blood and appearance of HBc-IgG.[13]

Table 24.1: Phases of Hep-B virus infection[14]

Phase	HBsAg	HBeAg	Anti-HBe	ALT pattern	HBV-DNA	Treatment
Immune tolerant	Positive	Positive	Negative	Normal	>20,000 IU/mL	Less responsive
Immune clearance	Positive	Positive	Negative	Elevated	>20,000 IU/mL	Better response
Inactive disease	Positive	Negative	Positive	Normal	<200 IU/mL	Follow-up required
HBeAg –ve CHB	Positive	Negative	Positive	Normal Elevated	Undetectable; >2 x 10³	Follow-up; treatment
Resolved HBV infection	Negative	Negative	Positive	Normal	Undetectable	Follow-up

HBeAg is found in serum early during acute HBV infection. The finding of HBeAg in the serum of an HBV carrier indicates a high level of viral replication and greater infectivity. Persistence of HBeAg reactivity three or more months after the onset of illness indicates a high likelihood of transition to chronic HBV infection. Patients with HBeAg-positive chronic hepatitis B have been shown to be having persistently high serum HBV DNA levels.

The measurement of serum HBV DNA by quantitative polymerase chain reaction (PCR) technique is important in selecting patients for antiviral therapy and in monitoring their response during therapy. Response to conventional interferon therapy is less likely seen with very high levels of HBV-DNA. In a patient on antiviral therapy, reappearance of DNA in blood suggests drug resistance. In post-liver transplant patients on lamivudine therapy high rate of recurrence is especially seen in those with very high pre-treatment HBV-DNA levels. Even after recovery from acute hepatitis B, small amounts of HBV-DNA can be detected in serum and peripheral mononuclear cells.

These different phases of chronic HBV infection have different serological patterns hence the diagnosis and management of chronic HBV infection cannot be done on the basis of a single serological test but done collectively (Table 24.1).

Treatment

Initial Management[4]

❏ Proper history and physical examination.
❏ Assess severity of liver disease: Liver function tests, prothrombin time, and α-fetoprotein.
❏ Assess HBV replication: HBeAg; Anti-HBe, HBV DNA-PCR
❏ Rule out concomitant disease: HCV, HDV.
❏ Screen for hepatitis A and vaccinate if anti-HAV negative.
❏ Screen all family members and vaccinate those households who are HBsAg negative.
❏ Baseline ultrasound.

Important Definitions in Management (Table 24.2)

Table 24.2: Important definitions in management

Terminology	Definition
Biochemical response	Normalization of ALT levels
Serological response for HBeAg	Defined as HBeAg loss and seroconversion to anti-HBe
Serological response for HBsAg	Defined as loss of HBsAg and development of anti-HBs antibodies
Virological response (VR)	Undetectable levels of HBV DNA (as determined by PCR assay) after 3–6 months of treatment for NA-treated patients or HBV DNA<2000 IU/mL after 6 months at the end of treatment for IFN-treated patients
Sustained virological response (SVR)	VR persisting at least 12 months after cessation of treatment
Virologic breakthrough	HBV DNA level increase of more than 1 log 10 IU/mL during therapy

(Adapted from ESPGHAN guidelines 2013[15]

Treatment Endpoints

The goal of anti-HBV therapy in children is to reduce the risk of progressive liver disease, cirrhosis, and HCC and hence to improve long-term survival and quality of life. The ideal end point of treatment is sustained HBsAg clearance but it occurs in a minority of treated subjects.[15] HBsAg clearance in patients stops disease progression and reduces the risk of HCC. When HBsAg seroclearance is not achieved, sustained suppression of viral replication (undetectable HBV DNA levels), associated with anti-HBe seroconversion in originally HBeAg-positive patients, is an acceptable end point.[15] In the absence of off-therapy viral suppression, undetectable HBV DNA under long-term antiviral therapy is the next desirable end point.

Factors Influencing the Choice of Agents

Various factors influence the choice of drug for treatment of chronic hepatitis B. These include serum ALT level, serum HBV DNA level and liver histology at baseline. The cost of treatment, likelihood of adverse effects, age and other co-morbid conditions also contribute in deciding the treatment. Interferon and nucleoside analogs are the two major class of drugs used for treatment of chronic hepatitis B. Each has advantages and disadvantages, and no one therapy is suitable for all patients.

Guidelines for the Management of Hepatitis B

American Association for the Study of Liver Diseases (AASLD), Asian-Pacific Association for the Study of the Liver and recently ESPGHAN[15] has published clinical practice guidelines for the management of chronic hepatitis B. In general, all these published guidelines recommend treatment for patients who have both biochemical evidence of liver injury and serum HBV DNA levels in excess of 20,000 IU/mL. Nucleoside analog therapy is the only recommended therapy in patients with decompensated cirrhosis (Flow chart 24.1).

Antiviral Agents

Interferons: Interferon has direct immune modulatory properties. It enhances HLA class I antigen expression on the surface of infected hepatocytes and augments CD8+ cytotoxic T cell (CTL) activity. Interferon has the advantage that it has a relatively short course of treatment (6 months to 1 year) and has not been associated with drug resistance. The major disadvantages of interferon relate to its poorer acceptance because of side effects such as flu-

Flow chart 24.1: Treatment of chronic Hep-B*

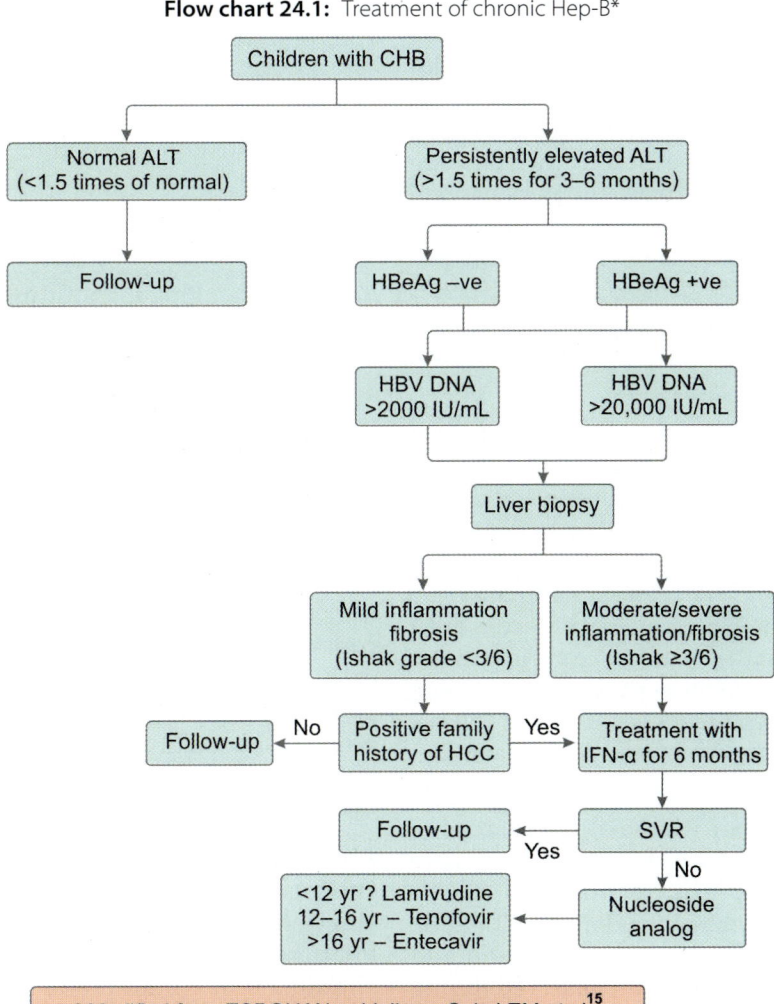

* Modified from ESPGHAN guidelines. Sokal EM et al[15]

like illness, behavioral disorders; ocular complications like retinitis, optic neuritis/neuropathy and thyroid disturbance (hypothyroidism) and leukopenia. However, children tolerate interferon better than adults. IFN is recommended from 12 months of age onwards.

The recommended dose for interferon is 0.1 MU/kg or 5 to 10 MU/m^2 subcutaneously three times a week for 6 months. The duration of treatment can be extended up to 12 months. Pegylated interferon alpha has been found to be more potent than conventional or standard interferon and requires once weekly dosing. Doses of 1.0 μg per kg of body weight of peginterferon alfa-2b and 180 μg/1.73m^2 of peginterferon alfa-2a given once weekly have been studied in clinical trials.[15] Presently trials for PEF-IFN (Phase-III trials) are undergoing in children (age 2–18 years) and as of now, it is not FDA approved for treatment of children with CHB.

Nucleoside and nucleotide analogs: These acts as competitive inhibitors of the viral reverse transcriptase and DNA polymerase by replacing natural nucleosides during the synthesis of HBV DNA. These are the only available drugs for the management of chronic Hep-B patients with decompensated cirrhosis, in whom the use of interferon can lead to worsening liver failure and severe infections.

The major disadvantage of using these drugs is that due to its mechanism of action of partially suppressing viral replication, the treatment duration becomes prolonged to more than a year and prolonged monotherapy is associated with increased risk of development of drug resistance. With these agents, HBsAg clearance rarely occurs after one year of treatment. In 25% of cases, post-withdrawal serum ALT flares have been seen.

Lamivudine: This drug is potent inhibitor of viral replication. The major advantage is that it is convenient to administer and it is free of severe adverse effects. Its drawback is its prolonged duration of therapy and relatively poor seroconversion rate when used for one year which improves when used for two years. Resistance to this drug increases with the duration of therapy. Resistance is even more commonly encountered (90% at four years) in patients coinfected with HIV because of the early use of lamivudine in HAART regimens. It is recommended for ≥3 years of age. The dose is 3 mg/kg/day as a single daily dose (Maximum dose—100 mg).

Adefovir dipivoxil: Adefovir dipivoxil is the acyclic phosphonate nucleotide analog of adenosine monophosphate. HBeAg seroconversion was slightly lower than those achieved with lamivudine for 52 weeks. A rise in the frequency of HBeAg seroconversion and nondetectability of HBV DNA has been observed during the second year of adefovir treatment. As with lamivudine,

the resistance to this drug also increases with the duration of therapy. Presently, it is recommended for use in children above 12 years of age. The dose is 10 mg/day once daily dose.

Adefovir has been shown to be effective in patients with lamivudine-resistant HBV. Adefovir-resistant mutants, on the other hand, remain susceptible to lamivudine, and adefovir resistance has been shown to occur more frequently when lamivudine is discontinued in lamivudine-resistant patients than when lamivudine is continued. Adefovir has the disadvantage of potential nephrotoxicity.

Tenofovir disoproxil fumarate: Tenofovir is an acyclic nucleotide inhibitor of HBV polymerase and HIV reverse transcriptase. Tenofovir has been recently approved for use in children more than 12 years of age. Phase III trials for children 2 to 12 years are undergoing with a dose of 8 mg/kg (Maximum dose 300 mg/day). Its antiviral activity against HBV has been reported to be significantly greater than that of adefovir in lamivudine-resistant and treatment-naïve patients. Resistance to tenofovir has not occurred after two years of treatment in either HBeAg-positive or HBeAg-negative patients.

Newer Drugs

Entecavir: Recommended for ≥16 years of age. Phase III trials for children 2 to 16 years are undergoing. The advantage is that it has a low resistance rates and can be given orally.[15] Dose in adults is 0.5–1 mg/day.

Telbivudine: Phase 1 studies in children have been completed. Not yet approved for children.

In patients on therapy with nucleoside analogs, serum HBV-DNA levels are checked three monthly. Those who do not have at least 1-log 10 reduction in DNA levels in three months may be considered as primary treatment failures and candidates for alternative therapy. Similarly virological breakthrough may be detected by monitoring regular HBV-DNA levels on therapy.

The common reasons for virological breakthrough are poor adherence to therapy or resistance. One must consider alternative nucleosides therapy in patients with drug resistance, keeping in mind the cross-resistance pattern of the drugs. Experience in adults suggests that sequential monotherapy may result in multidrug resistant HBV. Therefore, adding a second drug is preferred rather than switching to another agent.

Combination therapies: The benefit of different combinations of doses and schedules for interferon and lamivudine has been controversial. Comparisons between interferon versus lamivudine plus interferon have been conducted in children and adults but there has been no significant differences in the outcome measured.

Further larger studies are undergoing to test the various combination therapies with new antivirals for treatment of chronic hepatitis B (CHB) infection in children.

Prevention

Passive Immunization

Immune globulin is an important tool for the prevention of HBV infection. When an individual is exposed to a person with acute hepatitis, immune globulin treatment should be given as soon as feasible; it should be given within 2 weeks of exposure. It should not be given if the delay is greater than 14 days.[4]

Postexposure prophylaxis with HBIG has been recommended for administration following: (1) Perinatal exposure of an infant born to an HBsAg-positive woman (discussed later); (2) Sexual exposure to an HBsAg-positive person; (3) Accidental percutaneous or mucosal exposure to HBsAg-positive products, or (4) Household contact.[4]

Active Immunization

Vaccination is the most effective measure to prevent hepatitis B transmission in highly endemic areas. For term newborns, various regimens have been described but recent recommendations are for 0, 1 and 6 months schedule because this regimen has a higher efficacy as compared to others. Efficacy with this regimen is more than 95%. For preterms <2 kg birth dose is not counted and they have to be given 3 more doses as per the schedule. Postvaccination testing for a protective concentration of anti-HBs is recommended only for high-risk populations and immune-compromised individuals and is not recommended routinely. Dose of vaccine is 10 µg for children <18 years of age and 20 µg for adults. The recombinant and plasma vaccines are well tolerated. The vaccine in adults should be given in deltoid and not in gluteal region for better immunogenicity. In children middle 1/3rd of anerolateral thigh is preferred. The most common adverse effect noted is transient pain and low grade fever. Other effects, such as fatigue, headache, nausea, skin rash can occur very rarely.

Preventing Perinatal Transmission

Because of the high-risk of the development of chronic HBV infection following perinatal exposure, careful attention to immune-prophylaxis in the immediate newborn period remains essential. In most cases, transmission of HBV from an infected woman to her offspring occurs at the time of delivery. Therefore, immediate treatment of the infant born to an HBsAg-positive mother, using HBIG and HBV vaccine, can abort acquisition and significantly reduce the rate of chronic HBV infection. Treatment is predictably effective in modifying the infection and preventing the carrier state if instituted within 48 hours of delivery.

If the maternal HBsAg status is not known, it is not necessary to delay treatment until results of the serologic screening document maternal HBsAg positivity and prophylaxis should be started immediately. A single dose of Hep specific Ig (0.5 mL) and 0.5 mL of recombinant vaccine should be given in separate thighs. This dose of vaccine should be counted as the 1st dose of the schedule and further 2 doses are given as scheduled.

Breastfeeding has been shown not to contribute significantly to HBV transmission from infected mothers to infants who have received proper immunoprophylaxis. In the absence of cracked or bleeding nipples, breastfeeding of properly immunized infants is not contraindicated.

HEPATITIS C

Chronic hepatitis C is defined as evidence of chronic infection for >6 months with ongoing liver injury.

Viral Characteristics

HCV is a small virus, 30–60 nm in diameter that contains a single-stranded RNA genome that is translated into a single polypeptide, which is cleaved by viral and host enzymes. Hepatitis C virus replicates in infected cells, mainly hepatocytes. The viral genome encodes only 9 proteins, including RNA polymerase.[4]

The HCV genome contains a highly conserved five noncoding region followed by core and envelope structural regions and five nonstructural regions. Structural elements consist of core protein, envelope protein E1, and envelope protein E2, which is a major target of the host immune response. The E2 region contains two hypervariable regions, which may allow HCV to evade the host immune response.

Genotypes

Six main genotypes (Type 1–6) of HCV along with about 100 subtypes have been described. Each genotype differs in its amino acid sequence by 30–34%. Genotype 6 is primarily in Asia. Genotypes 1–3 have a worldwide distribution, genotypes 4 and 5 are found mainly in Africa.[16] In the United States, genotype 1 accounts for around 74% (57% 1a, 17% 1b) of HCV infections; genotype 2 for about 15%, genotype 3 for about 7%, genotype 4 for about 1%, and genotype 6 for 3%. In India the most common genotype is 3. Genotyping of HCV is particularly important in treating a patient, as genotypes 1 and 4 are relatively resistant to treatment.[4]

Epidemiology

HCV infection is estimated to affect 0.1% to 2% of children in the United States. Studies in India in children regarding the prevalence are lacking. In India, seroprevalence has been reported to be 0.87%. HCV is the etiological agent in about 20% of patients with chronic hepatitis in northern India in adults. Transmission of infection is by contaminated blood or body fluids. At one time HCV infection accounted for the majority of transfusion-associated hepatitis, but presently the risk of acquiring HCV infection by transfusion of blood or blood products is reduced. Presently, the primary mechanism of HCV infection in children is mother-to-infant transmission (vertical transmission).[17]

Perinatal Transmission

At present, materno-fetal transmission of HCV is the most common route of *childhood* infection. Of infants born to anti-HCV-positive women, 5–6% (range, 0–25%) acquires HCV. High maternal HCV viral load (>600,000 IU/mL) increases the chance of mother-to-infant HCV transmission. It is not known exactly when mother-to-infant HCV transmission takes place.[18]

Fetal scalp vein monitoring, prolonged rupture of membranes and fetal anoxia around the time of delivery may enhance the risk of infection. Most studies have shown no differences in infection rates between infants delivered vaginally and cesarean-delivered infants. Elective cesarean section is not required for HCV-monoinfected women because it confers no reduction in the rate of mother-to-infant HCV transmission. With vaginal delivery, large vaginal tears should be avoided.[19]

Concomitant HIV infection increases the risk of HCV transmission 2- to 3-fold. Of infants born to women coinfected with HCV and HIV, the rate of perinatal infection is in the range of 5–36%. Recent studies have shown this effect to be somewhat less prominent, perhaps because greatly effective antiretroviral therapy decreases HCV load during pregnancy.

The role of breastfeeding in the transmission of HCV has been evaluated in several studies.[20,21] Breastfeeding is not considered to be contraindicated in women who are infected with HCV. The HCV-infected women who wish to breastfeed their infants should be counselled accordingly. As in the case of Hep-B, it is better to avoid breastfeeding if the nipples are bleeding or if mastitis is present.

Pathogenesis

In persons in whom chronic HCV develops, the relatively weak response of cytotoxic lymphocytes is insufficient to clear viremia. However, this response is sufficient to cause damage through the elaboration of cytokines in the liver. Studies in humans and chimpanzees support the idea that a vigorous CD4 and CD8 T-cell response against multiple regions of HCV is necessary for elimination of HCV infection.[4]

Besides host factors that determine the innate ability to ward off HCV infection, the ability of the HCV to suppress IFN signaling and to downgrade the host's immune response are crucial to viral propagation.

Approximately, 10^{10} viral genomes are produced each day in a chronically infected person. The RNA polymerase of HCV is greatly error prone. Because of this high error rate of the HCV RNA polymerase, many variant viruses known as "quasispecies" are produced and confer a survival advantage to HCV.[17]

Natural History of HCV Infection in Infants and Children

HCV infection acquired in infancy can have several different patterns of outcome: (1) Spontaneous resolution of infection is an important outcome. It is still not clear whether children are more likely than adults to clear HCV infection. Little data is presently available about the long-term course of these children. (2) Some infants develop chronic Hep-C (CHC) but achieve spontaneous resolution during the first few years of childhood, generally by 7 years. This pattern of early spontaneous resolution may occur irrespective of the mode of transmission of infection. (3) Long-term course is mild for those who do not have spontaneous resolution of CHC in infancy. Most of these children are clinically well and have little inflammation in liver biopsy and near normal serum aminotransferases.[17]

Approximately 6% to 12% of older children experience spontaneous resolution with some reports showing higher proportions[22] with majority being clinically well. In a large European study (N = 224) most children had mild chronic hepatitis on liver biopsy and cirrhosis was only seen in 1 of 224. Only 14% of children in this study were symptomatic.[23]

Chronic Hep-C is a slowly progressive disease in children and cirrhosis has been reported in only 1–2% of children with CHC.

Spontaneous clearance is rare and more likely to be seen in genotype 3. Severity of the disease is increased in patients with high body mass index (BMI), chronic transfusions and co-infection with HIV or HBV.

Diagnosis

Serologic Assay

Enzyme immunoassay (EIA): The usefulness of first-generation enzyme immunoassay (EIA), which detected antibody directed against an HCV-related antigen is limited because of lack of sensitivity of this test. This was especially problematic early in the course of HCV infection where viral RNA could be detected by PCR in serum or liver tissue of patients well in advance of detectable antibody.[17] Equally problematic was the high rate of false positivity of this test which was seen in patients with autoimmune hepatitis (attributed to hypergammaglobulinemia in these patients).

The inherent limitations of these first-generation assay led to the development of second- and third-generation immune assays that incorporated additional structural and nonstructural antigens of the HCV, including antigens from the viral core. The specificity and sensitivity of the third-generation EIAs in patients with chronic liver disease due to HCV infection are around 98% and 97%, respectively.[24] In the past, qualitative tests were used for diagnosis but quantitative tests are now recommended for diagnosis in patients with positive anti-HCV antibody tests due to greater sensitivity of these tests.

Nucleic Acid-Based Detection Technology
Amplification of HCV nucleic acid sequences with PCR is a technique for the detection of viremia during acute and chronic HCV infection. Most EIA positive patients with liver disease (>90%) are HCV RNA positive by PCR, suggesting that testing for HCV RNA by PCR may be more appropriate to confirm infection.

Nucleic acid detection is superior to antibody testing in establishing the diagnosis of HCV infection in patients who lack HCV antibody. HCV RNA tests can be detected in serum as early as 1 to 2 weeks after exposure to the virus and weeks before the antibody tests become positive.[25] A positive HCV RNA is predictive of the presence of liver disease inpatients who are anti-HCV positive but have a normal ALT level.[17]

Therefore, PCR detection of HCV RNA is useful in diagnosis of acute infection even before the development of antibodies. In immune-compromised patients it helps in diagnosing infection as antibody assays are unreliable in these patients. These tests help in distinguishing resolved from persistent in fection and are also useful in measuring response to treatment.

If both antibody test and HCV RNA test are positive then the child has either acute or chronic HCV. If the antibody test is positive and the HCV RNA test is negative, this indicates resolution of HCV infection. If the antibody test is negative but the HCV RNA test is positive then it could be either early acute Hep-C infection or chronic HCV infection in an immune-compromised person or a false-positive HCV RNA test. If two HCV RNA tests are negative at an interval of 6 months then the individual does not have chronic HCV infection.

HCV Genotyping

HCV genotyping is indicated in patients considered for treatment as the duration of therapy is determined by HCV genotype (as discussed subsequently). Genotyping can be performed by direct sequence analysis, by reverse hybridization, or by use of restriction fragment length polymorphism (RFLP).

Treatment

The natural history of Hep-C in children is not clear. The progression to fibrosis/cirrhosis and severe disease is rare in children, therefore, the options of follow-up without treatment until adulthood may be considered valid. On the other hand since the treatment is well tolerated by children and it is known in adults that the response to treatment is better with less severe disease, it may be justified to treat and allow definite resolution in a subgroup of patients. However, all children with evidence of fibrosis on liver biopsy or persistently elevated serum aminotransferase must be considered for therapy.

Goals of therapy include eradicating virus infection and preventing end stage liver disease and its complication including HCC (Table 24.3).[17]

PEG-IFN a and ribavirin are the first line treatment option for CHC in adults and children 3 to 17 years of age as per the AASLD recommendations.[26]

Table 24.3: Definitions used in the management of CHC[17]	
Terminology	Definition
Rapid virological response (RVR)	Undetectable serum HCV RNA (<50 IU/mL) after 4 weeks of treatment
Complete early virological response (CEVR)	Undetectable HCV RNA (<50 IU/mL) after 12 weeks of treatment
Early virological response (EVR)	At least a 2 log decrease in serum HCV RNA from baseline after 12 weeks of treatment
End of treatment response (ETR)	Undetectable serum HCV RNA (<50 IU/mL) at the conclusion of treatment
Sustained virologic response (SVR)	Undetectable serum HCV RNA (<50 IU/mL) 24 weeks after the end of treatment
Nonresponse	Detectable serum HCV RNA at 24 weeks of treatment without any significant decrease in serum HCV RNA level
Relapse	Detection of serum HCV RNA after an end of treatment response had been achieved

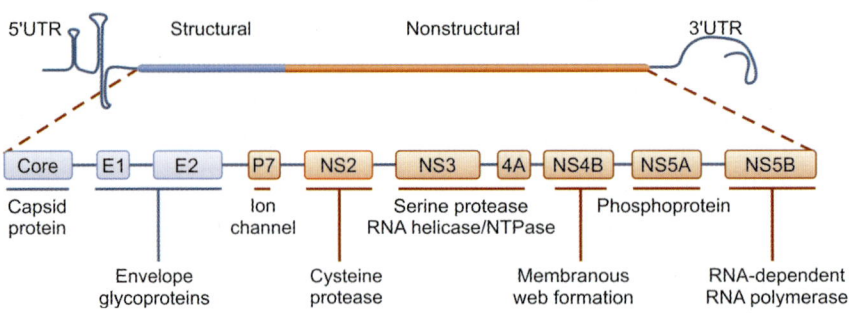

Fig. 24.3: HCV genome

This combination treatment has demonstrated superiority in achieving sustained virological response (SVR) and reducing relapse rates, over IFN-α alone as shown in multiple smaller open-labeled and large blinded, multicenter pediatric studies.[27,28]

IFN dosing is thrice a week while PEG-IFN is given as once weekly dose. Presence of genotype 2 and 3 and a lower viral load with genotype 1 (<6,00,000 IU/mL) are predictors of high virological response to therapy. Dose of PEG-IFN-α-2a is 180 µg/1,73 m^2/week subcutaneously and PEG-IFN-α-2b is 60 µg/m^2/week given subcutaneously.

Ribavirin is an oral nucleoside analog with broad activity against viral pathogens and has immunomodulatory effects. The mechanism of action of ribavirin is not clear and it has been shown to have some direct activity against HCV replication. Its use leads to rapid and lethal mutation of virions or depletion of intracellular GTP, which is necessary for viral RNA synthesis. Dose of ribavirin is 15 mg/kg/day orally in two divided doses. Addition of ribavirin to IFN improves SVR and ETR. The main side effect with this drug is hemolytic anemia which manifests generally during the first month of treatment. Dose reduction is recommended in such instances. Alternatives include use of GM-CSF, synthetic erythropoietin or use of blood products.

The recommended length of therapy is 48 weeks of treatment for genotypes 1 or 4 and 24-week duration of treatment for genotypes 2 or 3 in children.[17] If HCV-RNA does not become undetectable by 24 weeks, there is also no evidence that prolonged treatment improves clinical outcome (i.e. cirrhosis, HCC, SVR).[29] The patients who achieve RVR within 4 weeks or EVR in 12 weeks tend to have higher SVR. The efficacy of PEG-IFN and ribavirin therapy in children has been shown to be 80–100% in genotype 3 and less than 50–60% in genotype 1. The response to treatment is generally better in those who acquire infection via parenteral transmission rather than vertical transmission.

The newer therapy includes: (1) Direct acting agents (DAA); (2) Host cofactor inhibitors such as—cyclophilin inhibitors, miR122 antagonists, HMG CoA reductase (statins). The DAA includes (a) NS3/4A serine protease inhibitors (e.g. Telaprevir/Boceprevir); (b) NS5B RNA polymerase inhibitors (e.g. Sofosbuvir); (c) NS5A, and (d) NS4B inhibitors (Fig. 24.3).

In adults triple therapy using oral telaprevir/boceprevir (NS3/4A serine protease inhibitors), recently approved by FDA for use in adults with CHC, along with PEG-IFN and ribavirin in genotype 1 has increased the SVR to 70–80% and reduced the duration of therapy in a great proportion of patients. Side effects with telaprevir and boceprevir include anemia, thrombocytopenia, rash, pruritus and less frequently neutropenia.

Recently, a new oral drug sofosbuvir (NS5B RNA-dependent RNA polymerase inhibitor) has been approved in adults. It can be given as a combination therapy with IFN and ribavirin. The recommended treatment regimen depends on the viral genotype and patient characteristics. For genotypes 1 or 4, the recommended treatment regimen is 12 weeks of triple therapy with sofosbuvir, peginterferon-alfa, and ribavirin. A 12-week course of dual therapy with sofosbuvir and ribavirin is recommended for patients with HCV genotype 2 infection, and 24 weeks of the dual therapy is recommended for patients with genotype 3 infection. It is not recommended as a monotherapy. No serious side effects have been noted with this drug.

The future therapy may use a combination of oral therapeutic agents with excellent response. So one may debate whether the treatment in children with CHC and no fibrosis should be delayed till the availability of newer oral options.

Prevention

Unlike Hep-B there is no vaccine available for Hep-C as of now. There is a strong need of vaccine in view of huge global burden with significant morbidity, mortality and expensive treatment. Hepatitis C vaccine development has been difficult for the reasons that the various genotypes of HCV along with its high mutation rates make it difficult to develop something that would be effective against all types. Finally, to date, scientists have not been able to develop a good model or medium for testing vaccines. In spite of the barriers, the search for an effective vaccine continues. The vaccines options are both for prophylaxis and therapeutic. No therapeutic vaccine has reached a phase III clinical trials despite all efforts over the last three decades.

Other measures that can be taken to prevent HCV infection:

❑ Patient education and creating awareness in patients, family members and general population regarding the precautions.

❑ Strict and proper screening of all blood products in every blood bank before issue.

REFERENCES

1. Hepatitis B: World Health Organization Fact Sheet 204. 2000 : World Health Organization.
2. McMahon BJ, Alward WL, Hall DB, Heyward WL, Bender TR, Francis DP, et al. Acute hepatitis B virus infection: relation of age to the clinical expression of disease and subsequent development of the carrier state. J Infect Dis. 1985;151:599-603.
3. Tassopoulos NC, Papaevangelou GJ, Sjogren MH, Roumeliotou-Karayannis A, Gerin JL, Purcell RH. Natural history of acute hepatitis B surface antigenpositive hepatitis in Greek adults. Gastroenterology. 1987;92:1844-50.
4. Hochman JA, Balistreri F. Acute and chronic viral hepatitis. In: Suchy FJ, Sokol RJ, Balistreri FW (Eds). Liver diseases in children. 3rd Ed. New York: Cambridge University Press, 2007. pp. 382-424.
5. Ganem D, Prince AM. Mechanisms of disease: Hepatitis B virus infection – natural history and clinical consequences. N Engl J Med. 2004;350:1118-29.
6. Yuen MF, SablonE,Wong DKH, et al. Role of hepatitis B virus genotypes in chronic hepatitis B exacerbation. Clin Infect Dis. 2003;37:593-7.
7. Yen-Hsuan N, Chang MH, Wang KJ, et al. Clinical relevance of hepatitis B virus genotype in children with chronic infection and hepatocellular carcinoma. Gastroenterology. 2004;127:1733-8.
8. Janssen HL, van Zonneveld M, SenturkH, et al. Pegylated interferon alpha-2b alone or in combination with lamivudine for HbeAg-positive chronic hepatitis B: a randomised trial. Lancet 2005;365:123-9.
9. Hsu HY, Chang MH, Liaw SH, et al. Changes of hepatitis B surface antigen variants in carrier children before and after universal vaccination in Taiwan. Hepatology. 1999;30:1312-7.
10. Bonino F, Brunetto MR, Rizzetto M, et al. Hepatitis B virus unable to secret E antigen. Gastroenterology. 1991;100:1138-41.
11. Ganem D, Prince AM. Mechanism of disease: hepatitis B virus infection – natural history and clinical consequences. N Eng IJ Med 2004;350:1118-29.
12. Tong MJ, Thursby M, Rakela J, et al. Studies on the maternal infant transmission of the viruses which cause acute hepatitis. Gastroenterology. 1981;80:999-1003.
13. Hoofnagle JH, Di Bisceglie AM. Serologic diagnosis of acute and chronic viral hepatitis. Semin Liver Dis. 1991;11:73-83.
14. Sherman M, Shafran S, et al. Management of chronic hepatitis B: Consensus guidelines. Can J Gastroenterol. 2007; 21(C).
15. Sokal EM, et al. Management of chronic hepatitis B in childhood: ESPGHAN clinical practice guidelines. J Hepatol. 2013.
16. Report of World Health Organization. Global surveillance and control of hepatitis C. J Viral Hepatol. 1999;6:35-47.
17. Mack CI, et al. NASPGHAN Practice Guidelines: Diagnosis and Management of Hepatitis C Infection in Infants, Children, and Adolescents. JPGN. 2012;54:6.
18. Bortolotti F, Resti M, Giacchino R, et al. Changing epidemiologic pattern of chronic hepatitis C virus infection in Italian children. J Pediatr. 1998;133:378-9.
19. Centers for Disease Control and Prevention. Recommendations for prevention and control of hepatitis C virus (HCV) infection and HCV-related chronic disease. MMWR. 1998;47(no. RR-19):1-39.
20. National Institutes of Health. National Institutes of Health consensus development conference statement: management of hepatitis C 2002. Hepatology. 2002;36:(5 suppl 1):S3-20.
21. American Academy of Pediatrics. Hepatitis C. In: Pickering LK, (Ed). Red book: 2003 report of the Committee on Infectious Diseases. 26th ed. Elk Grove Village, IL: American Academy of Pediatrics, 2003:336-40.
22. Iorio R, Giannattasio A, Sepe A, et al. Chronic hepatitis C in childhood: an 18-year experience. Clin Infect Dis. 2005;41:1431-7.
23. Jara P, Resti M, Hierro L, et al. Chronic hepatitis C virus infection in childhood: clinical patterns and evolution in 224 white children. Clin Infect Dis. 2003;36:275-80.
24. deLeuw P, Sarrazin C, Zeuzem S. How to use virological tools for the optimal management of chronic hepatitis C. Liver Int. 2011;31(suppl)1:3-12.
25. Mukherjee S, Lin J, Bronze MS. Hepatitis C virus (HCV) assays are used to evaluate for HCV infection. Medscape. 2011;1996209.
26. Ghany MG, Strader DB, Thomas DL, et al. Diagnosis, management, and treatment of hepatitis C: an update. Hepatology. 2009; 49:1335-74.
27. Gonzalez-Peralta RP, Kelly DA, Haber B, et al. International Pediatric Hepatitis C Therapy Group Interferon alfa-2b in combination with ribavirin for the treatment of chronic hepatitis C in children: efficacy, safety, and pharmacokinetics. Hepatology. 2005;42:1010-8.
28. Schwarz KB, Gonzalez-Peralta RP, Murray KF, et al. The combination of ribavirin and peginterferon is superior to peginterferon and placebo for children and adolescents with chronic hepatitis C. Gastroenterology. 2011;140:450-8.
29. Di Bisceglie AM, Shiffman ML, Everson GT, et al. HALT-C Trial Investigators. Prolonged therapy of advanced chronic hepatitis C with low-dose peginterferon. N Engl J Med. 2008;359:2429-41.

Chapter

25

Autoimmune Hepatitis

M Geetha

INTRODUCTION

Autoimmune hepatitis (AIH) is a progressive inflammatory immunological disease more commonly seen in females. It was first described by Jan Waldenstrom, in a female patient with chronic hepatitis. Later, it came to be known as "lupoid hepatitis" when it was seen that some of these cases of chronic hepatitis also had features of SLE and and LE test was positive.[1,2] However, this term was discarded following the discovery of complement-fixing autoantibodies to cytoplasmic antigens indicating an autoimmune pathology. In 1965 Mackay et al. designated the term "autoimmune hepatitis" and this was endorsed by the scientific community. The disease is characterized by chronic hepatitis, circulating autoantibodies and raised IgG with no know etiologyz.[3] In children the disease is known to have a more aggressive course than in adults. Hence, it is imperative that an early and definite diagnosis is made and treatment initiated, in order to minimise the liver damage and improve the long-term outcome. Autoimmune liver diseasein children includes autoimmune hepatitis (AIH), autoimmune sclerosing cholangitis (ASC) and *de novo* AIH after liver transplantation.[4]

EPIDEMIOLOGY

Female preponderance is seen both in adults and children. About 75% of children with AIH are females. The actual prevalence of AIH even among adults is not well documented. This is primarily because the diagnosis of AIH was uncertain in many cases until the IAIHG scoring system was introduced in 1993. Subsequent to the introduction of the IAIHG scoring, the number of cases being reported started rising. An Alaskan study on adult population reported a prevalence of 35.9 case per 100,000 population.[5] This was twice as high as that of a Norwegian population based study published earlier. In United Kingdom, a study done in a tertiary referral center, showed an annual incidence of 3.0 per 100,000 population.[6] In

Asia, reports from Japan showed an incidence between 0.08 and 0.15 cases per 100,000 people per year.[7]

The corresponding statistics in children is as yet unknown. At King's College Hospital, a tertiary pediatric hepatology referral center, there has been a seven-fold increase in incidence of both types of AIH over the last decade accounting for approximately 10% of the referrals. Even though there must have been a referral bias in the patients attending a tertiary center, the consensus is that there seems to be an increasing incidence in AIH.

GENETICS

Most of the genetic information on AIH comes from studies on HLA genes which are believed to play a dominant role in the predisposition to autoimmune hepatitis. The strongest associations are found in the HLA-DRB1 locus of the major histocompatability complex (MHC) which presents the antigen to the immune system and stimulates a response.

From studies done in Europe, it has been shown that AIH type I in adults is associated with HLA DRB1*03 and HLA DRB1*04 genes.[8,9-11] However, studies in children have shown an association with the DRB1*03 gene only. In fact, presence of the DRB1*04 gene is found to be protective in children.[12] AIH patients who are DRB1*03 gene positive tend to have a higher incidence of mortality and are more likely to require liver transplantation.[13,14] Type II AIH is more commonly associated with HLA DRB1*07[15] and rarely with HLA DRB1*03.[15] A study stated that DRB1*1301 which predisposes to AIH type I in South America is also associated with prolonged hepatitis A viral infection.[16,17] In Northern Europe, HLA DRB1*0301 is associated with autoimmune sclerosing cholangitis. Some studies have shown a genetically determined isolated partial deficiency of C4 to be associated with pediatric AIH both type I and II.[18]

A number of polymorphisms are found to be associated with AIH in various studies. These include polymorphisms of cytotoxic T lymphocytic antigen 4 (CTLA-4)[19,20] (which is seen in North American and North European patients but not in South American[21] or Japanese[22] patients), tumour necrosis factor α TNFA*2.[23] Fas: tumor necrosis factor receptor superfamily (TNFRSF) at position _670 (TNFRSF6);[24,25] interleukin (IL)-2, -4, and -6;[26] and vitamin D receptor (VDR).[27,28] A point mutation in tyrosine phosphatase CD45 has also been associated with AIH.[29,30]

In addition to the known association between AIH and APECED (autoimmune polyendocrinopathy-cadidiasis-ectodermal dystrophy), a polymorphic variant and heterozygous mutation to an autoimmune regulator gene (AIRE) resulting in release of autoreactive lymphocytes into the circulation has been reported to predispose to childhood AIH.[31-33]

PATHOGENESIS

The exact etiology is as yet unknown. Genetic susceptibility-both within and outside the MHC complex, deficient cellular regulators and molecular mimicry are some of the pathogenic mechanisms described. Very little is known about the actual pathogenic process and it is difficult to sift out which is the primary event and which a secondary effect.

Environmental triggers, especially viruses have long been suspected to be the triggers of AIH but there is no conclusive evidence to prove this theory. Different theories have been put forward to explain the flooding of liver with inflammatory cells based on studies in mouse models. CD4 cells have been implicated in this regard. An autoantigen is postulated to start off the process by being presented to Th0 or CD4 helper cells through HLA class II molecules. When the Th0 cells get activated, it differentiates into differentiating phenotypes, based on the prevailing cytokines and triggers an immune response. Th0 cells get differentiated into Th1 or Th2 in the presence of IL-12 and into Th17 in the presence of IL-β and IL-6. Th1 cells produce IL-2 and IF-γ, which in turn activate CD8 cells which produce IFN-γ and TNF-α. These, on recognition of an antigen/MHC class I complex, cause cytotoxicity.[34] IFN-γ promotes macrophage activation and contributes to natural killer (NK) cell killing.[35] Th17 cells produce proinflammatory cytokines IL-17, IL-22 and TNF-α and also induce IL-6 secretion thereby enhancing Th17 activation. In the presence of IL-4, Th0 cells differentiate into Th2 and these then produce IL-4, IL-10 and IL-13 which result in antibody production by B-lymphocytes. Th1 and Th2 cells oppose each other. Sets of cells with CD4+, CD25+ called T reg are regulatory cells that are responsible for regulating the response generated. When this is disrupted, the autoimmune process continues unchecked. Th17, which is produced in presence of TGF-β

and IL-6 also plays a role in inflammation. Some defects in T reg cells have been identified in AIH type I at diagnosis and also during relapse. These CD4+, CD25+ T reg cells modulate CD8+ production and they are reduced in number in AIH type I allowing the autoimmune process to continue unchecked.[36] This deficiency may be genetically mediated and some studies have demonstrated that it can be corrected by adoptive transfer of cells.[37]

In normal liver, natural killer T cells (NKT) causes apoptosis of altered hepatocytes and thereby regulates cytokine production.[38] They have both immune stimulating and inhibiting capabilities depending on the intrinsic signalling factors and also play a role in the differentiation of T reg cells.[39] A deficiency of NKT cells in seen in AIH.

Molecular Mimicry

This principle of molecular mimicry may account for the mechanism of liver injury by various environmental triggers, viruses, drugs, etc. It is one of the most studied theories in animal models and is postulated to be responsible for the development of de novo AIH after liver transplant and also recurrent AIH after transplant.[40] It can also cause multiple autoimmune conditions in the same patient.[40] Due to the nonspecificity of the T-cell antigen receptors, multiple antigens which share the same epitopes can stimulate the production of T cells which in turn cause damage to the liver cells.[41,42] Antigen stimulated plasma cells results in the production of autoantibodies which may cross react with liver antigens.[43,44]

In a study, about 35% of patients with AIH were found to have IgG4 staining in the plasma cells in the liver tissue.[45] These patients however, did not have raised serum IgG4 although total IgG was high. IgG4 has only a low affinity to complement and hence is not thought to play a role in the pathogenesis.[46]

TYPES

Autoimmune hepatitis has been classified into two subtypes based on the antibody profile. These are as follows:

Type I: This affects mostly older children and adults. It is the most common type worldwide and accounts for about 2/3rds of the cases of autoimmune hepatitis diagnosed. It usually presents around puberty. It is characterized by the presence of smooth muscle antibody (SMA) and/or antinuclear antibody (ANA). Data from King's College, London show that patients with this type of AIH tend to have more advanced disease at diagnosis compared to type II. Table 25.1 presents differences between type I and type II AIH.

Table 25.1: Classification of autoimmune hepatitis

Variable	Type I autoimmune hepatitis	Type II autoimmune hepatitis
Characteristic autoantibodies	• Antinuclear antibody • Smooth muscle antibody • Antiactin antibody • Autoantibodies against soluble liver antigen and liver pancreas antigen • Atypical perinuclear antineutrophil cytoplasmic antibody	Antibody against liver-kidney microsome 1 Antibody against liver cytosol 1
Geographic variation	Worldwide	Worldwide; rare in North America
Age at presentation	Any age	Predominantly childhood and young adults
Sex of patients	Females in about 75% of cases	Females in approximately 95% cases
Association with other autoimmune diseases	Common	Common
Clinical severity	Broad range	Generally severe
Histopathological features at presentation	Broad range	Generally advanced
Treatment failure	Infrequent	Frequent
Relapse after drug withdrawal	Variable	Common
Need for long-term maintenance	Variable	Approximately 100%

Source: Edward L Krawitt. Autoimmune Hepatitis. N Eng J Med. 354;1:54-66.

Type II: This is mainly a paediatric condition and affects younger children, even infants. It is characterized by presence of liver kidney microsomal antibody (anti-LKM-1) and/or Liver cytosol antibody (anti-LC-1). Type II AIH tends to have an acute presentation unlike type I. Raised IgG is seen in most cases although in 40% cases it is normal. IgA deficiency is seen in 45% of Type II AIH.[12,47] It is more common in Northern Europe and South America and rare in North America.

Though the presence of SMA and LKM are usually mutually exclusive, sometimes both can occur together. In this situation, the behavior pattern of the disease is like type II AIH.

A type III AIH was described but later abandoned. It was used to refer to patients who had features of AIH along with positive antibodies to soluble liver antigen (anti-SLA) and absence of ANA and anti-LKM antibodies.[48]

In both types of AIH, approximately 20% of patients have other autoimmune disorders like autoimmune thyroiditis, vitiligo, type I diabetes mellitus, Graves' disease, inflammatory bowel disease, nephrotic syndrome, etc. Type II AIH can also be part of the autoimmune polyendocrinopathy—candidiasis—ectodermal dysplasia (APECED) syndrome,[49] a condition which has no HLA association or female preponderance.

A small proportion of patients with autoimmune hepatitis may be negative for all presently known antibodies and are termed "seronegative" AIH.[50-52] In such cases, diagnosis is based on the typical biopsy findings, raised IgG, presence of other autoimmune conditions and exclusion of other known etiologies of liver disease. Testing for other rare antibodies like anti-LKM-3 or anti-actin may sometimes be useful in such cases. Their response to treatment is similar to the seropositive cases.

CLINICAL PATTERNS OF PRESENTATION

AIH can have a spectrum of manifestations ranging from asymptomatic transaminitis to decompensated liver disease. However, the three major clinical patterns of presentation described are:[12]

- *Acute hepatitis*: Forty percent of patients present in this manner and the clinical features and course of the disease is indistinguishable from acute viral hepatitis. The usual symptoms are jaundice, anorexia, vomiting, dark urine and progressive deterioration clinically and in laboratory profile. A small percentage can also present as fulminant hepatic failure wherein liver transplantation may be the only treatment option. This is more common in type II AIH.
- *Chronic hepatitis:* In 25–40% of patients, the presentation is insidious, with symptoms of fatigue, arthralgia, relapsing jaundice, headache, anorexia, amenorrhoea and weight loss which can last months or years. Hence, they can present later in the disease with severe liver dysfunction. This is commonly seen in type I AIH.
- *Cirrhosis with portal hypertension*: Some patients present for the first time with variceal bleeding, encephalopathy or end-stage liver disease.

NATURAL HISTORY

Most observations on the natural history are from studies done in the 1970s when the diagnosis of AIH could not be made with certainty. These studies have reported a 5 and 10 years survival rate to be 50% and 10%, respectively. With treatment this has been shown to improve to 80% and 93%, respectively.[53,54] Nearly 50% of children have cirrhosis at the time of diagnosis and nearly 70% need long-term treatment.[12] About 15% nevertheless progress to end-stage liver disease and require liver transplantation.

AUTOANTIBODIES

Autoantibodies form an important aspect of the diagnostic armamentarium for AIH. Although not pathognomonic, they aid in diagnosis and in differentiating type I and type II AIH. The presence of autoantibodies and more specifically their titre is critical in making a diagnosis of AIH. However, autoantibody titers do not correlate closely with severity of liver damage and can vary even during the course of the disease.[55]

The 2004 Consensus Statement from the Committee for Autoimmune Serology of the International Autoimmune Hepatitis Group (IAIHG) provides guidelines on how to test for these diseases.[56] They recommend that routine screening of antibodies should be done on freshly prepared rodent samples of liver, stomach and kidney tissues. This helps in simultaneous detection, of ANA, SMA, LKM-1, AMA and anti-LC-1. The first dilution recommended before titration is 1:40 in adults and 1:20 in children for ANA and ASMA and 1:10 for LKM-1.[56] This difference is to avoid a large number of false-positivity. Healthy adults and children are known to have some amount of autoantibodies in their blood and this is more in adults than in children. Hence, the cutoff levels in children are much lower than in adults and even lower for anti-LKM. Many laboratories perform this test with a minimum dilution of 1/40 to begin with, and children with a titre of 1/20 are likely to be missed. Since, a lot hinges on the antibody titers, it is important that the laboratories doing the tests follow the IAIHG guidelines in determining the cutoff. If the cutoff titers are raised to 1:80 or 1:160, it results in a lot of "false-negatives" eliminating the need for repeat testing and thereby saving on costs for the laboratory but at the expense of more testing or delayed diagnosis for the patient. This can affect the ultimate outcome in the child.[57]

The conventional autoantibodies associated with AIH are antinuclear antibody (ANA), smooth muscle antibody (SMA) and liver–kidney microsomal antibody type I (LKM-1). However, even these standard antibodies are not exclusive to this disease. They may be present in a number of other conditions like chronic viral hepatitis,[58,59] drug-induced hepatitis,[60,61] Wilson's disease,[62] and nonalcoholic steatohepatitis.[63,64] Other nonstandard antibodies described in AIH are anti-liver cytosol antibody type I (LC-1), pANCA, anti-ASGPR, and SEPSECS autoantibody (SLA/LP). Most of these antibodies are nonspecific. Only SEPSECS (SLA/LP) autoantibodies are disease-specific but are found in less than 30% of cases.

Genetic predisposition may have a role in the expression of autoantibodies and can partly explain its sporadic occurrence.

Antinuclear Antibody (ANA)

This was the first autoantibody to be associated with AIH leading to its early labelling as "lupoid hepatitis". However, it is one of the most nonspecific antibodies and can be seen in a number of other conditions. In a freshly prepared rodent substrate, ANA positivity shows up as nuclear staining of the kidneys, stomach, and the liver. In the liver, the staining pattern maybe homogenous (more common) or speckled (coarsely or finely). The speckled pattern is more commonly seen in younger children and is associated with a higher level of transaminases when compared with the homogenous pattern.[65] In AIH for a more clearer definition of the nuclear pattern, human epithelial cells (Hep2) with larger nuclei can be used. However, it is preferable not to use human epithelial cells for screening purposes because serum positivity to these nuclei can be seen in the healthy population—both children and adults. It can also be assessed by enzyme immunoassay. It is seen alone or along with SMA in 67% patients with AIH type I.[55]

Smooth Muscle Antibody (SMA)

SMA was first detected by Johnson et al in 1965[66] and later confirmed by Whittingham et al.[67] It may be present alone or in conjunction with ANA in type I AIH. They are directed against the components of the cytoskeleton like actin, tubulin, vimentin, desmin and skeletin. Of these, the antibody to the F–actin microfilament is specific for AIH but the test is not standardized. This is detected by indirect immunofluoroscence on murine stomach and kidneys.

Liver Kidney Microsomal Type I Antibody

LKM antibody was first described by the Deborah Doniach group.[68,69] This is the main serological marker for AIH -2. For unknown reasons, this antibody is rare in North America. It has been described more commonly from Northern Europe and especially in children. The target antigen is located not in the microsome but in the endoplasmic reticulum. Based on the immunofluorescence pattern, the condition in which it is seen and the type of antigen, these antibodies are subclassified as LKM-1, LKM-2, and LKM-3.[70] The LKM-1 antibody seems to be directed against the Cytochrome P-450 protein CYP2D6, and this was described first by Alvarez et al.[71-73] LKM-2 antibodies which were seen in hepatitis caused by the diuretic tienilic acid[74] and LKM-3 was found in patients with chronic hepatitis D.[75] A fourth LKM antibody has been described in patients with the autoimmune polyendocrinopathy-candidiasis—ectodermal dysplasia (APECED).[76] Some authors have stated that anti-LKM-1 has been frequently misinterpreted as AMA especially by the immunofluorescence method.[77,78] Since both AMA and PBC are rare in children, a closer look is warranted if a pediatric patient tests positive for AMA.[79]

Anti-LC-1

These are specific to AIH-2 and are much more common in patients <20 years of age. They were originally described by Martini et al. in AIH—occurring either alone or in association with anti-LKM1.[80] The molecular target of this antibody is formiminotransferase cyclodeaminase enzyme (FTCD).[81,82] These antibodies are the only ones to target a liver–specific antigen. Concentrations of this antibody seem to fluctuate with serum aminotransferase levels thereby suggesting a role in the pathogenesis of liver injury. Presence of this antibody indicates an aggressive course.[80]

Anti-SLA/LP

The antibodies-antisoluble liver antigen (SLA) and anti-liver pancreas antigen (LP) were described independently by two German groups. Subsequently they were found to target the same antigen and was hence called anti-SLA/LP antibodies.[48,83,84] It is seen in about 50% of patients with AIH-1, AIH-2 and ASC, and defines a severe clinical course. This was initially characterized as type III AIH, but this classification was later abandoned. The target protein is UGA suppressor transfer (t)RNA)-associated protein also called t-RNP associated protein. SLA/LP antibodies are detected by radioimmunoassay and ELISA and not by indirect immunofluorescence.[85] AIH patients who are positive for this have a tendency to relapse after withdrawal of steroids.[86] This has recently been renamed as SEPSECS (Sep (O phosphoserine) tRNA synthase).[87]

Peripheral Antineutrophil Cytoplasmic Antibody (pANCA)

There are three types of pANCA—cytoplasmic ANCA (cANCA), perinuclear ANCA (pANCA), and atypical perinuclear (pANNA). The one found in AIH is pANNA and it is seen in type I AIH and ASC and not in type II AIH.[88] It does not have any diagnostic or prognostic significance. The reactant for this antibody in AIH and other gastrointestinal diseases is not the usual myeloperoxidase but has been speculated to be lactoferrin or elastase,[89] or high mobility group protein (HMG).[90] It is detected in Immunofluoroscence by using neutrophils as substrate.

Antibodies to the Asialoglycoprotein Receptor (Anti-ASGP-R)

These antibodies were first identified in the 1980s by radioimmunoassays and ELISA. These antibodies are directed against the transmembrane glycoprotein on the hepatocyte surface. Their presence correlates with disease activity and its disappearance indicates treatment response. Persistence of the antibody after steroid withdrawal may herald a relapse.[91,92] They are not specific for AIH.

Antibodies to Saccharomyces Cerevisiae (ASCA)

Antibodies to *Saccharomyces cerevisiae* have been described in association with Crohn's disease. Recently, they have been found to be positive in about 20% of patients with PSC and also about 20% of patients with PBC and AIH. Its significance, however, has not been established.

Antimitochondrial Antibody (AMA)

AMA is the hallmark for the diagnosis of primary biliary cirrhosis (PBC) which is rare in children. If a pediatric patient tests positive for AMA, a second–look is warranted as, anti-LKM can sometimes be mistaken for AMA.

Autoantibodies may, in the future, be useful as biological probes to identify the specific antigen which triggers the autoimmune response. This may prove invaluable in the better understanding of the disease and in the development of targeted therapies.

LIVER BIOPSY

In all cases of suspected AIH, a liver biopsy is recommended and should be done unless there is a significant contraindication.[93] This is an important test both for establishing the diagnosis, to rule out other pathologies in the liver, for guiding the treatment and also for the long-term follow-up of the patient. Liver biopsy allows disease staging and assessment of inflammation and fibrosis which in turn helps in prognostication. In "seronegative hepatitis", the liver biopsy picture helps make a diagnosis. Also, it may be useful in identifying overlap conditions like PSC, PBC. In situations where liver biopsy is contraindicated, if all other tests strongly point to a diagnosis of AIH, treatment should not be withheld for want of a tissue diagnosis.

There is no histological finding pathognomonic of autoimmune hepatitis. The characteristic feature is a mononuclear cell infiltrate invading the limiting plate—called interface hepatitis or piecemeal necrosis. There can be spillover of the inflammatory cells into the hepatic lobule and hepatic regeneration with "rosette" formation.[94] An abundance of plasma cells is usually seen along with a large number of eosinophils but an absence of plasma cells does not preclude the diagnosis. The biliary tree is usually sparred except in overlap syndromes when ductopenia and destructive cholangitis is seen.[95] A varying amount of fibrosis is usually present in most cases which indicate a chronic stage. In advanced cases, regenerative nodules are also seen.

In patients with an acute liver failure like presentation, a liver biopsy will shows submassive necrosis with less fibrosis. When in remission, the biopsy shows inflammation confined to the portal areas alone with minimal inflammation elsewhere. The cirrhosis and fibrosis earlier noted may even be reversed.[96-98]

IMAGING

Ultrasonography of the abdomen can detect complications like ascites and portal hypertension. Autoimmune sclerosing cholangitis (ASC) can occur along with AIH and the only indication of this may be a raised alkaline phosphatise or γ-glutamyl transferase. Hence, more recently, pediatric gastroenterologists have advocated the need for cholangiography at the time of diagnosis of AIH in cases with raised γ-GT[4] to rule out PSC.

DIAGNOSTIC CRITERIA

AIH is a condition which has no pathognomonic clinical feature or diagnostic test. The varied presentation of AIH and the fact that it mimics viral hepatitis, make it difficult to diagnose. The International Autoimmune Hepatitis Group (IAIHG) in 1993, established a set of clinical, biochemical, immunological and histological criteria for standardizing the diagnoses of autoimmune hepatitis. In 1999,[51] it was revised but this was found to be so cumbersome that it could be applied only in epidemiological studies and not in a clinical setting. In 2008, a simplified scoring system was introduced by Hennes et al. to allow its usage in clinical practice. This included four criteria: autoantibody detection, IgG levels, liver histology, and exclusion of viral hepatitis. It also included negative scoring for infections like hepatitis B and C and Wilson's disease. A score of 7 points or more was classified as "definite AIH" (sensitivity 75.5% and specificity 100%) and 6 points as "probable AIH" (sensitivity 91% and specificity 94%). On scoring 7 points or more (definite AIH), the median overall sensitivity was 75.5% and the median overall specificity was 100%.

However, all these studies were all done on adult population. The simplified scoring system, when applied to children, was found to have some limitations. One of the limitations is that these criteria are not sufficient to diagnose a case of fulminant hepatic failure due to AIH.[99] Another limitation is that the cutoff for antibody titers is 1:40, which may miss out many children with AIH in whom titers of 1:20 itself is significant. Also neither scoring system distinguishes between AIH and ASC which can be done only with a cholangiogram. Hence, some authors have now recommended that cholangiogram be done at the beginning of the work-up to ascertain if PSC is present or not (Table 25.2).[93,100]

TREATMENT

Anti-inflammatory or immunosupressive therapy has been the mainstay for both types of AIH in adults and in children. The goals of treatment are to reduce hepatic inflammation and induce remission, improve symptoms and prolong survival.[101] Response to treatment has been excellent in children and the 10-year survival rates, among treated patients, is estimated to be >80% (Flow chart 25.1). In adults, there is a debate about starting treatment for transaminitis, given the side-effect profile. Children, however, tend to have a more aggressive disease and it is recommended to start treatment in all cases.[12,102,103] About 44-80% of pediatric cases have cirrhosis at the time of diagnosis but, even in this group, with appropriate treatment, the prognosis is good.[94,104]

Table 25.2: Simplified diagnostic criteria for AIH		
Category	Parameter	Score 1 or 2 for each category
Autoantibodies	ANA or SMA 1:40	1
	ANA or SMA ≥1:80	2
	LKM ≥ 1:40	2
	SLA positive	2
IgG*	>Upper limit of normal	1
	>1.1 Upper limit of normal	2
Histology	Compatible with AIH	1
	Typical of AIH	2
Absence of viral hepatitis	Yes	2

Probable AIH = 6 points; Definite AIH =≥7 points; Maximum possible points = 8 points
ANA, antinuclear antibody; SMA, smooth muscle antibody; LKM, liver kidney microsomal antibody; SLA, soluble liver antigen
* For patients without IgG levels use serum globulins: normal range – 0 points
Source: Hennes et al. Simplified criteria for the diagnosis of Autoimmune hepatitis. Hepatology. 2008;48:1540-8.

About 8-19.8% of AIH present as fulminant hepatitis wherein establishing a rapid diagnosis is not feasible. Even if diagnosed and started on steroids, only 1/3rd of patients respond and the rest end up in liver transplantation. The decision to start on steroids arbitrarily is controversial as the fear of worsening sepsis is a deterring factor.

STANDARD TREATMENT

Initial treatment with prednisolone alone or in combination with azathioprine is mandatory in all children with histological evidence of hepatitis with or without fibrosis or cirrhosis. Prednisolone is started at a dose of 2 mg/kg/day (max 60 mg/day). Once adequate response is seen, it can be gradually decreased by 5–10 mg every two weeks, with weekly monitoring and maintained at the minimum possible dose. If the transaminases do not reduce by atleast 80% during the first 6–8 weeks of treatment with steroids, azathioprine should be added, starting with 0.5 mg/kg/day and then increasing it up to 2 mg/kg/day. Alternatively, azathioprine can be initially started along with steroids, especially in type II AIH. Although transaminases may start decreasing with treatment, complete normalization takes approximately 6 months in AIH-1 and 9 months in AIH 2.[12] Once a patient goes into remission, the steroids are gradually tapered and stopped and maintenance

dose of azathioprine is continued. Patients with type II AIH do not tolerate withdrawal of steroids and have to be maintained on low-dose steroids and azathioprine. A trial of medication withdrawal can be attempted in Type I AIH sometime after sustained remission is achieved, and a liver biopsy shows histological remission.[100,105] Patients with type II AIH invariably relapse if treatment is discontinued and this should not be attempted. Liver biopsy is essential because the histological resolution may lag behind the biochemical resolution and the biochemical tests may not reflect the histological status accurately.[94,106,107] Most patients relapse within six months of stopping treatment.

In patients who are unable to maintain stable remission with azathioprine or who are intolerant to azathioprine, rescue treatment with mycophenolate mofetil, or calcineurin inhibitors like tacrolimus, or cyclosporine should be considered, failing which liver transplantation is the only option.

Corticosteroids

Prednisolone

Prednisolone (or prednisone) is started at a dose of 1–2 mg/kg/day and then tapered based on the biochemical response over 4–8 weeks. The goal of the initial therapy is to effect an 80% reduction in transaminases level. Once the minimum dose is achieved, the daily maintenance dose is stabilized at 2.5–5 mg/day.[93,108] It is generally preferred to give it as a small daily dose than as alternate day therapy as this has a better control on disease activity and is associated with less frequent relapses.[12] This, in turn, minimises the need for high-dose steroid pulses during relapses and ultimately, has a less detrimental effect on the linear growth of the child.[109] Also, alternate day therapy, though effective in achieving biochemical and laboratory control, does not achieve adequate histological control.[110] The side effects of steroids are well known and include cushingoid features, dorsal hump, striae, weight gain, acne, hirsutism, osteopenia, diabetes, cataract, and hypertension.

Budesonide

Budesonide has recently been proposed as a "topical" steroid in the treatment of AIH. The proposed benefit of budesonide is that it undergoes extensive first pass metabolism (80–90%) in the liver and, hence, can exert its maximum effect on the liver without the systemic side effects. However, it cannot be used in cirrhotics. A study in children comparing azathioprine with either prednisolone or budesonide showed that budesonide combination, was effective in inducing remission (though slightly inferior compared to the prednisolone combination) and had

Flow chart 25.1: Algorithm for treatment of AIH in children*

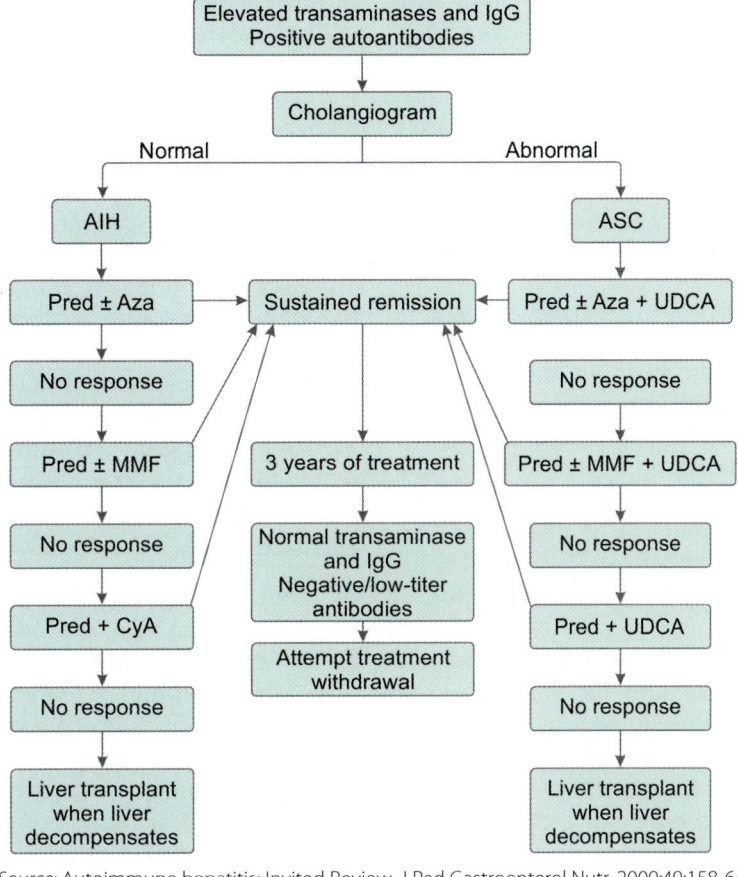

(*Source:* Autoimmune hepatitis; Invited Review. J Ped Gastroenterol Nutr. 2009;49:158-64.)

lesser sideeffects.[111] It may, in time, be considered an alternative to prednisolone.

Azathioprine

Azathioprine is added to corticosteroid therapy as a steroid sparing agent. The timing of addition of azathioprine varies in different centres. Some centers like Kings College Hospital of London, start it when the side effects of steroids appear or when the transaminases stop decreasing on steroids alone. Some others start it from the beginning. Yet, others start it only when the patient relapses after tapering the steroids. Whatever the regime, about 85% of patients ultimately go on to azathioprine.[4] The starting dose of Azathioprine is 0.5 mg/kg/day and can be increased, if well tolerated, to 2.0–2.5 mg/kg/day, until biochemical control is achieved.

Azathioprine is a prodrug of mercaptopurine. In the body, mercaptopurine and 6-MP undergo methylation catalyzed by thiopurine methyltransferase which converts this into the active form- 6-thioguanine. This blocks de novo purine nucleotide synthesis within the cell cycle, reducing

lymphocyte production. For patients, who are homozygous for a mutation of thiopurine methyltransferase and have low enzyme activity, this drug is contraindicated as it can produce complications, including death. Patients who are heterozygous are at intermediate risk. Hence, it is safer to perform the test for the enzyme before starting a patient on azathioprine[112] though this is not mandatory. If this testing is unavailable or unaffordable, the alternative is to monitor the blood counts and determine the enzyme activity if cytopenia occurs or if higher than usual doses are required. It has been observed that those intolerant to azathioprine are able to tolerate 6-MP without side effects indicating that the hepatotoxicity is not due to thiopurine methytransferase deficiency alone.[113] The side effects are pancreaitis, bone marrow suppression and flu-like syndrome.

Mycophenolate Mofetil

This drug acts by inhibition of inosine monophosphate dehydrogenase thereby inhibiting de novo purine synthesis and blocking both T-cell and B-cell proliferation. Among both adults and children, it is seen to be useful in those patients who are unresponsive or intolerant to azathioprine. The dose is 20 mg/kg twice daily along with prednisolone. The side effects are nausea, diarrhoea, headache, hair loss, vomiting, dizziness and neutropenia. A study on "difficult-to-treat" children[114] with AIH demonstrated a 70% response with an acceptable safety profile. However, patients with ASC do not seem to respond as well as AIH alone. More studies in a pediatric population are required before it can be recommended as a second line drug. A major limiting factor is its higher cost.

Cyclosporine

This drug acts by blocking the transcription of cytokines like IL-2, thereby interfering with helper T cell activation. The major limiting factor in the use of cyclosporine is its side effects like hypertension, nephrotoxicity, and risk of malignancy. There have been some studies on the use of cyclosporine in pediatric patients both for inducing remission in naive patients and also in patients with frequent relapses. One study showed induction of remission within six months of therapy[115] and another study demonstrated its safety when used for 3 years.[116] However, the American Association for Study of Liver Diseases recommends that further studies on larger groups of children for a longer duration is required to establish safety and efficacy of cyclosporine. Until this is available cyclosporine cannot be recommended as a standard drug.

Tacrolimus

This is a calcineurin inhibitor which acts by inhibiting the expression of IL-2 receptor and the expansion of T-CD-4 lymphocytes. It can be tried as a rescue drug in patients who do not respond to the first line therapy. Studies in children are scarce and children who are on this drug need careful monitoring for side effects like seizures and nephrotoxicity. There have been some studies implicating calcineurin inhibitors in the development of de novo AIH after transplantation.[117-119] Therefore, its role in the treatment of AIH is not clear.

TREATMENT DECISIONS: WHEN TO START TREATMENT

Among adult population, there has been some controversy regarding the initiation of treatment in asymptomatic patients with only mild transaminitis. Since the natural history of such patients is not known, it has been debated if they need to be started on medication at all, given the severe sideeffects of the drugs, patient's existing comorbidities and the possibility of spontaneous remissions. However, in children, in view of the long duration of disease and the risk of eventual cirrhosis in untreated cases, it seems reasonable to treat all patients with evidence of autoimmune hepatitis. Another argument in favor of treatment, is the study in adults, which showed that untreated patients underwent slower recovery and had lower survival rates (67 vs 98%) than treated patients.[120] The mild variety of AIH described in adults is not very commonly reported in children.[12,102,103,121] Hence, all children diagnosed with AIH at any stage of the disease need to be started on treatment without delay. The only exceptions are those presenting with fulminant hepatitis and those with cirrhosis and decompensation wherein medical treatment may not suffice and the child will require liver transplantation. Azathioprine is a better drug for maintenance compared to steroids and children who require long-term treatment should be started on this if not otherwise contraindicated.[12,102,103,121-123]

Monitoring

In the first 4–8 weeks of treatment, weekly LFTs are required to fine tune the medication. Thereafter, it can be done once in 4–6 weeks. Monitoring of antibody titres is not recommended in adults but in children, IgG levels and antibody levels seem to correlate with disease activity and are useful indices to monitor.[124] For patients on azathioprine measurement of serum levels of the metabolites 6-thioguanine and 6-mercaptopurine is not done routinely but can be done to identify compliance and drug toxicity.[125] It can also give an indication if therapeutic levels are obtained in blood though, what constitutes "therapeutic level" for AIH has not been determined.

When to Stop Treatment

Autoimmune hepatitis is known to go into sustained remission on starting treatment and this has prompted clinicians to attempt withdrawal of drugs in patients. In adults, this is done when the therapeutic goal has been reached, i.e. when the laboratory indices (transaminases, IgG and γ-globulin) are all normal for a minimum period of 12 months, and, a liver biopsy does not show much inflammation.[105,126-129] Liver biopsy is essential because the histological resolution may lag behind the biochemical resolution and the biochemical tests may not reflect the histological status accurately.[94,106,107] In children, the target goals are the same as in adult but include serum antibodies titres <1:20 for at least a year when on low dose steroids.[124] Some authors feel that it is not advisable to reduce steroids till remission is maintained for at least 3 years in children,[130] and also advise against withdrawal around the time of puberty as these are the times when relapses are common.[131] Drug withdrawal is done slowly over 6 weeks under close monitoring. Achievement of the end points, however, does not protect against a relapse. A high degree (60–80%) of relapse is seen, especially in children.[12,102-104,123,132] Only 20–30% of children tolerate withdrawal of medication in the long run. These patients need life-long annual check-ups to monitor for relapse. In the King's series, 20% of type I AIH achieved long-term remission but none in type II AIH achieved it.[12]

RELAPSE

A patient is deemed to have had a relapse when recurrence of symptoms or transaminitis occurs after medication have been stopped. In adolescents, noncompliance is an important cause.[133] It can also occur while on decreasing dose of steroids in 40% of cases. In a proven case of AIH, a repeat biopsy is not required to diagnose a relapse and treatment can be started immediately. The treatment consists of a similar protocol as for induction and most patients respond to this. Patients who frequently relapse are more prone to develop cirrhosis. Hence, it is always advisable to continue medication in these patients once remission is achieved, preferably with azathioprine.

TREATMENT FAILURE

Patients who do not respond within six months of initiating adequate therapy or who deteriorate while on treatment are deemed treatment failures. They require higher dose of prednisolone and azathioprine and if this is unsuccessful, rescue treatment with MMF, tacrolimus or cyclosporine may be tried. If no response is seen, these patients must be considered for liver transplantation.

PROGNOSIS

The prognosis of children who respond to immunosuppressive treatment is good. Prior to the introduction of immunosupression it was seen that nearly 40% of symptomatic patients used to succumb to the disease within six months of diagnosis. Those who survived, developed cirrhosis and portal hypertension and died of complications or of end stage disease after 10 years of diagnosis. Immunosupression has vastly improved the survival and decreased the morbidity for this condition and is definitely indicated once a diagnosis is established. The course of the disease is fluctuating with flares and spontaneous remissions. Even in patients who may have cirrhosis at presentation, the survival is better with treatment. However, inspite of good disease control, about 8.5% of patients develop end-stage liver disease and require liver transplantation.[12]

Those who present with acute liver failure have a worse prognosis. In this setting, in many instances, the diagnosis is difficult to arrive at. The autoimmune markers take some time to be done and liver biopsy may not be possible due to coagulopathy. If the child is not encephalopathic, and the diagnosis is somewhat certain, immunosuppressants may benefit the child. In the King's series only one out of six such children benefitted and survived without a transplant.[12] Most cases require liver transplantation.

All patients with AIH should receive vaccination for hepatitis B, and hepatitis A (if susceptible)[134] and this must be done preferably before the start of immunosupression to ensure better response.

TRANSPLANTATION

This is indicated in AIH in two settings—children who present with acute liver failure and those who present with end-stage liver disease. Even children with seemingly stable disease on immunosuppression, can later on deteriorate and require liver transplantation. Overall 8.5% of patients develop end-stage liver disease 8–14 years after diagnosis and require liver transplant.[12] The outcome for those transplanted for AIH was comparable with those transplanted for non AIH causes. Both the American and European registry showed similar survival rates. Though a greater degree of immunosupression was done in these patients fearing an increase in rejection, no such complication was noted, nor was there an increase in the incidence of infections. A combination of tacrolimus and prednisolone was the preferred combination in most centers.[135]

POST-TRANSPLANT RECURRENT AIH

AIH can recur in the transplanted liver at a mean rate of 30%[136,137] in both children and adults, at a mean time of approximately 4.6 years after transplant.[135,138-140]

The criteria[135,139,141] for recurrence include (i) Elevation of serum AST and ALT levels, (ii) persistence of autoantibodies, (iii) hypergammaglobulinemia or raised IgG levels, (iv) compatible histological findings, (v) exclusion of other etiologies and (vi) response to steroids.

The risks for recurrence include inadequate immuno-supression, and this increases after discontinuation of steroids. Other risk factors are type I AIH and HLA DRB1*03 or DRB1*04.[139,142] Treatment of recurrent AIH includes reintroduction of prednisolone and adjustment of the dose of calcineureine inhibitors. Alternatively, azathioprine and steroids also produce good results.

POST LIVER TRANSPLANTATION DE NOVO AIH

This was initially reported in children but was later observed both in adults and children.[143,144] It refers to the development of a steroid responsive hepatitis after liver transplantation done for non-autoimmune conditions and occurs in about 6–10% of transplanted patients.[145] The pathogenesis of this phenonmenon was suggested in studies on mice, who were on immunosuppressant agents following bone marrow transplantation. The immunosupressants seemed to interfere with the maturation of T lymphocytes resulting in the development of auto-aggressive T-cell clones.[117-119] It has been speculated that the development of this condition may be related to the HLA alleles of the donor which in turn are known to be associated with AIH.[144,146] It is characterized by high IgG and positive autoantibodies—ANA, SMA or LKM-1 antibody. Atypical LKM antibody positivity (staining only the renal tubules) has also been described. These patients may present with transaminitis and a picture similar to acute rejection. However, they do not respond to standard anti-rejection therapy and hence establishing a diagnosis by liver biopsy is essential to prevent graft loss. Liver biopsy findings are typical of autoimmune hepatitis with interface hepatitis and multilobular collapse. These patients respond very well to treatment with prednisolone and azathioprine, as for classical AIH, along with a reduction in calcineurin inhibitor dose. If response is poor, retransplantation should be considered.

AUTOIMMUNE SCLEROSING CHOLANGITIS (ASC)

In paediatrics, children with features of autoimmune hepatitis, (including elevated titers of autoantibodies—ANA and SMA, elevated IgG and interface hepatitis), along with sclerosing cholangitis, are referred to as ASC.[102] In short, it is clinically and histologically, AIH type I along with radiological changes of sclerosing cholangitis. It was earlier classified as one of the overlap syndromes. ASC is said to have similar prevalence as AIH Type I in childhood.[102] Also evolution from AIH to ASC has also been seen, suggesting that it is a spectrum of the same disease.[102] Presence of HLA DRB1*1301 confers susceptibility to ASC.

In a study, all children with features of AIH underwent cholangiogram at presentation and approximately 50% were found to have bile duct changes, though less advanced than the adult PSC.[102] 25% had abnormal cholangiogram but no histological features to suggest bile duct involvement and the diagnosis of ASC was made based on the cholangiographic findings. Liver function tests do not help differentiate AIH from ASC but the alkaline phosphatase/aspartate transaminase levels and, in children, gGT are raised.It should be suspected when patients with AIH present with cholestatic symptoms or respond poorly to steroids alone. Inflammatory bowel disease is seen in 16% and should be looked for.

Treatment for ASC is the same as for AIH. However, the bile duct disease does not respond as well as the parenchymal problem. UDCA is generally added in a dose of 15 mg/kg/day, based on its benefit in adult PSC (primary sclerosing cholangitis),[147] but its benefit in children is not clear. High dose UDCA was reported by the Mayo group to have a deleterious effect in adults is no longer advocated.[148] Monitoring is done as for AIH, but the prognosis is worse than children with AIH. A 7-year-survival of 100% was reported[102] though 15% required transplant. Recurrence after transplant has also been reported in about 70%.

OVERLAP SYNDROME

This term has been proposed to indicate patients with AIH (diagnosed as per the criteria) and another disorder such as, PBC,PSC or chronic viral hepatitis. Such patients have conventional antibodies (ANA, ASMA, anti-LKM, pANCA) in unusual combinations, e.g. AMA and SMA or LKM-1. In pediatric age group, AIH-PSC overlap is more common and this is designated as ASC.

MANAGEMENT

Management of overlap syndrome is based on the predominant manifestation of the disease. EASL guidelines has recommended the option of either starting a combination of UDCA and steroids or starting only UDCA and adding steroids if the biochemical response is not adequate in three months. A steroid-sparing agent should be considered in patients requiring long-term immunosupression.

CONCLUSION

Autoimmune hepatitis is probably underdiagnosed in children due to the insidious symptoms and lack of standardized laboratory tests. However, it should be looked for and excluded in all cases of transaminitis or liver dysfunction so as to enable early diagnosis and prompt institution of treatment, which can prevent and to a certain extent reverse damage to the liver. In advanced cases liver transplantation may be the only option available. In the future, better immunosupressants with targeted action may produce more sustained remission with lesser side effects, thereby, improving the morbidity and mortality associated with this disease.

REFERENCES

1. Cowling DC, Mackay IR, Taft LI. Lupoid hepatitis. Lancet. 1956;271(6957):1323-6.
2. Mackay IR, Taft LI, Cowling DC. Lupoid hepatitis and the hepatic lesions of systemic lupus erythematosus. Lancet. 1959;1(7063):65-9.

3. Vergani DM-vD. Autoimmune Hepatitis. 3rd ed. Textbook of Hepatology: From Basic science to clinical practice. Oxford, UK: Blackwell Publication. 2007;pp.1089-101.

4. Mieli-Vergani, GD Vergani. Autoimmune liver diseases in children—what is different from adulthood? Best Pract Res Clin Gastroenterol. 2011;25(6):783-95.

5. Hurlburt KJ, et al. Prevalence of autoimmune liver disease in Alaska Natives. Am J Gastroenterol. 2002;97(9):2402-7.

6. Whalley S, et al. Hepatology outpatient service provision in secondary care: a study of liver disease incidence and resource costs. Clin Med. 2007;7(2):119-24.

7. Toda G, et al. Present status of autoimmune hepatitis in Japan-correlating the characteristics with international criteria in an area with a high rate of HCV infection. Japanese National Study Group of Autoimmune Hepatitis. J Hepatol. 1997;26(6):1207-12.

8. Donaldson PT. Genetics in autoimmune hepatitis. Semin Liver Dis. 2002;22(4):353-64.

9. Strettell MD, et al. Allelic basis for HLA-encoded susceptibility to type 1 autoimmune hepatitis. Gastroenterology. 1997;112(6):2028-35.

10. Doherty DG, et al. Allelic sequence variation in the HLA class II genes and proteins in patients with autoimmune hepatitis. Hepatology. 1994;19(3):609-15.

11. Montano-Loza AJ, Carpenter HA, Czaja AJ. Clinical significance of HLA DRB103-DRB104 in type 1 autoimmune hepatitis. Liver Int. 2006;26(10):1201-8.

12. Gregorio GV, et al. Autoimmune hepatitis in childhood: a 20-year experience. Hepatology. 1997;25(3):541-7.

13. Czaja AJ, et al. Associations between alleles of the major histocompatibility complex and type 1 autoimmune hepatitis. Hepatology. 1997;25(2):317-23.

14. Czaja AJ, et al. Significance of HLA DR4 in type 1 autoimmune hepatitis. Gastroenterology. 1993;105(5):1502-7.

15. Ma Y, et al. Polyclonal T-cell responses to cytochrome P450IID6 are associated with disease activity in autoimmune hepatitis type 2. Gastroenterology. 2006;130(3):868-82.

16. Fainboim L, et al. Protracted, but not acute, hepatitis A virus infection is strongly associated with HLA-DRB*1301, a marker for pediatric autoimmune hepatitis. Hepatology. 2001;33(6):1512-7.

17. Pando M, et al. Pediatric and adult forms of type I autoimmune hepatitis in Argentina: evidence for differential genetic predisposition. Hepatology. 1999;30(6):1374-80.

18. Vergani D, et al. Genetically determined low C4: a predisposing factor to autoimmune chronic active hepatitis. Lancet. 1985;2(8450):294-8.

19. Agarwal K, et al. Cytotoxic T lymphocyte antigen-4 (CTLA-4) gene polymorphisms and susceptibility to type 1 autoimmune hepatitis. Hepatology. 2000;31(1):49-53.

20. Djilali-Saiah I, et al. CTLA-4/CD 28 region polymorphisms in children from families with autoimmune hepatitis. Hum Immunol. 2001;62(12):1356-62.

21. Bittencourt PL, et al. Cytotoxic T lymphocyte antigen-4 gene polymorphisms do not confer susceptibility to autoimmune hepatitis types 1 and 2 in Brazil. Am J Gastroenterol. 2003;98(7):1616-20.

22. Umemura T, et al. Association of cytotoxic T-lymphocyte antigen 4 gene polymorphisms with type 1 autoimmune hepatitis in Japanese. Hepatol Res. 2008;38(7):689-95.

23. Pociot F, et al. Association of tumor necrosis factor (TNF) and class II major histocompatibility complex alleles with the secretion of TNF-alpha and TNF-beta by human mononuclear cells: a possible link to insulin-dependent diabetes mellitus. Eur J Immunol. 1993;23(1):224-31.

24. Hiraide A, et al. Fas polymorphisms influence susceptibility to autoimmune hepatitis. Am J Gastroenterol. 2005;100(6):1322-9.

25. Agarwal K, Czaja AJ, Donaldson PT. A functional Fas promoter polymorphism is associated with a severe phenotype in type 1 autoimmune hepatitis characterized by early development of cirrhosis. Tissue Antigens. 2007;69(3):227-35.

26. Fan LY, et al. Genetic association of cytokines polymorphisms with autoimmune hepatitis and primary biliary cirrhosis in the Chinese. World J Gastroenterol. 2005;11(18):2768-72.

27. Vogel A, Strassburg CP, Manns MP, Genetic association of vitamin D receptor polymorphisms with primary biliary cirrhosis and autoimmune hepatitis. Hepatology. 2002;35(1):126-31.

28. Fan L, et al. Genetic association of vitamin D receptor polymorphisms with autoimmune hepatitis and primary biliary cirrhosis in the Chinese. J Gastroenterol Hepatol. 2005;20(2):249-55.

29. Vogel A, Strassburg CP, Manns MP. 77 C/G mutation in the tyrosine phosphatase CD45 gene and autoimmune hepatitis: evidence for a genetic link. Genes Immun. 2003;4(1):79-81.

30. Esteghamat F, et al. C77G mutation in protein tyrosine phosphatase CD45 gene and autoimmune hepatitis. Hepatol Res. 2005;32(3):154-7.

31. Vogel A, et al. Autoimmune regulator AIRE: evidence for genetic differences between autoimmune hepatitis and hepatitis as part of the autoimmune polyglandular syndrome type 1. Hepatology. 2001;33(5):1047-52.

32. Djilali-Saiah I, et al. Linkage disequilibrium between HLA class II region and autoimmune hepatitis in pediatric patients. J Hepatol. 2004;40(6):904-9.

33. Lankisch TO, et al. AIRE gene analysis in children with autoimmune hepatitis type I or II. J Pediatr Gastroenterol Nutr. 2009;48(4):498-500.

34. Ichiki Y, et al. T cell immunity in autoimmune hepatitis. Autoimmun Rev. 2005;4(5):315-21.

35. Schroder K, et al. Interferon-gamma: an overview of signals, mechanisms and functions. J Leukoc Biol. 2004;75(2):163-89.

36. Longhi MS, et al. Impairment of CD4(+)CD25(+) regulatory T-cells in autoimmune liver disease. J Hepatol. 2004;41(1):31-7.

37. Longhi MS, et al. Expansion and de novo generation of potentially therapeutic regulatory T cells in patients with autoimmune hepatitis. Hepatology. 2008;47(2):581-91.

38. Zhang C, Zhang J, Tian Z. The regulatory effect of natural killer cells: do "NK-reg cells" exist? Cell Mol Immunol. 2006;3(4):241-54.

39. Nowak M, Stein-Streilein J. Invariant NKT cells and tolerance. Int Rev Immunol. 2007;26(1-2):95-119.

40. Vergani D, et al. Pathogenesis of autoimmune hepatitis. Clin Liver Dis. 2002;6(3):727-37.

41. Doherty DG, et al. Structural basis of specificity and degeneracy of T cell recognition: pluriallelic restriction of T cell responses to a peptide antigen involves both specific and promiscuous interactions between the T cell receptor, peptide, and HLA-DR. J Immunol. 1998;161(7):3527-35.

42. Bogdanos DP, et al. Multiple viral/self immunological cross-reactivity in liver kidney microsomal antibody positive hepatitis

C virus infected patients is associated with the possession of HLA B51. Int J Immunopathol Pharmacol. 2004;17(1):83-92.

43. Kammer AR, et al. Molecular mimicry of human cytochrome P450 by hepatitis C virus at the level of cytotoxic T cell recognition. J Exp Med. 1999;190(2):169-76.

44. Albert LJ, Inman RD. Molecular mimicry and autoimmunity. N Engl J Med. 1999;341(27):2068-74.

45. Chung H, et al. Identification and characterization of IgG4-associated autoimmune hepatitis. Liver Int. 2010;30(2):222-31.

46. Shimosegawa T, Kanno A. Autoimmune pancreatitis in Japan: overview and perspective. J Gastroenterol. 2009;44(6):503-17.

47. Homberg JC, et al. Chronic active hepatitis associated with antiliver/kidney microsome antibody type 1: a second type of "autoimmune" hepatitis. Hepatology. 1987;7(6):1333-9.

48. Manns M, et al. Characterisation of a new subgroup of autoimmune chronic active hepatitis by autoantibodies against a soluble liver antigen. Lancet. 1987;1(8528):292-4.

49. Ahonen P, et al. Clinical variation of autoimmune polyendocrinopathy-candidiasis-ectodermal dystrophy (APECED) in a series of 68 patients. N Engl J Med. 1990;322(26):1829-36.

50. Johnson PJ, McFarlane IG. Meeting report: International Autoimmune Hepatitis Group. Hepatology. 1993;18(4):998-1005.

51. Alvarez F, et al. International Autoimmune Hepatitis Group Report: review of criteria for diagnosis of autoimmune hepatitis. J Hepatol. 1999;31(5):929-38.

52. Gassert DJ, et al. Corticosteroid-responsive cryptogenic chronic hepatitis: evidence for seronegative autoimmune hepatitis. Dig Dis Sci. 2007;52(9):2433-7.

53. Feld JJ, et al. Autoimmune hepatitis: effect of symptoms and cirrhosis on natural history and outcome. Hepatology. 2005;42(1):53-62.

54. Roberts SK, Therneau TM, Czaja AJ. Prognosis of histological cirrhosis in type 1 autoimmune hepatitis. Gastroenterology. 1996;110(3):848-57.

55. Czaja AJ. Behavior and significance of autoantibodies in type 1 autoimmune hepatitis. J Hepatol. 1999;30(3):394-401.

56. Vergani D, et al. Liver autoimmune serology: a consensus statement from the committee for autoimmune serology of the International Autoimmune Hepatitis Group. J Hepatol. 2004;41(4):677-83.

57. Giorgina MieliVergani, et al. Autoimmune Hepatitis. Journal of Pediatric Gastroenterology and Nutrition. 2009;49:158-64.

58. Czaja AJ, et al. Genetic predispositions for the immunological features of chronic active hepatitis. Hepatology. 1993;18(4):816-22.

59. Czaja AJ, et al. Immunologic features and HLA associations in chronic viral hepatitis. Gastroenterology. 1995;108(1):157-64.

60. Maddrey WC, Boitnott JK. Drug-induced chronic liver disease. Gastroenterology. 1977;72(6):1348-53.

61. Seeff LB. Drug-induced chronic liver disease, with emphasis on chronic active hepatitis. Semin Liver Dis. 1981;1(2):104-15.

62. Dhawan A, et al. Wilson's disease in children: 37-year experience and revised King's score for liver transplantation. Liver Transpl. 2005;11(4):441-8.

63. Hay JE, et al. The nature of unexplained chronic aminotransferase elevations of a mild to moderate degree in asymptomatic patients. Hepatology. 1989;9(2):193-7.

64. Czaja AJ, et al. Host- and disease-specific factors affecting steatosis in chronic hepatitis C. J Hepatol. 1998;29(2):198-206.

65. Czaja AJ, et al. Patterns of nuclear immunofluorescence and reactivities to recombinant nuclear antigens in autoimmune hepatitis. Gastroenterology. 1994;107(1):200-7.

66. Johnson GD, Holborow EJ, Glynn LE. Antibody to smooth muscle in patients with liver disease. Lancet. 1965;2(7418):878-9.

67. Whittingham S, et al. Smooth muscle autoantibody in "autoimmune" hepatitis. Gastroenterology. 1966;51(4):499-505.

68. Rizzetto M, Bianchi FB, Doniach D. Characterization of the microsomal antigen related to a subclass of active chronic hepatitis. Immunology. 1974;26(3):589-601.

69. Rizzetto M, Swana G, Doniach D. Microsomal antibodies in active chronic hepatitis and other disorders. Clin Exp Immunol. 1973;15(3):331-44.

70. Manns MP, Obermayer-Straub P. Cytochromes P450 and uridine triphosphate-glucuronosyltransferases: model autoantigens to study drug-induced, virus-induced, and autoimmune liver disease. Hepatology. 1997;26(4):1054-66.

71. Gueguen M, et al. Anti-liver kidney microsome antibody recognizes a cytochrome P450 from the IID subfamily. J Exp Med. 1988;168(2):801-6.

72. Manns MP, et al. Major antigen of liver kidney microsomal autoantibodies in idiopathic autoimmune hepatitis is cytochrome P450db1. J Clin Invest. 1989;83(3):1066-72.

73. Zanger UM, et al. Antibodies against human cytochrome P-450db1 in autoimmune hepatitis type II. Proc Natl Acad Sci U S A. 1988;85(21):8256-60.

74. Smith MG, et al. Hepatic disorders associated with liver-kidney microsomal antibodies. Br Med J. 1974;2(5910):80-4.

75. Crivelli O, et al. Microsomal autoantibodies in chronic infection with the HBsAg associated delta (delta) agent. Clin Exp Immunol. 1983;54(1):232-8.

76. Clemente MG, et al. Two cytochromes P450 are major hepatocellular autoantigens in autoimmune polyglandular syndrome type 1. Gastroenterology. 1998;114(2):324-8.

77. Bogdanos DP, Baum H, Vergani D. Antimitochondrial and other autoantibodies. Clin Liver Dis. 2003;7(4):759-77,vi.

78. Czaja AJ, Manns MP, Homburger HA. Frequency and significance of antibodies to liver/kidney microsome type 1 in adults with chronic active hepatitis. Gastroenterology. 1992;103(4):1290-5.

79. Gregorio GV, et al. A 12-year-old girl with antimitochondrial antibody-positive autoimmune hepatitis. J Hepatol. 1997;27(4):751-4.

80. Martini E, et al. Antibody to liver cytosol (anti-LC1) in patients with autoimmune chronic active hepatitis type 2. Hepatology. 1988;8(6):1662-6.

81. Lapierre P, et al. Formiminotransferase cyclodeaminase is an organ-specific autoantigen recognized by sera of patients with autoimmune hepatitis. Gastroenterology. 1999;116(3):643-9.

82. Muratori L, et al. Distinct epitopes on formiminotransferase cyclodeaminase induce autoimmune liver cytosol antibody type 1. Hepatology. 2001;34(3):494-501.

83. Stechemesser E, Klein R, Berg PA. Characterization and clinical relevance of liver-pancreas antibodies in autoimmune hepatitis. Hepatology. 1993;18(1):1-9.

84. Wies I, et al. Identification of target antigen for SLA/LP autoantibodies in autoimmune hepatitis. Lancet. 2000;355(9214):1510-5.

85. Strassburg CP, Manns MP. Autoantibodies and autoantigens in autoimmune hepatitis. Semin Liver Dis. 2002;22(4):339-52.

86. Czaja AJ, Donaldson PT, Lohse AW. Antibodies to soluble liver antigen/liver pancreas and HLA risk factors for type 1 autoimmune hepatitis. Am J Gastroenterol. 2002;97(2):413-9.

87. Palioura S, et al. The human SepSecS-tRNASec complex reveals the mechanism of selenocysteine formation. Science. 2009;325(5938):321-5.

88. Zauli D, et al. Anti-neutrophil cytoplasmic antibodies in type 1 and 2 autoimmune hepatitis. Hepatology. 1997;25(5):1105-7.

89. Lindgren S, et al. Anti-neutrophil cytoplasmic antibodies in patients with chronic liver diseases: prevalence, antigen specificity and predictive value for diagnosis of autoimmune liver disease. Swedish Internal Medicine Liver Club (SILK). J Gastroenterol Hepatol. 2000;15(4):437-42.

90. Sobajima J, et al. High mobility group (HMG) non-histone chromosomal proteins HMG1 and HMG2 are significant target antigens of perinuclear anti-neutrophil cytoplasmic antibodies in autoimmune hepatitis. Gut. 1999;44(6):867-73.

91. Czaja AJ, et al. Frequency and significance of antibodies to asialoglycoprotein receptor in type 1 autoimmune hepatitis. Dig Dis Sci. 1996;41(9):1733-40.

92. McFarlane IG, et al. Antibodies to liver-specific protein predict outcome of treatment withdrawal in autoimmune chronic active hepatitis. Lancet. 1984;2(8409):954-6.

93. Manns MP, et al. Diagnosis and management of autoimmune hepatitis. Hepatology. 2010;51(6):2193-213.

94. Ferreira AR, et al. Effect of treatment of hepatic histopathology in children and adolescents with autoimmune hepatitis. J Pediatr Gastroenterol Nutr. 2008;46(1):65-70.

95. Carpenter HA, Czaja AJ. The role of histologic evaluation in the diagnosis and management of autoimmune hepatitis and its variants. Clin Liver Dis. 2002;6(3):685-705.

96. Dufour JF, DeLellis R, Kaplan MM. Reversibility of hepatic fibrosis in autoimmune hepatitis. Ann Intern Med. 1997;127(11):981-5.

97. Cotler SJ, Jakate S, Jensen DM. Resolution of cirrhosis in autoimmune hepatitis with corticosteroid therapy. J Clin Gastroenterol. 2001;32(5):428-30.

98. Czaja AJ, Carpenter HA. Decreased fibrosis during corticosteroid therapy of autoimmune hepatitis. J Hepatol. 2004;40(4):646-52.

99. Mileti E, Rosenthal P, Peters MG. Validation and modification of simplified diagnostic criteria for autoimmune hepatitis in children. Clin Gastroenterol Hepatol. 2012;10(4):417-21 e1-2.

100. Czaja AJ, Freese DK, American Association for the Study of Liver, Diagnosis and treatment of autoimmune hepatitis. Hepatology. 2002;36(2):479-97.

101. Alvarez F. Autoimmune hepatitis and primary sclerosing cholangitis. Clin Liver Dis. 2006;10(1):89-107,vi.

102. Gregorio GV, et al. Autoimmune hepatitis/sclerosing cholangitis overlap syndrome in childhood: a 16-year prospective study. Hepatology. 2001;33(3):544-53.

103. Maggiore G, et al. Treatment of autoimmune chronic active hepatitis in childhood. J Pediatr. 1984;104(6):839-44.

104. Saadah OI, Smith AL, Hardikar W. Long-term outcome of autoimmune hepatitis in children. J Gastroenterol Hepatol. 2001;16(11):1297-302.

105. Czaja AJ, Carpenter HA. Histological features associated with relapse after corticosteroid withdrawal in type 1 autoimmune hepatitis. Liver Int. 2003;23(2):116-23.

106. Sogo T, et al. Intravenous methylprednisolone pulse therapy for children with autoimmune hepatitis. Hepatol Res. 2006;34(3):187-92.

107. Al-Chalabi T, Heneghan MA. Remission in autoimmune hepatitis: what is it, and can it ever be achieved? Am J Gastroenterol. 2007;102(5):1013-5.

108. Mieli-Vergani, Vergani GD. Autoimmune hepatitis in children. Clin Liver Dis. 2002;6(3):623-34.

109. Czaja AJ, et al. Treatment challenges and investigational opportunities in autoimmune hepatitis. Hepatology. 2005;41(1):207-15.

110. Summerskill WH, et al. Prednisone for chronic active liver disease: dose titration, standard dose, and combination with azathioprine compared. Gut. 1975;16(11):876-83.

111. Woynarowski M, et al. Budesonide versus prednisone with azathioprine for the treatment of autoimmune hepatitis in children and adolescents. J Pediatr. 2013;163(5):1347-53 e1.

112. Krawitt EL. Autoimmune hepatitis. N Engl J Med. 2006;354(1):54-66.

113. Pratt DS, Flavin DP, Kaplan MM. The successful treatment of autoimmune hepatitis with 6-mercaptopurine after failure with azathioprine. Gastroenterology. 1996;110(1):271-4.

114. Aw MM, et al. Mycophenolate mofetil as rescue treatment for autoimmune liver disease in children: a 5-year follow-up. J Hepatol. 2009;51(1):156-60.

115. Alvarez F, et al. Short-term cyclosporine induces a remission of autoimmune hepatitis in children. J Hepatol. 1999;30(2):222-7.

116. Cuarterolo M, et al. Follow-up of children with autoimmune hepatitis treated with cyclosporine. J Pediatr Gastroenterol Nutr. 2006;43(5):635-9.

117. Bucy RP, et al. Cyclosporin A-induced autoimmune disease in mice. J Immunol. 1993;151(2):1039-50.

118. Cooper MH, et al. The induction of pseudo-graft-versus-host disease following syngeneic bone marrow transplantation using FK 506. Transplant Proc. 1991;23(6):3234-5.

119. Hess AD, et al. Cyclosporine-induced autoimmunity: critical role of autoregulation in the prevention of major histocompatibility class II-dependent autoaggression. Transplant Proc. 1993;25(5):2811-3.

120. Czaja AJ. Features and consequences of untreated type 1 autoimmune hepatitis. Liver Int. 2009;29(6):816-23.

121. Maggiore G, et al. Autoimmune hepatitis associated with anti-actin antibodies in children and adolescents. J Pediatr Gastroenterol Nutr. 1993;17(4):376-81.

122. Roberts EA. Autoimmune hepatitis. Indian J Pediatr. 1995;62(5):525-31.

123. Yachha SK, et al. Autoimmune liver disease in children. J Gastroenterol Hepatol. 2001;16(6):674-7.

124. Gregorio GV, et al. Organ and non-organ specific autoantibody titres and IgG levels as markers of disease activity: a longitudinal

study in childhood autoimmune liver disease. Autoimmunity. 2002;35(8):515-9.

125. Rumbo C, et al. Azathioprine metabolite measurements in the treatment of autoimmune hepatitis in pediatric patients: a preliminary report. J Pediatr Gastroenterol Nutr. 2002;35(3):391-8.

126. Montano-Loza AJ, Carpenter HA, Czaja AJ. Improving the end point of corticosteroid therapy in type 1 autoimmune hepatitis to reduce the frequency of relapse. Am J Gastroenterol. 2007;102(5):1005-12.

127. Verma S, et al. Factors predicting relapse and poor outcome in type I autoimmune hepatitis: role of cirrhosis development, patterns of transaminases during remission and plasma cell activity in the liver biopsy. Am J Gastroenterol. 2004;99(8):1510-6.

128. Czaja AJ, et al. Corticosteroid-treated chronic active hepatitis in remission: uncertain prognosis of chronic persistent hepatitis. N Engl J Med. 1981;304(1):5-9.

129. Miyake Y, et al. Persistent normalization of serum alanine aminotransferase levels improves the prognosis of type 1 autoimmune hepatitis. J Hepatol. 2005;43(6):951-7.

130. Kanzler S, et al. Duration of immunosuppressive therapy in autoimmune hepatitis. J Hepatol. 2001;34(2):354-5.

131. Mieli-Vergani, Vergani GD. Autoimmune paediatric liver disease. World J Gastroenterol. 2008;14(21):3360-7.

132. Alvarez F. Treatment of Autoimmune Hepatitis: Current and Future Therapies. Curr Treat Options Gastroenterol. 2004;7(5):413-420.

133. Kerkar N, et al. Prospective analysis of nonadherence in autoimmune hepatitis: a common problem. J Pediatr Gastroenterol Nutr. 2006;43(5):629-34.

134. Worns MA, et al. Incidence of HAV and HBV infections and vaccination rates in patients with autoimmune liver diseases. Am J Gastroenterol. 2008;103(1):138-46.

135. Vogel A, et al. Long-term outcome of liver transplantation for autoimmune hepatitis. Clin Transplant. 2004;18(1):62-9.

136. Seaberg EC, et al. Liver transplantation in the United States from 1987-1998: updated results from the Pitt-UNOS Liver Transplant Registry. Clin Transpl. 1998;pp.17-37.

137. Wiesner RH, et al. Acute hepatic allograft rejection: incidence, risk factors, and impact on outcome. Hepatology. 1998;28(3):638-45.

138. Birnbaum AH, et al. Recurrence of autoimmune hepatitis in children after liver transplantation. J Pediatr Gastroenterol Nutr. 1997;25(1):20-5.

139. Manns MP, Bahr MJ. Recurrent autoimmune hepatitis after liver transplantation-when non-self becomes self. Hepatology. 2000;32(4 Pt 1):868-70.

140. Czaja AJ. Autoimmune hepatitis after liver transplantation and other lessons of self-intolerance. Liver Transpl. 2002;8(6):505-13.

141. Kotlyar DS, Campbell MS, Reddy KR. Recurrence of diseases following orthotopic liver transplantation. Am J Gastroenterol. 2006;101(6):1370-8.

142. Duclos-Vallee JC, et al. A 10 year follow up study of patients transplanted for autoimmune hepatitis: histological recurrence precedes clinical and biochemical recurrence. Gut. 2003;52(6):893-7.

143. Miyagawa-Hayashino A, et al. Outcome and risk factors of de novo autoimmune hepatitis in living-donor liver transplantation. Transplantation. 2004;78(1):128-35.

144. Heneghan MA, et al. Graft dysfunction mimicking autoimmune hepatitis following liver transplantation in adults. Hepatology. 2001;34(3):464-70.

145. Kerkar N, et al. De-novo autoimmune hepatitis after liver transplantation. Lancet. 1998;351(9100):409-13.

146. Salcedo M, et al. Response to steroids in de novo autoimmune hepatitis after liver transplantation. Hepatology. 2002;35(2):349-56.

147. Johnson PJ, McFarlane IG, Williams R. Azathioprine for long-term maintenance of remission in autoimmune hepatitis. N Engl J Med. 1995;333(15):958-63.

148. Lindor KD, et al. High-dose ursodeoxycholic acid for the treatment of primary sclerosing cholangitis. Hepatology. 2009;50(3):808-14.

Chapter

26

Wilson's Disease

Dinesh Banur

INTRODUCTION

Wilson's disease (WD) also known as hepatolenticular degeneration is an autosomal recessive condition effecting 1 in 30000 individuals worldwide.[1-3] It was first described in 1912 by "Kinnear Wilson" as a familial lethal neurological disease accompanied by chronic liver disease leading to cirrhosis.[4]

The basic problem in Wilson's disease is a genetic defect blocking the natural excretion of absorbed copper from the liver. It is the most common metabolic liver disease.[5]

PATHOGENESIS AND METABOLISM OF COPPER

Copper is a essential trace element and has an integral role in the formation of metallo proteins. Just like vitamins, copper in small amounts is required for many critical metabolic pathways.[6] An average diet typically provides 2–5 mg/day of copper (Recommended intake is 0.63mg/day).[7-9]

Copper is absorbed from the duodenum and proximal small intestine and transported to liver through portal circulation. Liver utilizes some copper for metabolic needs, synthesizing copper-containing protein ceruloplasmin, and rest of the excess copper is excreted in bile. Ceruloplasmin is the major carrier for copper in the blood, accounting for 90% of the circulating copper in normal individuals. Liver is intimately connected in regulating plasma concentration of copper (Fig. 26.1).

PATHOGENESIS

The gene, *ATP7B* responsible for Wilson's disease is located on the chromosome 13. It encodes for P-type adenosine triphosphatase (ATPase) expressed in hepatocytes, which is responsible for transmembrane transport of copper within hepatocytes and also incorporating copper into ceruloplasmin.

In a steady state ATPase is localized to trans-Golgi network. With elevated copper concentration inside hepatocyte, ATPase is redistributed to vesicular compartment of cytoplasm facilitating excretion of copper in bile.[10-11]

Absent or reduced function of ATP7B protein leads to decreased hepatocellular excretion of copper into bile and formation of ceruloplasmin.[12-14] This leads to, excessive copper accumulation in the tissues, especially in the liver and brain causing hepatic and neurological manifestation of Wilson's (Fig. 26.1).

There are more than 300 mutations of *ATP7B* have been identified, some of which are rather characteristic of geographical regions and ethnic population, e.g. Sardinian, Icelandic, Korean, Japanese, Taiwanese, Spanish and in the Canary Islands, Eastern European, Chandigarh group, Kolkata group, Vellore group, etc.[15-25] There are total of 51 mutations of ATP7B have been documented in India, including 34 novel mutations. C813A is the common mutation in India.[5] Mutation analysis can be focused on this location while screening these population. However, there is no convincing genotype-phenotype correlation.

Mutation analysis looking into whole gene sequencing should be performed in patients whom the diagnosis is difficult. Haplotype analysis or specific testing for known mutations can be used for family screening of first-degree relatives of patients with WD.

CLINICAL FEATURES

Wilson disease is a multisystem disorder presents between 5–55 years of age.[26] Children and young adults present with liver disease unlike older adults, who present with neurological symptoms. Symptoms at any age are frequently nonspecific. The clinical manifestations of WD are summarized in Table 26.1.[26]

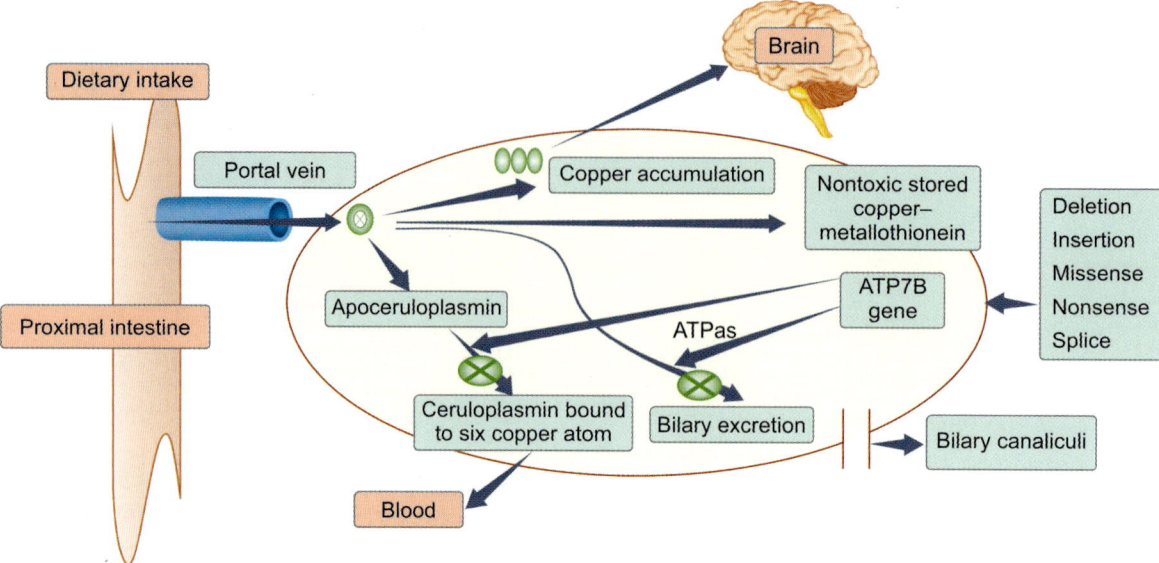

Fig. 26.1: Copper metabolism and pathogenesis of Wilson's disease

Table 26.1: Clinical features of Wilson's disease[26,40-58]

Hepatic
- Asymptomatic hepatomegaly
- Isolated splenomegaly
- Persistently elevated serum aminotransferase activity (AST, ALT)
- Fatty liver
- Acute hepatitis
- Resembling autoimmune hepatitis
- Cirrhosis: compensated or decompensated
- Acute liver failure

Neurological
- Movement disorders (tremor, involuntary movements)
- Inability to perform activities requiring good hand-eye coordination. Handwriting may deteriorate, and cramped small handwriting (micrographia)
- Drooling, dysarthria, rigid dystonia, pseudobulbar palsy
- Dysautonomia
- Migraine headaches, insomnia, seizures
- Psychiatric
- Depression, neurotic behaviors, psychosis
- Personality changes—changes in behavior, deterioration in schoolwork

Other Systems
- Ocular: Kayser-Fleischer rings (on slit lamp examination), sunflower cataracts
- Cutaneous: lunulae ceruleae
- Renal abnormalities: aminoaciduria and nephrolithiasis
- Skeletal abnormalities: premature osteoporosis and arthritis
- Cardiomyopathy, dysrhythmias
- Pancreatitis
- Hypoparathyroidism
- Menstrual irregularities; infertility, repeated abortions
- Coombs-negative hemolytic anemia
- Recurrent/low grade or chronic anemia
- One needs to consider excluding Wilson's disease, in a cause of unexplained hepatic, neurologic, or psychiatric symptoms

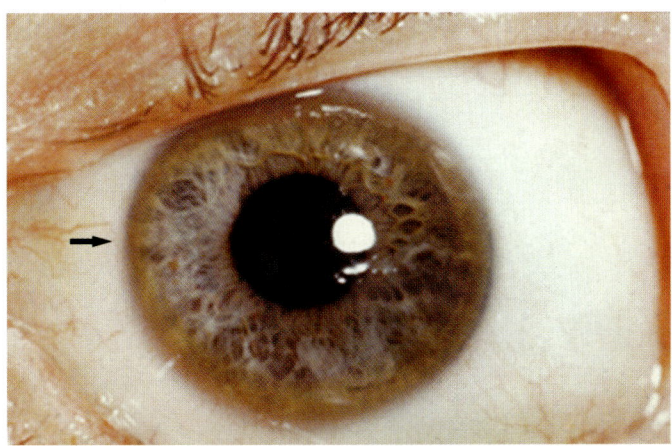

Fig. 26.2: Kayser-Fleischer ring: Band of golden brownish pigment near limbus (arrow)

The spectrum of liver disease encountered in patients can be highly variable, ranging from asymptomatic with only biochemical abnormalities to acute liver failure.

Kayser-Fleischer Ring[63]—are due to deposition of copper in Descemet's membrane usually visible by slit lamp examination. When visible to naked eyes, they appear as a band of golden-brownish pigment near the limbus (Fig. 26.2). KF rings not entirely specific for WD, it is present in only 50% of patients with hepatic manifestation. It gradually disappears with effective medical treatment.[58,64-66] It is more common in patients with neurological manifestations rather than liver disease.[67] Its reappearance in a patient on treatment suggests noncompliance.

DIAGNOSIS

A combination of clinical findings and biochemical testing is usually necessary to establish the diagnosis of WD (Table 26.2).[26] At present genetic diagnosis is expensive and not universally available and sometimes inconclusive.

Ceruloplasmin is an acute phase reactant and its values have to be interpreted cautiously in a setting of acute inflammation, hyperesotrogenemia, end-stage renal disease, protein loosing enteropathy. Subnormal ceruloplasmin has a very low positive predictive value and should not be used alone in diagnosis of WD.[27]

The 24-hour urinary excretion of copper reflects the amount of nonceruloplasmin bound copper in the circulation. Overlap has also been reported in children with autoimmune hepatitis and heterozygotes.[28-29]

The earlier liver biopsy findings in WD include microvesicular and macrovesicular steatosis, focal hepato-cellular necrosis. With progression of the disease parenchymal damage sets in leading to fibrosis and macronodular cirrhosis. Apoptosis of hepatocytes

Table 26.2: Diagnostic algorithm for Wilson's disease
*Classical Wilson's disease[3,59]
• Ophthalmologic slit lamp examination for Kayser-Fleischer ring[60]
• Ceruloplasmin levels <20 mg/dL (0.2 g/L)[61]
• 24-hour urine Cu >40 µg (0.6 µmol)/or urinary copper excretion post-D-penicillamine administration- 1600 microgram copper/24 hours (>25 µmol/24 hours)[58,62]
↓
• Liver biopsy for histology and histochemistry and copper quantification
• If the liver has >250 µg/g dry weight of copper on a adequate biopsy size specimen of 1–2 cm biopsy core length, Wilson disease is confirmed
• If the copper levels <50 µg/g/dry weight, diagnosis of Wilson is excluded
↓ If the quantity of copper is inderminate
Genetic testing

*Half of the patient does not meet the classical criteria of Wilson's disease[2]

is a prominent feature with acute liver failure due to WD. Detection of copper in hepatocytes by routine histochemical evaluation is highly variable. The absence of histochemically identifiable copper does not exclude WD, and this test has a poor predictive value for screening for WD. The most striking alterations are increased intracristal space with dilatation of the tips of the cristae, creating a cystic appearance. In the absence of cholestasis, these changes are considered to be essentially pathognomonic of WD.[30-39] Transjugular biopsy can be considered in high risk patient with decompensated liver disease.

Family Screening for Wilson's Disease

It is important to diagnose Wilson disease as early as possible, since severe liver damage can occur before there are any signs of the disease making a liver transplant necessary. All siblings of the patient with Wilson's disease should be screened with genetic testing. If genetic testing is indertminate or unavailable, one should consider investigations as described in Flow chart 26.1.

First-degree relatives of any patient newly diagnosed with WD must be screened for WD as per the algorithm (Flow chart 26.1). Treatment should be initiated for all individuals greater than 3 years old identified by family screening.

Flow chart 26.1: Family screening for Wilson's disease

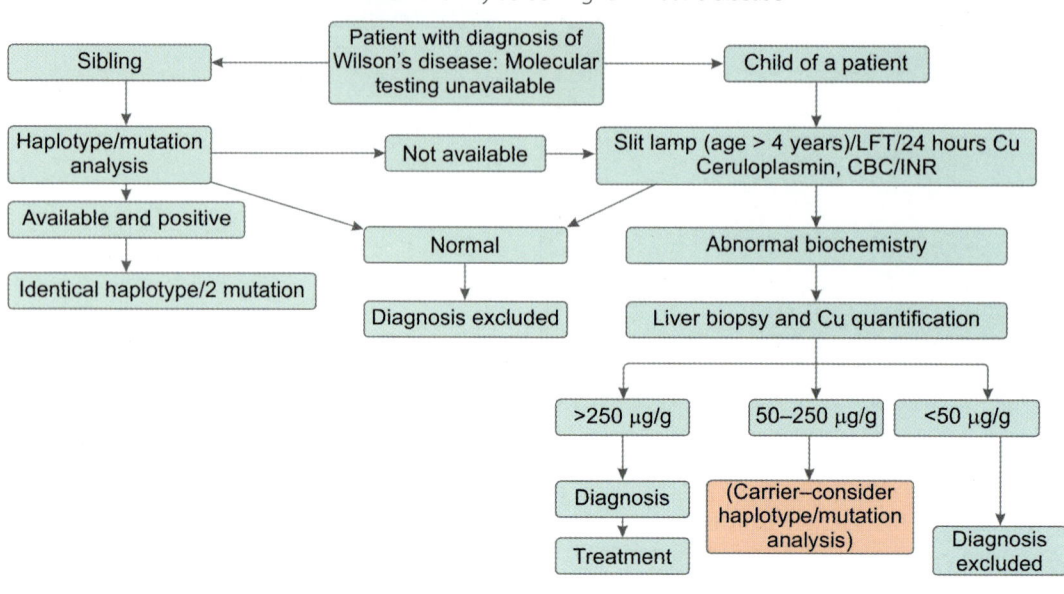

Table 26.3: Diagnosis of Wilson's disease in patients presenting with acute liver failure

- Coombs-negative hemolytic anemia with features of acute intravascular hemolysis
- Coagulopathy unresponsive to parenteral vitamin K administration
- Rapid progression to renal failure
- Relative modest rises in serum aminotransferases (typically <2000 IU/L) from the beginning of clinical illness; AST levels > ALT
- Normal or markedly subnormal serum alkaline phosphatase (ALP: bilurubin ratio < 4)
- Female: male ratio of 2:1
- Sibling with Wilson's disease

Acute Liver Failure and Wilson's Disease

Diagnosis of WD in the setting of acute liver failure could be challenging. There are some constellations of features which point towards WD (Table 26.3).[64,68-74]

TREATMENT

The mainstay of treatment for WD remains life-long pharmacologic therapy. Liver transplantation, which corrects the underlying hepatic defect in WD, is reserved for severe or resistant cases.

Choice of therapy and dosage of medication is determined by whether there is clinically-evident disease, presence of neurological involvement or presymptomatic cases detected by screening.

All patients presenting with neurological WD should undergo detailed neurological evaluation and brain imaging preferably with MRI prior to treatment.

The most commonly used medications include D-pencillamine (DP), trientine (triethylene tetramine dihydrochloride or 2-2-2-tetramine, also known as trien), and zinc. Individual mechanism of action, dosage and indications are summarized in Table 26.4.

Both D-penicillamine and trientine promotes copper excretion by the kidneys. Whether trientine is a weaker chelator of copper than penicillamine is controversial.[75-76] Ammonium tetrathiomolybdate (TM) is a very strong decoppering agent remains an experimental therapy.

The efficacy of simultaneous use of chelators and zinc as primary therapy over chelator therapy alone requires future studies.

Once disease symptoms or biochemical abnormalities have stabilized, typically in 2–6 months after initiation of therapy, maintenance dosages of chelators or zinc therapy can be used for treatment.[77]

It is important to councel patient to comply with life-long therapy as failure could lead to recurrent symptoms and liver failure, the latter requiring liver transplantation for survival. No matter how well a patient appears, treatment should never be terminated indefinitely, as there is a risk of intractable hepatic decompensation.[78]

Once treatment is initiated, patients needs to be regularly monitored for optimal treatment to ensure that they are not over or under treated. Certain urinary and serum biochemical markers guide the optimal drug treatment (Table 26.5).

Children presenting with decompensated cirrhosis with no encephalopathy can be treated with induction regimen consisting of alternating two doses of zinc (25 mg) and trientine (10 mg/kg) per day with 6 hours between the doses. Failure respond to this treatment should prompt one to refer for liver transplantation.[79-81]

Table 26.4: Pharmacological therapy for Wilson's disease

Medication	D-Pencillamine[97-103]	Trientine *	Zinc
Mechanism of action	Chelator	Chelator	Reduces absorption (metallothionein inducer)
Cost factor	Reasonable cost	Expensive	Cheap
Treatment indication	For Initial treatment at diagnosis	• For Initial treatment at diagnosis • Intolerance /side effects with DP • History of renal disease	• Initial treatment for asymptomatic or pre-symptomatic WD[87-91] • Cotreatment • Maintenance treatment
Dosage and administration	20 mg/kg/day in 2–3 divided doses, 1 hour before or 2 hours after food[94,95]	20 mg/kg/day in 2–3 divided doses, 1 hour before or 2 hours after food Avoid coadministering with iron Reduce by 25% when clinically stable	< 50 kg—75 mg/day in three divided doses Older children 150 mg/day in three divided doses[92-93] Reduce by 25% when clinically stable
Side effects	Worsening of neurological symptoms at onset of treatment Early: Fever, rash, marrow suppression, proteinuria, lymphadenopathy Late: Nephotoxicity, lupus, skin lesions Very late: Myasthenia, loss of taste, ploymyositis, retinitis, hepatotoxicity	Less worsening of neurological symptoms Less side effects compared to DP Hemorrhagic gastritis, loss of taste, and rashes.[96]	Neurological worsening uncommon Gastric discomfort Leukopenia Increased lipase and amylase

*Not easily available in India

Table 26.5: Treatment targets and monitoring of treatment

	Zinc	D-Pencillamine /Trientine
Initial treatment	U Cu 100–500 µg/day S free Cu >25 µg/dL	U Cu >500 µg/day S free Cu >25 µg/dL
Good control	U Cu <75 µg/day S free Cu <15 µg/dL	U Cu 200–500 µg/day S free Cu <15 µg/dL
Noncompliance/inadequate dose	U Zn <2 mg/day	U Cu < 200 µg/day S free Cu >15 µg/dL
Over treatment	U Cu <25 µg/day S free Cu<5 µg/dL Anemia, leukpenia, increased ferritin	U Cu <25 µg/day S free Cu< 5 µg/dL Anemia, leukopenia, increased ferritin (sign of excessive copper depletion)

Many side effects are reported with medications used for the treatment of WD. Patient needs to be regularly monitored for the side effects (Table 26.6) and treatment should be discontinued or changed to alternate medications at the onset.

Antioxidants, mainly vitamin E, may have a role as adjunctive treatment. Serum and hepatic vitamin E levels have been found to be low in WD.[82-86]

Foods with very high concentrations of copper (shellfish, nuts, chocolate, mushrooms, and organ meats) generally should be avoided. Copper containers or cookware should not be used to store or prepare foods or drinks

Liver Transplantation and Wilson's Disease

Liver transplant is indicated in Wilson disease patients presenting with acute liver failure, and decompensated cirrhosis unresponsive to therapy.[105,106] The mortality without liver transplant is close to 100% in children

Table 26.6: Monitoring parameters for children on chleator therapy

Clinical
- Liver functions, neurological, and psychiatric worsening
- KF rings annually

Biochemical
- Complete blood count, liver function test, urine dipsticks
- Initially once every 3 days for 15 days
- Then weekly, biweekly, monthly, and subsequently, 6 monthly

Urinary cooper, serum-free copper
- Initially 3 monthly for year
- Later 1–2 times per year

Some suggest liver biopsy every 3 years to asses fibrosis[104]

Table 26.7: New Wilson's index for predicting mortality,[81] children with a score >11 died without transplantation, whereas all those with a score <11 survived

Score	Bilirubin (µmol/L)	INR	AST (IU/L)	WBC (10⁹/L)	Albumin (g/L)
0	0–100	0–1.29	0–100	0–6.7	>45
1	101–150	1.3–1.6	101–150	6.8–8.3	34–44
2	151–200	1.7–1.9	151–300	8.4–10.3	25–33
3	201–300	2.0–2.4	301–400	10.4–15.3	21–24
4	>301	>2.5	>401	>15.4	<20

presenting with fulminant hepatic failure and encephalopathy. These children should be urgently listed for transplant. A scoring system devised by King's College (Table 26.7) can be used as a guide for assessment of patients for transplantation especially when presenting with acute liver failure without encephalopathy. This scoring system helps one to make decision whether to transplant subjecting children to lifelong immunosuppressant's, who perhaps would have got better with chelation therapy alone.[81]

Although it has been suggested that liver transplantation should also be considered in those patients on chelation therapy who do not achieve normal liver function after 3 months of treatment, the results have been variable with different centres.[81,107]

While awaiting for transplantation, plasmapheresis, hemofiltration, or dialysis may be considered to protect the kidneys from copper mediated tubular damage.[108-111]

Liver transplantation corrects the hepatic metabolic defects and may normalise extrahepatic copper metabolism.[112] Successful living donor transplantation is possible when the donor is a family member heterozygous for WD.[113-115] The one- and five-year patient survival post-transplant in children is 90.1% and 89%.[106]

Individuals with decompensated liver disease and neurological manifestations have improved after trans-plantation.[116] Liver transplantation is not recommended as a primary treatment for neurologic WD as liver disease should be stabilized by medical therapy in most of these individuals as outcomes with liver transplantation are not always beneficial.[117-121] Furthermore, patients with neurological or psychiatric disease due to WD may have poorer outcomes and also difficulties with adherence to medical regimens after liver transplantation.[121]

REFERENCES

1. Frydman M. Genetic aspects of Wilson's disease. J Gastroenterol Hepatol. 1990;5:483-90.
2. Schilsky M. Wilson disease: Genetic basis of copper toxicity and natural history. Semin Liver Dis. 1996;16:83-95.
3. Sternlieb I. Perspectives on Wilson's disease. Hepatology. 1990;12:1234-9.
4. Wilson SAK. Progressive lenticular degeneration: a familial nervous disease associated with cirrhosis of the liver. Brain. 1912;34:295-507.
5. Pediatric Liver Study Group of India. Metabolic liver diseases in childhood: Indian scenario. Indian J Pediatr. 1999;66:S97-103.
6. Pena MM, Lee J, Thiele DJ. A delicate balance: Homeostatic control of copper uptake and distribution. J Nutr. 1999;129:1251-60.
7. Leverton RM, Binkley ES. The copper metabolism and requirement of young women. J Nutr. 1944;27:43-52.

8. Tompsett SL. The copper and "inorganic" iron contents of human tissues. Biochem J. 1935;29:480-6.

9. Tompsett SL. The excretion of copper in urine and faeces and its relation to the copper content of the diet. Biochem J. 1934;28:2088-91.

10. Hung IH, Suzuki M, Yamaguchi Y, et al. Biochemical characterization of the Wilson's disease protein and functional expression in the yeast Saccharomyces cerevisiae. J Biol Chem. 1997;272:21461-46.

11. Schaefer M, Roelofsen H, Wolters H, et al. Localization of the Wilson's disease protein in human liver. Gastroenterology. 1999;117:1380-5.

12. Bull PC, Thomas GR, Rommens JM, Forbes JR, Cox DW. The Wilson disease gene is a putative copper transporting P-type ATPase similar to the Menkes gene. Nat Genet. 1993;5:327-37.

13. Tanzi RE, Petrukhin K, Chernov I, Pellequer JL, Wasco W, Ross B, et al. The Wilson disease gene is a copper transporting ATPase with homology to the Menkes disease gene. Nat Genet. 1993;5:344-50.

14. Yamaguchi Y, Heiny ME, Gitlin JD. Isolation and characterization of a human liver cDNA as a candidate gene for Wilson disease. Biochem Biophys Res Commun. 1993;197:271-7.

15. Thomas GR, Jensson O, Gudmundsson G, Thorsteinsson L, Cox DW. Wilson disease in Iceland: a clinical and genetic study. Am J Hum Genet. 1995;56:1140-6.

16. Kim EK, Yoo OJ, Song KY, Yoo HW, Choi SY, Cho SW, et al. Identification of three novel mutations and a high frequency of the Arg778Leu mutation in Korean patients with Wilson disease. Hum Mutat. 1998;11:275-8.

17. Nanji MS, Nguyen VT, Kawasoe JH, Inui K, Endo F, Nakajima T, et al. Haplotype and mutation analysis in Japanese patients with Wilson disease.Am J Hum Genet. 1997;60:1423-29.

18. Wan L, Tsai CH, Tsai Y, Hsu CM, Lee CC, Tsai FJ. Mutation analysis of Taiwanese Wilson disease patients. Biochem Biophys Res Commun. 2006;345:734-8.

19. Margarit E, Bach V, Gomez D, Bruguera M, Jara P, Queralt R, et al. Mutation analysis of Wilson disease in the Spanish population—identification of a prevalent substitution and eight novel mutations in the ATP7B gene. Clin Genet. 2005;68:61-8.

20. Deguti MM, Genschel J, Cancado EL, Barbosa ER, Bochow B, Mucenic M, et al. Wilson disease: novel mutations in the ATP7B gene and clinical correlation in Brazilian patients. Hum Mutat. 2004;23:398.

21. Caca K, Ferenci P, Kuhn HJ, Polli C, Willgerodt H, Kunath B, et al. High prevalence of the H1069Q mutation in East German patients with Wilson disease: rapid detection of mutations by limited sequencing and phenotype-genotype analysis. J Hepatol. 2001;35:575-81.

22. Firneisz G, Lakatos PL, Szalay F, Polli C, Glant TT, Ferenci P. Commonmutations of ATP7B in Wilson disease patients from Hungary. Am J Med Genet. 2002;108:23-8.

23. Kumar S, Thapa BR, Kaur G, Prasad R. Identification and molecular characterization of 18 novel mutations in the ATP7B gene from Indian Wilson disease patients: Genotype. Clin Genet. 2005;67:443-5.

24. Gupta A, Aikath D, Neogi R, Datta S, Basu K, Maity B, et al. Molecular pathogenesis of Wilson disease: Haplotype analysis, detection of prevalent mutations and genotype-phenotype correlation in Indian patients. Hum Genet. 2005;118:49-57.

25. Santhosh S, Shaji RV, Eapen CE, Jayanthi V, Malathi S, Chandy M, et al. ATP7B mutations in families in a predominantly Southern Indian cohort of Wilson's disease patients. Indian J Gastroenterol. 2006;25:277-82.

26. Roberts EA, Michael L. Schilsky, Diagnosisis and treatment of Wilsons disease an Update, AASLD practice guidelines, Hepatology. 2008;47:2089-110.

27. Cauza E, Maier-Dobersberger T, Polli C, Kaserer K, Kramer L, Ferenci P. Screening for Wilson's disease in patients with liver diseases by serum ceruloplasmin. J Hepatol. 1997;27:358-62.

28. Tu JB, Blackwell RQ. Studies on levels of penicillamine-induced cupriuresis in heterozygotes of Wilson's disease. Metabolism. 1967;16:507-13.

29. LaRusso NF, Summerskill WH, McCall JT. Abnormalities of chemical tests for copper metabolism in chronic active liver disease: differentiation from Wilson's disease. Gastroenterology. 1976;70:653-5.

30. Ludwig J, Moyer TP, Rakela J. The liver biopsy diagnosis of Wilson's disease. Methods in pathology. Am J Clin Pathol. 1994;102:443-6.

31. Langner C, Denk H. Wilson disease. Virchows Arch. 2004;445:111-8.

32. Stromeyer FW, Ishak KG. Histology of the liver in Wilson's disease: a study of 34 cases. Am J Clin Pathol. 1980;73:12-24.

33. Strand S, Hofmann WJ, Grambihler A, Hug H, Volkmann M, Otto G, et al. Hepatic failure and liver cell damage in acute Wilson's disease involve CD95 (APO-1/Fas) mediated apoptosis. Nat Med. 1998;4:588-93.

34. Goldfischer S, Sternlieb I. Changes in the distribution of hepatic copper in relation to the progression of Wilson's disease (hepatolenticular degeneration). Am J Pathol. 1968;53:883-901.

35. Geller SA, Petrovic LM, Batts KB, Ferrell LM, Cohen C, Lewin K, et al. Histopathology of end-stage Wilson disease [Abstract]. Mod Pathol. 2000;13:184A.

36. Sternlieb I. Mitochondrial and fatty changes in hepatocytes of patients with Wilson's disease. Gastroenterology. 1968;55:354-67.

37. Feldmann G, Groussard O, Fauvert R. L'ultrastructure he'patique au cours de la maladie de Wilson [Hepatic ultrastructure in Wilson's disease].Biol Gastroenterol. 1969;2:137-60.

38. Sternlieb I. Fraternal concordance of types of abnormal hepatocellular mitochondria in Wilson's disease. Hepatology. 1992;16:728-32.

39. Phillips MJ, Poucell S, Patterson J, Valencia P. The Liver. An Atlas and Text of Ultrastructural Pathology. New York, NY: Raven Press; 1987.

40. Saito T. Presenting symptoms and natural history of Wilson disease. Eur J Pediatr. 1987;146:261-5.

41. Scott J, Gollan JL, Samourian S, Sherlock S. Wilson's disease, presenting as chronic active hepatitis. Gastroenterology. 1978;74:645-51.

42. Schilsky ML, Scheinberg IH, Sternlieb I. Prognosis of Wilsonian chronic active hepatitis. Gastroenterology. 1991;100:762-67.

43. Milkiewicz P, Saksena S, Hubscher SG, Elias E. Wilson's disease with superimposed autoimmune features: report of two cases and review. J Gastroenterol Hepatol. 2000;15:570-4.

44. Azizi E, Eshel G, Aladjem M. Hypercalciuria and nephrolithiasis as a presenting sign in Wilson disease. Eur J Pediatr. 1989;148:548-9.

45. Nakada SY, Brown MR, Rabinowitz R. Wilson's disease presenting as symptomatic urolithiasis: a case report and review of the literature. J Urol. 1994;152:978-9.

46. Chu CC, Huang CC, Chu NS. Recurrent hypokalemic muscle weakness as an initial manifestation of Wilson's disease. Nephron. 1996;73:477-9.

47. Golding DN, Walshe JM. Arthropathy of Wilson's disease. Study of clinical and radiological features in 32 patients. Ann Rheum Dis. 1977;36:99-111.

48. Factor SM, Cho S, Sternlieb I, Scheinberg IH, Goldfischer S. The cardiomyopathy of Wilson's disease. Myocardial alterations in nine cases. Virchows Arch Pathol Anat. 1982;397:301-11.

49. Kuan P. Cardiac Wilson's disease. Chest. 1987;91:579-83.

50. Hlubocka Z, Maracek Z, Linhart A, Kejrova E, Pospisilova L, Martasek P, et al. Cardiac involvement in Wilson disease. J Inherit Metab Dis. 2002;25:269-77.

51. Weizman Z, Picard E, Barki Y, Moses S. Wilson's disease associated with pancreatitis. J Pediatr Gastroenterol Nutr. 1988;7:931-3.

52. Carpenter TO, Carnes DL Jr, Anast CS. Hypoparathyroidism in Wilson's disease. N Engl J Med. 1983;309:873-7.

53. Walshe JM. Pregnancy in Wilson's disease. Q J Med. 1977;46:73-83.

54. Klee JG. Undiagnosed Wilson's disease as cause of unexplained miscarriage. Lancet. 1979;2:423.

55. Kaushansky A, Frydman M, Kaufman H, Homburg R. Endocrine studies of the ovulatory disturbances in Wilson's disease (hepatolenticular degeneration). Fertil Steril. 1987;47:270-3.

56. Tarnacka B, Rodo M, Cichy S, Czlonkowska A. Procreation ability in Wilson's disease. Acta Neurol Scand. 2000;101:395-8.

57. Cairns JE, Williams HP, Walshe JM. "Sunflower cataract" in Wilson's disease. Br Med J. 1969;3:95-6.

58. Gow PJ, Smallwood RA, Angus PW, Smith AL, Wall AJ, Sewell RB. Diagnosis of Wilson's disease: an experience over three decades. Gut. 2000;46:415-9.

59. Steindl P, Ferenci P, Dienes HP, Grimm G, Pabinger I, Madl C, et al. Wilson's disease in patients presenting with liver disease: a diagnostic challenge. Gastroenterology. 1997;113:212-8.

60. Fleischer B. Ueber einer der "Pseudosclerose" nahestehende bisher unbekannte Krankheit (gekennzeichnet durch Tremor, psychische Stoerungen, braeunlicke Pigmentierung bestimmter Gewebe, insbesondere Such der Hornhauptperipherie, Lebercirrhose). Deutsch Z Nerven Heilk. 1912;44:179-201.

61. Scheinberg IH, Gitlin D. Deficiency of ceruloplasmin in patients with hepatolenticular degeneration (Wilson's disease). Science. 1952;116:484-5.

62. Martins da Costa C, Baldwin D, Portmann B, Lolin Y, Mowat AP, Mieli-Vergani G. Value of urinary copper excretion after penicillamine challenge in the diagnosis of Wilson's disease. HEPATOLOGY. 1992;15:609-15.

63. Fred H, van Dijk H. Images of Memorable Cases: Case 9. Connexions, December 8, 2008. http://cnx.org/content/m15007/1.3/

64. Emre S, Atillasoy EO, Ozdemir S, Schilsky M, Rathna Varma CV, Thung SN, et al. Orthotopic liver transplantation for Wilson's disease: a single-center experience. Transplantation. 2001;72:1232-6.

65. Medici V, Trevisan CP, D'Inca R, Barollo M, Zancan L, Fagiuoli S, et al. Diagnosis and management of Wilson's disease: results of a single center experience. J Clin Gastroenterol. 2006;40:936-41.

66. Merle U, Schaefer M, Ferenci P, Stremmel W. Clinical presentation, diagnosis and long-term outcome of Wilson's disease: a cohort study. Gut. 2007;56:115-20.

67. Taly AB, Meenakshi-Sundaram S, Sinha S, Swamy HS, Arunodaya GR. Wilson disease: Description of 282 patients evaluated over 3 decades. Medicine (Baltimore). 2007;86:112-21.

68. Roche-Sicot J, Benhamou JP. Acute intravascular hemolysis and acute liver failure associated as a first manifestation of Wilson's disease. Ann Intern Med. 1977;86:301-3.

69. Hamlyn AN, Gollan JL, Douglas AP, Sherlock S. Fulminant Wilson's disease with haemolysis and renal failure: copper studies and assessment of dialysis regimens. Br Med J. 1977;2:660-2.

70. McCullough AJ, Fleming CR, Thistle JL, Baldus WP, Ludwig J, McCall JT, et al. Diagnosis of Wilson's disease presenting as fulminant hepatic failure. Gastroenterology. 1983;84:161-7.

71. Rector WG Jr, Uchida T, Kanel GC, Redeker AG, Reynolds TB. Fulminant hepatic and renal failure complicating Wilson's disease. Liver. 1984;4:341-7.

72. Enomoto K, Ishibashi H, Irie K, Okumura Y, Nomura H, Fukushima M, et al. Fulminant hepatic failure without evidence of cirrhosis in a case of Wilson's disease. Jpn J Med. 1989;28:80-4.

73. Ferlan-Marolt V, Stepec S. Fulminant Wilsonian hepatitis unmasked by disease progression: report of a case and review of the literature. Dig Dis Sci. 1999;44:1054-8.

74. Berman DH, Leventhal RI, Gavaler JS, Cadoff EM, Van Thiel DH.Clinical differentiation of fulminant Wilsonian hepatitis from other causes of hepatic failure. Gastroenterology. 1991;100:1129-34.

75. Wiggelinkhuizen M, Tilanus ME, Bollen CW, Houwen RH. Systematic review: clinical efficacy of chelator agents and zinc in the initial treatment of Wilson disease. Aliment Pharmacol Ther. 2009;29(9):947-58.

76. Sarkar B, Sass-Kortsak A, Clarke R, Laurie SH, Wei P. A comparative study of in vitro and in vivo interaction of D-penicillamine and triethylene- tetramine with copper. Proc R Soc Med. 1977;70(Suppl 3):13-8.

77. Kaushansky A, Frydman M, Kaufman H, Homburg R. Endocrine studies of the ovulatory disturbances in Wilson's disease (hepatolenticular degeneration). Fertil Steril. 1987;47:270-3.

78. Walshe JM, Dixon AK. Dangers of non-compliance in Wilson's disease. Lancet. 1986;1:845-7.

79. Santos Silva EE, Sarles J, Buts JP, Sokal EM. Successful medical treatment of severely decompensated Wilson disease. J Pediatr. 1996;128:285-7.

80. Askari FK, Greenson J, Dick RD, Johnson VD, Brewer GJ. Treatment of Wilson's disease with zinc. XVIII. Initial treatment of the hepatic

decompensation presentation with trientine and zinc. J Lab Clin Med. 2003;142:385-90.

81. Dhawan A, Taylor RM, Cheeseman P, De Silva P, Katsiyiannakis L, Mieli-Vergani G. Wilson's disease in children: 37-Year experience and revised King's score for liver transplantation. Liver Transpl. 2005;11:441-8.

82. von Herbay A, de Groot H, Hegi U, Stremmel W, Strohmeyer G, Sies H. Low vitamin E content in plasma of patients with alcoholic liver disease, hemochromatosis and Wilson's disease. J Hepatol. 1994;20:41-6.

83. Sokol RJ, Twedt D, McKim JM Jr, Devereaux MW, Karrer FM, Kam I, et al. Oxidant injury to hepatic mitochondria in patients with Wilson's disease and Bedlington terriers with copper toxicosis. Gastroenterology. 1994;107:1788-98.

84. Ogihara H, Ogihara T, Miki M, Yasuda H, Mino M. Plasma copper and antioxidant status in Wilson's disease. Pediatr Res. 1995;37:219-26.199.

85. Sinha S, Christopher R, Arunodaya GR, Prashanth LK, Gopinath G, Swamy HS, et al. Is low serum tocopherol in Wilson's disease a significant symptom? J Neurol Sci. 2005;228:121-3.

86. Nagasaka H, Inoue I, Inui A, Komatsu H, Sogo T, Murayama K, et al. Relationship between oxidative stress and antioxidant systems in the liver of patients with Wilson disease: hepatic manifestation in Wilson disease as a consequence of augmented oxidative stress. Pediatr Res. 2006;60:472-7.

87. Marcellini M, Di Ciommo V, Callea F, Devito R, Comparcola D, Sartorelli MR, et al. Treatment of Wilson's disease with zinc from the time of diagnosis in pediatric patients: a single-hospital, 10-year follow-up study. J Lab Clin Med. 2005;145:139-43.

88. Alexiou D, Hatzis T, Koutselinis A. Maintenance treatment of Wilson's disease with oral zinc. Apropos of a child treated for 4 years. Arch Fr Pediatr. 1985;42:447-9.

89. Brewer GJ, Dick RD, Yuzbasiyan-Gurkan V, Johnson V, Wang Y. Treatment of Wilson's disease with zinc. XIII: therapy with zinc in presymptomatic patients from the time of diagnosis. J Lab Clin Med. 1994;123:849-58.

90. Mizuochi T, Kimura A, Shimizu N, Nishiura H, Matsushita M, Yoshino M. Zinc monotherapy from time of diagnosis for young pediatric patients with presymptomatic Wilson disease. J Pediatr Gastroenterol Nutr. 2011 Oct;53(4):365-7.

91. Shimizu N, Fujiwara J, Ohnishi S, Sato M, Kodama H, Kohsaka T, et al. Effects of long-term zinc treatment in Japanese patients with Wilson disease: efficacy, stability, & copper metabolism, Transl Res. 2010;156(6):350-7.

92. Brewer GJ, Dick RD, Johnson VD, Fink JK, Kluin KJ, Daniels S. Treatment of Wilson's disease with zinc XVI: Treatment during the pediatric years. J Lab Clin Med. 2001;137:191-8.

93. Brewer GJ, Dick RD, Johnson VD, Brunberg JA, Kluin KJ, Fink JK. Treatment of Wilson's disease with zinc: XV Long-term follow-up studies. J Lab Clin Med. 1998;132:264-78.

94. Schuna A, Osman MA, Patel RB, Welling PB, Sundstrom WR. Influence of food on the bioavailability of penicillamine. J Rheumatol. 1983;10:95-7.

95. Kukovetz WR, Beubler E, Kreuzig F, Moritz AJ, Nimberger G, Werner- Breitnecker L. Bioavailability and pharmacokinetics of D-penicillamine. J Rheumatol. 1983;10:90-4.

96. Epstein O, Sherlock S. Triethylene tetramine dihydrochloride toxicity in primary biliary cirrhosis. Gastroenterology. 1980;78:1442-5.

97. Falkmer S, Samuelson G, Sjolin S. Penicillamine-induced normalization of clinical signs, and liver morphology and histochemistry in a case of Wilson's disease. Pediatrics. 1970;45:260-8.

98. Walshe JM. Copper chelation in patients with Wilson's disease. A comparison of penicillamine and triethylene tetramine dihydrochloride. Q J Med. 1973;42:441-52.

99. Sass-Kortsak A. Wilson's disease. A treatable liver disease in children. Pediatr Clin North Am. 1975;22:963-84.

100. Grand RJ, Vawter GF. Juvenile Wilson disease: histologic and functional studies during penicillamine therapy. J Pediatr. 1975;87:1161-70.

101. Sternlieb I. Copper and the liver. Gastroenterology. 1980;78:1615-28.

102. Czlonkowska A, Gajda J, Rodo M. Effects of long-term treatment in Wilson's disease with D-penicillamine and zinc sulphate. J Neurol. 1996;243:269-73.

103. Merle U, Schaefer M, Ferenci P, Stremmel W. Clinical presentation, diagnosis and long-term outcome of Wilson's disease: a cohort study. Gut. 2007;56:115-20.

104. Cope-Yokoyama S, Finegold MJ, Sturniolo GC, Kim K, Mescoli C, Rugge M, Medici V, Wilson disease: histopathological correlations with treatment on follow-up liver biopsies. World J Gastroenterol. 2010;16(12):1487-94.

105. Sokol RJ, Francis PD, Gold SH, Ford DM, Lum GM, Ambruso DR. Orthotopic liver transplantation for acute fulminant Wilson disease. J Pediatr. 1985;107:549-52.

106. Arnon R, Annunziato R, Schilsky M, Miloh T, Willis A, Sturdevant M, et al. Liver transplantation for children with Wilson disease: comparison of outcomes between children and adults, Clin Transplant. 2011;25(1):E52-60.

107. Robles R, Parrilla P, Sicilia J, Ramirez P, Bueno FS, Rodriguez JM, et al. Indications and results of liver transplants in Wilson's disease. Transplant Proc. 1999;31:2453-4.

108. Rakela J, Kurtz SB, McCarthy JT, Krom RA, Baldus WP, McGill DB, et al. Postdilution hemofiltration in the management of acute hepatic failure: a pilot study. Mayo Clin Proc. 1988;63:113-8.

109. Rakela J, Kurtz SB, McCarthy JT, Ludwig J, Ascher NL, Bloomer JR, et al. Fulminant Wilson's disease treated with postdilution hemofiltration and orthotopic liver transplantation. Gastroenterology. 1986;90:2004-7.

110. Sarles J, Lefevre P, Picon G. Plasma exchange for fulminant Wilson disease. Eur J Pediatr. 1992;151:310.

111. Morgan SM, Zantek ND. Therapeutic plasma exchange for fulminant hepatic failure secondary to Wilson's disease. J Clin Apher. 2012 Nov;27(5):282-6.

112. Groth CG, Dubois RS, Corman J, Gustafsson A, Iwatsuki S, Rodgerson DO, et al. Metabolic effects of hepatic replacement in Wilson's disease. Transplant Proc. 1973;5:829-33.

113. Asonuma K, Inomata Y, Kasahara M, Uemoto S, Egawa H, Fujita S, et al. Living related liver transplantation from heterozygote genetic carriers to children with Wilson's disease. Pediatr Transplant. 1999;3:201-5.

114. Komatsu H, Fujisawa T, Inui A, Sogo T, Sekine I, Kodama H, et al. Hepatic copper concentration in children undergoing living related liver transplantation due to Wilsonian fulminant hepatic failure. Clin Transplant. 2002;16:227-32.

115. Wang XH, Cheng F, Zhang F, Li XC, Kong LB, Li GQ, et al. Livingrelated liver transplantation for Wilson's disease. Transpl Int. 2005;18:651-6.

116. Eghtesad B, Nezakatgoo N, Geraci LC, Jabbour N, Irish WD, Marsh W, et al. Liver transplantation for Wilson's disease: a single-center experience. Liver Transpl Surg. 1999;5:467-74.

117. Guarino M, Stracciari A, D'Alessandro R, Pazzaglia P. No neurological improvement after liver transplantation for Wilson's disease. Acta Neurol Scand. 1995;92:405-8.

118. Kassam N, Witt N, Kneteman N, Bain VG. Liver transplantation for neuropsychiatric Wilson disease. Can J Gastroenterol. 1998;12:65-8.

119. Brewer GJ, Askari F. Transplant livers in Wilson's disease for hepatic, not neurologic, indications. Liver Transpl. 2000;6:662-4.

120. Senzolo M, Loreno M, Fagiuoli S, Zanus G, Canova D, Masier A, et al. Different neurological outcome of liver transplantation for Wilson'sdisease in two homozygotic twins.Clin Neurol Neurosurg. 2007;109:71-5.

121. Medici V, Mirante VG, Fassati LR, Pompili M, Forti D, Del Gaudio M, et al. Liver transplantation for Wilson's disease: The burden of neurological and psychiatric disorders. Liver Transpl. 2005;11:1056-63.

Chapter

27 — Metabolic Disorders in the Infant

Suresh Vijay

INTRODUCTION

Inherited metabolic disorders (IMDs) are a disparate group of around 700 disorders that are individually rare and occur due to single-gene defects in specific metabolic pathways in the body. Each inherited metabolic defect leads to a 'metabolic block', which leads to organ dysfunction, either due to a downstream deficiency of essential metabolic products or due to an upstream excess of the metabolic substrate or both. IMDs can occur due to such defects in enzymes, cofactors or the transport of metabolites. Most IMDs present with typical biochemical abnormalities and clearly discernable clinical phenotypes that help identify them without much delay. However, the severity of the metabolic defect may be variable and a high index of suspicion is essential in order to diagnose IMDs.

The altered metabolic milieu may affect a single organ or may have systemic effects. Organs or organ systems that have a high metabolic rate and/or high energy requirement, such as the brain, the liver and the heart or those with a high turnover of cell products, such as the bone marrow or the growing skeleton, are particularly susceptible to the effects of such metabolic abnormalities.

The liver is one of most metabolically active organs in the body. It is host to numerous synthetic and detoxification pathways and is inextricably linked to almost all vital chemical reactions in the body required to sustain life and maintain health. Therefore, IMDs involving the liver can have wide-ranging effects on the body.

Early identification and initiation of therapy is essential to increase the prospects of a good outcome. Newborn screening and early treatment is available for several metabolic disorders affecting the liver in the newborn period. Prenatal diagnosis is almost always possible all IMDs and genetic counseling can be offered to inform further reproductive choices for the parents and the extended family.

METABOLIC LIVER DISEASE[1]

In order to understand the liver disorders that occur due to IMDs, a classification based on clinical presentation can help the clinician consider potential diagnoses and plan investigations judiciously.

IMDs that affect the liver can be considered mainly under the following presentations:
- Prolonged neonatal jaundice
- Acute liver failure
- Organomegaly and associated symptoms
- Hydrops fetalis

Prolonged Neonatal Jaundice

Jaundice is the most common symptom of liver disease in the newborn period. Unconjugated neonatal jaundice is almost always physiological and resolves spontaneously within a few days after birth. There are numerous causes of prolonged neonatal jaundice (jaundice lasting beyond 14 days of age). IMDs may present either with prolonged conjugated or unconjugated jaundice or both (Table 27.1). The differential diagnosis of prolonged neonatal jaundice is extensive and urgent investigation is necessary. The presence of hypoglycemia or encephalopathy usually suggests the existence of a metabolic or endocrine problem in the newborn period. Metabolic causes of liver disease in the newborn period are often associated with early failure to thrive and abnormalities of acid–base balance. Basic biochemical investigations can often indicate the likelihood of inherited metabolic disease and also guide further investigations. Metabolic investigations will almost always be required in neonates with prolonged jaundice (Table 27.2). However, such investigation has to be carefully targeted and they may not always be easily available. Even if they are available, metabolic investigations are often invasive and expensive.

Table 27.1: Etiology of conjugated hyperbilirubinemia in infancy

Some inherited metabolic disorders that cause conjugated hyperbilirubinemia in infancy
- Classical galactosemia
- Tyrosinemia type 1
- Citrin deficiency
- Niemann-Pick disease type C
- Wolman disease
- Zellweger syndrome
- Congenital disorders of glycosylation (CDGs)

Other causes
- Alpha-1-antitrypsin deficiency
- Cystic fibrosis
- Progressive familial intrahepatic cholestasis (types 1–3)
- Bile acid synthetic disorders
- ARC syndrome
- Bilirubin metabolism defects—Dubin-Johnson syndrome and Rotor syndrome

Table 27.2: Initial metabolic investigations for prolonged neonatal jaundice

Blood
- Plasma glucose
- Plasma lactate
- Plasma amino acids
- Ammonia
- Plasma acylcarnitine analysis
- Galactosemia screen—Gal-1-PUT (In newborns who have been transfused - Gal-1-P)

Urine
- Reducing substances
- Sugar chromatography
- Organic acid analysis

Usually liver synthetic dysfunction and complications in other organ systems, such as encephalopathy may occur before the investigations for prolonged jaundice are performed. The possibility of IMDs should be considered early in the investigation of neonatal jaundice, at the same time as other causes with a view to excluding them.

Classical Galactosemia[2,3]

Galactosemia occurs due to the autosomal recessive inherited deficiency of the enzyme galactose-1-phosphate uridyl transferase (Gal-1-PUT). Affected neonates present in the latter half of the first week to the second week of life with poor weight gain, mixed conjugated and unconjugated jaundice and if untreated, rapidly progress to encephalopathy and liver dysfunction. Affected neonates are prone to gram-negative sepsis and multiorgan failure may prove fatal. Nuclear cataracts may be present and provide a clue to the diagnosis.

Investigation

- As soon as the possibility of galactosemia is considered, breastfeeding and milk feeds should be discontinued and supportive therapy provided for liver dysfunction
- Red cell GAL-1-PUT enzyme assay ('galactosemia screen') should be requested urgently
- If the neonate has been transfused, the GAL-1-PUT assay cannot be performed until 3 months after transfusion. Instead, serum galactose-1-phosphate and urine galactitol should be measured in such neonates
- Urine is frequently analyzed for reducing substances in jaundiced neonates. However, it is not reliable. Glycosuria (clinistix positive) and galactosuria (clinitest positive and clinistix negative) have to be differentiated and both of which may be present in galactosaemia due to renal Fanconi syndrome
- Mutation analysis of the GALT gene will confirm the diagnosis and provide information regarding the likely severity of the enzyme defect and therefore the prognosis.

Treatment

- After treatment of the acute liver dysfunction, life-long dietary restriction of galactose is essential. Calcium supplementation may be required if dietary intake is insufficient
- Cataracts almost always resolve if treatment is initiated early, but may sometimes require surgical removal.

Prognosis

Early diagnosis and treatment is lifesaving. In the survivors, despite normal life expectancy, long-term neurodevelopmental outcome remains poor even with satisfactory dietary management.

Hereditary Tyrosinemia Type 1 (HT1)

This autosomal recessive disorder results from an inherited deficiency of the enzyme—fumaryl acetoacetase (FAA). The neonatal form usually presents with jaundice, liver failure, encephalopathy and hypotonia. Milder variants may present later with renal Fanconi syndrome, rickets, failure to thrive, and liver dysfunction leading rapidly to cirrhosis. Hepatocellular carcinoma can occur if the condition is untreated.

Diagnosis and Management[4]

- Plasma urine or organic acid analysis to identify succinylacetone (diagnostic)
- Increased δ aminolevulinic acid (δ ALA) in urine

- Elevated γ GT and alpha-fetoprotein (AFP)
- Plasma amino acid analysis—elevated tyrosine.

Treatment

- Immediate institution of life-long dietary restriction of tyrosine and phenylalanine
- 2-(2-nitro-fluoro-methylbenzoyl)-1, 3-cyclohexanedione (NTBC) is a very specific and effective treatment for tyrosinaemia type I. It minimizes the risk of hepatocellular carcinoma, if treatment is commenced early in the neonatal period or infancy and continued for life.

Outcome

Long-term neurological outcome is generally poor, even with satisfactory and early initiation of treatment. Life-long monitoring for hepatocellular carcinoma is essential and liver transplantation can be lifesaving. Without early diagnosis and treatment, the mortality is high. Death usually occurs from acute liver failure and sepsis. Unless treatment with NTBC is commenced early in the neonatal period or infancy, hepatocellular carcinoma, and neurological complications lead to reduced life expectancy.

Citrin Deficiency/Citrullinemia Type II[5-7]

Citrin deficiency occurs due to an autosomal recessive defect in the mitochondrial aspartate transporter. The neonatal form of citrin deficiency can manifest with intrahepatic cholestasis (NICCD). Other forms occur in older children, such as failure to thrive and dyslipidemia caused by citrin deficiency (FTTDCD) and in adults as recurrent hyperammonemia with neuropsychiatric symptoms in citrullinemia type II (CTLN2). Classically, citrin deficiency is characterized by an unusual fondness for protein-rich and/or lipid-rich foods and aversion to carbohydrate-rich foods.

Neonates and infants may present with poor growth, transient intrahepatic cholestasis and hepatomegaly. Other features are, a diffuse fatty liver and parenchymal cellular infiltration associated with hepatic fibrosis on biopsy, variable liver synthetic dysfunction and hypoglycemia. NICCD is usually mild and resolves during infancy. It may then recur in its CTLN2 form in adulthood.

Investigations

- Plasma ammonia may be elevated, but not always
- Galactosuria may be present
- Elevated plasma citrulline is usually indicative of NICCD

- Plasma or serum threonine-to-serine ratio may be elevated
- Mutation analysis of the SLC25A13 gene is diagnostic.

Treatment

- Reduced carbohydrate, high protein-high fat ('modified Atkins') diet
- Clinical monitoring for life as the CTLN2 form can manifest in adulthood.

Outcome

- Long-term outcome is generally good, although some neonates die of infection or liver failure.

Niemann-Pick Disease Type C[8]

Niemann-Pick disease type C (NPC) is a lipid storage disease that can present at any age, from infancy to adulthood. This occurs due to an autosomal recessive inherited defect in intracellular trafficking of cholesterol, which plays an essential role in cell-signaling, neurological structure and function. Neonates usually present with prolonged conjugated jaundice and may develop acute liver failure with ascites and/or respiratory failure from infiltration of the lungs. Infants may also present without liver or pulmonary disease, but with neurological features such as hypotonia and developmental delay. The neonatal jaundice is transient, resolves spontaneously and does not recur. Other variants that present in childhood and adult life predominantly present with progressive neurological features.

Splenomegaly and rarely hepatomegaly may be present. Many infants succumb in the neonatal period. Of those who survive, some are hypotonic and delayed in psychomotor development, whereas in others the neurological features may completely resolve, only to present with neurologic disease many years later. Children who present mainly with hypotonia and delayed development usually do not have vertical supranuclear gaze palsy (VSGP) at the onset but this develops after a variable period along with other signs of neurological regression.

Investigations

- Serum chitotriosidase might be elevated, but pseudodeficiency occurs in about 5% of the normal population. Normal chitotriosidase activity therefore does not exclude NPC
- Demonstration of impaired cholesterol esterification in fibroblasts
- Positive Filipin staining in cultured fibroblasts demonstrating accumulation of unesterified cholesterol

❏ Molecular genetic testing of *NPC1* and *NPC2* genes
❏ Plasma oxysterol analysis is becoming increasing available as a diagnostic tool
❏ Biopsy of the bone marrow, spleen, and liver are not required, but may demonstrate foamy cells (lipid-laden macrophages and sea-blue histiocytes).

Treatment

❏ No effective treatment is available
❏ Miglustat is a form of substrate—deprivation therapy that is licenced for use in NPC, though the long-term benefits are unclear.

Outcome

Long-term outlook for the neonatal form of NPC is generally poor, resulting in death in infancy in most and progressive neurological deterioration through childhood in a small proportion. In a small minority, complete resolution of symptoms is followed by recurrence of neurological features in later life.

Wolman Disease (Lysosomal Acid Lipase (LAL) Deficiency)[9-11]

Wolman disease (WD) is a rare cause of liver disease and occurs at the most severe end of the spectrum of lysosomal acid lipase (LAL) deficiency, an autosomal recessive inherited defect. Milder phenotypes may present later in life, as cholesterol ester storage disease (CESD). This enzyme deficiency results in defective lysosomal hydrolysis of both, esterified cholesterol and triglycerides from lipoproteins leading to their accumulation in most tissues. WD can sometimes present in the fetal period with hepatomegaly, ascites, hydrops fetalis and adrenal calcification. But the typical presentation occurs in the first weeks of life with abdominal distention, massive hepatosplenomegaly and ascites. Calcification of the adrenal glands is nearly always diagnostic of WD. Foamy histiocytes in bone marrow biopsy may also be found, indicating abnormal storage of lipids. Vomiting, diarrhea, steatorrhea and failure to thrive often precede developmental arrest and neurological regression. Babies become anaemic, jaundiced, and cachectic before death ensues, usually in infancy.

Investigations

Confirmation of the diagnosis is by:
❏ Enzyme analysis in white blood cells or skin fibroblasts
❏ Mutation analysis of the LAL gene.

Treatment

❏ Prenatal diagnosis is possible
❏ There is no specific treatment available for Wolman disease at present
❏ Early bone marrow transplant may lead to prolonged survival
❏ Clinical trials of recombinant enzyme replacement therapy and gene therapy are promising.

Outcome

At present, the prognosis for WD is poor. Survival beyond infancy is rare. New therapies are on the horizon and offer hope.

Zellweger Syndrome[12]

Zellweger syndrome (ZS) is the most severe form of peroxisomal biogenesis disorders (PBDs) and is inherited in an autosomal recessive fashion. It is also known as cerebrohepatorenal syndrome. In addition to early-onset liver dysfunction, characteristic craniofacial dysmorphic features often makes a clinical diagnosis possible— flattened facies, large anterior fontanell, open sutures, prominent high forehead, flattened occiput, up-slanting palpebral fissures, epicanthic folds, broad nasal bridge, macrocephaly or microcephaly, high arched palate, micrognathia, and redundant skinfolds in the neck. Severe neurological abnormalities, such as severe developmental delay, hypotonia, and neonatal seizures are characteristic.

Radiological abnormalities, such as chondrodysplasia punctata and subcortical renal cysts may be present. Liver disease presents as failure to thrive, hepatomegaly, jaundice, and coagulopathy. Cataracts, glaucoma, pigmentary retinopathy, nystagmus, corneal clouding and optic nerve hypoplasia along with severe sensorineural hearing loss are almost always present. Genital abnormalities are also frequent.

Investigations

❏ Plasma very-long-chain fatty acid (VLCFA) analysis— increased very long chain fatty acids and VLCFA ratios— C22/C24, C22/C26
❏ Red cell plasmalogen analysis will demonstrate decreased plasmalogen synthesis
❏ Reduced docosahexaenoic acid (DHA)
❏ Mutation analysis of the PEX genes

Treatment

❏ There is no effective treatment or cure for PBDs
❏ Supportive treatment of liver dysfunction and seizures may be required

- Supplementation of DHA, vitamin K, bile acids—cholic and chenodeoxycholic acid
- Dietary restriction of phytanic acid may be attempted in milder forms of ZS.

Outcome

Despite supportive treatment, prognosis is poor, with most dying during infancy. Death usually occurs due to respiratory tract infections or intractable epilepsy.

Congenital Disorders of Glycosylation (CDG)[13]

Congenital disorders of glycosylation (CDG) are a group of more than 29 different inherited disorders in the synthesis of N-linked oligosaccharides. Onset of symptoms is usually in the neonatal period or infancy. This large group of separate disorders with Protean features—severe developmental delay, hypotonia, hypoglycemia and dysmorphism. Cyclical vomiting, severe hypoglycemia, failure to thrive, hepatic fibrosis, and protein-losing enteropathy, occasionally associated with coagulation disturbances without neurologic involvement, are characteristic of CDG-Ib, which is the most common type of CDG. Most CDGs are inherited in an autosomal recessive manner.

Investigations

- Transferrin isoelectric focusing (T-IEF) may help in making a diagnosis of CDG
- Further investigations, such as analysis of lipid-linked oligosaccharides (LLO), enzyme analysis, and mutation analysis will be required to characterize the exact nature of the underlying defect.

Treatment

- There is no specific treatment available for CDGs except for CDG 1b
- Prenatal diagnosis may be possible if the deleterious mutations are known
- CDG1b is the only CDG for which specific treatment is available. Mannose supplementation is effective in rapidly correcting protein-losing enteropathy, hypoalbuminemia, hypoglycemia, and coagulation defects.

ACUTE LIVER FAILURE

Acute liver failure presents with unexpected acute liver dysfunction and coagulopathy. Symptoms, such as encephalopathy, jaundice, organomegaly are usually

Table 27.3: Metabolic and other causes of liver failure

Metabolic causes of liver failure
- Galactosemia
- Tyrosinemia type I
- Hereditary fructose intolerance
- Mitochondrial hepatopathy
- Long chain fatty acid oxidation defects
- Urea cycle defects

Other metabolic causes of liver failure
- Bile salt synthetic disorders
- Valproate toxicity
- Wilson's disease

present in acute liver failure due to inherited metabolic disease. Early recognition and supportive treatment is essential, while the underlying cause is investigated without delay. Specific treatment may be available for certain metabolic causes of liver failure, such as galactosemia and tyrosinemia (Table 27.3). Most infants succumb to liver failure before effective treatment can be administered. Liver transplantation may be the only option in severe cases. The presence of multisystem involvement, as in most mitochondrial diseases, may preclude transplantation.

Hereditary Fructose Intolerance (HFI) (Aldolase B deficiency)

HFI is an autosomal recessive condition, which occurs due to a deficiency of the enzyme aldolase B in the liver. It should not be confused with fructose malabsorption or a gastrointestinal 'intolerance'. Neonates with HFI are typically well until they are offered food that contains fructose. Rapid metabolic decompensation follows ingestion of fructose. Acute liver failure presents with vomiting, hypoglycaemia, failure to thrive, cachexia, hepatomegaly, jaundice, coagulopathy, coma, renal Fanconi syndrome, and severe metabolic (and lactic) acidosis.

Rapid resolution of symptoms (especially hypoglycemia and lactic acidosis) follows exclusion of fructose in the diet.

Investigations

- Increased plasma urate, lactic acidosis, liver failure and hypoglycemia with a history of fructose ingestion are typical
- Fructose challenge tests can be dangerous and unnecessary
- Mutation analysis in the ALDOB gene is confirmatory
- Liver biopsy for enzyme analysis in hepatocytes may not be required, as mutation analysis is less invasive.

Treatment

❑ Symptoms resolve rapidly with removal of fructose containing food from the diet
❑ Life-long fructose free diet.

Outcome

Death and multiorgan damage can occur unless HFI is diagnosed and treated early. Prompt recognition and life-long dietary fructose restriction leads to rapid and lasting resolution of all the complications. With effective treatment long-term outcome is favorable. Fructose-containing medications, infusions and foods may cause life-threatening recurrence of acute metabolic decompensation.

Mitochondrial Liver Disease[14,15]

The liver has the highest metabolic activity of any organ system in the body and therefore the highest concentration of mitochondria in each cell. Most pathways of intermediary metabolism and synthesis are dependent on mitochondrial metabolism. Neonatal–onset mitochondrial liver disorders usually present with multi-organ involvement. The symptoms and signs are non-specific and mitochondrial disease may not be considered early in the differential diagnosis of liver failure. Lactic acidosis, severe hypoglycemia, elevated liver enzymes and conjugated bilirubinemia are common features of mitochondrial hepatopathy. However, some of these features may not always be present. Hepatosplenomegaly is uncommon. Intrauterine growth retardation, lactic acidosis, hypoglycemia, coagulopathy, and cholestasis, especially in conjunction with neurological symptoms and/or renal tubulopathy increase the likelihood of mitochondrial disease. The absence of lactic acidosis does not exclude mitochondrial disease. Mitochondrial liver disease may occur due to mutations in mitochondrial DNA (maternal inheritance), such as Pearson syndrome or due to mutations in nuclear DNA, e.g. mitochondrial depletion syndrome caused by BCS1L, DGUOK, MPV17, POLG1 mutations.

Investigations

❑ Liver or skeletal muscle biopsy may be required for mitochondrial respiratory function studies
❑ Mitochondrial DNA depletion studies
❑ Specific genetic studies if clinical presentation is classical, e.g. Alpers disease, Pearson disease
❑ Magnetic resonance spectroscopy (MRS) may identify raised lactate in the brain.

Treatment

❑ There are no specific treatments available for mitochondrial disorders
❑ Management is symptomatic and supportive
❑ Liver transplantation has to be considered carefully as multiorgan involvement often leads to poor overall outcome
❑ Prenatal diagnosis, preimplantation genetic diagnosis (PGD) and egg donation are among the reproductive options available to affected couples.

Defects of Long Chain Fatty Acid Metabolism (LCFAODs)[16,17]

LCFAODs are inherited in an autosomal recessive manner and occur due to genetic defects in the transport and function of enzymes that catalyze beta-oxidation of long-chain fatty acids within the mitochondria. As with almost all IMDs, the neonatal form is almost always severe and milder variants may present at any age. LCFAODs are rare but are generally treatable. It is, therefore, vital that the diagnosis is made early and treatment commenced without delay. Without prompt treatment life-threatening complications ensue rapidly. Fatty liver of pregnancy and HELLP syndrome are more frequent in mothers carrying foetuses affected with a long-chain fatty acid oxidation defect (LCFAOD), than in the general population.

Disorders of Transport across the Mitochondrial Membranes

❑ Carnitine palmitoyl transferase I (CPTI) deficiency
This presents with neonatal hypoketotic hypoglycemia, hypertriglyceridemia and lipemia. Hepatomegaly is frequently present at diagnosis
❑ The neonatal form of carnitine palmitoyl transferase II deficiency
The severe neonatal form is often fatal and presents with hypoketotic hypoglycemia, cardiomyopathy, hypotonia, and congenital abnormalities.

Long-chain Fatty Acid Oxidation Defects (LCFAODS)

❑ The neonatal form of long-chain hydroxy acyl CoA dehydrogenase (LCHAD) deficiency and trifunctional protein (TFP) deficiency.
In its severe form, this disorder presents with neonatal encephalopathy, acidosis, cardiomyopathy, and arrhythmia and liver disease. Neonatal mortality is high. Severe congenital defects are common. Milder forms may show

failure to thrive from an early age with repeated attacks of lactic acidosis and hypoketotic hypoglycemia often triggered by intercurrent infections and starvation. Survivors and those with a milder form of the condition continue to have long-term problems despite treatment such as retinopathy, peripheral neuropathy and nephropathy.

□ **Very long-chain acyl CoA dehydrogenase deficiency (VLCADD)**
  Clinical presentation and management are very similar to that of LCHAD.

Investigations

□ Blood: Plasma free carnitine and acylcarnitine analysis are often diagnostic.
□ Urine: Organic acid analysis may indicate/ support the diagnosis.
□ Confirmation of diagnosis by mutation analysis may be required in certain cases, e.g. the common mutation (E474Q) causing the LCHAD deficiency and this helps to differentiate it from TFP deficiency, which is very similar in biochemical basis and acylcarnitine profile.

Treatment

Though the treatment of individual LCFAODs may vary slightly, the general principles of management are:
□ Prevention of metabolic decompensation
□ Provision of plan for emergency management during illness
□ Low-fat diet
□ Medium-chain triglyceride and essential fatty acid supplementation
□ Overnight continuous feeds in infants with short fasting tolerance.

Outcome

The severe, early onset forms of LCFAODs are incompatible with life. They are often diagnosed postmortem during investigation of sudden unexplained infant death. The early diagnosis and management of survivors of neonatal forms of these disorders can lead to a favourable outcome for survival and quality of life. Life-long dietary management will be required and symptoms such as muscle fatigue and rhabdomyolysis may occur during times of illness or metabolic stress. However, these complications can usually be foreseen and prevented.

ISOLATED ORGANOMEGALY OR WHEN ASSOCIATED WITH OTHER CLINICAL FEATURES

Organomegaly at birth or during the neonatal period would be unusual in most forms of inherited metabolic disease. Enlargement of visceral organs, such as the liver, spleen and occasionally the kidneys usually becomes more obvious over the first 2 years of life. Most IMDs that present with organomegaly also have other clinical manifestations. It is usually the other ('extrahepatic') clinical features that draw attention to the underlying metabolic disease. Often, hepatomegaly and splenomegaly are noted incidentally during thorough physical examination in an apparently well child or for an unrelated health issue.

Glycogen Storage Disorders (GSDs/Hepatic Glycogenoses)

GSDs I and III typically present with symptoms, such as hypoglycemia and lactic acidosis, when the interval between feeds increases during infancy. They may also present with an incidental finding of hepatomegaly. The more severe forms can present during the neonatal period with lactic acidosis with or without concurrent hypoglycemia. The GSDs VI and IX are more likely to be diagnosed due to hepatomegaly but may also often have unrecognised hypoglycemia at diagnosis. GSD IV presents with progressive liver dysfunction in addition to hypoglycemia and is one of the few IMDs that cause liver cirrhosis. Chronic energy deficiency often results in poor linear growth and delayed diagnosis. Asymptomatic hypoglycemia may lead to developmental delay.

Glycogen Storage Disease Type Ia (Glucose-6-Phosphatase Deficiency)[18]

GSD type Ia is inherited in an autosomal recessive manner and presents with poor tolerance of fasting, growth retardation and hepatomegaly resulting from accumulation of glycogen and fat in the liver.

GSD type Ia accounts for nearly 80% of patients of GSD type I. The disease may manifest in the neonatal period with hepatomegaly or more commonly in early infancy with symptoms of hypoglycemia with increasing intervals between feeds. Hepatomegaly, growth retardation, osteopenia, and osteoporosis due to persistent lactic acidosis, a typical full or round face, nephromegaly (hence 'hepatorenal glycogenosis') are frequent features. Epistaxis may occur due to platelet dysfunction.

In type GSD Ib (20% of patients with GSD type I), there is an increased susceptibility to infections and inflammatory bowel disease, due to neutrophil dysfunction).

Investigations

□ Hypoglycemia, increased plasma lactic acid, short fasting tolerance
□ Increased plasma uric acid, serum triglycerides, and cholesterol

- Mutation analysis is the investigation of choice to confirm the diagnosis and identify the type of GSD type I, which is of crucial importance
- Liver biopsy will indicate glycogen storage, and enzyme analysis may be required if genetic testing is not available.

Treatment

- Prevention of hypoglycemia—frequent feeds, overnight nasogastric tube feeds, and uncooked corn starch (UCCS)
- Gastrostomy may be required in GSD Ia but should be avoided in GSD Ib, as neutrophil dysfunction could lead to poor healing and complications
- Hyperuricemia will require treatment with allopurinol and hepatic complications
- G-CSF for neutropenia in GSD Ib
- Liver (GSD Ia/Ib) and/or bone marrow transplantation (in GSD Ib).

Glycogen Storage Disease Type III (GSDIII) (Glycogen Debrancher Deficiency)[19]

GSD III is a recessive disorder that usually presents in early childhood. Clinical features can be fairly similar to GSD I—hepatomegaly, growth retardation and hypoglycemia. Progressive muscle weakness is common in GSD III (though this can also be present in GSD I). Hypotonia and hypertrophic cardiomyopathy are features of the GSDIIIa phenotype. The liver is predominantly affected in the GSDIIIb phenotype.

Investigation

- Hypoglycemia, usually without lactic acidemia
- Hypertriglyceridemia and elevated liver enzymes (CK)
- Liver biopsy is rarely indicated but will show glycogen accumulation
- Mutation analysis to confirm the diagnosis.

Treatment

- Prevention of hypoglycemia, as in GSD I
- Overnight nasogastric or gastrostomy feeds
- Uncooked corn starch (UCCS).

Glycogen Storage Disease type IV (Glycogen Brancher Deficiency)[20]

GSD IV is a recessively inherited, severe and progressive form of glycogen storage disease. Typically, children develop hepatomegaly, hypotonia, and developmental delay during early infancy. Cirrhosis with portal hypertension and ascites eventually ensues, leading to death in early childhood. A static hepatic phenotype and neuromuscular presentations are also known.

Investigation

- Liver biopsy might shows accumulation of abnormal glycogen (amylopectin)
- Enzyme assay in liver biopsy specimens, blood, skin fibroblasts.

Treatment

- Liver transplant can be life saving, as cirrhosis often leads to reduced life expectancy.

Prognosis for Hepatic GSDs

GSD I, III and IV may be identified in infancy, although diagnosis is usually made in the first years of life. The prognosis is generally good, as long as symptoms, such as hypoglycemia are recognised early and treated effectively. Complications involving the bones, heart, muscle and kidneys can affect long-term outcome and quality of life. Short stature, obesity and psychological problems are common in later in life. Children with GSDIV are likely to suffer from complications of cirrhosis and malignancy, unless liver transplantation is performed early. Adenomas and malignancy also occur later in life in other hepatic glycogenosis.

Mucopolysaccharidoses (MPS)[21]

The mucopolysaccharidoses arise due to specific inherited enzyme deficiencies resulting in abnormal lysosomal storage of complex carbohydrate molecules—glycosaminoglycans (GAGs). All the disorders are inherited in an autosomal recessive manner except for MPS II, which is an X-linked recessive disorder (Table 27.4).

Each MPS subtype generally presents with a typical constellation of clinical features with considerable overlap. Hepatomegaly, splenomegaly, and symptoms, such as recurrent upper airway obstruction, are conductive deafness due to serous otitis media are common in MPS disorders and usually precede the diagnosis by months or years. Hepatomegaly and splenomegaly may only be identified in infancy by an astute clinician and the diagnosis is usually made in the second year of life. Dysmorphism (coarse facial features, short-neck, large tongue), skeletal abnormalities (dysostosis multiplex), kyphoscoliosis, short stature, joint stiffness become gradually apparent. Facial dysmorphism is almost never

Table 27.4: Mucopolysaccharidoses

Disorder	GAG storage material	Deficient enzyme	Genetic inheritance
MPS I (Hurler, Hurler–Scheie, Scheie syndromes)	Dermatan sulfate, heparan sulfate	α-L-iduronidase	Autosomal recessive
MPS II (Hunter syndrome)	Dermatan sulfate, heparan sulfate	Iduronate-2-sulfatase	X-linked recessive
MPS III A, B, C, D (Sanfilippo syndrome)	Heparan sulfate	A: Heparan N-sulfatase B: α-N-acetylglucosaminidase C: Acetyl-CoA: α-glucosaminide acetyltransferase D: N-acetylglucosamine 6-sulfatase	Autosomal recessive
MPS IV A, B (Morquio syndrome)	A: Keratan sulfate, chondroitin sulfate	A: Galactose 6-sulfatase	Autosomal recessive
	B: Keratan sulfate	B: β-galactosidase	
MPS VI (Maroteaux–Lamy syndrome)	Dermatan sulfate, chondroitin sulfate	Arylsulfatase B	Autosomal recessive
MPS VII (Sly syndrome)	Dermatan sulfate, heparan sulphate, chondroitin sulfate	β-Glucuronidase	Autosomal recessive
MPS IX	Hyaluronic acid	Hyaluronidase	Autosomal recessive

present at birth. MPS IV is associated with joint laxity and extreme short stature. Indeed, MPS disorders should always be considered in the differential diagnosis of short limbed dwarfism and skeletal dysplasia. Stenotic and regurgitant cardiac valve defects, obstructive and restrictive lung defects are frequent. Corneal clouding is a feature of MPS I, MPS IV, and MPS VI. Progressive storage of GAGs in the brain leads to developmental delay in almost all MPS disorders and neurological regression especially in MPS II and MPS III. MPS VII has been reported to present with hepatomegaly and cholestatic jaundice. Multiple sulfatase deficiency (MSD) may present in the neonatal period with similar dysmorphic features which may be clinically indistinguishable from MPS disorders.

Investigations

- ❑ Urine: Glycosaminoglycans and oligosaccharide electrophoresis.
- ❑ Blood: Enzyme analysis in white cells.
- ❑ Radiology: Skeletal survey.

Treatment

Symptomatic and supportive interventions as indicated
- ❑ Bone marrow transplantation might be the best treatment option in severe forms of MPS I (Hurler

Syndrome), especially if performed before the second birthday.
- ❑ Intravenous recombinant enzyme replacement therapy (ERT) is currently available for MPS I, MPS II, MPS IV and MPS VI. While intravenous ERT might help reduce storage of GAGs in some organ systems, improve stamina and quality of life, it does not cross the blood–brain barrier and hence does not treat the CNS manifestations
- ❑ Gene therapy and alternative routes of ERT administration are undergoing clinical trials.

Outcome

ERT is available for MPS I, II, VI and improves the life expectancy and quality of life. However, this form of therapy is prohibitively expensive and cannot be considered to be cost-effective. Progressive neurological and cardio-respiratory complications shorten the life-expectancy in most MPS disorders.

Gaucher Disease (Glucocerebrosidase Deficiency)[22]

Gaucher disease (GD) is an autosomal recessive, inherited lysosomal storage disorder caused by a deficiency of the enzyme, glucocerebrosidase. There are 3 main types of GD—types I–III.

Type I GD is known as non-neuronopathic GD, while type II and type III are known as neuronopathic GD.

GD type I is the chronic and non-neurological form associated with organomegaly (spleen, liver), bone complications (bone pain, osteonecrosis, pathological fractures) and pancytopenia.

GD type II, the early–onset, severe, acute neurological form presents with rapidly progressing brainstem dysfunction, organomegaly and death before the second birthday.

GD type III, the subacute neurological form, affects infants, children or adolescents and is characterized by progressive neurological regression (strabismus, nystagmus, oculomotor apraxia, epilepsy and ataxia) along with the systemic manifestations seen in GD type I.

Investigations

- White cell enzyme assay will confirm glucerebrosidase deficiency
- Chitotriosidase, a nonspecific indicator of macrophage activation is increased
- Bone marrow examination: Gaucher-like cells may be demonstrated.

Treatment

- Enzyme replacement therapy is available for GD type I and type III
- GD III is associated with progressive neurological disease. Bone marrow transplantation should be considered in those with GD type III, and significant neurological involvement
- Substrate deprivation therapy (Miglustat) may be a treatment option for GD type I (and GD type III) in specific circumstances.

Prognosis

The prognosis is good in GD type I with normal life expectancy while receiving regular ERT. In GD type II, death usually occurs before the second birthday. GD type III is associated with reduced life expectancy, though survival into the third and fourth decade is well known (Table 27.5).

Niemann-Pick Disease A and B (NPC A and B)[23]

Niemann-Pick disease type A and B (NPC A and B) are autosomal recessive inherited lysosomal storage disorders that occur due to the deficiency of the enzyme spingomyelinase. They are biochemically and clinically distinct from Niemann-Pick disease type C (NP-C) which is an autosomal recessive disorder of cholesterol trafficking.

Niemann-Pick disease type A (NP-A) is the very severe end of the spectrum of spingomyelinase deficiency. In

Table 27.5: Metabolic disorders that present with organomegaly in infancy

Isolated hepatomegaly
- Glycogen storage diseases I, III, IV
- Mucopolysaccharidoses (not at birth, but later appears in infancy)
- Fatty acid oxidation defects—CPT I deficiency
- Hereditary fructose intolerance

Isolated splenomegaly
- Non-neuronopathic—Gaucher disease (type I)
- Neuronopathic—Gaucher disease (types II, III)
- Niemann-Pick disease—type A, B, C

Hepatosplenomegaly
- Mucopolysaccharidoses (MPS) (presentation unusual in infancy)

Other disorders
- Urea cycle defects (argininosuccinic aciduria)

addition to hepatosplenomegaly, infants present with failure to thrive, and rapidly progressive neurological regression, hypotonia, liver failure and death before the second birthday.

Niemann-Pick disease type B (NP-B) is the mild subtype of spingomyelinase deficiency, and presents with insidious onset of hepatosplenomegaly, which is usually identified incidentally during routine physical examination or with a protuberant abdomen in childhood. NP-B is associated with growth retardation, recurrent bruising due to thrombocytopenia from splenic sequestration, infiltrative lung disease causing respiratory symptoms such as cough, breathlessness (usually misdiagnosed as bronchial asthma) and bone disease. The central nervous system is spared and the absence of neurological features clearly differentiates NP-B from NP-A, which is always associated with severe neurological regression. Patients with NP-B have normal life expectancy though they suffer significant morbidity.

Investigations

- Full blood count—anemia, thrombocytopenia
- Abdominal ultrasound examination
- CT-Scan of the chest—will show infiltrative lung disease
- Plasma chitotriosidase is almost always elevated (though normal chitotriosidase does not exclude the condition as pseudodeficiency is known to occur in about 5% of the population)
- Enzyme assay in leukocytes confirms the enzyme deficiency
- Mutation analysis will provide further confirmation.

Treatment

- Symptomatic treatment.
- There is no specific treatment available, although ERT is currently undergoing clinical trial.

Prognosis

NP-B is associated with normal life-expectancy though significant morbidity. Infants with NP-A, however suffer from severe rapid neurological regression that almost always leads to death in the first two years of life.

Other Disorders

Urea Cycle Enzyme Defects (UCEDs)

Urea cycle enzyme defects (UCEDs) are inherited disorders of nitrogen detoxification, which takes place mainly in the liver. In severe, early onset variants, hyperammonemic coma presents within hours or days after birth. The duration and severity of hyperammonemia strongly correlates with long-term brain damage. In milder, later onset variants, symptoms can be variable—ranging from asymptomatic adults with normal neurological function to those with recurrent episodes of hyperammonemia and learning difficulties. All UCEDs are inherited in an autosomal recessive fashion except OTC deficiency, which is an X-linked recessive disorder (Table 27.6).

There may be no abnormal clinical features during times of health. Hyperammonemic encephalopathy and liver dysfunction often occur during times of illness and metabolic stress. Hepatomegaly is a feature of ASA but not usually of other UCEDs. Arginase deficiency may present in the neonatal period with hyperammonemia but more typically presents with progressive spastic diplegia. Females with OTC deficiency may also present with clinical features similar to that in males, due to lyonization. Late onset forms of UCEDs are generally milder, though death and disability can occur at any age without early diagnosis and treatment.

Investigations

- ❏ Plasma amino acids
  - The most likely UCED can be identified with a fair degree of certainty, based on the plasma quantitative amino acid profile. Increased plasma glutamine and glutamic acid reflect hyperammonemia. Reduced citrulline indicates a proximal UCED while a raised citrulline indicates a more distal defect
- ❏ Urine organic acids
  - Increased orotic acid suggests the likelihood of OTC deficiency. Absence of urinary orotic acid may indicate the likelihood of a more proximal UCED such as CPS or NAGS
- ❏ Urine amino acids
  - Shows increased argininosuccinic acid in ASA and glutamine in most UCEDs
- ❏ Liver function tests
- ❏ Skin biopsy—enzyme assay to confirm the diagnosis
- ❏ Mutation analysis—will help confirm the diagnosis and genetic counseling.

Treatment

- ❏ The principle of management of UCEDs is essentially a combination of a low protein diet and ammonia – scavenging medications, such as sodium benzoate, sodium phenylbutyrate and supplementation of either L-arginine or L-citrulline
- ❏ Emergency management regimens may help prevent further metabolic decompensation during illness or metabolic stress
- ❏ Haemofiltration or dialysis may be required to rapidly treat severe hyperammonemia
- ❏ Liver transplantation may remove the need for life-long dietary protein restriction and medications
- ❏ Gene therapy and hepatocyte transplantation are being developed.

Table 27.6: Classical urea cycle enzyme disorders		
Inheritance	Enzyme	Urea cycle enzyme defect
AR	N-Acetylglutamate synthetase (NAGS)	N-Acetylglutamate synthase deficiency
AR	Carbamoyl phosphate synthetase I (CPS1)	Carbamoyl phosphate synthetase I deficiency
XR	Ornithine transcarbamylase (OTC)	Ornithine transcarbamylase deficiency
AR	Argininosuccinic acid synthetase (ASS)	Citrullinemia
AR	Argininosuccinase acid lyase (ASL)	Argininosuccinic aciduria (ASA)
AR	Arginase (ARG)	Arginase deficiency

Abbreviations: AR, autosomal recessive inheritance; XR, X-linked recessive inheritance.

Outcome

All the urea cycle disorders are treatable, although the long-term outcome tends to be generally poor in the early onset variants. Prenatal diagnosis may allow termination of an affected fetus or early presymptomatic treatment, which could lead to improved outcomes. Prevention of episodes of hyperammonemia is essential. Liver transplantation should be offered, where available, and is likely to be successful in all UCEDs except perhaps in arginase deficiency. ASA is associated with a poor long-term outcome even if severe hyperammonemia is prevented.

HYDROPS FETALIS

Mucolipidosis (I-cell Disease or MLII)[24]

Mucolipidosis II (or I-cell disease) (MLII) is a rare autosomal recessive lysosomal storage disease arising due to autosomal recessive, inherited N-acetylglucosamine 1-phosphotransferase deficiency. This leads to the defective mannose-6–phosphate mediated lysosomal targeting of many lysosomal enzymes. Clinical and radiological signs are varied and similar to those in mucopolysaccharidoses. However, MLII presents earlier than the MPS disorders. It can present in the antenatal period or at birth with hydrops fetalis, during the neonatal period with multiple congenital abnormalities, cardiac failure, ascites, fractures and hypophosphatemia mimicking rickets. The disorder is fatal during childhood because of cardiorespiratory failure, arrthymia, and infections. Gingival hypertrophy, enlarged tongue, coarse facies, hirsutism, congenital hernias, joint stiffness, dysostosis multiplex, hepato-splenomegaly, corneal opacities, deafness, developmental delay, and growth retardation are characteristic (Table 27.7).

Investigation

Investigation of unexplained hydrops fetalis should always include glycosaminoglycan and oligosaccharide electrophoresis in urine. Urine oligosaccharide analysis will demonstrate increased excretion in MLII.

White cell enzymes will show generalized increase in lysosomal enzymes (hydrolases).

Enzyme assay and mutation analysis will confirm the diagnosis.

Treatment

No specific treatment is available. Supportive treatment includes management of cardiac failure and treatment of hypophosphatemia.

Outcome

It is highly unusual for infants with MLII to survive beyond their second birthday.

CONCLUSION

Though IMDs that cause liver disease are individually rare, they should be considered early in the differential diagnosis. Awareness of the clinical features of IMDs and a high index of suspicion will enable early diagnosis. Prompt investigation and treatment are essential in order to save life and prevent disability. Though some IMDs remain untreatable at present, there are several others for which empirical and specific treatments are available. Understanding the genetic basis and prenatal testing may enable genetic counseling and inform reproductive options. Early postnatal treatment before the onset of symptoms may lead to better outcome in many IMDs. Liver transplantation offers a lasting solution for several IMDs that cause severe liver disease.[25] Newborn screening and newer interventions, such as prenatal genetic diagnosis (PGD), gene therapy, and hepatocyte transplantation have raised expectations of improved outcome for IMD related liver disease in the future.

Table 27.7: Metabolic causes of hydrops and neonatal ascites
Lysosomal storage disorders
• Mucolipidosis type II (I-cell disease)
• Mucopolysaccharidosis VII
• Gaucher disease
• Wolman disease
• Niemann-Pick type A and C
• GM I gangliosidosis
• Sialic acid storage disease
• Sialidosis type II
Other IMDs that can cause hydrops fetalis
• Hereditary tyrosinemia type 1
• Congenital disorders of glycosylation

REFERENCES

1. McKiernan P. Metabolic liver disease. Clin Res Hepatol Gastroenterol. 2012;36(3):287-90.
2. Bosch AM. Classical galactosaemia revisited. J Inherit Metab Dis. 2006;29(4):516-25.
3. Walter JH, JE Collins, JV Leonard. Recommendations for the management of galactosaemia. UK Galactosaemia Steering Group. Arch Dis Child. 1999;80(1):93-6.
4. de Laet C, et al. Recommendations for the management of tyrosinaemia type 1. Orphanet J Rare Dis. 2013;8:8.
5. Hutchin T, et al. Neonatal intrahepatic cholestasis caused by citrin deficiency (NICCD) as a cause of liver disease in infants in the UK. J Inherit Metab Dis. 2009;32(Suppl 1):S151-5.
6. Ohura T, et al. Clinical pictures of 75 patients with neonatal intrahepatic cholestasis caused by citrin deficiency (NICCD). J Inherit Metab Dis. 2007;30(2):139-44.

7. Saheki T, et al. Citrin deficiency and current treatment concepts. Mol Genet Metab. 2010;100(Suppl 1): S59-64.

8. Patterson MC, et al. Recommendations for the diagnosis and management of Niemann-Pick disease type C: an update. Mol Genet Metab. 2012;106(3):330-44.

9. Grabowski G. Therapy for lysosomal acid lipase deficiency: replacing a missing link. Hepatology. 2013;58(3):850-2.

10. Zhang B, AF Porto. Cholesteryl ester storage disease: protean presentations of lysosomal acid lipase deficiency. J Pediatr Gastroenterol Nutr. 2013;56(6):682-5.

11. Balwani M, et al. Clinical effect and safety profile of recombinant human lysosomal acid lipase in patients with cholesteryl ester storage disease. Hepatology. 2013;58(3):950-7.

12. Steinberg SJ, et al. Peroxisome Biogenesis Disorders. Zellweger Syndrome Spectrum. 1993.

13. Jaeken J. Congenital disorders of glycosylation (CDG): it's (nearly) all in it! J Inherit Metab Dis. 2011;34(4):853-8.

14. Lee WS, RJ Sokol. Liver disease in mitochondrial disorders. Semin Liver Dis. 2007;27(3):259-73.

15. Fellman V, H Kotarsky. Mitochondrial hepatopathies in the newborn period. Semin Fetal Neonatal Med. 2011;16(4):222-8.

16. Spiekerkoetter U, PA Wood. Mitochondrial fatty acid oxidation disorders: pathophysiological studies in mouse models. J Inherit Metab Dis. 2010;33(5):539-46.

17. Spiekerkoetter U, et al. Current issues regarding treatment of mitochondrial fatty acid oxidation disorders. J Inherit Metab Dis. 2010;33(5):555-61.

18. Bali DS, Chen YT, Goldstein JL. Glycogen Storage Disease Type I. 1993.

19. Kishnani PS, et al. Glycogen storage disease type III diagnosis and management guidelines. Genet Med. 2010;12(7):446-63.

20. Magoulas PL, El-Hattab AW. Glycogen Storage Disease Type IV. 1993.

21. Muenzer J. Overview of the mucopolysaccharidoses. Rheumatology (Oxford). 2011;50(Suppl 5):v4-12.

22. Pastores GM, Hughes DA. Gaucher Disease. 1993.

23. McGovern MM, Schuchman EH. Acid Sphingomyelinase Deficiency. 1993.

24. Leroy JG, Cathey S, Friez MJ. Mucolipidosis II. 1993.

25. McKiernan P. Liver transplantation and cell therapies for inborn errors of metabolism. J Inherit Metab Dis. 2013;36(4):675-80.

Chapter 28

Metabolic Disorders in the Older Child

Wikrom Karnsakul, Kathleen B Schwarz

Metabolic disorders include defects in bile acid synthesis, progressive familial intrahepatic cholestasis (PFIC 1–3), Alagille syndrome, storage disorders affecting the liver, cystic fibrosis liver disease and disorders of heme metabolism and the liver. The first three are characterized by chronic cholestasis whereas storage diseases (especially glycogen storage disease on which we are focusing) typically present with hepatomegaly and the metabolic defects secondary to the aberrant enzyme, particularly hypoglycemia. In contrast, cystic fibrosis liver disease and disorders of heme metabolism are multi-system diseases with cirrhosis being the ultimate consequence of the hepatic involvement. Each section will begin with a common clinical scenario.

DEFECTS IN BILE ACID SYNTHESIS

CLINICAL SCENARIO

Saudi Arabian parents who were first cousins had three children with progressive liver disease starting in the neonatal period. The first affected child, a girl, was jaundiced from the first week of life with pale stools and dark urine. She had loose stools and never developed pruritus. Her growth and mental development in infancy were normal. Laboratory testing showed increased direct bilirubin, alkaline phosphatase and aminotransferases. At 18 months physical examination was remarkable for hepatosplenomegaly and a normal facies. A liver biopsy showed giant cell hepatitis and bridging fibrosis with normal intrahepatic bile ducts. She died following a gastrointestinal hemorrhage at 19 months. The second child, a boy, had a similar course. A liver biopsy at 6 weeks showed giant cell hepatitis. He remained jaundiced but had no pruritus and only mild steatorrhea. His developmental progress was normal. At the age of 3 years, 9 months he had a second biopsy. Canalicular bile plugs, neocholangiolar proliferation and micronodular cirrhosis were present. He succumbed to hemorrhage following the biopsy. The third child presented with neonatal cholestasis and pale stools. At the age of 3 months his physical examination was remarkable for moderate jaundice and hepatomegaly. Laboratory examination revealed results similar to that of his sister; in addition values for

Contd...

CLINICAL SCENARIO (CONTD...)

plasma 25 hydroxy-vitamin D and vitamin E were very low. 72 hours fecal fat was increased. Analysis of serum bile acids was remarkable for the absence of cholic and chenodeoxycholic acid, suggestive of an inborn error of bile acid synthesis. Examination of the urine by fast atom bombardment mass spectroscopy showed abnormal bile acids consistent with 3β-hydroxy-C27-steroid dehydrogenase oxidoreductase deficiency.[1,2] The child was treated with cholic and chenodeoxycholic acids and supplemental fat-soluble vitamins. The cholestasis gradually resolved and the child thrived.

The two primary acidic bile acids (cholic and chenodeoxy- cholic acids) are formed from cholesterol and there are many different enzymes involved in this pathway. The first genetic defect to be described in this pathway was the rare lipid storage disorder—cerebrotendinous xanthomatosis.[3,4] This disorder is caused by several different mutations in the sterol 27-hydroxylase enzyme. The presentation is in adult life with xanthomas, premature atherosclerosis and dementia. However, recently Setchell et al[5] described a patient with neonatal cholestasis who had a mutation in this enzyme.

There are currently seven known genetic defects of bile acid malabsorption and the clinical presentation is quite variable. Some present with neonatal cholestasis progressing to giant cell hepatitis and cirrhosis whereas others are characterized by fat-soluble vitamin deficiency and neurologic disease. The seven defects include 3β-hydroxy-C_{27}-steroid dehydrogenase oxidoreductase deficiency which was the first to be described,[1] Δ^4-3-oxosteroid 5β-reductase deficiency, oxysterol 7α hydroxylase deficiency, 2-methylacyl-CoA racemase deficiency, sterol 27-hydroxylase deficiency, bile acid-CoA: amino acid N-acyltransferase deficiency, and cholesterol 7α-hydroxylase deficiency.[3] These diseases are all rare and only about 100 patients with any of them have been described, accounting for ~2% of all cases of unexplained liver disease.[3]

The age at diagnosis can be quite variable and the diseases should be suspected with unexplained late onset cholestasis. The phenotype is determined by the type of enzyme defect. If a patient has a defect involving an enzyme responsible for catalyzing reactions in the steroid nucleus, he/she usually presents with varying degrees of hyperbilirubinemia, elevations in serum aminotransferases and on clinical examination, hepatosplenomegaly. However, for patients with a defect involving modifications to the cholesterol side-chain the presentation is usually fat-soluble vitamin malabsorption and/or neurological disease.[3]

The major take-home lesson regarding this family of defects is that the presentation varies from neonatal to late onset cholestasis which can evolve to fatal cirrhotic liver disease unless diagnosed and treated. The diseases should be suspected when serum bile acids and gamma-glutamyl-transpeptidase are normal in a cholestatic patient. Diagnosis is confirmed by examination of the urine with fast atom bombardment mass spectroscopy. Treatment for most of these defects should be undertaken with the primary bile acids cholic and chenodeoxycholic acid since the liver injury is thought to be secondary to their absence as well as the presence of toxic metabolites. Cholic and chenodeoxycholic acid are necessary to stimulate bile acid dependent bile flow. Therapy with these bile acids is assessed both clinically and by the disappearance of toxic bile acid metabolites from the urine. Chronic administration of cholic acid in patients with primary bile acid synthetic defects has been shown to be safe and can preserve liver function, thus avoiding the need for liver transplantation.[6]

PROGRESSIVE FAMILIAL INTRAHEPATIC CHOLESTASIS (PFIC)— TYPES 1, 2, AND 3

CLINICAL SCENARIO

A 17-year-old Pakistani male presented with a history of liver transplantation 12 years earlier for severe cholestasis and pruritus despite partial external biliary diversion. Given that serum gamma-glutamyl transpeptidase (GGT) was normal it was thought that his liver disease was most consistent with PFIC 2 but genetic testing had not been performed. He presented to the emergency department at age 17 years with a history of rising total bilirubin over the preceding 7 days in association with pruritus, diarrhea, nausea and vomiting. Total serum bilirubin rose from 0.5, 1.9, 2.5, to 2.7 mg/dL over this time period. Total serum bilirubin was 3.0 mg/dL and GGT was normal. AST was mildly elevated. He was admitted to the hospital. Over the next month the bilirubin slowly rose to a peak of 22 mg/dL. Percutaneous liver biopsy showed minimal portal inflammation, moderate lobular canalicular bile plugging and no evidence of acute or chronic cellular rejection.

Contd...

CLINICAL SCENARIO (CONTD...)

Imaging studies showed mild intrahepatic ductal dilatation. He underwent endoscopic retrograde cholangiography which demonstrated a stricture at the hepatic-jejunostomy and a biliary stent was placed. However serum bilirubin only fell slightly. Given the lack of response to biliary stenting and the normal GGT, the diagnosis of antibody-mediated recurrent PFIC 2 [bile salt export pump (BSEP) deficiency] was entertained. Genetic studies revealed a homozygous splice site mutation in the ABCB11 gene: c.1639 (-2) A>C, predictive of PFIC 2. Immunostaining of the liver explant revealed an absence of BSEP; the liver graft revealed normal BSEP. Serum anti-BSEP antibody was positive at 1:1280. The patient was treated with plasmapheresis to remove the antibody, intravenous gamma-globulin to replace amounts lost in the plasmapheresis, and an anti-CD20 monoclonal antibody to prevent B cells from synthesizing the anti-BSEP antibody. One year later the patient is clinically well with normal laboratory values.[7]

Normal bile formation is dependent on hepatocanalicular transporters and deficiency of these transporters leads to cholestatic liver disease. Deficiency of ATP8B1 (FIC1), a P4 P-type ATPase, which is essential for a proper composition of the canalicular membrane, is the cause of PFIC 1.[9] ATP8B 1 translocates phosphatidyl-serine from the outer to the inner leaflet of plasma membranes, causing the outer leaflet to be enriched in phosphatidylcholine, sphingomyelin and cholesterol.[10,11] PFIC 1, also called Byler's disease, is characterized by progressive cholestatic liver disease sometimes accompanied by extrahepatic manifestations such as diarrhea. Liver biopsy generally shows bland cholestasis with coarse granular bile visible by electron microscopy. Deficiency of this enzyme is also characteristic of BRIC 1 which is a milder syndrome with intermittent cholestasis.

ABCB 11 (BSEP) ABCB 11 deficiency (PFIC 2, BRIC 2) causes a spectrum of intrahepatic cholestasis. BSEP is the major bile salt export pump and patients with PFIC 2 suffer from progressive cholestasis, pruritus and in some cases cholelithiasis. Liver biopsy shows peri-portal fibrosis and bile duct proliferation. Ultrastructural examination of the liver shows amorphous canalicular bile. Deficiency of this enzyme also causes a milder phenotype (BRIC 2: episodic cholestasis and pruritus). In patients with BRIC 2, in between episodes there are no symptoms. In both PFIC 1 and PFIC 2, serum bile acids are elevated but GGT is normal.

Patients with ABCB 4 (MDR 3), ABCB 4 deficiency (PFIC 3) exhibit progressive intrahepatic cholestasis, and high serum GGT concentrations secondary to defective transport of phosphatidylcholine into bile. Pruritus is less prominent than in PFIC 1 and 2. Liver biopsy shows fibrosis and marked bile duct proliferation.

Management strategies for these diseases have been nicely summarized by Stapelbroek et al.[8] Oral rifampicin can decrease pruritus in PFIC 1 and 2 whereas ursodeoxycholic acid can be effective in some patients with PFIC 3. Partial external biliary diversion usually decreases pruritus in patients with PFIC 1 and 2 but liver transplantation is sometimes necessary in those with PFIC 1 and 2 who do not benefit from biliary diversion. Patients with PFIC 3 often develop severe symptoms requiring liver transplantation. However, more specific therapies are currently being developed including nuclear receptors as a target, using chaperones to enhance the expression of the mutated transporter protein and mutation-specific therapies. These rational therapies hold considerable future promise.

ALAGILLE SYNDROME (AGS)

CLINICAL SCENARIO

A 9-year-old male with AGS, presented for evaluation for liver transplantation. The medical history revealed neonatal cholestasis diagnosed at an outside hospital led to the performance of a Kasai hepatic portoenterostomy on the basis of presumed biliary atresia. The other significant medical problem in the neonatal period was pulmonary atresia with tetralogy of Fallot. At 2 months he was referred for evaluation for liver transplantation given that the cholestasis did not improve post-Kasai. Review of the liver biopsies from the outside hospital was done by an experienced liver pathologist who commented that "This is a challenging case. The liver biopsy shows mild periductular fibrosis but the histological findings are not diagnostic of classic biliary atresia. The portal plate sections do show small-sized bile ducts suggesting at least a biliary hypoplasia. The biopsy does not show significant bile duct loss or atrophy to strongly suggest Alagille syndrome. However, the bile duct paucity seen in Alagille syndrome often takes time to develop and the biopsy, while certainly not diagnostic, could be consistent with Alagille syndrome."

In the ensuing 9 years, he underwent multiple cardiothoracic surgical procedures to correct the tetralogy of Fallot and pulmonary atresia. Genetic evaluation demonstrated a mutation in the Jagged 1 gene consistent with AGS. At age of 9 years, he had short stature and diminished muscle mass, typical AGS facies with frontal bossing, hypertelorism and triangular chin, pruritus, hyper-cholesterolemia with xanthomata, growth failure and was dependent on gastrostomy-tube feeding. He had a history of significant muscle weakness due to a low phosphorus secondary to vitamin D deficiency despite extremely high-dose vitamin D supplementation. He had fractured his right humerus four years earlier while throwing a baseball. Progressive thrombocytopenia and splenomegaly were consistent with evolving portal hypertension. Careful re-evaluation of his cardiac status was the initial step before serious consideration of liver transplantation could be undertaken.

Alagille syndrome is an autosomal dominant disorder due to mutations in the gene *JAG1*, occurring in 1:100,000 live births.[12] Although neonatal cholestasis is the main feature presenting to the pediatrician, there are other features which form the syndrome including congenital heart disease (most commonly peripheral pulmonic stenosis, but pulmonary atresia, tetralogy of Fallot, atrial septal defect and ventricular septal defect have all been reported). There is a peculiar characteristic facies, butterfly vertebrae and ocular embryotoxon. Liver biopsy shows bile duct paucity but as noted by the clinical scenario above, the histopathologic pattern in early infancy may not be fully developed. For this reason the liver disease is sometimes confused with biliary atresia in young infants but performance of the Kasai in young infants with AGS appears to worsen outcome and should be avoided.[13]

AGS is essentially a vasculopathy as suggested by the fact that Jagged 1 is predominately expressed in the vasculature, disruption of the Jagged 1 gene in mice leads to lethal cardiac defects and non-cardiac vascular defects such as renal artery stenosis and intracerebral vascular anomalies are frequently observed.[14] Prognosis depends principally on the evolution of cardiac and liver disease. Although hepatocellular carcinoma is rare it has been reported in young children with AGS.

Evaluation of a child with AGS for liver transplantation should be done with great care. Common indications for consideration of liver transplantation in children with AGS include a poor quality of life secondary to refractory pruritus, generalized xanthomata, fractures and severe growth retardation. End stage liver disease is uncommon. Evaluation for transplant should include careful assessment of cardiac performance preoperatively with dynamic stress tests to mimic the hemodynamic changes which occur during liver transplantation.[15,16]

STORAGE DISORDERS AFFECTING THE LIVER

CLINICAL SCENARIO

A 13-month-old male infant was found to have hepatomegaly during a visit to his pediatrician. The Bangladeshi parents (who were first cousins) noted irritability and diaphoresis since birth and reported that they had to feed him every few hours during the night to control his fussiness. Laboratory tests showed a non-fasting glucose of 91 mg/dL, AST and ALT at approximately 30 times normal values and an otherwise normal hepatic function panel. Lactate and uric acid were normal but cholesterol and triglyceride were significantly elevated. Creatine kinase (CK), tested because of a history of delayed gross motor function, was 10 times the normal value. Fasting serum glucose was 57 mg/dL.

Contd...

CLINICAL SCENARIO (CONTD...)

Percutaneous liver and thigh muscle biopsies were performed after a 6 hour fast. The liver biopsy showed markedly distended glycogen laden hepatocytes and portal and focal septate fibrosis. Glycogen content in the thigh muscle was 6.4% (normal 0.94 +/− 0.55%) and the debranching enzyme activity was 0 micro mol/min/gram tissue (normal 0.28 +/− 0.08). These findings were consistent with GSD TYPE IIIa. The patient was treated with frequent administration of uncooked corn starch and a high protein diet. His hypoglycemia, elevated serum aminotransferases, lipid profile and hepatomegaly were significantly improved at the 2-year follow-up visit but the gross motor function gradually worsened, with CK values rising over time.

Deficient activity of enzymes in hepatocytes or reticuloendothelial systems can result in abnormal storage of substances in these organs particularly in the liver. In this section the focus is glycogen storage diseases (GSD). Other storage disorders affecting the liver will not be discussed here including nonalcoholic fatty liver disease, fibrinogen storage disease, lysosomal storage disorders, Gaucher, Fabry, Niemann-Pick diseases, mucopolysaccharidoses, Wolman disease and cholesteryl ester storage disease.

GSDs are metabolic disorders with a wide spectrum of presenting features depending on their individual enzyme deficiencies (Table 28.1). The lack of these enzymes leads to abnormal synthesis, degradation, and storage of glycogen in different organs.[17-22] The principal storage depots for glycogen are the liver and skeletal muscle. Hypoglycemia is the primary consequence of liver involvement.[17-22] A mutation in a single gene is responsible for defective synthesis of specific enzymes; however, there is phenotypic variation with differences in age at presentation of symptoms, morbidity, and mortality.

In GSD TYPE 0, deficiency in glycogen synthase results in a significant reduction in liver glycogen stores (aglycogenosis). Dietary carbohydrate is converted to lactate rather than being stored as glycogen in the liver. While fasting, hypoglycemia leads to lethargy, pallor, nausea, vomiting, and, rarely, seizures. Hyperglycemia, glycosuria, and lactic acidosis occur postprandially mimicking diabetes. Developmental delay, short stature and osteopenia may be observed in some children.[17-22]

In GSD TYPE I (von Gierke disease, hepatorenal glycogenosis), affected children have defect in glycogenolysis and gluconeogenesis leading to severe hypoglycemia and lactic acidosis, hypertriglyceridemia, and hyperuricemia since birth.[17-29] Severe hypoglycemic tremors, irritability, hyperventilation, cyanosis, apnea, convulsions, sweating, and pallor often start in early infancy. Symptoms improve over time with nocturnal feeds and introduction of corn starch in older children. They also have a tendency for epistaxis due to impaired platelet function. Older children may develop eruptive xanthomata, rickets, anemia, chronic renal disease due to hyperuricemia, and renal stones. Short stature is common and gout may be present in affected children and adults. Children with GSD TYPE Ib could have persistent or cyclic neutropenia with predisposition to recurrent oral mucosal ulceration, gingivitis, progressive periodontal disease, and otitis media. The presentation also could mimic that of inflammatory bowel disease.[28,29]

GSD TYPE III is secondary to deficiency of the glycogen debrancher enzyme (Cori disease, Forbes disease, limit dextrinosis, debrancher enzyme disease). The disease is responsible for about 25% of all GSD cases.[17-22,30,31] Glucose residues which are released from glycogen require both glycogen phosphorylase and glycogen debranching enzyme. When there is absence or a deficiency in the debrancher enzyme, glycogenolysis is halted at the outermost branch points. Accumulation of abnormal glycogen (phosphorylase limit dextrin) occurs in affected organs (liver, heart, skeletal muscle, leukocytes in GSD TYPE IIIa; liver in GSD TYPE IIIb). The symptoms include hepatomegaly, hypoglycemia, short stature, and dyslipidemia.[17-22,30,31] Hypoglycemia, hepatomegaly and elevated liver function tests may improve after puberty; however, progressive muscle weakness and distal muscle wasting may eventually become the predominant feature during adulthood. Osteoporosis is explained by poor nutrition, lactic acidosis, and hypogonadism.[30]

GSD TYPE IV or a deficiency in amylo-1,4 to 1,6-transglucosidase (Andersen disease, brancher deficiency, amylopectinosis, glycogen branching enzyme deficiency) is a rare autosomal recessive disease and accounts for less than 1% of GSDs. With this type, glycogen cannot undergo branching and resembles an amylopectin-like structure—polyglucosan, accumulated in several organ tissue types, including liver, skeletal muscle, amniocytes, fibroblasts, and leukocytes. Clinical features vary and in the classic form, affected children appear to be asymptomatic at birth. By 18 months of age, they rapidly develop failure to thrive, portal hypertension, hepatosplenomegaly, and cirrhosis. Death occurs by 3 to 5 years of age.[17-22, 32-34]

Children with GSD secondary to liver glycogen phosphorylase (GSD TYPE VI or Hers disease), phosphorylase activation system defects (GSD TYPE IX) and cyclic 3′,5′-AMP-dependent kinase defect (GSD TYPE X) have a benign course with a good prognosis in older children and adulthood; cirrhosis is rare.[17-22,35]

GSD TYPE XI is secondary to a deficiency in the glucose transporter 2 (Fanconi-Bickel syndrome, GLUT2 deficiency). GLUT2 is the most important glucose transporter in hepatocytes, pancreatic beta-cells, enterocytes, and renal tubular cells. Both glucose and galactose utilization are impaired, because both of these are dependent on GLUT2 for exportation from affected cells. Impaired export results in hepatorenal glycogen accumulation and proximal tubule dysfunction. Symptoms manifest between 3 and 10 years of age with fasting hypoglycemia, postprandial hyperglycemia, hypophosphatemic rickets with osteoporosis, marked growth retardation, delayed puberty and hepatomegaly.[36]

Early recognition would allow prompt diagnosis of specific defects and pave the way for treatment to improve quality of life, reducing the damaging effects on the targeted organs and possibly extending the child's lifespan.[17-22] Unique clinical features give a clue to the recognition since early infancy particularly in GSD TYPE 0, I, III, IV and XI (Table 28.1). Hepatomegaly is often noted at the diagnosis or follow-up in all types of GSD except GSD TYPE 0. Splenomegaly manifests as a complication of portal hypertension in children with GSD with an early presentation in children with GSD TYPE IV. Galactose intolerance is present in GSD TYPE XI. Renal Fanconi syndrome could complicate GSD TYPE I and XI.

Table 28.1: Enzyme defects, genetics, special clinical features of glycogen storage disease

Storage disease types/ gene sequencing	Inheritance	Enzyme deficiency	Liver histopathology (glycogen/fat/ fibrosis)	Cardiac muscle/ skeletal muscle/ neurological
GSD 0, GYS2, 12p12.2	AR*	Glycogen synthase	-/+/-	
GSD I			+/±/±	-/-/-
GSD 1a, G6PC,17q21	AR	Glucose-6-phosphatase translocase/ transporter (liver, kidney, intestine)		-/-/-
GSD 1b, SLC37A4, 11q23	AR	Glucose-6-phosphatase translocase/ transporter (liver)		-/-/-
GSD 1c, SLC37A4, 11q23-24.2	AR	Phosphatase translocase/transporter (liver)		-/-/-
GSD III, AGL, 1p21	AR	Amylo-1-6-glucosidase	+/±/±	
GSD III a	AR	Phosphorylase limit dextrin accumulation		+/+/-
GSD III b	AR	Phosphorylase limit dextrin accumulation		-/-/-
GSD III c	AR	Glucosidase activity loss		
GSD III d	AR	Transferase activity loss		
GSD IV, GBE1, 3p12	AR	Amylo-1,4 to 1,6-transgluosidase	+/-/+ EM: fibrillar material that resembles amylopectin	-/-/+
GSD VI, PYGL,14q21-q22	AR	Liver glycogen phosphorylase E (liver, leukocytes, and erythrocytes)	+/±/-	-/-/-
GSD IX				
GSD IX, α subunit, PHKA2, Xp22.2-22.1	X linked		+/±/-	-/-/-
GSD IX, beta subunit, PHKB, 16q12-q13	AR		+/+/-	-/+/+
GSD IX, gamma subunit, PHKG2,16p12.1	AR		+/+/+	-/+/+
GSD X, PGAM2, 17q23-24	AR	Cyclic 3',5'AMP-dependent kinase	+/±/-	-/+/-
GSD XI, 3q26.1-q26.3	AR	Glucose transporter 2	+/±/±	-/-/-

+ typically present, - typically absent, ± may not be present in all cases
*AR (autosomal recessive)

Investigations to specifically diagnose GSD often require analysis of liver tissues for confirmation of the presence of abnormal glycogen storage. Histochemical staining (PAS and PAS-diastase) allows qualitative assessment of glycogen content which should be minimal after fasting preoperatively in a normal individual without GSD (except GSD TYPE 0). Therefore, the first investigation can be obtaining the quantitative content of glycogen on liver and muscle histology. Once abnormal glycogen storage is identified, further subsequent enzyme analysis can be determined. Careful preparation of the tissue is required as the routine formalin fixation could cause up to 70% loss of glycogen due to the soluble nature of the predominant form of glycogen in the hepatic/muscle cytoplasm.

Quantitative GSD screening is offered at commercial laboratories to quantify the glycogen-glycogen content of liver or muscle. Specific enzyme assays can be assessed: glucose-6-phosphatase (liver only), debrancher enzyme (liver or muscle), total phosphorylase activity (liver or muscle), GSD TYPE Ia (liver), GSD IIIa (liver or muscle), GSD TYPE IIIb (liver only), GSD TYPE VI (liver) and GSD TYPE IX (liver, red blood cells from blood, muscle, heart).[1-6,15] This initial screen will cover the most common glycogen storage diseases. Quantitative analysis of glycogen in these organ tissues and the suspected enzyme assays and an evaluation of gene mutation and sequencing of the gene responsible for a specific GSD must be done on snap-frozen liver or skeletal muscle tissue. The tissue should be maintained at –70°C until it reaches the appropriate reference laboratory. Electron microscopy may be needed if certain types of GSDs are suspected. Unique histologic and ultrastructural features are characteristic of different types of GSDs but most helpful in GSD TYPE IV with the presence of amylopectin (Table 28.1).[17-22,32-34] Gene mutation analysis can be performed through genetic consultation (Table 28.1).

Current treatment is directed towards efforts to prevent the effects or partially ameliorate the sequelae of abnormal glycogen storage. For infants and older children with GSD TYPE 0, I, III, and XI their symptoms are rapidly ameliorated with low simple sugar and protein-rich meals at 3–6 hour intervals throughout the day and night[17-23,26-27] and/or bedtime feeding of uncooked cornstarch under guidance of a nutrition specialist.[17-22.] Increased protein during meals provides the substrate for gluconeogenesis, and a reduction of carbohydrate diet reduces postprandial hyperglycemia, glycosuria, and lactic acidosis in those children. Following such dietary restrictions results in improvement of hepatomegaly with decreased glycogen content and promotes growth. Individuals with GSD TYPE VI, VIII, IX, and X usually have a rather benign course but may still require same approach based on their defect in gluconeogenesis or glycogenolysis depending on their enzyme deficiencies. Treatment is directed towards avoiding prolonged fasting and ingestion of a bedtime snack to avoid early morning hypoglycemia in these milder types.

Aggressive management is required to stabilize glucose homeostasis, replace renal loss of solutes including phosphorus, and supplementation with vitamin D in children with GSD TYPE I and XI, to reverse cirrhosis in GSD TYPE IX and to delay the development of hepatic adenomata in GSD TYPE I and III.[17-22,35] Galactose restriction is important in GSD TYPE XI to avoid cataract development. However, even untreated, GSD TYPE XI may be compatible with survival into adulthood. When children with GSD TYPE I, III, or IV may develop chronic liver disease, liver transplantation may be indicated.[36]

CYSTIC FIBROSIS

CLINICAL SCENARIO

A 7-year-old boy presented with a history of feeding intolerance, chronic constipation and distal intestinal obstruction syndrome was diagnosed during an admission prior to his 8th birthday. Hepatosplenomegaly was noted at physical examination as a coincidental finding. Abdominal sonogram confirmed that his liver was enlarged with coarse texture indicating a manifestation of cirrhosis. Laboratory findings were significant for thrombocytopenia suggestive of a process of hypersplenism from portal hypertension. Work-up for causes of cirrhosis showed a pilocarpine iontophoresis sweat chloride of 122 mEq/L. Analysis of cystic fibrosis transmembrane conductance regulator (CFTR) genotypes showed that the boy was homozygous for CFTR ΔF508. Over the following one year, he had several episodes of hematemesis. Upper endoscopy revealed high grades of esophageal varices. Several sessions of band ligation were performed to treat such lesions. Although his synthetic liver functions remained intact, portal hypertension appeared to be his only predominant liver problem. Parents inquired about the need of liver transplantation.

Cystic fibrosis (CF) is a multiorgan disorder with an incidence of 1:2000 among Caucasians. Mutations in the CFTR gene results in CFTR dysfunctions in chloride channels of affected organs, such as lungs, pancreas, gastrointestinal tract, and sweat glands. Based on CF mutation database greater than 1300 mutations were reported.[37] Cystic fibrosis associated liver disease (CFLD) has been more identified as an early complication in the first decade of life.[38] No specific genotype and phenotype correlation has been currently identified.[38] The pathophysiology of CFLD is unclear. Several factors have been mentioned including a change in bile acid metabolism, drug induced liver disease, cytokine production, toxins from bacterial organisms, malnutrition (vitamin and essential fatty acid deficiencies) and bile duct obstruction.[39,40] CFTR protein is present only in biliary epithelia in the liver. Bile plugs secondary from reduced chloride secretion could result in bile duct obstruction which subsequently leads to focal biliary fibrosis and cirrhosis.[41-42] Evidently not all CF patients develop CFLD and ongoing research proposed that perhaps modifier genes could be responsible for hepatic presentation.[43]

CF patients develop liver disease with different degrees and patterns of liver involvement from asymptomatic abnormal liver enzymes (up to or more than 50%) cirrhosis with clinical presentation of chronic liver disease in 4% of CF patients depending on various studies.[40,42,44-49] Advanced liver disease mostly manifests in adolescents and young adults with CF with incidence ranging 4–10% of all CF population.[46,49,50]

Infants with CF could manifest as neonatal cholestasis which could be associated with bowel surgery, parenteral nutrition, infection. The natural history is still unclear and it is not known which factors increase the risk to develop cirrhosis.[51]

It is unusual for CF patients with liver disease to manifest as acute liver failure. Most children with liver disease rather have insidious or chronic progression as hepatic steatosis, focal biliary cirrhosis, multilobular cirrhosis. CFLD is often first recognized as a coincidental finding on physical or radiologic examination or as abnormal liver function tests. Biliary tract anomalies are uncommon.

Liver biopsy is not routinely performed to diagnose CFLD as the finding likely does not impact management nor does it aid in predicting cirrhosis progression. When another liver disease is suspected and liver histopathology is required for such a diagnosis, liver biopsy could be considered. There are several research studies using non-invasive tools to monitor progression of liver fibrosis including laboratory biomarkers, doppler liver ultrasound, shear-wave ultrasound, and transient elastography. Currently, there is no single use in clinical practice in patients with CFLD.

Treating the complications of portal hypertension promptly is crucial in CF patients with advanced liver disease as no effective therapy is proven to alter the course of progression to cirrhosis.[50] Treatment with ursodeoxycholic acid (UDCA) was only conducted in short-term clinical trials noted to improve bile-flow, an elevation of aminotransferase values, and benign liver histopathology with less inflammation and bile duct proliferation; however, there were no long-term outcome clinical trials.[52-54] A 10-year prospective study in CFLD patients with UDCA demonstrated an improvement of the sonographic finding of the liver.[55] Possible mechanisms of UDCA action include improved bile acid-dependent

bile flow, enriched hydrophilic bile acids in the bile acid pools, ATP release and purinergic-stimulated increases in secretion, immunomodulatory and cytoprotective effects, stimulation of bicarbonate and chloride secretion.[56-59] The recommendation from the Cystic Fibrosis Foundation Hepatobiliary Disease Consensus Group is to use UCDA in patients with CFLD.[60] Beta-blockers usually used as a prophylaxis in chronic liver disease patients with portal hypertension to prevent variceal bleeding is contraindicated in CF patients due to risks of pulmonary exacerbations with increased bronchospasm.[42,50] When CFLD patients fail to respond to endoscopic therapy for variceal hemorrhage, surgical or transjugular intrahepatic portosystemic shunts are indicated; however, increased risk of encephalopathy has been noted.[61]

Most patients with CFLD maintain hepatocellular function for decades. The care should target on recognition and management of complications of portal hypertension. Liver transplantation (LT) should be reserved for those who develop synthetic liver failure and resistant variceal hemorrhage or intractable ascites. The timing of LT is challenging as it could be influenced by several factors, such as pulmonary status, nutritional status, and cardiac function. Therefore, LT should be considered before the deterioration of lung function.[46] The best outcomes are seen in patients without severe lung involvement, and pulmonary status may improve post–liver transplant.[42,62-64] The 1-year patient survival rate following LT for CFLD ranges from 75% to 100%.[42,63-65] The United Network for Organ Sharing (1987–2009) reported 294 CF patients (210 children), 265 (90.1%) received an LT and 29, a combined liver and lung transplantation (L-LT). Patient survival in adult LT was 80%, 74%, and 67% at 1, 3, and 5 years respectively, and for combined lung and liver transplant was 72%, 61.4%, and 61.4%. Patient survival for pediatric LT was 85%, 82%, and 74% at 1, 3, and 5 years, and for L-LT, 83%, 83%, and 83% respectively with comparable graft and patient survival.[66] Worsening pulmonary disease is related to late mortality.

DISORDERS OF HEME METABOLISM AND THE LIVER

CLINICAL SCENARIO

A 13-year-old Caucasian girl was diagnosed with hemochromatosis (HC) at age 3 years because of a strong family history of HC. Genetic studies showed homozygosity for the C282Y mutation. Routine phlebotomy was performed (100 mL monthly) since the diagnosis. She had not yet menstruated. She did not have hepatomegaly or any abnormality of liver function tests. She avoided dietary iron and vitamin C. At the visit at 13 years of age, her serum iron level was 240 µg/dL, (27–164), TIBC

Contd...

Contd...

CLINICAL SCENARIO (CONTD...)

259 µg/dL (271–448), transferrin saturation 93% (8–52%), and ferritin 136 µg/L (10–143). Complete blood count showed a hemoglobin 12.9 g/dL, MCV 90. Although treatment of children with HC with C282Y/C282Y is controversial, her mother insisted on the therapy given a strong history of significant liver disease in her other family members with HC. The diet was reviewed for a compliance issue. She was referred to a HC geneticist to rule out other HC related gene mutations. The phlebotomized volume was increased as the most recent values of transferrin saturation and ferritin showed iron overload despite phlebotomy. At a follow-up a year later, her hepatic function panel was normal, hemoglobin 13.2 g/dL, transferrin saturation 61% and ferritin 19 µg/L. The phlebotomized volume was recommended to be adjusted per her menstruation history.

Table 28.2: Disorders of iron metabolisms of the liver in the older child

Hereditary iron overload:
- Hemochromatosis from HFE (C282Y homozygous or C282Y/H63D), TFR2, HJV or HAMP related
- Ferroportin disease
- Aceruloplasminemia
- A (hypo) transferrinemia
- H-ferritin-related iron overload
- Survivor from neonatal hemochromatosis
- Tyrosinemia
- Zellweger syndrome

Hereditary hemolytic diseases that leads to iron overload:
- Thalassemia
- Sideroblastic anemia
- Sicke cell disease
- Other chronic hemolytic anemias

Acquired iron overload:
- Dieta related
- Transfusion related
- Chronic liver disease such as Wilson disease, hepatitis B and C, steatohepatitis, cystic fibrosis
- Porphyria cutanea tarda
- Miscellaneous
- Iron overload in sub-Saharan Africa

Adapted from
1. Pietrangelo A. Hereditary hemochromatosis—a new look at an old disease. N Engl J Med. 2004;350:2383-97.
2. Pietrangelo A. Non-HFE hemochromatosis. Hepatology. 2004;39:21-9.

In this section we will review only disorders leading to iron overload (hereditary hemochromatosis, HC) in older children and young adults. Disorders associated with hereditary iron-loading anemia (thalassemia and other diseases with hemolytic anemia), acquired iron overload such as dietary/parenteral/transfusion iron overload, chronic liver disease, hepatitis C, chronic hemodialysis, porphyria cutanea tarda, and iron overload in sub-Saharan Africa, and neonatal hemochromatosis are classified in Table 28.2 will not be discussed in detail.

Hemochromatosis (HC) is an autosomal recessive disorder of iron metabolism resulting in tissue iron overload and multiorgan involvement including cirrhosis, endocrinopathy and cardiomyopathy.[67] The disorder is caused by a mutation of HC related genes, HFE (C282Y and H63D) with a high frequency in population of European descent, "non-HFE" genes including hepcidin (HAMP gene), hemojuvelin (HJV), transferrin receptor 2 (TfR2) and ferroportin. Hepcidin, modulated by HFE, TfR2 and HJV is responsible in mobilizing iron depending on the body's iron status.

Individuals with mutations in HAMP gene manifest hemochromatosis in the second or third decade of life, as a result of defect in their hepcidin production and inability to inhibit iron absorption from the intestine despite saturated body's iron status. HAMP, therefore, has a negative impact on the cellular regulation of iron efflux by affecting the availability of ferroportin cell surface (Table 28.2).[67]

These "non-HFE" forms of HC are not very common disordered compared to HFE-related HC (HHC) but they could share a similar presentation (HC-1).[67] The approach of HFE form of HC can be used for evaluation and diagnosis of the "non-HFE" forms as well.[67]

Individual with early-onset primary iron overload most likely have juvenile form of HC (JH) with hypogonadotropic hypogonadism and cardiac involvement being prominent symptoms.[68-70] Only fewer than than 50 cases have been reported at a much younger age in the second decade of life. Most of these cases are from HJV mutations[71] and to a lessor degree with HAMP mutations.[72] The plasma iron pool in JH (HJV and HAMP-related HC) is rapidly expanded compared with the late-onset forms (HHC and TfR2 related HC) due to an increase in iron transfer from enterocytes and reticuloendothelial (RE) macrophages to the blood compartment.[67] *TfR2 mutations is rare* and only few pedigrees from non-Northern Europeans have been reported.[73]

While all other HCs are autosomal recessive inherited disorders, ferroportin disease (FD) associated with ferroportin (FPN) mutation is of autosomal dominant inheritance.[74,75] FD causes progressive iron retention predominantly in reticuloendothelial cells of liver and spleen with a profile of serum ferritin being inappropriately high when compared with serum transferrin saturation. Patients with FD usually have marginal anemia and mild organ disease. The loss of FPN function is believed to cause significant iron recycling by reticuloendothelial macrophages processing and releasing a large quantity of iron from lysis of senescent erythrocytes.[74]

Aceruloplasminemia caused by a mutation in ceruloplasmin (CP) gene is a rare autosomal recessive disorder. Its ferroxidase activity helps release iron from cells.[76-78] The disorder leads to iron accumulation in the basal ganglia, dentate nucleus, hepatocytes, RE cells and pancreatic islet cells. Despite severe iron overload, patients with CD have mild liver disease.[79]

A(hypo)transferrinemia presents with severe anemia due to an impaired plasma iron transport and delivery to bone marrow.[80] Tissue iron overload is a result of compensatory intestinal iron uptake and is thought to be caused by a mutation in the regulatory region of H ferritin.[81]

Management generally consists of periodic therapeutic phlebotomy to treat all forms of HC except aceruloplasminemia and a(hypo)transferrinemia (chelation with desferoxamine is recommended to prevent anemia). Symptomatic children should initially have 5–8 mL/kg of weekly blood letting until the serum ferritin is less than 300 µg/L and thereafter for maintenance therapy biannually to quarterly to keep the serum ferritin below 50 µg/L and transferrin saturation below 50%.[82,83] A more aggressive schedule may be required in JH forms.

The appropriate age to test children at risk of developing HC is still controversial. It is not recommended to test HFE gene for children age less than 18 years.[84]

REFERENCES

1. Clayton PT, Leonard JV, Lawson AM, et al. Familial giant cell hepatitis associated with synthesis of 3β,7α-dihydroxy- and 3β,7α,12α-trihydroxy-5-cholenoic acids. J Clin Invest. 1987;79:1031-8.
2. Schwarz M, Wright AC, Davis DL, et al. The bile acid synthetic gene 3 beta-hydroxy-Delta(5)-C(27)-steroid oxidoreductase is mutated in progressive intrahepatic cholestasis. J Clin Invest. 2000;106(9):1175-84.
3. Setchell KDR, Heubi JE. Defects in Bile Acid Biosynthesis: Diagnosis and Treatment. Journal of Pediatr Gastroenterol and Nutr. 2006;43:S17YS22.
4. Van Bogaert L, Scherer HJ, Epstein E. Une forme cerebrale de la cholesterinose generalisee. Paris: Masson et Cie, 1937.
5. Setchell KDR, O`Connell N, Russell DW, et al. A unique case of cerebrotendinous xanthomatosis presenting in infancy with cholestatic liver disease further highlights bile acid synthetic defects as an important category of metabolic liver disease. In: Den Haeg (Ed). XVI International Bile Acid Meeting. Biology of Bile Acids in Health and Disease. The Netherlands; 2000,p.13.
6. Gonzales E, Gerhardt MF, Fabre M, Setchell KD, Davit-Spraul A, Vincent I, et al. Oral cholic acid for hereditary defects of primary bile acid synthesis: a safe and effective long-term therapy. Gastroenterology. 2009;137:1310-20.e1-3.
7. Lin HC, Alvarez L, Laroche G, Melin-Aldana H, Pfeifer K, Schwarz K, et al. Rituximab as therapy for recurrence of bile salt export pump deficiency after liver transplantation. Liver Transplantation; 2013. in press.
8. Stapelbroek JM, van Erpecum KJ, Klomp LWJ, and Houwen RHJ. Liver disease associated with canalicular transport defects: Current and future therapies. Hepatol. 2010;52:258-71.
9. Ujhazy P, Ortiz D, Misra S, Li S, Moseley J, Jones H, et al. Familial intrahepatic cholestasis 1: studies of localization and function. Hepatology. 2001;34:768-75.
10. Paulusma CC, Folmer DE, Ho-Mok KS, de Waart DR, Hilarius PM, Verhoeven AJ, et al. ATP8B1 requires an accessory protein for endoplasmic reticulum exit and plasma membrane lipid flippase activity. Hepatology. 2008;47:268-78.
11. Pomorski T, Lombardi R, Riezman H, Devaux PF, van MG, Holthuis JC. Drs2p-related P-type ATPases Dnf1p and Dnf2p are required for phospholipid translocation across the yeast plasma membrane and serve a role in endocytosis. Mol Biol Cell. 2003;14:1240-54.
12. Vajro P, Ferrante L, Paolella G. Alagille syndrome: An overview. Clinics and Research in Hepatology and Gastroenterology. 2012; 36,275-7.
13. Kaye AJ, Rand EB, Munoz PS, Spinner NB, Flake AW, Kamath BM. Effect of Kasai procedure on hepatic outcome in Alagille syndrome. J Pediatr Gastroenterol Nutr. 2010;51(3):319-21.
14. Emerick KM, Krantz ID, Kamath BM, Darling C, Burrowes DM, Spinner NB, et al. Intracranial vascular abnormalities in patients with Alagille syndrome. J Pediatr Gastroenterol Nutr. 2005;41(1):99-107.
15. Kamath BM, Schwarz KB, Hadzic N. Alagille syndrome and liver transplantation. J Pediatr Gastroenterol Nutr. 2010;50:11-5.
16. Lykavieris P, Hadchouel M, Chardot C, Bernard O. Outcome of liver disease in children with Alagille syndrome: a study of 163 patients. Gut. 2001;49:431-5.
17. Ozen H. Glycogen storage diseases: new perspectives. World J Gastroenterol. 2007;13:2541-53.
18. Di Mauro S, Bruno C. Glycogen storage disease of muscle. Curr Opin Neurol Neurosurg. 1998;11:477-84.
19. Wolfsdorf JI, Weinstein DA. Glycogen storage diseases. Rev Endocrinol Metab Disorders. 2003;4:95-102.
20. Wolsdorf JI, Holm IA, Weinstein DA. Glycogen storage disease: phenotypic, genetic, and biochemical characteristics, and therapy. Endocrinol Metab Clin. 1999;28:802-24.
21. Jevon GP, Dimmick JE. Histopathologic approach to metabolic liver disease: part 1. Pediatr Dev Pathol. 1998;1:179-99.
22. Roy A, Finegold MJ. Biopsy diagnosis of inherited liver disease. Surg Pathol Clin. 2010;3:743-68.
23. Koeberl DD, Kishnani PS, Chen YT. Glycogen storage disease types I and II: treatment updates. J Inherit Metab Dis. 2007;30:159-64.
24. Janecke AR, Mayatepek E, Utermann G. Molecular genetics of type I glycogen storage disease. Mol Genet Metab. 2001;73:117-25.

25. Chou JY, Matern D, Mansfield BC, Chen Y-T. Type I glycogen storage disease: disorders of the glucose-6-phosphatase complex. Curr Mol Med. 2002;2:121-43.

26. Chou JY. The molecular basis of type I glycogen storage diseases. Curr Mol Med. 2001;1:25-44.

27. Viega-da-Cunha M, Gerin I, Van Schaftingen E. How many forms of glycogen storage disease type I? Eur J Pediatr. 2000;159:314-8.

28. Yamaguchi T, Ihara K, Matsumoto T, et al. Inflammatory bowel disease-like colitis in glycogen storage disease type1b. Inflammatory Bowel Dis. 2001;7(2):128-32.

29. Karasawa Y, Kobayashi M, Nakano Y, et al. A case of glycogen storage disease type 1a with multiple hepatic adenomas and G72T mutation in glucose-6-phosphatase gene, and a comparison with other mutations previously reported. Am J Gastroenterol. 1998;93(9):1550-53.

30. Kishnani PS, Austin SL, Arn P, Bali DS, Boney A, Case LE, et al. ACMG. Glycogen storage disease type III diagnosis and management guidelines. Genet Med. 2010;12:446-63.

31. Demo E, Frush D, Gottfried M, et al. Glycogen storage disease type III-hepatocellular carcinoma a long-term complication? J Hepatol. 2007;46:492-8.

32. Moses SW, Parvari R. The variable presentations of glycogen storage disease type IV: a review of clinical, enzymatic and molecular studies. Curr Mol Med. 2002;177-88.

33. Vucic S, Pamphlett R, Wills EJ, Yiannikas C. Polyglucosan body disease myopathy: an unusual presentation. Muscle Nerve. 2007;35:536-9.

34. Raben N, Dannon M, Lu N, et al. Surprises of genetic engineering: a possible model of polyglucosan body disease. Neurology. 2001;56:1739-45.

35. Tsilianidis LA, Fiske LM, Siegel S, Lumpkin C, Hoyt K, Wasserstein M, et al. Aggressive therapy improves cirrhosis in glycogen storage disease type IX. Mol Genet Metab. 2013;109:179-82.

36. Sokal E. Liver transplantation for inborn errors of liver metabolism. J Inherit Metab Dis. 2006;29:426–430.

37. Rowe SM, Miller S, Sorscher EJ. Cystic fibrosis. N Engl J Med 2005;352:1992-2001. CF Mutation Database, http://www.genet.sickkids.un.ca/cftr.

38. Colombo C, Battezzati PM, Crosignani A, Morabito A, Costantini D, Padoan R, et al. Liver disease in cystic fibrosis: A prospective study on incidence, risk factors, and outcome. Hepatology. 2002;36:1374-82.

39. Strandvik B. Hepatobiliary disease in cystic fibrosis. In: Kelly D (Ed). Diseases of the Liver and Biliary System in Children. Volume 1. 2nd ed. Malden, MA: Blackwell Publishing, Ltd.; 2004:197-210.

40. Jonas MM. The role of liver transplantation in cystic fibrosis re-examined. Liver Transpl. 2005;11:1463-5.

41. Molmenti EP, Squires RH, Nagata D, Roden JS, Molmenti H, Fasola CG, et al. Liver transplantation for cholestasis associated with cystic fibrosis in the pediatric population. Pediatr Transplant. 2003;7:93-7.

42. Colombo C, Russo MC, Zazzeron L, Romano G. Liver disease in cystic fibrosis. J Pediatr Gastroenterol Nutr. 2006;43(suppl 1):S49-S55.

43. Gabolde M, Hubert D, Guilloud-Bataille M, Lenaerts C, Feingold J, Besmond C. The mannose binding lectin gene influences the severity of chronic liver disease in cystic fibrosis. J Med Genet. 2001;38:310-1.

44. Feigelson J, Anagnostopoulos C, Poquet M, Pecau Y, Munck A, Navarro J. Liver cirrhosis in cystic fibrosis—therapeutic implications and long-term follow-up. Arch Dis Child. 1993;68:653-7.

45. Psacharopoulos HT, Howard ER, Portmann B, Mowat AP, Williams R. Hepatic complications of cystic fibrosis. Lancet. 1981;2:78-80.

46. Lindblad A, Glaumann H, Strandvik B. Natural history of liver disease in cystic fibrosis. Hepatology. 1999;30:1151-8.

47. Ling SC, Wilkinson JD, Hollman AS, McColl J, Evans TJ, Paton JY. The evolution of liver disease in cystic fibrosis. Arch Dis Child 1999;81:129-32.

48. Noble-Jamieson G, Barnes N, Jamieson N, Friend P, Calne R. Liver transplantation for hepatic cirrhosis in cystic fibrosis. J R Soc Med. 1996;89 (suppl 27):31-7.

49. Scott-Jupp R, Lama M, Tanner MS. Prevalence of liver disease in cystic fibrosis. Arch Dis Child. 1991;66:698-701.

50. Sokol RJ, Durie PR. For the Cystic Fibrosis Foundation Hepatobiliary Disease Consensus Group. Recommendations for management of liver and biliary tract disease in cystic fibrosis. J Pediatr Gastroenterol Nutr. 1999;28(suppl 1):S1-S13.

51. Gaskin KJ, Waters DL, Howman-Giles R, de Silva M, Earl JW, Martin HC, et al. Liver disease and common-bile-duct stenosis in cystic fibrosis. N Engl J Med. 1988;318(6):340-6.

52. Colombo C, Battezzati PM, Podda M, Bettinardi N, Giunta A. Ursodeoxycholic acid for liver disease associated with cystic fibrosis: a double-blind multicenter trial. The Italian Group for the Study of Ursodeoxycholic Acid in Cystic Fibrosis. Hepatology. 1996;23(6):1484-90.

53. Cotting J, Lentze MJ, Reichen J. Effects of ursodeoxycholic acid treatment on nutrition and liver function in patients with cystic fibrosis and long-standing cholestasis. Gut. 1990;31(8):918-21.

54. Galabert C, Montet JC, Lengrand D, Lecuire A, Sotta C, Figarella C, Chazalette JP. Effects of ursodeoxycholic acid on liver function in patients with cystic fibrosis and chronic cholestasis. J Pediatr. 1992;121(1):138-41.

55. Nousia-Arvanitakis S, Fotoulaki M, Economou H, Xefteri M, Galli-Tsinopoulou A. Long-term prospective study of the effect of ursodeoxycholic acid on cystic fibrosis-related liver disease. J Clin Gastroenterol. 2001;32(4):324-8.

56. Shimokura GH, McGill JM, Schlenker T, Fitz JG. Ursodeoxycholate increases cytosolic calcium concentration and activates Cl— currents in a biliary cell line. Gastroenterology. 1995;109(3):965-72.

57. Colombo C, Castellani MR, Balistreri WF, Seregni E, Assaisso ML, Giunta A. Scintigraphic documentation of an improvement in hepatobiliary excretory function after treatment with ursodeoxycholic acid in patients with cystic fibrosis and associated liver disease. Hepatology. 1992;15(4):677-84.

58. Heuman DM. Hepatoprotective properties of ursodeoxycholic acid. Gastroenterology. 1993;104(6):1865-70.

59. Nathanson MH, Burgstahler AD, Masyuk A, Larusso NF. Stimulation of ATP secretion in the liver by therapeutic bile acids. Biochem J. 2001;358(Pt 1):1-5.

60. Sokol RJ, Durie PR. Recommendations for management of liver and biliary tract disease in cystic fibrosis. Cystic Fibrosis Foundation Hepatobiliary Disease Consensus Group. J Pediatr Gastroenterol Nutr. 1999;28 (Suppl) 1:S1-13.

61. Shun A, Delaney DP, Martin HC, Henry GM, Stephen M. Portosystemic shunting for paediatric portal hypertension. J Pediatr Surg. 1997;32:489-93.

62. Fridell JA, Bond GJ, Mazariegos GV, Orenstein DM, Jain A, Sindhi R, et al. Liver transplantation in children with cystic fibrosis: a long-term longitudinal review of a single center's experience. J Pediatr Surg. 2003;38:1152-6.

63. Mack DR, Traystman MD, Colombo JL, Sammut PH, Kaufman SS, Vanderhoof JA, et al. Clinical denouement and mutation analysis of patients with cystic fibrosis undergoing liver transplantation for biliary cirrhosis. J Pediatr. 1995;127:881-7.

64. Milkiewicz P, Skiba G, Kelly D, Weller P, Bonser R, Gur I. Transplantation for cystic fibrosis: outcome following early liver transplantation. J Gastroenterol Hepatol. 2002;17:208-13.

65. Mekeel KL, Langham MR Jr, Gonzalez-Perralta R, Reed A, Hemming AW. Combined en bloc liver pancreas transplantation for children with CF. Liver Transpl. 2007;13:406-9.

66. Desai CS, Gruessner A, Habib S, Gruessner R, Khan KM. Survival of cystic fibrosis patients undergoing liver and liver-lung transplantations. Transplant Proc. 2013;45:290-2.

67. Pietrangelo A. Hereditary hemochromatosis—a new look at an old disease. N Engl J Med. 2004;350:2383-97.

68. Camaschella C, Piperno A. Hereditary hemochromatosis: recent advances in molecular genetics and clinical management. Haematologica. 1997;82:77-84.

69. Roetto A, Totaro A, Cazzola M, Cicilano M, Bosio S, D'Ascola G, et al. Juvenile hemochromatosis locus maps to chromosome 1q. Am J Hum Genet. 1999;64:1388-93.

70. De Gobbi M, Roetto A, Piperno A, Mariani R, Alberti F, Papanikolaou G, et al. Natural history of juvenile haemochromatosis. Br J Haematol. 2002;117:973-9.

71. Papanikolaou G, Samuels ME, Ludwig EH, MacDonald ML, Franchini PL, Dubé MP, et al. Mutations in HFE2 cause iron overload in chromosome 1q-linked juvenile hemochromatosis. Nat Genet. 2004;36:77-82.

72. Roetto A, Papanikolaou G, Politou M, Alberti F, Girelli D, Christakis J, et al. Mutant antimicrobial peptide hepcidin is associated with severe juvenile hemochromatosis. Nat Genet. 2003;33:21-2.

73. Pietrangelo A. Non-HFE hemochromatosis. Hepatology. 2004;39:21-9.

74. Pietrangelo A. The ferroportin disease. Blood Cells Mol Dis. 2004;32,131-8.

75. Montosi G, Donovan A, Totaro A, Garuti C, Pignatti E, Cassanelli S, et al. Autosomal-dominant hemochromatosis is associated with a mutation in the ferroportin (SLC11A3) gene. J Clin Invest. 2001;108:619-23.

76. Yoshida K, Furihata K, Takeda S, Nakamura A, Yamamoto K, Morita H, et al. A mutation in the ceruloplasmin gene is associated with systemic hemosiderosis in humans. Nat Genet. 1995;9:267-72.

77. Harris ZL, Takahashi Y, Miyajima H, Serizawa M, MacGillivray RT, Gitlin JD. Aceruloplasminemia: molecular characterization of this disorder of iron metabolism. Proc Natl Acad Sci USA. 1995;92:2539-43.

78. Goode CA, Dinh CT, Linder MC. Mechanism of copper transport and delivery in mammals: review and recent findings. Adv Exp Med Biol. 1989;258:131-44.

79. Miyajima H, Takahashi Y, Kamata T, Shimizu H, Sakai N, Gitlin JD. Ann Neurol. Use of desferrioxamine in the treatment of aceruloplasminemia. 1997;41:404-7.

80. Hayashi A, Wada Y, Suzuki T, Shimizu A. Studies on familial hypotransferrinemia: unique clinical course and molecular pathology. Am J Hum Genet. 1993;53:201-13.

81. Kato J, Fujikawa K, Kanda M, Fukuda N, Sasaki K, Takayama T, et al. A mutation, in the iron-responsive element of H ferritin mRNA, causing autosomal dominant iron overload. Am J Hum Genet. 2001;69:191-7.

82. Tavill AS. American Association for the Study of Liver Diseases; American College of Gastroenterology; American Gastroenterological Association. Diagnosis and management of hemochromatosis. Hepatology. 2001;33:1321-8.

83. Escobar GJ, Heyman MB, Smith WB, Thaler MM. Primary hemochromatosis in childhood. Pediatrics. 1987;80:549-54.

84. Delatycki MB, Powell LW, Allen KJ. Hereditary hemochromatosis genetic testing of at-risk children: what is the appropriate age? Genet Test. 2004;8:98-103.

Chapter 29

Nonalcoholic Fatty Liver Disease

Vidyut Bhatia

INTRODUCTION

Nonalcoholic fatty liver disease (NAFLD) has recently emerged as the leading cause of chronic liver disease in children.[1-3] The increasing incidence of NAFLD is a mirror of the worldwide annual increment of obese individuals.

DEFINITION

NAFLD is an important cause of fatty liver, occurring when fat is deposited (steatosis) in the liver. NAFLD is defined by hepatic fat infiltration >5% hepatocytes, as assessed by liver biopsy, in the absence of evidence of viral, autoimmune or drug-induced liver disease.[4] It includes a spectrum of liver disease ranging from intrahepatic fat accumulation (steatosis) to various degrees of necrotic inflammation and fibrosis [non-alcoholic steatohepatitis (NASH)].

EPIDEMIOLOGY

NAFLD is the most common liver disease in the United States.[3] It is thought to affect nearly 30 million people, 8.6 million of who have the more severe form of the disease, NASH.[5] The estimates of prevalence of NAFLD vary from 3–10% of all children.[1] The variation is in part due to the difference in population characteristics, method used for estimation and lifestyle. It has been estimated that nearly 1% of 2–4 years old, and 17% of children aged 15–19 years old have NAFLD.[6] In addition, almost 40% of obese children may also have NAFLD.[1]

There are very few population-based studies available but the one published from the United States shows that the prevalence of elevated ALT levels (>30 IU/L) was between 7.4–11.5%.[7] Elevated ALT levels were also present in 12.4% of male subjects compared with 3.5% of female subjects. The prevalence of fatty liver (as defined as >5% of hepatocytes containing macrovesicular fat), when adjusted for multiple factors like age, gender, race, and ethnicity was estimated to be nearly 10% in an autopsy-based study of children dying from unnatural causes.[6] Another study has shown the prevalence to be between 6–10%.[8]

Children with NAFLD typically have slightly elevated liver enzyme values in the absence of other causes of steatosis. Therefore, elevated levels of these enzymes, even though they do not indicate the extent of intrahepatic damage, are used as surrogate markers to screen for pediatric NAFLD. Alternatively, body mass index and ultrasonography are also be used for screening for NAFLD.[9]

Children are at particular risk of complications and poor prognosis since the time period to which they are exposed is the longest. They are susceptible to all the known complications that can be associated with any long-standing liver disease including the need for liver transplant in adulthood. A long-term study over 20 years amongst children [66 children with NAFLD (mean age 13.9 years)] with a total of 409.6 person-years of follow-up, presenting to a tertiary care center found that the risk for undergoing a liver transplant was higher in these children.[16] The metabolic syndrome was present in 29% children at the time of NAFLD diagnosis with 83% presenting with at least one feature of the metabolic syndrome viz. obesity, hypertension, dyslipidemia and/or hyperglycemia. Among adults, NAFLD has become the third leading indication for liver transplantation in the western hemisphere.

RISK FACTORS

Most children with NAFLD are in their early adolescent years. But the roots of development of this disease may lie at a very young age. This is because changing life styles and food habits of children. Males may be at a higher risk as shown by the epidemiological studies where it was shown that they are affected twice as often as females. Obese children, as alluded to earlier are at the greatest risk for developing NAFLD. In addition, presence of co-morbidities like Type 2 diabetes or pre-diabetes, the metabolic syndrome, or hyperlipidemia increases the risk of developing NAFLD.[2]

NATURAL HISTORY AND PATHOGENESIS

The natural history and prognosis of NAFLD in children is still uncertain, owing to the relative paucity of published data with long-term follow-up. It has been reported that, in susceptible individuals, NAFLD can evolve to cirrhosis and hepatocellular carcinoma in adulthood, with the consequent need for liver transplantation.[16] Both genetic and environmental factors appear to contribute in the development and progression of the disease. The '2-hit' hypothesis of NAFLD pathogenesis promulgated in earlier papers has been modified several times; in most patients, however, NAFLD appears to begin with lipid accumulation, or steatosis, which is in turn, determined by obesity and insulin resistance. Ensuing progression to steatohepatitis and fibrosis then depends on other factors such as free fatty acids, inflammatory cytokines and adipokines, oxidative stress and mitochondrial dysfunction in a complex interaction with genetic factors.

SYMPTOMS

In children, NAFLD is generally asymptomatic. In most such cases, the disease is suspected when blood tests show abnormalities during a routine checkup. Some children though can experience right-sided abdominal pain, fatigue, or constipation.

On examination, one may find obesity, especially in truncal, an enlarged liver, and signs of insulin resistance such as acanthosis nigricans. The examination may be completely normal in many cases.

HISTOPATHOLOGY AND SCORING SYSTEMS

Evidence of steatosis in >5% of hepatocytes is the essential criterion for diagnosing NAFLD both in adults and children. Classical histological findings that characterize NAFLD in children are: steatosis, ballooning, inflammation and fibrosis.[10] The way to differentiate between adult and pediatric NAFLD is to see the distribution of steatosis. In adults, the distribution of steatosis can be seen predominantly in the acinar zone 3 (perivenular zone), whereas in children, it starts in the acinar zone 1 (periportal zone) or sometimes may be azonal in distribution. The adult pattern of NASH has been seen in children too in which steatosis has a zonal distribution prevalent in zone 3, and is associated with lobular inflammation, ballooning

and perisinusoidal fibrosis. The presence of inflammatory infiltrate can be either in lobules or in portal tracts of the liver. Ballooning of the liver cells is an important major distinguishing feature of NASH that confers an increased risk of disease progression to the individual. Fibrosis of the liver occurs as a response to the insult of NASH. Like steatosis, the fibrosis pattern too is prevalent in acinar zone 1 in children.

Currently, there are three scoring systems to evaluate histological activity in NAFLD. The *Brunt score* is based on the semiquantitative assessment of macrovacuolar steatosis, ballooning, lobular and portal inflammation, generates three-tier grades of activity: mild or grade 1; moderate or grade 2; severe or grade 3.[11] The other scoring system is the *NASH–CRN system*, that generates a numeric score for grading the disease, the so-called NAFLD activity score (NAS).[12] NAS results from adding together the individual scores for steatosis (0–3), lobular inflammation (0–3), and ballooning (0–2), range from 0 to 8. A NAS score of 1 and 2 corresponds to 'not NASH', whilst a score >5 corresponds to 'definite-NASH'. Activity scores 3 and 4 are the borderline cases. Both scoring systems generate a numeric score for staging fibrosis: stage 1 (perisinusoidal fibrosis); stage 2 (portal- periportal fibrosis); stage 3 (bridging fibrosis); and stage 4 (cirrhosis).

Another score that has recently been developed is the *Pediatric NAFLD Histological Score* (PNHS).[13] The advantage of this score is that it takes into account the presence of portal inflammation. Histological features were scored: steatosis (0–3), lobular inflammation (0–3), ballooning (0–2), and PI (0–2). The authors have shown that there was a good correlation between PNHS scores and the presence of NASH, however, it needs further validation before it is used regularly.

ULTRASONOGRAPHY

Ultrasonography (USG) of the liver is the most commonly used imaging diagnostic modality since it is relatively inexpensive, safe, and accessible and is user-friendly. It can provide a good estimate of the degree, or the extent of hepatic steatosis that is present, based on a series of ultrasonographical characteristics.[14] A meta-analysis looking at the sensitivity and specificity of ultrasound for the detection of moderate-severe fatty liver, compared to histology (which is taken as the gold standard), found sensitivity to be 84.8% (95% confidence interval: 79.5–88.9) and specificity to be 93.6% (87.2–97.0). Recently, Shannon et al demonstrated that liver ultrasonography is a useful tool for quantifying steatosis in pediatric patients who have suspected NAFLD; ultrasonography scores strongly correlate with the grade of steatosis when conducting a liver biopsy.[9] However, the disadvantage of USG is that it cannot rule out the presence or absence of inflammation (steatohepatitis) or fibrosis. The other limitation of USG is that its diagnostic sensitivity decreases when the quantity of fat in the liver is <30% (i.e. in mild cases) or the individual has a BMI ≥40.

COMPUTED TOMOGRAPHY/ MAGNETIC RESONANCE IMAGING

Computed tomography (CT) though more specific is not used for the screening of fatty liver in children owing to radiation exposure and high costs. Magnetic resonance imaging (MRI) has the greatest accuracy to determine hepatic fat content, but is used mostly in research studies.[4]

TRANSIENT ELASTOGRAPHY

Transient elastography (TE) can be used to evaluate fibrosis in children. The results correlate well with liver fibrosis scores as determined by histopathology.[15] However, there is not enough data to support its regular use for non-invasively monitoring the liver disease progression in children.

TREATMENT

The approach to treatment of patients with NAFLD aims at decreasing the incidence of the known risk factors. This strategy calls for prevention and control of modifiable risk factors such as obesity and unhealthy lifestyle, along with primordial prevention by giving optimum care during pregnancy so as to prevent low birth weight babies and encouraging breastfeeding.[4] This can impact the overall health of these children and adolescents as well as the prevention and control of pediatric NAFLD and the related metabolic syndrome. NAFLD must be treated by gradual weight loss (approximately about one pound per week). It has been shown that even losing only 10% of the body weight benefits the liver disease in these children. Since a single strategy does not help, this should be achieved through a combination of both exercise and dietary changes. A practical goal would be to exercise 3 to 5 times per week for at least half an hour.[4] Exercise not only helps to burn stored energy, but also increases the body's metabolism. The point to be made while advising exercise as a beneficial measure is that it should consist of active play. Children become increasingly bored with simple exercise regimens unless a play factor is incorporated in their exercise regimen. Nutrition should be balanced. Sugar sweetened beverages should be restricted since fructose is present in very high quantities in these drinks and fructose is known to be directly converted to fat by the body's metabolic forces. Lean meats, poultry and fish, along with fresh fruits and vegetables and whole grains intakes need to be emphasized.

The incidence of NAFLD is likely to rise over time due to the combined epidemics of obesity and diabetes. Presently, there is no definitive treatment for NAFLD. Based on existing evidence, vitamin E is the only treatment recommended for NASH adults and that too those without diabetes or cirrhosis and with aggressive histology. Validation through randomized controlled trials is needed before its use can be endorsed in children.

To conclude, NAFLD is a growing health problem globally. It might evolve to NASH, cirrhosis and cause HCC at a later stage. This disease, which has increased because of changing lifestyles, eating habits and changes in food content starts to affect people from childhood. The important risk factors are obesity, insulin resistance, gender, ethnicity, genetic predisposition and some medical problems. Cirrhosis in children is rare but is reported. NAFLD does not have a proven treatment. Weight loss with community-based treatments is the most acceptable management. Exercise with active play and a diet with low glycemic index keeping in mind appropriate calorie intake is preferred. Drugs look promising but are not sufficient for children.

REFERENCES

1. Bellentani S, Scaglioni F, Marino M, Bedogni G. Epidemiology of non-alcoholic fatty liver disease. Dig Dis. 2010;28:155-61.
2. Tominaga K, Fujimoto E, Suzuki K, Hayashi M, Ichikawa M, Inaba Y. Prevalence of nonalcoholic fatty liver disease in children and relationship to metabolic syndrome, insulin resistance, and waist circumference. Environ Health Prev Med. 2009;14:142-9.
3. Welsh JA, Karpen S, Vos MB. Increasing prevalence of nonalcoholic fatty liver disease among United States adolescents, 1988-1994 to 2007-2010. J Pediatr. 2013;162:496-500 e1.
4. Giorgio V, Prono F, Graziano F, Nobili V. Pediatric nonalcoholic fatty liver disease: old and new concepts on development, progression, metabolic insight and potential treatment targets. BMC Pediatr. 2013;13:40.
5. Lazo M, Hernaez R, Eberhardt MS, Bonekamp S, Kamel I, Guallar E, et al. Prevalence of nonalcoholic fatty liver disease in the United States: the Third National Health and Nutrition Examination Survey, 1988-1994. Am J Epidemiol. 2013;178:38-45.
6. Schwimmer JB, Deutsch R, Kahen T, Lavine JE, Stanley C, Behling C. Prevalence of Fatty Liver in Children and Adolescents. Pediatrics. 2006;118:1388-93.
7. Fraser A, Longnecker MP, Lawlor DA. Prevalence of elevated alanine aminotransferase among US adolescents and associated factors: NHANES 1999-2004. Gastroenterology. 2007;133:1814-20.
8. Yuksel F, Turkkan D, Yuksel I, Kara S, Celik N, Samdanci E. Fatty liver disease in an autopsy series of children and adolescents. Hippokratia. 2012;16:61-5.

9. Shannon A, Alkhouri N, Carter-Kent C, Monti L, Devito R, Lopez R, et al. Ultrasonographic quantitative estimation of hepatic steatosis in children With NAFLD. J Pediatr Gastroenterol Nutr. 2011;53:190-5.

10. Schwimmer JB, Behling C, Newbury R, Deutsch R, Nievergelt C, Schork NJ, et al. Histopathology of pediatric nonalcoholic fatty liver disease. Hepatology. 2005;42:641-9.

11. Brunt EM, Janney CG, Di Bisceglie AM, Neuschwander-Tetri BA, Bacon BR. Nonalcoholic steatohepatitis: a proposal for grading and staging the histological lesions. Am J Gastroenterol. 1999;94:2467-74.

12. Kleiner DE, Brunt EM, Van Natta M, Behling C, Contos MJ, Cummings OW, et al. Design and validation of a histological scoring system for nonalcoholic fatty liver disease. Hepatology. 2005;41:1313-21.

13. Alkhouri N, De Vito R, Alisi A, Yerian L, Lopez R, Feldstein AE, et al. Development and validation of a new histological score for pediatric nonalcoholic fatty liver disease. J Hepatol. 2012;57:1312-8.

14. Hernaez R, Lazo M, Bonekamp S, Kamel I, Brancati FL, Guallar E, et al. Diagnostic accuracy and reliability of ultrasonography for the detection of fatty liver: a meta-analysis. Hepatology. 2011;54:1082-90.

15. Alkhouri N, Sedki E, Alisi A, Lopez R, Pinzani M, Feldstein AE, et al. Combined paediatric NAFLD fibrosis index and transient elastography to predict clinically significant fibrosis in children with fatty liver disease. Liver Int. 2013;33:79-85.

16. Feldstein A, Charatcharoenwitthaya P, Treeprasertsuk S, Benson J, Enders F, Angulo P. The natural history of nonalcoholic fatty liver disease in children: a follow-up study for up to 20 years. Gut. 2009;58(11):1538-44.

Chronic Liver Disease

B Sumathi

INTRODUCTION

Chronic liver disease accounts for at least 1 to 5% of pediatric admissions and is responsible for approximately 20% mortality in our country. The changing pattern of liver disease in our country is outlined in Table 30.1.[1] The signs and symptoms depend on the underlying stage of liver disease ranging from asymptomatic hepatosplenomegaly and growth retardation to acute complications of chronic liver failure namely gastrointestinal bleeding, altered mental status, ascites and renal dysfunction. Childhood liver disorders are distinct from that of adult population by way of etiology and mode of presentation. Now data are available for chronic hepatitis B and C managed with alpha interferon with reported remission rates varying from 20-58%. Oral chelation therapy and liver transplantation have radically affected the outcome of patients with Wilson's disease. Corticosteroids and immunosuppressive therapy are effective in reducing both morbidity and mortality due to autoimmune hepatitis. Dietary management like elimination, restriction, modifications have made an impact in disorders like Wilson's disease, galactosemia, tyrosinemia, hereditary fructose intolerance. The most important component of management of chronic liver diseases in childhood are nutritional management with prompt interventions for ascites, spontaneous bacterial peritonitis, portal hypertension and hepatic encephalopathy to have favorable outcome. With definitive etiological and histological assessment and institution of specific as well as supportive therapy, children with chronic liver disease may have prolonged survival with improved quality of life. Availability of liver transplant across the country definitely has made a favorable outcome in children with chronic liver disease.

DEFINITION

Chronic liver disease in children encompasses a wide spectrum of disorders, including infectious, metabolic, genetic, drug-induced, idiopathic, structural and autoimmune diseases with ongoing liver damage progressing to cirrhosis or end-stage liver disease. Chronicity of liver disease is determined either by duration of liver disease (typically >3–6 months) in pediatric population or by evidence of either severe liver disease or physical stigmata of chronic liver disease. The two most important causes of chronic liver disease in Indian infants are neonatal hepatitis and biliary atresia. Wilson disease and autoimmune liver disease are the most common causes in older children presenting with acute on chronic liver failure.

The spectrum of chronic liver disease includes compensated cirrhosis of any etiology, chronic hepatitis, nonalcoholic steatohepatitis (NASH), cholestatic liver disease, metabolic liver disease.

CAUSES OF CHRONIC LIVER DISEASE OTHER THAN NEONATAL CHOLESTASIS SYNDROME

Chronic Hepatitis

Chronic viral hepatitis (B, C), autoimmune hepatitis, sclerosing cholangitis, chronic drug induced hepatitis.

Table 30.1: Changing pattern of CLD in India, KEM Hospital, Pune[1]							
Liver disease	1980–84	85–89	90–94	95–99	2000–04	05–09	09+
ICC	37	22	4	2	1	1	0
Neonatal cholestasis	9	10	28	34	44	40	51
Metabolic	2	5	6	10	14	22	32
Chronic hepatitis	9	6	6	7	8	6	5
Wilson	2	4	5	7	14	16	21
Misc.	18	9	13	23	32	28	16
Total	77	56	62	83	113	113	125

Genetic/Metabolic Liver Disease

Glycogen storage disease (type III and IV), galactosemia, tyrosinemia, mucopolysaccharidosis, Gaucher's disease, Niemann Pick's disease, Wolman disease, alpha 1 antitrypsin deficiency.

Copper and Iron Storage Disease

Wilson's disease, Indian childhood cirrhosis (ICC), hemochromatosis.

Venous Congestion/Vascular Congestion

Budd-Chiari syndrome, congestive cardiac failure, constrictive pericarditis.

Miscellaneous

Nonalcoholic steatohepatitis (NASH), histiocytosis, nutritional cirrhosis.

Nonalcoholic Steatohepatitis

With resurgence of obesity in Indian children due to westernization of diets, sedentary life style, NASH is currently a cause of concern. Nonalcoholic fatty liver disease (NAFLD) is a spectrum of disorders that encompasses simple steatosis to more serious steatohepatitis that can progress to cirrhosis. The major association with NAFLD is obesity and as the prevalence of obesity in childhood and adolescent increases, fatty liver is recognized with greater frequency. The pathogenesis of NASH is the two hit hypothesis that includes disturbed lipid homeostasis, resistance to the effects of insulin, hyperinsulinemia and local toxic effects of triglycerides on hepatocytes. Fibrosis may be more common at the time of diagnosis of NAFLD in children and adolescents. Weight reduction leads to improvement in hepatic histology but may be difficult to achieve.

CLINICAL PRESENTATION OF CHRONIC LIVER DISEASE

1. Chronic liver disease with or without decompensation.
2. Asymptomatic presentation with hepatosplenomegaly.
3. Acute hepatitis like picture.
4. Acute on chronic liver disease.

The common presentation is characterized by insidious onset of abdominal distension, firm hepatosplenomegaly with or without ascites, growth retardation, muscle wasting, hematemesis, malena, jaundice, high colored urine, palmar erythema, pedal edema, cutaneous spiders, altered mental status.

SIGNS OF CHRONIC LIVER FAILURE

Comprises some or all of the following features in children
- General failure of health
- Growth retardation
- Jaundice
- Hyperdynamic circulation
- Recurrent infections
- GI bleed
- Hepatic encephalopathy
- Ascites
- Renal impairment
- Endocrine disturbances
- Disorders of coagulation

CLINICAL CLUES FOR ETIOLOGY

When to Suspect Inherited Disorders

- Family or sibling with liver disease, consanguineous parents
- Unexplained hepatomegaly without jaundice
- Dysmorphic facies, rickets, seizures, failure to thrive, respiratory symptoms
- Liver failure in infancy, severe uncorrectable coagulopathy.

General Examination

It should include:
- Eye—KF ring (Fig. 30.1), sunflower cataract—Wilson's disease
- Cherry red spot—lipid storage disease
- Chorioretinitis—TORCH infections, posterior embryotoxon—Alagille syndrome
- Palmar erythema (Fig. 30.2)
- Characteristic facies, e.g. Alagille syndrome (Fig. 30.3)
- Seborrheic dermatitis, draining ears, ear discharge, bony swellings, chronic cholestasis-histiocytosis
- Many signs of chronic liver disease can be made by simple clinical examination
- Jaundice (Recurrent or prolonged) with high colored urine
- Pale stool in obstructive cholestasis (Fig. 30.4)
- Pruritus
- Malnutrition, muscle wasting
- Firm hepatomegaly, splenomegaly with scar (Fig. 30.5)
- Anemia, clubbing, palmar erythema, cutaneous spider, xanthomas, edema of legs
- Ascites, dilated anterior abdominal veins (caput) (Fig. 30.6)
- Prominent back veins—BCS (Fig. 30.7)
- Clubbing, spider telangiectasia and hepatosplenomegaly, ascites, growth retardation

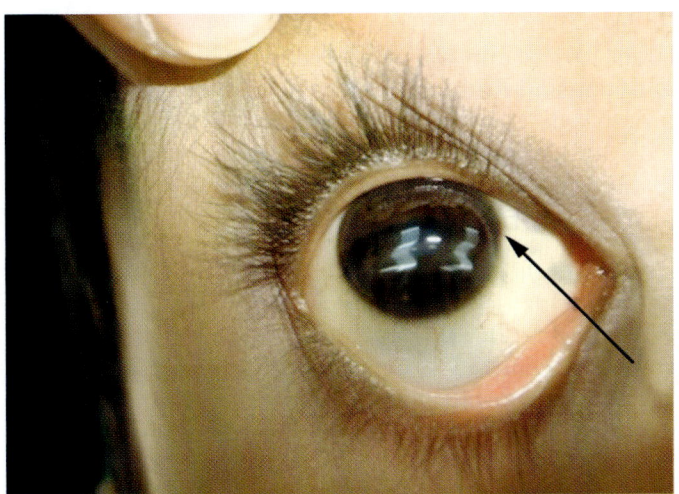

Fig. 30.1: KF ring in a boy with Wilson's disease

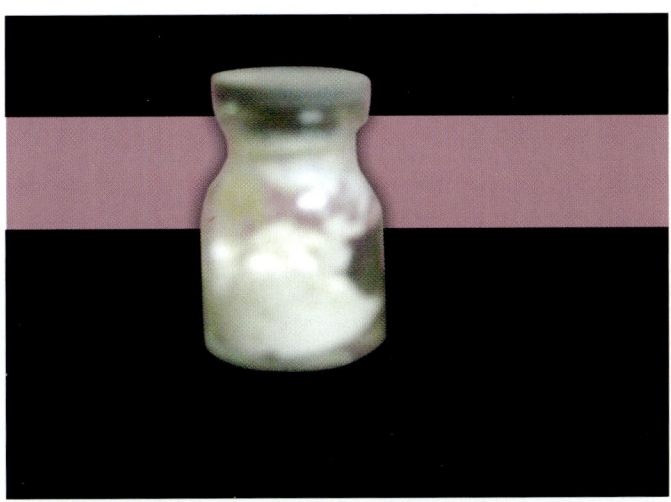

Fig. 30.4: White stool in a child with biliary atresia

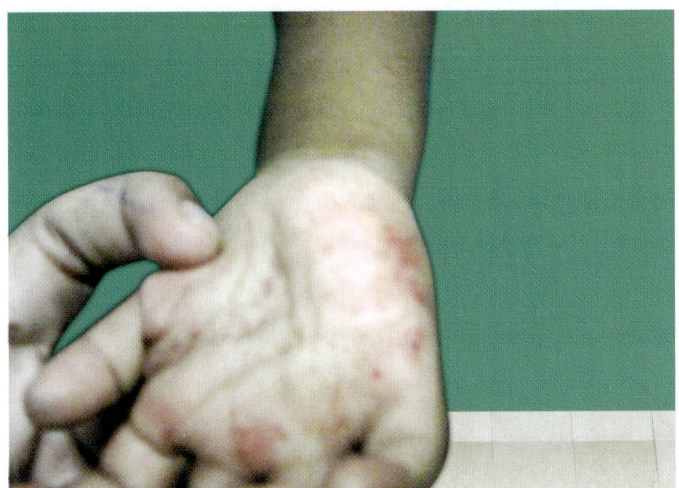

Fig. 30.2: Palmar erythema in a child with chronic liver disease due to histiocytosis

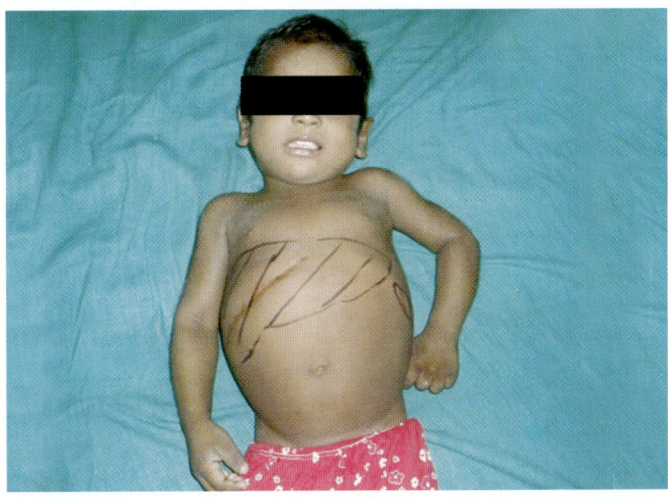

Fig. 30.5: Post-Kasai with secondary biliary cirrhosis and portal hypertension

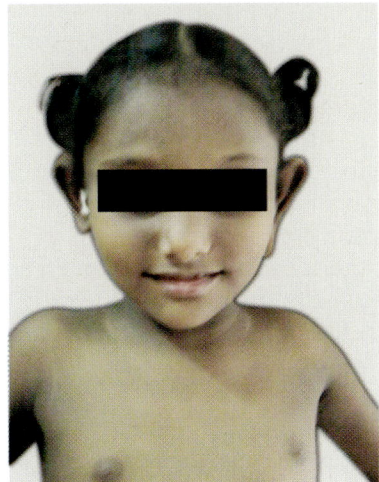

Fig. 30.3: Typical facies of Alagille syndrome

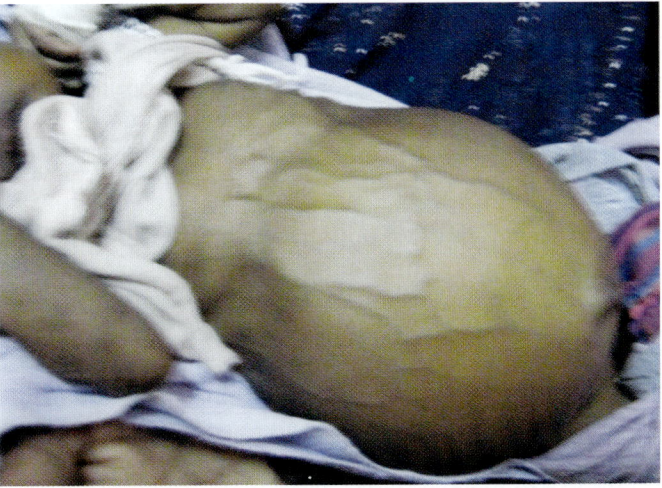

Fig. 30.6: Child with end stage liver disease showing ascites and distended veins

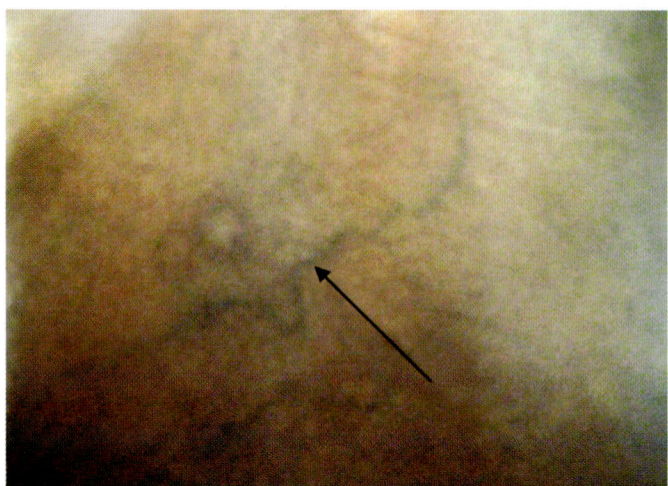

Fig. 30.7: Presence of back veins in Budd-Chiari syndrome

❑ Gynecomastia
❑ Hepatic encephalopathy
❑ Renal failure, hepatorenal syndrome
❑ Spontaneous bacterial peritonitis (ascites, fever, abdominal pain, diarrhea, ileus)
❑ Refractory ascites
❑ Bacterial infections.

COMPLICATIONS

Portal Hypertension

Clinical criteria of portal hypertension are firm hepatomegaly, splenomegaly and dilated anterior abdominal veins (Caput medusae). Portal hypertension is caused by increased resistance to portal blood flow and aggravated by an increased portal venous inflow secondary to increased splanchnic vasodilatation by local endothelial factors and humoral vasodilatators. Clinical importance of portal hypertension include development of gastroesophageal varices, variceal hemorrhage, ascites, renal dysfunction, portosystemic encephalopathy, hypersplenism and hepatopulmonary syndrome.[2]

Variceal Bleed[3]

Variceal bleed due to portal hypertension is another important complication of chronic liver disease commonly presenting as major upper GI bleed. Bleeding from esophagogastric varices is more common than bleeding from other sites of portosystemic collaterals and often major and recurrent. Prevention of portal hypertension bleed is classified as primary and secondary. The goal of primary prophylaxis is to identify varices and initiate primary prophylaxis with nonselective beta blockers.

Endoscopic variceal band ligation (EVL) is indicated in larger varices and is a very effective technique to control and prevent further bleeding. The goal of secondary prophylaxis is to prevent recurrence of further bleeding with drugs or endoscopic sclerotherapy or band ligation.

Hepatic Encephalopathy

Hepatic encephalopathy (HE) is a reversible neuropsychiatric complication of chronic liver disease which is clinically evident by disturbance in central nervous system function due to hepatic insufficiency and manifests as personality changes, intellectual impairment and depressed level of consciousness. The common pathogenic mechanism is usually caused by substances that under normal circumstances are efficiently metabolized by liver but retained in the circulation. Porto-systemic shunting plays a critical role through which the gut derived substances that are normally cleared by liver enter the systemic circulation, bypassing the liver. The clinical features of hepatic encephalopathy are attributed to altered astrocyte-neuronal communications, astrocyte swelling and cerebral edema. Accumulation of unmetabolized ammonia, disturbance of central glutamatergic, serotoninergic, noradrenergic pathways, production of false neurotransmitters, activation of central GABA/benzodiazepine receptors and altered cerebral metabolism are important in the pathogenesis of HE.[2] Precipitating factors include infection, inflammation, electrolyte disturbances, gastrointestinal bleed, excessive and inappropriate use of sedatives, therapeutic shunts, large volume paracentesis.

Clinical Grades of HE[4]

I. Mild confusion, euphoria, anxiety or depression
   - Shortened attention span
   - Slowing of ability to perform mental tasks
   - Reversal of sleep rhythm
II. Drowsiness, lethargy, gross deficits in ability to perform mental tasks
   - Obvious personality changes
   - Inappropriate behavior
   - Intermittent disorientation of time and place
   - Lack of sphincter control
III. Somnolent but arousable
   - Persistent disorientation of time and space
   - Unable to perform mental tasks
IV. Coma with (IVa) or without (IVb) response to painful stimuli.

The most characteristic neurological abnormality is flapping tremor which can be elicited in older children and adolescents.

RENAL COMPLICATIONS AND HEPATORENAL SYNDROME[2]

Renal impairment is most often due to functional abnormalities that occur in response to severe splanchnic arterial vasodilatation that triggers an intense homeostatic neurohumoral response with subsequent sodium, solute free water retention causing severe renal vasoconstriction. Hepatorenal syndrome (HRS) is the end spectrum of functional renal abnormalities. There are two types. Type 1 is an acute and rapidly progressive form with poor prognosis and type 2 is a more stable form with a slightly better prognosis.

ASCITES AND SPONTANEOUS BACTERIAL PERITONITIS

Ascites is the most common application in children with cirrhosis. Ascites formation is mostly associated with events occurring in the arterial vascular compartment and in the kidneys. The pathogenetic mechanism causing accumulation of ascetic fluid in the peritoneal cavity in cirrhotics is splanchnic arterial vasodilatation secondary to portal hypertension inducing forward increase in capillary pressure because of great inflow of blood at high pressure into splanchnic microcirculation with subsequent leakage of fluid into the peritoneal cavity.[5]

Spontaneous bacterial peritonitis (SBP) is spontaneous infection of previously sterile ascitic fluid without an apparent intra-abdominal infection. SBP has a prevalence of 10 to 30% among patients with ascites.[6,7]

Bacterial translocation occurs due to increased gut permeability resulting from disruption of the gut mucosal barrier, bacterial overgrowth, intestinal hypomotility and decrease in host immune defenses. Gram-negative aerobic bacteria derived from gut from the family of *Enterobacteriaceae*, namely *Escherichia coli* is the most common organism followed by nonenteric organisms from skin, urinary tract and upper respiratory tract.

EVALUATION

Proper history taking including family history of liver disease, consanguinity, drug intake and thorough physical examination forms an important step in evaluation.

- ❑ Assessment of nutritional status with height, weight, BMI in absence of ascites, skin fold thickness.
- ❑ Complete hemogram, ESR,
- ❑ Blood sugar, renal function tests, serum electrolytes
- ❑ Liver function tests, GGT
- ❑ Prothrombin time, blood ammonia,

- ❑ Upper GI endoscopy to look for varices, portal hypertensive changes
- ❑ USG abdomen
- ❑ Liver biopsy
- ❑ Etiological investigations
- ❑ Hepatobiliary scintigraphy
- ❑ Viral markers for hepatitis B and C
- ❑ Antinuclear antibody, antismooth muscle antibody. Anti-LKm antibody for autoimmune liver disease.
- ❑ Wilson's disease work-up—KF ring by slit-lamp examination, serum ceruloplasmin, serum copper, 24 hours urine copper.
- ❑ Aminoaciduria, glycosuria, phosphaturia, uricosuria in Wilson's disease.
- ❑ Fasting blood sugar, pyruvate and lactate, triglycerides, uric acid for GSD.
- ❑ Serum bile acids for PFIC
- ❑ TORCH screening
- ❑ Doppler study of portal and hepatic venous system for portal hypertension and Budd-Chiari syndrome.

Investigations for Complications

Serum ascetic albumin gradient (SAAG) is a simple and best test to classify ascites into portal hypertensive and nonportal hypertensive. Value > 1.1 is indicative of portal hypertension with 97% accuracy.

USG abdomen with Doppler—increased liver echoes, dilated portal vein, presence of collaterals with or without ascites.

Polymorpholeukocytes more than 250 cells/cu mm in ascitic fluid is suggestive of SBP.

CT scan and MRI can give accurate information as angiography and useful in planning for liver transplant.

Fibroscan is another new modality that can be used for assessing hepatic fibrosis, though only limited data is available in children.

Liver Biopsy

Before planning for liver biopsy, coagulation profile, platelet count and bleeding time are mandatory.

Liver biopsy can be either USG guided percutaneous biopsy, transvenous biopsy, a laparoscopic procedure or an open surgical biopsy. Interpretation of liver histology needs to be made by an experienced pediatric liver pathologist. Special stains for copper, glycogen storage diseases, neonatal iron storage disease are needed. Specimen need to be transported in alcohol in suspected glycogen storage disease.

For glycogen storage disease biopsy specimen should be fixed in alcohol. Glycogen often accumulates to such an extent the hepatocytes are swollen appearing as plant cell. Type IV is associated with the accumulation of abnormal glycogen molecule, amylopectin appearing as homogenous, slightly eosinophilc or even colorless in the hepatocytes which is intense PAS positive and diastase resistance but digested with pectinase.

AAT, liver histology will show characteristic eosinophilic globules in the hepatocytes which are PAS positive and diastase resistant.

Wilson's disease—steatosis, periportal glycogenated nuclei, Mallory-hyaline will be evident. Special copper stains will show excess copper in the hepatocytes.

TREATMENT

The primary objective of treatment is to minimize further liver damage by treating the cause, preventing complications and ensuring optimal growth and development.

General treatment include nutritional rehabilitation, adequate vitamin supplementation

Dietary management includes salt restriction in presence of fluid retention, avoidance of protein of animal origin in encephalopathy. Children with hepatic encephalopathy should be admitted in an intensive care unit. Supportive measures include intravenous fluid therapy with maintenance of electrolyte balance. Children should be nursed with head end elevation and handled minimally. Grade 1 encephalopathy is an indication for elective mechanical ventilation.

Protein restriction is not recommended, even in the presence of encephalopathy and in fact, adequate protein supplementation contributes to an improved overall nutritional status, promoting faster recovery. A high energy to nitrogen ratio, which is characteristic of casein based and vegetable based diets reduces gluconeogenesis and has anabolic effects on utilization of dietary proteins. Oral lactulose is useful in reducing the production of ammonia in the colon.

The risk of gastrointestinal bleeding from stress ulceration can be reduced by oral sucralfate, H_2 blockers or proton pump inhibitors. Coagulopathy can be corrected with parenteral vitamin K, fresh frozen plasma, factor VII C concentrate.

MANAGEMENT OF VARICEAL BLEED[3,8]

Volume replacement and airway maintenance is an important first step in management.

The time frame for the acute bleeding episode should be 120 hours (5 days)

Ht (or Hb) is measured at least every 6 hours for the first 2 days, 12 hours for days 3–5. The transfusion target should be a hematocrit of 24% or a hemoglobin of 8 g/dL.

Medical Therapy

In acute variceal bleeding, vasoactive drugs must be started even before endoscopy, and should be maintained for up to 5 days. The choice of vasoactive drug depends on availability. The drugs that are used are terlipressin, somatostatin and octreotide. Vasopressin along with nitroglycerin may be used. Sengstaken-Blakemore tube can be used in acute setting if adequate size is available.

Emergency endoscopic procedures like EST or EVL can be done in controlling active bleed after initial stabilization. Newer endoscopic technique like endoloop to tackle bleeding esophageal varices has been tried in adults. Tissue adhesive (e.g. N-butylcyanoacrylate) is recommended for acute gastric variceal bleeding.

Secondary Prophylaxis

For secondary prophylaxis, endoscopic therapy is effective. There is insufficient evidence to recommend beta-blockers, however, can be given as it reduces the rebleed rate. EVL followed with EST is as effective as EST alone and is preferable as it requires fewer sessions with less complications as well as low recurrence of varices.

Surgical Modalities

Emergency devascularization may benefit in acute uncontrolled bleed. Shunt surgeries have the disadvantage of precipitating encephalopathy in cirrhotics.

Radiological Method

Angiography with transcatheteral embolization of feeding vessel can be done for uncontrollable acute bleed with failed endotherapy.

Management of Ascites

Management of ascites include bed rest, low sodium diet and diuretics with spironolactone, furosemide. The dose of furosemide is 1–2 mg/kg/dose to a maximum dose of 6 mg/kg. Spironolactone is an aldosterone antagonist that inhibits aldosterone secretion and sodium retention and the dose 1–3 is mg/kg/day in 3–4 divided doses. Combination with spironolactone is preferred to monotherapy because of high efficacy, less side effects in cirrhotic ascites. Gradual weight loss and negative sodium balance is an optimum criteria for response to therapy. Therapeutic paracentesis is indicated in case of tense ascites with plasma volume expansion by synthetic colloids or albumin. Patients unresponsive to low sodium diet plus adequate diuretics are likely to have refractory ascites. Treatment options include large volume paracentesis, transjugular intrahepatic portosystemic shunts and liver transplantation.

SPONTANEOUS BACTERIAL PERITONITIS

Antibiotic therapy with either cefotaxime or ceftriaxone must be started once the diagnosis of spontaneous bacterial peritonitis (SBP) is made. Antibiotics prophylaxis with quinolones is indicated in case of GI bleed or following an attack of SBP.

Specific Treatment

Copper chelators with oral D penicillamine, zinc, trientene for Wilsons disease along with dietary management. Antiviral therapy with lamuvudine and interferons in selected cases. NTBC for tyrosinemia.

Children with chronic cholestatic liver disease require regular supplementation with fat-soluble vitamins, twice the RDA of water-soluble vitamins along with micronutrients.

DIET IN CHRONIC LIVER DISEASE

Diseases Requiring Dietary Elimination

Dietary copper intake should be restricted and foods such as shell-fish, dried fruits, chocolates, mushroom and liver should be avoided in children with Wilson's disease. In children with hemochromatosis, iron containing multivitamin preparations and eating liver, spinach and molasses should be avoided. In infants with galactosemia, withdrawal of milk and milk products from diet to prevent worsening of liver disease is mandatory.

Liver Diseases Requiring Diet Modification

In children with glycogen storage disease (GSD), continuous source of glucose to prevent hypoglycemia may be achieved by continuous nasogastric nocturnal glucose drip or by raw cornstarch feeds in the evening. Similar dietary measures may be required in the milder form of GSD Type III with debrancher enzyme deficiency. In hereditary fructose intolerance (HFI), dietary restriction of sucrose and fructose is essential. Tyrosinemia of acute type leads to death in infancy, irrespective of dietary management. The chronic type may benefit from restriction of aromatic amino acids and growth may be normalized and hepatomegaly may be prevented or ameliorated. Hepatocellular carcinoma is, however, not preventable.

The only definitive treatment for end stage liver disease is liver transplantation.

REFERENCES

1. IAP speciality series on pediatric gastroenterology, 2nd edition, Jaypee Publisher, 2013.
2. Schiff"s Disease of liver, 10th edition, Volume 1, Wolters Kluwer Publishers, New Delhi, 2009.
3. de Franchis R. Evolving Consensus in Portal Hypertension Report of the Baveno IV Consensus Workshop on methodology of diagnosis and therapy in portal hypertension. J Hepatol. 2005;43:167-76.
4. Sherlock S. Disease of liver and biliary system. 11th edition, Blackwell Publishers, 2002.
5. Runyon BA. Ascites and Spontaneous Bacterial Peritonitis. Sleisenger and Fordtran, 7th edition, Gastrointestinal and Liver Disease, pathophysiology/diagnosis/management, Vol 2, Philadelphia, WB Saunders. 2002;1517-42.
6. Rimola A, Garcia-Tsao G, Navasa M, et al. Diagnosis, treatment and prophylaxis of spontaneous bacterial peritonitis: a consensus document. J Hepatol. 2000;32:142-53.
7. Larcher VF, Manolaki N, Vegnent A, et al. Spontaneous bacterial peritonitis with chronic liver disease: clinical features and etiologic factors. J Pediatr. 1985;106:907-12.
8. Rodriguez- Perez F, Groszmann RJ. Pharmacologic treatment of portal hypertension. Gastroenterol Clin North Am. 1992;21:15-40.

Chapter
31

Surgical Disorders of the Hepatobiliary System

Sujit Chowdhary

BILIARY ATRESIA

Biliary atresia is potentially disastrous disease of new-borns which usually gets recognized in early infancy. It presents with persistent jaundice and clay-colored stools in a well-baby. It is the result of progressive obliterative cholangiopathy with secondary liver cirrhosis leading to liver failure. The obliterative process is usually thought to start at the caudal end of the bile duct and progress cranially towards the liver. The onset of the disease is usually perinatal and the effect becomes obvious anywhere between 2–6 weeks. The incidence of the disease has been variously estimated as 1: 15,000, but no reliable data on epidemiology is available from India.[1]

Since the disease starts as an obiliterative cholangiopathy in the common bile duct near its opening in the duodenum and progresses cranially it was postulated that early diagnosis, excision of the bile duct cranially until the porta will remove the entire obliterated biliary tree and expose normal biliary canaliculi at the porta hepatis. In that case portoenterostomy may lead to resolution of the disease. Since the etiology, evolution, natural history and progression is poorly understood, that does not happen in all cases. The first series of such operations were reported by Kasai from Japan.[2]

Although the Kasai portoenterostomy has become accepted as the standard initial operation for biliary atresia, only less than 50% respond to this surgery in the best of circumstances and most of long-term survivors develop complications.[3]

Etiology

The exact etiology is uncertain, it is postulated that the common form of the disease is the result of perinatal viral infection. There is also a possibility of this disease being a developmental disease in a small subset either due to an inherited genetic defect or without. In this small subset, the disease is associated with a range of other associated abnormalities like malrotation, polysplenia, preduodenal portal vein, interrupted inferior vena cava, etc.[4] The development of the liver from the hepatic diverticulum of the foregut and fusion with the developing parenchyma in the septum transverse undergoes a differentiation abnormality. In the absence of a reliable animal model much more remains to be understood about the etiopathogenesis of the disease.

Classification

The disease starts in the intrauterine life of the baby and continues to progress after the birth of the baby. On the basis of various patterns of the obliteration of the extrahepatic biliary duct, as observed on the intraoperative cholangiogram and intraoperative findings, the disease has been classified. The main categories are types I, II, and III and are defined as atresia at the site of the common bile duct (CBD), at the site of the hepatic duct, and up to the porta hepatis, respectively. Most patients have type III. Cystic dilatation at the distal end of a patent duct is seen in some cases of type I biliary atresia.

In the early stage of the disease, liver may appear normal. However, after the first three months of life, the liver is enlarged, firm, and splenomegaly may be present. The gallbladder may be small and filled with white mucus, or it may be completely atretic. The biliary tracts contain inflammatory and fibrous cells surrounding miniscule ducts that are probably remnants of the original embryonic duct system. The liver parenchyma is fibrotic and shows signs of cholestasis. The proliferation of biliary neoductules is characteristic with bile plugs. This process develops into end-stage cirrhosis if good drainage cannot be achieved. These early changes are often nonspecific and may be confused with neonatal hepatitis and metabolic disease.

Diagnosis

The cardinal signs and symptoms of biliary atresia are jaundice, clay-colored stools, and hepatomegaly in an otherwise well baby. The stool which initially may be pigmented begins to turn acholic in later weeks. As the disease progresses and secondary liver cirrhosis starts to set in, all features of liver failure, malabsorption, etc. starts appearing.

In any baby with raised serum bilirubin and, disproportionate rise in conjugated fraction biliary atresia must be an important differential diagnosis. A repeat serum bilirubin within two weeks with a complete liver function test will demonstrate no significant fall in bilirubin with increase in the liver enzymes particularly alkaline phosphatase and gamma-glutamyl transferase. The coagulation parameters may be deranged. A basic ultrasound examination in fasting and postfeed state will reveal nonvisualized gallbladder in the majority.

A HIDA scan will reveal good uptake of dye in the liver from the blood with nonexcretory pattern.[5] It is usually done after 3–5 days of enzyme induction with phenobarbitone, although there is no hard evidence to suggest this is of any real benefit.

A needle liver biopsy should be used to assess secondary changes in the liver and helps in diagnosis and staging the development of liver cirrhosis. However, it is not the diagnostic test, as it reflects secondary changes in liver, consequent to disease process starting in the extrahepatic biliary tree progressing to porta hepatis. It can be used to almost conclusively eliminate biliary atresia from differential diagnosis if there is absence of bile plugs and proliferating bile ductules on biopsy.[6] It is also helpful in diagnosing the extremely rare diagnosis of biliary hypoplasia.

The diagnostic test for biliary atresia is an intraoperative cholangiogram by a minilaparotomy in the right subcostal region. In more than 50% cases of biliary atresia, the gallbladder is completely atretic, precluding any cholangiography. The atretic gallbladder is the confirmatory evidence of the disease. In the other half the obliterative process has not lead to complete atresia of the gallbladder, allowing the lumen to accept a small feeding tube for cholangiography and confirmation of the diagnosis. In order to make sense of the cholangiogram, the cholangiogram in a normal baby, and baby with cirrhotic liver without biliary atresia should be understood in the first instance. If the cholangiogram is feasible after a minilaparotomy, it will demonstrate block at different levels of the biliary tree depending on the evolution of the disease.

Treatment

Biliary atresia has no medical treatment. The treatment of the disease is surgical, depending on the evolution of the disease. If the disease has been diagnosed early, treatment is portoenterostomy with success rates around only 40% to 50%.[7,8] Liver transplant is the definitive surgical treatment in those babies who have failed to improve after portoenterostomy or have got a diagnosis after 100 days. Portoenterostomy is successful in only 40%, provided diagnosis is made before 60 days and an experienced surgeon operates in an established tertiary center. It is important to appreciate that in these 40% babies both the baby and family are spared major surgery with lifelong medication following liver transplant. There should be every effort to delete unnecessary tests after 60 days, as the postoperative results fall steeply after every week's delay beyond sixty days.[9]

The preoperative preparation of the baby entails hydration, correction of coagulation, gut preparation, intravenous antibiotics, etc. for at least 48–72 hours before surgery. It is the quality of preoperative preparation which will define the outcome of surgery and incidence of postoperative cholangitis. Postoperative cholangitis is a major morbidity after successful surgery which requires preoperative steps to reduce the incidence and postoperative failures.

The surgery is started by a minilaparotomy no more than an inch incision in the subcostal area, which can confirm the anatomy of the gallbladder and extrahepatic biliary architecture. Intraoperative cholangiogram is performed to demonstrate the anatomy. It is important to be aware that in a vast majority it may not be technically feasible as the gallbladder may be totally atretic, which itself confirms the diagnosis. At this stage, the laparotomy is extended to proceed to portoenterostomy. The entire liver has to be exteriorized after incising the ligaments. The dissection starts from gallbladder bed skeletoning the hepatic arteries and excising the entire atretic biliary structures progress craniad into porta hepatis. The portal vein has to dissected ligating minor tributaries so that the entire fibrotic triad in the porta hepatis can be excised and anastomosed to Roux loop. The success of operation depends on the extent of the disease process and quality of surgery. If the disease is in evolution or obliterative cholangiopathy has extended cranially beyond the porta, no amount of dissection will help other than liver transplantation.

The postoperative care in these babies is similar to any other baby with major intestinal and hepatobiliary surgery. A short course of steroids in the postoperative period is used by some to improve outcome by its cholerectic effect and reducing scarring at anastomosis. Fat-soluble vitamins (A, D, E, and K) and formula feeds enriched with medium-chain triglycerides are also used.

Postoperative cholangitis is the most frequent morbidity which leads to fever, decreased quantity and quality of bile, elevations in serum bilirubin and deterioration of liver function.[10] The risk for repeated attacks remains in the first two years of life. It requires aggressive surveillance, hospital treatment to prevent failures in a potentially curable situation. Other complications are late decompensation, portal hypertension, gastrointestinal bleeding, etc. Each of these require specific treatment strategies. In the group where the initial portoenterostomy has failed with progressive liver failure, liver transplantation is the treatment.[11]

Outcome

In a baby with biliary atresia, if portoenterostomy is offered earlier than 60 days in a tertiary center, at least 25% will remain asymptomatic. Another 15% will need supportive treatment with mild icterus and not progress to liver transplantation.

Various centers from all over the world have reported variable results.[12,13] That reflects varying health standards in the countries. Indian results are discouraging with persisting delay in diagnosis and late referral.[14] There is a delay in Kasai portoenterostomy as late as 75 days even at our own center. A comparative chart (Table 31.1) shows the results reported from various units around the world.

In our experience of 40 babies with extrahepatic biliary atresia over the last 8 years, 55% had good bile flow in the immediate post-Kasai period. There was no intra- or perioperative mortality. One baby was re-explored for peritonitis, and found to have perforation in the Roux limb. Postoperative recurrent cholangitis was the most common morbidity. The four-year survival with the native liver was 40% and 30% were jaundice free. In our babies only 50% were diagnosed before 60 days and 15 (37%) were between 60 and 90 days[5] (13%), babies were beyond 90 days. The four-year survival with native liver in less than 60 days group was 60%, whereas only one baby with Kasai done after 90 days survived at one year. Only three children from this series could afford a liver transplant.

Conclusion

Biliary atresia is a miserable disease, as by the time the diagnosis becomes clear to all, the chance for surgical treatment without transplantation is over. At that stage, the only treatment is liver transplantation, which involves major surgery on the baby and mother with lifelong medical support.

Every baby with obstructive jaundice at six weeks should have detailed evaluation in a center with experience in this disease, and reach operating room before 60 days.

Forty percent babies can hope to live normal lives without need for transplantation after confirmation of diagnosis, meticulous preoperative preparation, surgery and aggressive treatment of cholangitis in the first two years of life.

▌CHOLEDOCHAL CYST

Choledochal cyst is an abnormal cystic dilatation of the intra- or extrahepatic biliary ducts or both. It is characterized by a terminal narrow and sometimes obliterated opening into the duodenum or pancreatic duct. The obstruction to the flow of bile leads to a range of complications. This predisposes these babies to recurrent attacks of pancreatitis, jaundice, cholangitis and choledocholithiasis eventually leading to secondary biliary cirrhosis. This symptom complex subsequently in later life can even lead to malignant change in the dysplastic epithelium of the mucosal lining of the cyst. The treatment is cyst excision and bilioenteric bypass. It is curative in the vast majority; however, in cases with delay in treatment since birth, the recurrent attacks of inflammation in a structure surrounded by portal vein and hepatic artery, surgery is far more difficult, incomplete and prone to complications.

This condition is relatively uncommon, with an estimated incidence in western populations of 1 in 13,000 to 15,000 live births.[15] The incidence is higher in the Asians, with rates as high as 1 per 1000 live births; incidence being higher in Orientals.[16] In the developed world, majority of them are being diagnosed antenatally with treatment

Table 31.1: Outcome of Kasai portoenterostomy (PE)				
	No. of patients	Median age at PE	4 yr survival with native liver	4 yr overall survival
Japan 1989	108	–	62%	69%
France 2006	271	57 days	42%	87%
United States* 2006	104	61 days	55%	93%
Switzerland 2008	48	68 days	37%	91%
England 2011	424	54 days	46%	90%
Apollo 2013	40	74 days	40%	40%

* 2-year survival

in early infancy. The Indian studies have documented later diagnosis and treatment of the disease with various secondary complications.[17]

Etiology and Pathogenesis

The etiology of choledochal cyst is not clear and a number of theories have been proposed. The congenital weakness of the bile duct wall, a primary abnormality of proliferation during embryologic ductal development, and congenital obstruction have all been postulated. The most commonly accepted theory is Babbitt's "long common channel theory", who postulated that choledochal cysts result from pancreatobiliary malunion (PBMU), which allows reflux of pancreatic enzymes into the CBD, which leads to disruption of the duct walls.[18]

Clinical Presentation

Choledochal cysts commonly present in childhood with more than half of patients seen within the first decade of life. The classic triad of symptoms includes pain abdomen, palpable abdominal mass, and jaundice. Clinical manifestations differ according to the age at onset. Neonates detected antenatally are usually asymptomatic at birth but it has to be intervened early before the onset of complications. Young infants may have obstructive jaundice, nonpigmented stools, and hepatomegaly, resembling biliary atresia, and may even have advanced liver fibrosis. Young infants may also present with a large upper abdominal mass without jaundice. In young children, presenting symptoms can be divided roughly into two groups: a right upper quadrant mass with intermittent jaundice due to biliary obstruction, seen in patients with saccular choledochal cyst, and abdominal pain due to pancreatitis, which is characteristic of fusiform choledochal cyst (FFCC). In adolescence and adulthood, choledochal cyst has often been misdiagnosed for many years as cholelithiasis, cirrhosis, portal hypertension, hepatic abscess and biliary carcinoma.

Diagnosis

Imaging techniques confirm the diagnosis of choledochal cysts. Radiographic visualization of both biliary system and pancreatic duct prior to surgery helps in complete excision of choledochal cysts. So the diagnostic workup should be done for meticulous operative planning.

Abdominal ultrasonography (US) is the first investigation in patients who are suspected of having choledochal cyst. The diagnosis will be confirmed on US in most of the cases. Widespread availability of US has made possible the diagnosis of choledochal cyst antenatally and also incidentally in children.

MRCP avoids ionizing radiation, is noninvasive and has sensitivity as high as 90–100%.[19] MRCP with magnetic resonance imaging (MRI) can also image surrounding structures, stones, and malignancy. It provides anatomical detail superior to US.

Endoscopic retrograde cholangiopancreatography (ERCP) is not routinely done as it is an invasive procedure, which may cause cholangitis and pancreatitis, and it also exposes the children to risks of radiation. But, in the forme fruste and choledochocoele variants of choledochal cyst, ERCP has a specific diagnostic as well as therapeutic role.[20]

At times a combination of imaging modalities is needed for a complete and definitive diagnosis. Intraoperative cholangiography is a useful tool to delineate the entire biliary system before cyst excision and it should be done as a first step in the operative plan.

Classification and Treatment

The choledochal cysts have been classified based on the anatomical variants and each type has implications on the surgical management and long-term outcome. The cyst can present in five main anatomical variants with subtypes as per Figure 31.1. The classification was proposed by Alonso lej et al[21] and later modified by Todani et al to include two further subtypes.[22]

The type 1f or 1c is the most common variety, and is managed by cyst excision and hepaticojejunostomy or hepaticoduodenostomy; both approaches have their own merits. The choledochocoele is rare may be approached endoscopically or open intraduodenal deroofing. Caroli's disease or intrahepatic sacculation and dilatatation is prone to delayed complications. In case of delayed presentation with secondary complication of the cyst various approaches with initial percutaneous hepatic drainage, open drainage, cystojejunostomy, etc. have been used with good results.

A rare presentation may be with recurrent attacks of pancreatitis or choledocholithiasis without a significantly dilated bile duct (more than 10 mm). The characteristic hallmark of the disease is pancreaticobilary malunion with long common channel. This requires endoscopic retrograde cholangiopancreatography, and is perhaps one of the few absolute indications of ERCP in a child. In cases with mild dilatation (less than 10 mm), the diagnosis of form fruste was proposed by Lilly et al as the mild dilatation of common bile duct and simpler treatment like choleycytectomy and sphincterotomy, and failure of

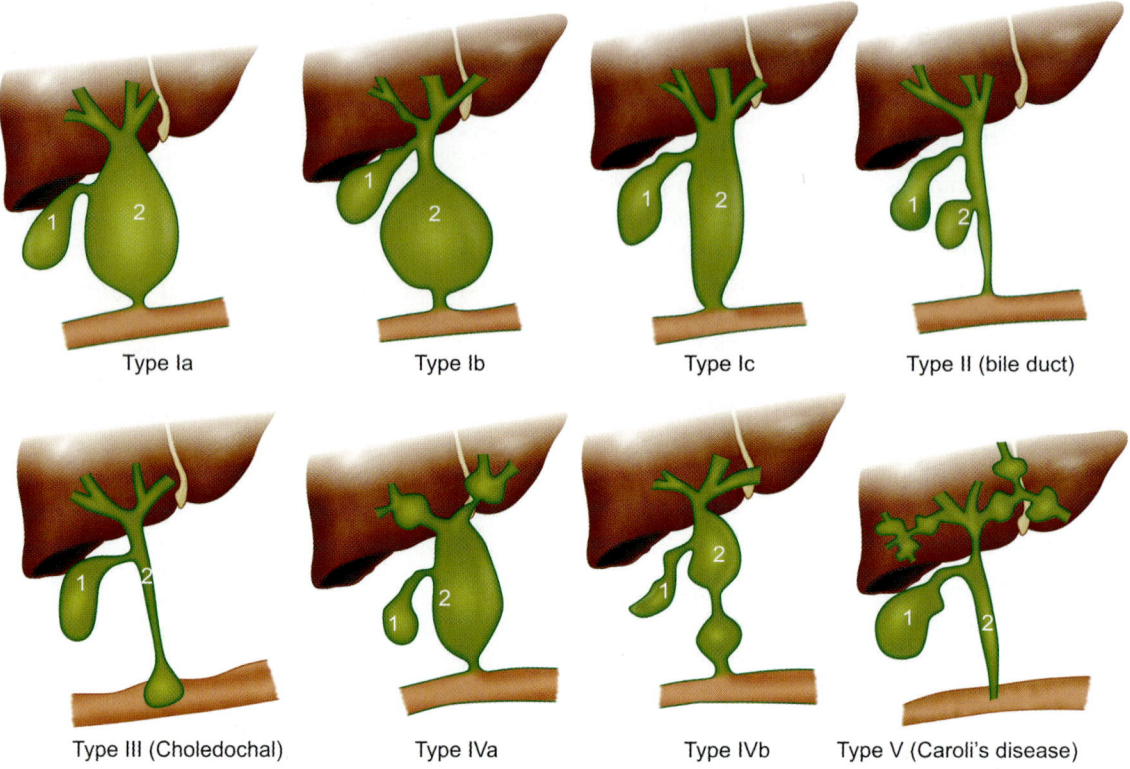

Type Ia   Type Ib   Type Ic   Type II (bile duct)

Type III (Choledochal)   Type IVa   Type IVb   Type V (Caroli's disease)

1—gallbladder; 2—common bile duct

Fig. 31.1: Classification of choledochal cyst

medical treatment with recurrent symptoms frustrates the clinician.[23]

The radical treatment of bile duct excision and bile diversion in forme fruste variant prevents premature activation of the pancreatic enzymes as the premature union of the bile duct with pancreatic duct and long common channel is the central pathology leading to all the symptoms. Biliary diversion is successful in preventing this cascade with complete relief of symptoms.

In our experience of 35 cases over a period of 8 years, male to female ratio was 1:3 and mean age at diagnosis was 7 years. Among our 35 patients 3 were of forme fruste variety and 5 had diagnosis in neonatal period. All underwent excision of cyst and Roux-en-Y hepaticojejunostomy, the youngest baby was 2 months old. There was no mortality and perioperative morbidity in three, which required re-exploration in one. One child developed anastomotic stricture eight years after surgery requiring redo-surgery. She had delayed diagnosis with secondary complication prior to initial surgery.

Outcome

There is a excellent short and mid-term outcome after cyst excision and biliary diversion. However, many studies have reported long-term complications of cholangitis, pancreatitis, portal hypertension, anastomotic stricture,

stone formation and even malignancy. Therefore, these patients need a life-long follow-up.

PORTAL HYPERTENSION

Portal hypertension occurs when there is increased portal resistance and/or increased portal blood flow. Normal portal pressure is between 5 and 10 mm Hg. Once portal pressure rises to 12 mm Hg or greater, complications such as bleeding esophageal varices, hypersplenism and ascites may occur.[24] Extrahepatic portal venous obstruction is the most common cause in children. Pediatric patients with portal hypertension constitute a heterogeneous population in terms of variety of liver diseases which can lead to this sequel. According to the level of obstruction the causes of portal hypertension are divided into three groups.

Prehepatic Obstruction

Portal vein thrombosis is the most common cause of portal hypertension in children accounting for nearly 50% of the cases.[25] The cause of extrahepatic portal venous thrombosis (EHPVO) is unknown in majority of cases, but congenital malformation of the portal vein or acquired thrombosis following umbilical sepsis, umbilical vein catheterization, pylephlebitis following intestinal infection and dehydration are some of the risk factors. It is usually detected early in the first decade, because of splenomegaly, gastrointestinal bleeding, or both. These babies typically have normal liver synthetic functions so the variceal bleeding is tolerated well.

INTRAHEPATIC OBSTRUCTION

Biliary atresia and choledochal cyst are two main causes of intrahepatic obstruction leading to portal hypertension. Children with biliary atresia tend to develop varices very early, with an estimated risk of bleeding of 15% before the age of two.[26] Other causes of intrahepatic portal hypertension in children are congenital hepatic fibrosis, focal biliary cirrhosis, α1-antitrypsin deficiency, chronic active hepatitis and complications secondary to irradiation or chemotherapy.

Suprahepatic Obstruction

Obstruction to the hepatic venous outflow (Budd-Chiari syndrome) is a rare cause of portal hypertension in children. Most of the patients have an associated thrombobophilic state.[27] These patients typically present with hepatomegaly and ascitis rather than variceal bleeding.

Clinical Presentation

In children with portal hypertension, approximately two-thirds present with hematemesis or melena, usually from rupture of an esophageal varix.[28] Other sites of collaterals are retroperitoneal, periumbilical, and hemorrhoidal, but they rarely cause significant bleeding. Splenomegaly and hypersplenism are the second most common finding in children with portal hypertension after gastrointestinal bleeding. In patients with portal hypertension, increased sodium retention and raised portal pressure may cause accumulation of fluid within the abdomen and the resultant ascites can cause respiratory compromise.

Treatment

Acute variceal bleeding is the most common and dramatic presentation of portal hypertension, with an associated mortality up to 20%, especially in patients with deranged liver function.[29] It is a life-threatening medical emergency and needs aggressive initial management and stabilization. Once stabilized, patients should be treated by direct approach of the varices, either with band ligation or sclerotherapy. Both are equally effective and choice of a procedure depends upon the expertise available but generally, endoscopic band ligation is preferred approach as it is easier and safe. In small number of cases where acute variceal bleeding cannot be controlled by all available means, surgical therapy is required as a last resort. The surgical procedures available are transection, devascularization, and portosystemic shunting. The first two techniques work by interrupting blood flow through the esophagus. Transjugular intrahepatic portosystemic shunt (TIPS) placement may be considered, but it has limited availability and is unsuitable for small children.

After the control of acute variceal bleeding further management is directed at the underlying pathology. For patients with good liver function and prehepatic cause for portal hypertension shunt surgery should be considered after first bleeding episode itself.[30] The shunt can be either total, partial or selective.

Nonselective shunts enable complete decompression of portal system by diverting total portal blood flow away from liver. These are end-to-side and side-to-side portacaval shunts, central lienorenal shunt, end-to-side mesocaval shunt and large diameter interposition portacaval and mesocaval shunts. Selective shunts like the splenorenal shunt divert blood of gastroesophageal-splenic segment and maintain blood flow in mesenteric segment which enables portal decompression with maintenance of hepatopetal portal perfusion, mesenteric venous pressure and hepatotropic factors. In 1998, Rex shunt was first described in which internal jugular vein graft is harvested and used to form a bypass between the SMV and the left portal vein located at the Rex recess of the liver.

In children with portal hypertension resulting from intraparenchymal liver disease and advanced cirrhosis liver transplantation needs to be considered.

CHOLELITHIASIS

Cholelithiasis is uncommon in children but with the increasing use of US more number of children is being identified . The prevalence of gallstone disease in children has been reported to be around 1.9%.[31]

It is believed that most of the childhood cholelithiasis is secondary to hemolytic disorders.[32] Hereditary spherocytosis, sickle cell anemia, and thalassemia are the most common hemolytic disorders resulting in the development of gallstones in children. These children typically have pigment stones. Our own experience and recent studies indicate that there has been an increase in the number of nonhemolytic cholelithiasis in children.[33,34]

Certain risk factors like obesity, family history of gallstones, abdominal surgery, IgA deficiency, cystic fibrosis, therapy with ceftriaxone, and Gilbert's disease have been associated with gallstone disease. Contrary to adults most of the stones in children are symptomatic. The symptoms are right upper quadrant abdominal pain and the diagnosis is made at ultrasonography.

The children can be divided into two groups—symptomatic and asymptomatic. The asymptomatic stones need periodic clinical and ultrasound evaluation for spontaneous resolution. If they persist beyond six months and are multiple, laparoscopic cholecystectomy is the treatment of choice. If the stones are symptomatic, surgery is necessary. In an asymptomatic single stone follow-up can be for longer without surgery. The risk of pancreatitis secondary to cholelithiasis is much more with multiple smaller stones.

Laparoscopic cholecystectomy is the gold standard and has a definite advantage over open cholecystectomy in terms of reduced pain, better cosmesis and shorter hospitalization.[35] In our experience of 41 cases of pediatric gallstone disease over 8 years, the mean age at diagnosis was 9 years. One child had hemolytic disorder, two had gallstones secondary to prolonged ceftriaxone therapy and the rest had idiopathic stones. In 3 children stones resolved spontaneously. Thirty-nine underwent laparoscopic cholecystectomy and one underwent laparoscopic splenectomy and laparoscopic cholecystectomy for gallstones secondary to hereditary spherocytosis.

Conclusion

Gallstone disease in children is being diagnosed earlier than ever before. After a period of observation, laparoscopic cholecystectomy is the treatment of choice.

▌ LIVER TUMORS

Liver tumors in childhood are rare and are typically not detected clinically until they reach a large size and often spread within the organ or metastasize elsewhere. Primary liver tumors comprise between 1% and 4% of all solid tumors in children.[36] Benign tumors account for 30 to 40% of these, with a majority of them being hemangiomas. Benign tumors of the liver in children include vascular tumors, hamartomas, adenomas, and focal nodular hyperplasia. Primary liver malignancies in children include hepatoblastoma, sarcomas, germ cell tumors, hepatocellular carcinoma and rhabdoid tumors.

Benign Tumors of the Liver

Infantile Hemangioendothelioma

Infantile hemangioendothelioma is the most common benign solid hepatic tumor in children. These vascular tumors are usually diagnosed based on the charecerestic appearance on CECT in the first 6 months of life and also is the most common liver tumor in the first year of life. Hemangiomas are characterized by a period of rapid growth followed by involution. Although benign in their pathology, these tumors are still associated with significant morbidity and mortality, leading to the classic triad of hepatomegaly, congestive heart failure, and anemia.[37] These children may also present with consumptive coagulopathy (Kasaback-Merrit syndrome) and bleeding.

On computed tomography (CT) with intravenous contrast, classically the lesions either enhance diffusely or rim enhancement is followed by gradual filling of the center of the lesion.

Treatment

Asymptomatic small lesions are simply monitored, and no specific therapy is instituted until symptoms occur.

Patients presenting with congestive heart failure, coagulopathy, or respiratory compromise are resuscitated and stabilized. Once stabilized, therapy is directed towards the hemangioma. Surgical resection is the most definitive treatment. In patients whose condition is thought to be too unstable for surgical intervention, trial of steroids or interferon-alfa can be done with some benefit.[38]

Patients who are asymptomatic or who become asymptomatic after conservative therapy must be monitored for complete resolution of their hemangioendothelioma. Surgical resection of any residual lesion should be considered.

Finally, in patients in whom other modes of treatment have failed, liver transplantation has been used as successful therapy for severe congestive heart failure or unremitting coagulopathy.

▌ MESENCHYMAL HAMARTOMA

The reason for the development of a mesenchymal hamartoma is unclear. Although most mesenchymal hamartomas have a characteristic multiseptated cystic appearance, which is rarely seen in other liver neoplasms, many are mixed solid and cystic or completely solid.[39] Laboratory studies are almost always normal, including liver function tests. The AFP level can be moderately elevated and it will return to normal after resection. Most of these lesions grow slowly and require resection, some remain stable in size or even involute but this is unusual. Complete excision of the lesion with a margin of normal liver is usually curative.

▌ FOCAL NODULAR HYPERPLASIA

Focal nodularhyperplasia (FNH) is not a neoplasm but a nonspecific hyperplasic reaction to vascular abnormalities. FNH and related lesions are uncommon, especially in young children. Symptomatic FNH are more frequent in children than in adults and the most frequent symptom is abdominal pain and rarely, weight loss and weakness. The etiology of FNH is not certain, but the evidence suggests that it may be a congenital vascular abnormality. Conservative management is possible, but resection is required if the child is symptomatic or if there is clear evidence of growth of the lesion.[40]

HEPATOCELLULAR ADENOMA

Hepatocellular adenomas (HCAs) are extremely rare during childhood. They are benign liver tumors soft, well-demarcated with little or no fibrous capsule. Most HCAs are diagnosed during the teenage years (the mean age at diagnosis is around 14 years). The two major concerns with HCA are hemorrhage and malignant transformation into HCC.

In patients who are receiving oral contraceptives or androgenic steroid therapy, the first step should be withdrawal of these medications. If discontinuation is not effective, then the adenoma should be surgically resected. This removes the potential for future hemorrhage or malignant degeneration.[41] HCAs which are frequently larger than 5 cm are resected or if the diagnosis of the hepatic lesion is uncertain, then surgical excision is immediately recommended.

MALIGNANT PRIMARY LIVER TUMORS

Malignant liver tumors account for slightly 1% of all pediatric malignancies. Two-thirds of liver tumors in children are malignant.[42] Unlike liver tumors in adults, in which the predominant histology is hepatocellular carcinoma, hepatoblastoma accounts for two-thirds of liver tumors in children. Other liver malignancies in children include sarcomas, germ cell tumors, and rhabdoid tumors, as well as the more familiar hepatocellular carcinoma.

HEPATOBLASTOMA

Hepatoblastoma is the most common primary malignant liver tumor of childhood. Hepatoblastoma is diagnosed in very young children with a peak in the newborn period reflecting the fact that these tumors develop prenatally, at an overall median age at diagnosis of 18 months.

Histologically, these tumors can be divided into epithelial or mixed epithelial/mesenchymal tissue. The majority of hepatoblastomas are epithelial and consist of a mixture of embryonal and fetal cell types. Approximately 5% of hepatoblastomas are of the small cell undifferentiated subtype, which is associated with a worse prognosis.[43]

Children tend to present with an abdominal mass. Serum alpha-fetoprotein is almost always elevated, often to extreme levels and thrombocytosis is common. Metastases occur almost exclusively in the lungs.

Almost all liver masses in children are surgically treated, either primarily or following systemic chemotherapy. CT and MRI are helpful in determining the amount of liver that will remain after the hepatectomy. Children generally lack other serious comorbidities, usually have an otherwise normal liver, and are, therefore, able to tolerate larger resections than adults. Although CT and MRI are very helpful in determining resectability, in many cases the final determination is made in the operating room.

The treatment of hepatoblastoma requires a combined-modality approach. The only chance for a long-term cure is complete resection of the primary tumor. Primary resection is preferred whenever the imaging studies indicate the potential for complete excision without endangering the patient. This avoids the toxicity of chemotherapy, including marrow suppression, mucositis, gastrointestinal dysfunction, and nutritional consequences.[44] A completely resected tumor, without the presence of metastatic disease, is deemed stage I.

For a tumor deemed unresectable at diagnosis or a patient with metastatic disease, current therapy consists of neoadjuvant chemotherapy followed by either resection or liver transplantation. Liver transplantation is recommended when complete tumor excision by partial hepatectomy is unlikely.

Another approach to the unresectable hepatoblastoma is the use of preoperative chemoembolization.[45] The dual blood supply of the liver from the hepatic arteries and branches of the portal vein makes hepatic artery chemoembolization feasible. Chemoembolization can convert unresectable tumor to resectable and also act as a bridge to transplantation, for recurrent tumors and for palliation.

UNDIFFERENTIATED EMBRYONAL SARCOMA

The third most common hepatic malignancy, after hepatoblastoma and hepatocellular carcinoma, is undifferentiated embryonal sarcoma. It may have an atypical presentation leading to delay in diagnosis.[46] These tumors occur in children 5–10 years of age and are mesenchymal in appearance. This is a very malignant tumor with a poor outcome.

The most common clinical presentation is either right upper quadrant or epigastric pain with or without a palpable abdominal mass. Occasionally, marked hepatomegaly is seen without a definite mass. Rarely, this tumor can even masquerade as a hepatic abscess or infection. Laboratory studies, including AFP level, are usually normal.

On ultrasound examination, the lesion appears predominantly solid. However, on CT and MRI, the lesion appears cystic without any significant solid component. Such a discrepancy between the two imaging techniques is highly suggestive of an undifferentiated embryonal sarcoma.

The only chance for cure is radical excision. Unfortunately, despite complete surgical resection of the tumor, many patients have recurrent disease, which suggests the need for postoperative chemotherapy. In patients in whom complete resection of the tumor is not possible despite chemotherapy, liver transplantation has been advocated as another possible means for complete excision.

HEPATOCELLULAR CARCINOMA

Hepatocellular carcinoma, the second most common malignancy of the liver in children, is markedly distinct from hepatoblastoma. Most cases of hepatocellular carcinoma are diagnosed after 10 years of age. Hepatocellular carcinoma is the most common hepatic malignancy of adolescents. Often, hepatocellular carcinoma is associated with known hepatic viral infection or cirrhosis, and while it can take decades for malignancy to develop, occasionally cases are seen in very young children. Although worldwide its incidence in childhood is falling, due to widespread immunization against hepatitis B,[47] it remains a difficult problem as chemotherapy has made little or no impact on survival and most tumors are unresectable. Predisposing factors include tyrosinemia and progressive familial intrahepatic cholestasis. Serum alpha-fetoprotein is often elevated, but usually not to extreme levels.

Most patients are initially seen with either an abdominal mass or abdominal pain. Other associated symptoms include nausea and vomiting, anorexia, malaise, and a significant weight loss. In case of focal small localized lesions, even laparoscopic resection may be feasible and curative.[48]

Complete surgical resection offers the only chance for a cure for HCC, as the tumor is chemoresistant. The outcome for patients with hepatocellular carcinoma, regardless of the treatment modality, is still not as good as the outcome for hepatoblastoma.

REFERENCES

1. Fischler B, Haglund B, Hjern A. A population-based study on the incidence and possible pre- and perinatal etiologic risk factors of biliary atresia. Journal of Pediatrics. 2002;141(2):217-22.
2. Kasai M, Suzuki S. A new operation for, 'non-correctable' biliary atresia: hepatic portoenterostomy. Shuiyutsu. 1959;13:733-9.
3. Hol L, van den Bos IC, Hussain SM, Zondervan PE, de Man RA. Hepatocellular carcinoma complicating biliary atresia after Kasai portoenterostomy. Eur J Gastroenterol Hepatol. 2008;20:227-31.
4. Davenport M, Tizzard SA, Underhill J, Mieli-Vergani G, Portmann B, Hadžić N. The biliary atresia splenic malformation syndrome: a 28-year single-center retrospective study. Journal of Pediatrics. 2006;149(3):393-400.
5. Takaya J, Nakano S, Imai Y, Fujii Y, Kaneko K. Usefulness of magnetic resonance cholangiopancreatography in biliary structures in infants: a four-case report. European Journal of Pediatrics. 2007;166(3):211-4.
6. Ashcraft K. Pediatric Surgery. 3rd edition. Saunders; 2000.
7. Davenport M, Ong E, Sharif K, et al. Biliary atresia in England and Wales: results of centralization and new benchmark. Journal of Pediatric Surgery. 2011;46(9):1689-94.
8. Wildhaber BE, Majno P, Mayr J, et al. Biliary atresia: Swiss national study, 1994–2004. Journal of Pediatric Gastroenterology and Nutrition. 2008;46(3):299-307.
9. Mieli-Vergani G, Portman B, Howard ER, Mowat AP. Late referral for biliary atresia—missed opportunities for effective surgery. Lancet. 1989;1(8635):421-3.
10. Lünzmann K, Schweizer P. The influence of cholangitis on the prognosis of extrahepatic biliary atresia. European Journal of Pediatric Surgery. 1999;9(1):19-23.
11. Cox KL, Berquist WE, Castillo RO. Paediatric liver transplantation: indications, timing and medical complications. Journal of Gastroenterology and Hepatology. 1999;14:S61-6.
12. Serinet MO, Broué P, Jacquemin E, et al. Management of patients with biliary atresia in France: results of a decentralized policy 1986–2002. Hepatology. 2006;44(1):75-84.
13. Santamaria ML, Gamez M, Murcia J, et al. Kasai operation in the age of liver transplantation. Healing or merely palliative technique? Cirugía Pediátrica. 2000;13(3):102-5.
14. Narasimhan KL, Chowdhary SK, Vaiphei K, Samujh R, Mahajan JK, Thapa BR, et al. Outcome of biliary atresia from Chandigarh: results of a prospective analysis. Indian Pediatr. 2001;38(10):1144-8.
15. Gigot J, Nagorney D, Farnell M, Moir C, Ilstrup D. Bile duct cysts: A changing spectrum of disease. J Hepatobiliary Pancreat Surg. 1996;3:405-11.
16. O'Neill JA Jr. Choledochal cyst. Curr Probl Surg. 1992;29:361-410.
17. Rao KL, Chowdhary SK, Kumar D. Choledochal cyst associated with portal hypertension. Pediatr Surg Int. 2003;19(11):729-32. Epub 2003 Dec 24.
18. Babbitt DP. Congenital choledochal cyst: New etiological concept based on anomalous relationships of the common bile duct and pancreatic bulb. Ann Radiol (Paris). 1969;12:231-40.
19. Park DH, Kim MH, Lee SK, Lee SS, Choi JS, Lee YS, et al. Can MRCP replace the diagnostic role of ERCP for patients with choledochal cysts.? Gastrointest Endosc. 2005;62:360-6.
20. Cory DA, Don S, West KW. CT cholangiography of a choledochocele. Pediatr Radiol. 1990;21:73-4.
21. Alonso-Lej F, Rever WB, Jr, Pessagno DJ. Congenital choledochal cyst, with a report of 2, and an analysis of 94, cases. Int Abstr Surg. 1959;108:1-30.
22. Todani T, Watanabe Y, Narusue M, Tabuchi K, Okajima K. Congenital bile duct cysts: Classification, operative procedures,

and review of thirty-seven cases including cancer arising from choledochal cyst. Am J Surg. 1977;134:263-9.

23. Lilly JR, Stellin GP, Karrer FM. Forme fruste choledochal cyst. J Pediatr Surg. 1985;20:449-51.

24. Reddy SI, Grace ND. Liver imaging. A hepatologist's perspective. Clin Liver Dis. 2002;6:297-310.

25. Sarin SK, Agarwal SR, "Extrahepatic portal vein obstruction," Seminars in Liver Disease. 2002;22(1):43-58.

26. Duch´e M, Ducot B, Tournay E, et al. "Prognostic value of endoscopy in children with biliary atresia at risk for early development of varices and bleeding. Gastroenterology. 2010;139(6):1952-60.

27. Valla DC. Primary Budd-Chiari syndrome. Journal of Hepatology. 2009;50(1):195-203.

28. Beppu K, Inokuchi K, Koyanagi N, Nakayama S, Sakata H, Kitano S, et al. Prediction of variceal hemorrhage by esophageal endoscopy. Gastrointest Endosc. 1981;27:213-8.

29. Ling SC. Should children with esophageal varices receive beta-blockers for the primary prevention of variceal hemorrhage? Canadian Journal of Gastroenterology. 2005;19(11):661-6.

30. Bismuth H, Franco D, Alagille D. Portal diversion for portal hypertension in children: The first ninety patients. Ann Surg. 1980;192:18-24.

31. Wesdorp I, Bosman D, de Graaff A, Aronson D, van der Blij F, Taminiau J. Clinical presentations and predisposing factors of cholelithiasis and sludge in children. J Pediatr Gastroenterol Nutr. 2000;31:411-7.

32. Holcomb GW Jr, Holcomb GW 3rd. Cholelithiasis in infants, children, and adolescents. Pediatr Rev. 1990;11:268-74.

33. Della Corte C, Falchetti D, Nebbia G, Calacoci M, Pastore M, Francavilla R, et al. Management of cholelithiasis in Italian children. A national multicenter study. World J Gastroenterol. 2008;14:1383-8.

34. Miltenburg DM, Schaffer R III, Breslin T, Brandt ML. Changing indications for pediatric cholecystectomy. Pediatrics. 2000;105(6):1250-3pmid:10835065

35. Chowdhary SK, Kandpal D. Minimal access surgery in children: a 5 year study. Indian Pediatr. 2012;49(12):971-4. Epub 2012 Jun 10.

36. Multerys M, Goodman MT, Smith MA, et al. Hepatic Tumors. In: Ries LAG, Smith MA, Gurney JG, et al (Eds). Cancer Incidence, Survival among Children,Adolescents: United States SEER Program 1975–1995. SEER Program, NIH Pub. No 99–4649. Bethesda, MD: National Cancer Institute, 1999:91-7.

37. Selby DM, Stocker JT, Waclawiw MA, et al. Infantile hemangioendothelioma of the liver. Hepatology. 1994;20:39-45.

38. Daller JA, Bueno J, Gutierrez J, Dvorchik I, Towbin RB, Dickman PS, et al. Hepatic hemangioendothelioma: clinical experience and management strategy. J Pediatr Surg. 1999;34(1):98-105; discussion 105-6.

39. Ye BB, Hu B, Wang LJ, et al. Mesenchymal hamartoma of liver: magnetic resonance imaging and histopathologic correlation. World J Gastroenterol. 2005;11:5807-10.

40. Okada T, Sasaki F, Kamiyama T, et al. Management and algorithm for focal nodular hyperplasia of the liver in children. Eur J Pediatr Surg. 2006;16:235-40.

41. Kishnani PS, Chuang TP, Bali D, et al. Chromosomal and genetic alterations in human hepatocellular adenomas associated with type Ia glycogen storage disease. Human Molecular Genetics. 2009;18(24):4781-90.

42. Weinberg AG, Finegold MJ. Primary hepatic tumors of childhood. Hum Pathol. 1983;14:512-37.

43. Haas JE, Feusner JH, Finegold MJ. Small cell undifferentiated histology in hepatoblastoma may be unfavorable. Cancer. 2001;92:3130-4.

44. Mueller BU, Lopez-Terrada D, Finegold MJ. Tumors of the liver. In: Pizzo PA, Poplack DG (Eds). Principles and Practice of Pediatric Oncology. 5th ed. Philadelphia, PA: Lippincott-Williams & Wilkins; 2006:887-904.

45. Arcement CM, Towbin RB, Meza MP, Gerber DA, Kaye RD, Mazariegos GV, et al. Intrahepatic chemoembolization in unresectable pediatric liver malignancies. In: Li JP, Chu JP, Yang JY, Chen (Eds). Pediatr Radiol. 2000;30:779-85.

46. Chowdhary SK, Trehan A, Das A, Marwaha RK, Rao KL. Undifferentiated embryonal sarcoma in children: beware of the solitary liver cyst. J Pediatr Surg. 2004;39(1):E9-12.

47. Chang MH, Chen CJ, Lai MS, et al. Universal hepatitis B vaccination in Taiwan and the incidence of hepatocellular carcinoma in children. Taiwan Childhood Hepatoma Study Group. N Engl J Med. 1997;336:1855-9.

48. Yeung CK, Chowdhary SK, Chan KW, Lee KH, Till H. Atypical laparoscopic resection of a liver tumour in a 4 year old girl. J Laparoendosc Adv Surg Tech. 2006;16(3):325-7.

Chapter

32

Drug-induced Liver Injury

Seema Alam, Sanjiv Verma

INTRODUCTION

Definition of drug-induced liver injury (DILI) is "liver injury caused by medications, herbs, or xenobiotics, leading to liver dysfunction when other common etiologies have been excluded".[1] It could be a prescribed 'drug' or bought over-the-counter. Herbs and herbal medications are included in the definition of DILI. Many are exposed to these 'herbs' whose safety profile has not been studied scientifically. "Herbs" and "folk remedies" are popular in other Asian countries also.[2]

EPIDEMIOLOGY

Drug-induced liver injury accounts for 4% of cases of new onset jaundice in the US.[1] Despite being a rare liver disease, DILI is responsible for considerable morbidity and mortality. Different regions have varying causes and outcome of DILI. Acetaminophen is common in the West, whereas complementary medicines are common in the Far East. Of the 1148 acute liver failure (ALF) cases, 133 (11.1%) had DILI in a multicentric prospective study at 23 centers in US.[3] Annual incidence of 12 lac/year has been reported from Korean university hospital.[2] It also is well recognized that adverse reactions from drugs including DILI are markedly underreported. In the study, the number of hepatic events was 16 times greater than the number spontaneously reported to the French authorities.[4] Incidence of DILI was 19.1% cases per 100,000 in Iceland. In 75% cases, DILI was caused by single medication. Dietary supplements were responsible for 16% of cases. Amoxicillin-claulanate, diclofenac, azathioprine and nitrofurantoin were the common drugs implicated.[5] In multicentric centric study from Europe and USA, acetaminophen was the most common cause of pediatric ALF present in 14% of the 348 children included.[6]

DILI is not uncommon cause of liver disease in children. Retrospectively (1997–2004) and prospectively (2005–2010)

collected Indian data revealed 39 (8.7%) children of the 450 cases of DILI. The median age was 16 years of these 22 boys and 17 girls. Antitubercular (n = 22), phenytoin (n = 10) and carbamazepine (n = 6) were the common drugs associated with DILI.[7] 30 children aged 2 to 18 years with suspected DILI were identified by DILIN (Drug-induced liver injury network) in a prospective longitudinal multicenter study between September 2004 and September 2009.[8] Mean age in this sample was 14 years; 70% were girls. Median time from drug initiation to symptom onset was 32 days.[8] In a survey done in UK, 1% adverse drug reactions records in children and adolescents were DILI and majority were in the adolescents. Drugs implicated were paracetamol, valproic acid, carbamazepine, methotrexate, minocycline, ceftriaxone, ciclosporin, basiliximab, erythromycin and voriconazole.[9] Among Chinese children, 31 cases of DILI accounted for 1.7% of the 1831 total cases treated from 2002 to June 2011. The pediatric DILI population included 20 males and 11 females, with an average age of 8.8+/–3.9 years old (range, 0.3–14.0). Antimicrobials were the most common cause (41.9%) of DILI, followed by the herbal medicine (29.0%) and antipyretic drugs (19.4%). A single drug was implicated in nine cases (29.0%), and two or more drugs were implicated in 71%[10]. In an Indian study, all the children (41%) who developed hypersensitivity features (skin rashes, fever, lymphadenopathy, and/or eosinophilia) presented earlier, had less severe disease and survived.[7] These included 3 children with Steven-Johnson syndrome.

It has been seen that, isoniazid exhibits the highest incidence rate of 606 per 100 000 persons. Of the 265 DILI cases, 41% were mild; 12% moderate and 17% exhibited severely decompensated liver disease. There was 3% mortality with no liver transplant.[8] Transplant-free survival (27%) was poor in a multicentric US ALF study with successful transplantation in 42.1%.[3] In another study, overall 90-day mortality of 17.3% was higher for antitubercular drugs vs others (21.5% vs 11.4%).[12] A single center analysis reveals, 90-day mortality of 22.7% for antitubercular drugs.[13] DILI accompanied by jaundice, encephalopathy, ascites, high INR or high creatinine were associated with high mortality.[13]

DEVELOPMENT OF DRUG METABOLISM IN LIVER

Liver is an important site of drug metabolism in humans. Varied sensitivity to many drugs can be explained by the developmental changes in liver's metabolic activity during fetal life and in perinatal period. Fetal liver has 30% of the total cytochrome P450 whereas the adult liver has 60%. Hence, there is a decreased capacity of fetal and newborn liver to metabolize, detoxify and excrete drugs. This also explains the lower incidence of DILI in newborns. Greater capacity of newborns to synthesize glutathione helps in inactivating many toxic metabolites. Cytochrome 450 increases with age in childhood but decreases in adulthood, hence it is more active in older children then in adults. That is why some of the drugs are needed in larger doses per kilogram weight in children.[14]

PATHOGENESIS

A three-step pathogenetic model (Fig. 32.1) of DILI mechanisms involves direct cell stress by drugs or their metabolites. This in turn, triggers immune reactions, which directly impair mitochondrial function. The second step is the mitochondrial permeability changes, which lead to third and final step of apoptosis or necrotic cell death.[15] The concept of adaptation is important in DILI where the injury reverses with the continuation of the drug. The

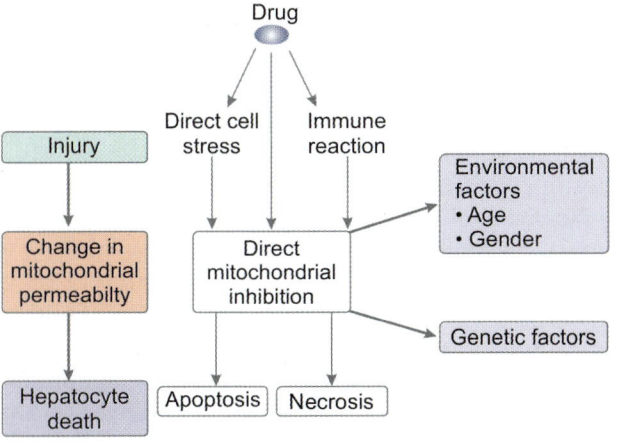

Fig. 32.1: Pathogenesis of the drug-induced liver injury

reasons for adaptation could be (1) Changes in phases 1, 2 or 3 which decrease the exposure of hepatocytes to the toxic chemical; (2) Oxidative stress caused by the toxic chemical and its effects on mitochondria can activate the expression of antioxidant genes; (3) Mitochondrial injury results in mitochondrial biogenesis; (4) Stress to endoplasmic reticulum induces an adaptive response to modulate stress.[16]

DIAGNOSIS OF DILI

Being a diagnosis of exclusion, DILI is a diagnostic dilemma for physicians. Moreover, there are no specific signs, symptoms and tests for DILI. Clinical profile can vary from just mild liver dysfunction to acute liver failure. The clinical history must include comprehensive details of the drug usage and its temporal association to the illness. Records of the 30 children identified as DILI revealed peak aspartate aminotransferase (AST) levels as 503 U/L, alanine aminotransferase (ALT) 727 U/L, alkaline phosphatise (ALP) 331 U/L, and total bilirubin of 3.9 mg/dL. Two-thirds of the children were seropositive for autoantibodies. Hepatocellular damage (78%) was the most common liver injury pattern, followed by cholestatic (13%), and mixed (9%).[7] The liver injury patterns represented among the 39 Indian children were: hepatocellular (25.8%), cholestasis (25.8%), and mixed hepatocellular-cholestatic (48.4%).[8] In the prospective collection of data in Iceland among adults, 42% had a hepatocellular, 32% had cholestatic, and 26% had mixed injury.[5]

A positive rechallenge, which is the gold standard for DILI, is unacceptably dangerous. The most widely used method is the Roussel Uclaf Causality Assessment Method (RUCAM) scale.[17] Two other scales have also been developed but are not very feasible (Table 32.1).[18,19] For the clinical characterization of DILI, the ratio of ALT to ALP was designated as the R value [R= (ALT/ULN of ALT)/ALP/ULN of ALP)]. Hepatocellular DILI was defined as R≥5, cholestatic as R≤2, and mixed as 2<R<5. Due to variations in the serum enzyme profile during disease progression, the time point for calculating the R value is important.[20] There are no clear recommendations regarding the timing of the enzymes values used. Many clinicians use enzyme values from the first analytical test showing elevations above normal to establish the R value, while others use peak values, which may or may not coincide with the initial analytical values. Genetic screening tests are a necessary requirement which can guide decision whether a particular patient can receive a certain potentially hepatotoxic drug. Genetics of idiosyncratic hepatotoxicity would be more complex.

Table 32.1: Three scales to determine attribution of causality

- Roussel Uclaf Casuality Assessment Method (RUCAM) scale: Most widely used and validated
  - Objective and consistent assessment but cumbersome[17]
  - 86% sens, 89% spec and PPV 93% and NPV 78% using a cut-off point of 5
- Clinical diagnostic scale or M and V scale[18]
  - Simple scoring system
  - Definite, probable, unlikely, and excluded
- Digestive diasease week-Japan (DDW-J scale)[19]
  - Recently proposed in Japan
  - In vitro drug lymphocyte stimulation test (DLST) evaluation

COMMONLY INCRIMINATED DRUGS IN CHILDREN

❑ Antitubercular drugs: In a report from a transplantation centers in US, hepatic failure with isoniazid (INH) was seen in 3.2 of 100,000 children treated for latent TB. Fourteen of 20 children (70%) had jaundice and nausea, followed by fatigue, loss of appetite, abdominal pain and vomiting with a mean AST and ALT of 1399 IU and 1030 IU/dL and mean total bilirubin of 13.7 mg/dL during a mean duration of INH therapy of 3.3 months. Five of these children were reported as hepatitis but the drug was not discontinued.[21] Even though discontinuation at the onset of symptoms does not assure recovery, but there is a need for increased awareness of hepatotoxicity risk. On comparative analysis of monitoring for DILI in a scheduled monthly manner or passive detection found none deaths of 111 in the former as against 3 of 162 in the latter group. It was further noted that scheduled monitoring reduced the hospitalization rate, improved the drug compliance and detection of asymptomatic liver dysfunction.[22] In a cohort of children with HIV on INH prophylaxis on two different dosing schedules of thrice weekly and daily, a total of 16/297 (5.4%) developed severe liver injury. But none developed hepatic failure. The incidence was not higher when combination of INH and antiretroviral therapy (ART) were compared with ART alone. The dosing schedules had no influence but the incidence was higher in those below 12 months of age and in those with higher CD4 levels.[23] In a study to determine the risk factors of DILI among Japanese children, multivariate analysis revealed age below 5 years and pyrazinamide were found to be associated with DILI due to antitubercular drugs.[24] Hence, in the high-risk cases such as infants or those on pyrazinamide, a scheduled biochemical monitoring and clinical monitoring as well as stopping the incriminating drug on early evidence of hepatoxicity

would definitely reduce the mortality in these cases. Scheduled biochemical monitoring in the first and second month of treatment would pick up majority of the asymptomatic cases. A meta-analysis reported that tuberculosis patients with slow acetylators had a higher risk of DILI than other acetylators. Screening of patients for the NAT2 genetic polymorphisms will be useful for prediction and prevention of DILI.[25]

❑ Amoxicillin-clavulanic acid is known to be more responsible for DILI then amoxicillin. In a prospective observational study done in 8 Spanish Hospitals, 11 children with DILI due to amoxicillin clavulanate combination were reported. Half of the children reported with anorexia, vomiting and pain abdomen. Seven (64%) required hospitalization with a mean hospital stay of 7.9 days (5–12 days). The transaminases became normal after 4 to 36 weeks: with a mean duration of 14 weeks. Mean dose of amoxicillin was 42 mg/kg/d. Clavulanic acid in a proportion of 250 mg amoxicillin/62.5 mg of clavulanic acid in 7/11 cases. Use of the combination was justified for 18% and in 82% amoxicillin alone could have been prescribed instead.[26] It is strongly felt that prescription of unnecessary drugs should be avoided.

❑ Anticonvulsants: Sodium valproate (VPA) toxicity is an uncommon but potentially fatal cause of idiosyncratic liver injury. Rare mutations in POLG, which codes for the mitochondrial DNA polymerase-γ (pol-γ), cause Alpers-Huttenlocher syndrome (AHS) which is a neurometabolic disorder associated with an increased risk of developing fatal VPA hepatotoxicity.

A prospective study[27] of subjects enrolled in the DILIN from 2004–2008 through five US centers revealed that heterozygous genetic variation in POLG was strongly associated with VPA-induced liver toxicity (OR 23.6, 95% CI 8.4–65.8). So there is impaired liver regeneration in VPA toxicity and prospective genetic testing of POLG will identify individuals at high-risk of this. The time from VPA exposure to liver failure can be between 2 and 3 months.[28] POLG mutations have been observed in every ethnic group studied to date and so POLG gene testing should be considered in any child or adolescent who presents with intractable seizures and has a history of psychomotor regression. In a Japanese study, it was suggested that glutathione S-transferase (GST) M1 null genotype was a risk factor for carbamazepine-induced mild hepatotoxicity.[29]

❑ Paracetomol and nonsteroidal anti-inflammatory drugs: Acetaminophen (APAP) is the leading worldwide cause of drug overdose and ALF. Single overdose ingestion and therapeutic misadventure may cause hepatotoxicity. This usually happens in the unfortunate alignment of circumstances, e.g. prolonged febrile illness, poor nutritional status coupled with poor intake, multiple round-the-clock doses of APAP, underlying (FAO defect, altered Cytochrome P-450). Early manifestations of APAP hepatotoxicity are nonspecific, but require prompt recognition by physicians. APAP hepatotoxicity is characterized by marked elevation of serum aminotransferase (often >3000 IU/L), which typically starts increasing within 24 to 36 hours, and peaks around 72 hours after overdose. The AST can be greater than 10,000 IU/L, usually more elevated than the ALT. The degree of aminotransferase elevation correlates roughly with the degree of hepatocellular damage. Maximal liver injury typically peaks between 3 and 5 days after ingestion, and may have jaundice, coagulopathy, and encephalopathy. Bilirubin and INR are less involved in APAP related hepatotoxicity. Acute ingestion of paracetomol in the range of 150 to 200 mg/kg in children older than 6 years (all APAP consumed within 8 hours) may be responsible for dose-related APAP related ALF. In a European study, among 600 (6.3 %) cases of DILI related ALF needing liver transplant, 187 had been exposed to drugs within 30 days, without overdose.[30] Of these 40 were exposed to an NSAID and 192 to paracetamol (half without overdose). For paracetamol, the event rate was 3.3 (95 % CI 2.6-4.1) without overdoses and 7.8 (95% CI 6.8–9.0) including overdoses. Event rates were 2.3 (95% CI 1.2–3.9) for ibuprofen, 1.9 (95% CI 0.8–3.7) for nimesulide and 1.6 (95% CI 0.6–3.4) for diclofenac. Non-overdose paracetamol-exposed liver failure was twice more common than NSAID-exposed liver failure.[31]

TREATMENT OF DILI

In majority of cases of DILI, discontinuation of the incriminated drug results in improvement of liver injury and some DILI cases improve without discontinuation of the drug. Therefore, careful evaluation is required keeping in mind the importance of the medication and the degree of liver damage. Hy's rule (elevation of AST or ALT more than 3×ULN or ALP more than 1.5×ULN in combination with more than 3×ULN elevated bilirubin) indicates serious liver injury in which case the suspected drug should be stopped. FDA (Food and Drug Administration) recently recommended discontinuing the drug in case of ALT > 8 × ULN, ALT > 5 × ULN for two weeks, ALT > 3 × ULN in association with serum bilirubin > 2 × ULN, > 1.5 × PT-INR, or symptoms of liver injury.[32] In hepatocellular DILI 50% decrease in serum ALT within 8 days of discontinuing the suspected drug is considered as the positive re-challenge which is also included in the RUCAM scale. Whereas, in cholestatic DILI improvement of biliary enzymes after

discontinuation of the suspected drug requires a longer period. Serious liver damage can be predicted using the standard acetaminophen toxicity nomogram (Fig. 32.2), but cannot be used to exclude possible toxicity due to multiple doses over time, when the time of ingestion is unknown, or when altered metabolism occurs such as in the alcoholic or fasting patient.[33] APAP toxicity should be treated with activated charcoal if presents within 3–4 hours of ingestion and N acetylcysteine should be started ideally within 6 hours but beneficial effects have been seen up to 48 hours of presentation. The therapeutic regimen for N acetylcysteine includes a loading dose of 150 mg/kg in 5% dextrose given over 15 minutes followed by 100 mg/kg administered over 16 hours. Corticosteroid therapy may or may not provide benefits in even hypersensitivity associated DILI cases.

Fortunately, majority of patients with symptomatic acute DILI, milder DILI and clinically significant DILI are expected to completely recover with supportive care after discontinuation of the suspect drug. In contrast, the prognosis is poor for severe DILI who progress to acute liver failure. Spanish hepatotoxicity registry revealed 5.7% incidence of chronic DILI.[34] To register and study the DILI cases caused by 'herbs', 'health foods or dietary supplements', or 'folk remedies', a reporting system on the lines of drug-induced liver injury network (DILIN) in the United States, should be established as soon as possible in all countries. There are reports of successfully treated DILI-related acute liver failure with high-volume plasma exchange without liver transplantation.[35]

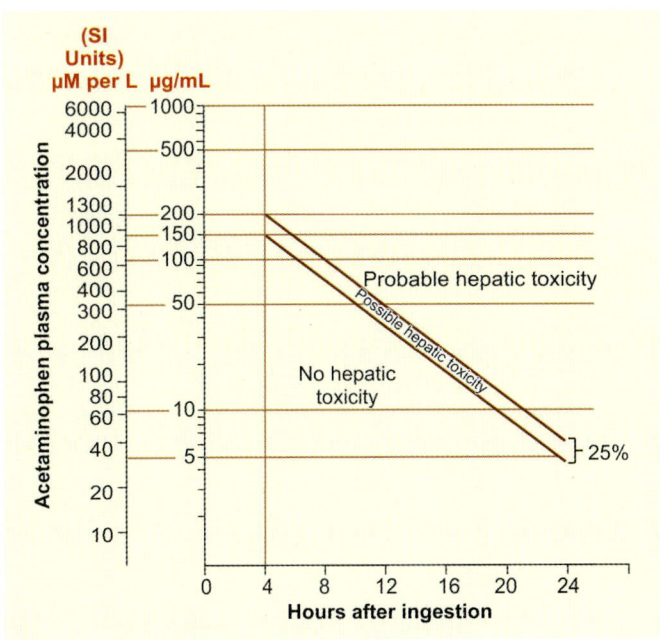

Fig. 32.2: Nomogram for the management of acetaminophen toxicity

LIVER TRANSPLANTATION IN DILI

It is recommended to refer patients with severe DILI to a transplant center, keeping in view their poor outcome. The prognosis of patients with APAP-induced ALF is better than other causes of ALF. Liver transplantation should be offered to those who are unlikely to survive without transplant.[36] Prothrombin time that continues to increase beyond 4 seconds after overdose, and with a peak prothrombin time greater than or equal to 180 seconds are associated with approximately 90% mortality without liver transplantation (LT). Nonhepatotoxic antituberculous therapy (cycloserine, ciprofloxacin, streptomycin, and ethambutol) and low-dose immunosuppressive therapy were started after successful liver transplantation for DILI due to antitubercular therapy.[37] Of the 17 children transplanted for VPA-ALF, 82% died within 1 year of LT. One-year survival probability was worse in VPA-ALF than non-VPA-DIALF (20% versus 69%, P < .0001). Median post-LT survival time for VPA-ALF was 2.8 months. Children who underwent LT for VPA-ALF had a significantly lower survival probability than children with non-VPA-DIALF. Current data suggest that VPA-ALF in children represents an "unmasking" of mitochondrial disease. VPA-ALF should be a contraindication for LT, even in the absence of a documented mitochondrial disease.[38]

REFERENCES

1. Vuppalanchi R, Liangpunsakul S, Chalasani N. Etiology of new-onset jaundice: how often is it caused by idiosyncratic drug-induced liver injury in the United States? Am J Gastroenterol. 2007;102:558-62.

2. Suk KT, Kim DJ, Kim CH, Park SH, Yoon JH, Kim YS, et al. A prospective nationwide study of drug-induced liver injury in Korea. Am J Gastroenterol. 2012;107(9):1380-7.

3. Reuben A, Koch DG, Lee WM. Acute Liver Failure Study Group. Drug-induced acute liver failure: results of a US multicenter, prospective study. Hepatology. 2010;52(6):2065-76.doi:10.1002/hep.23937. Epub 2010 Oct 14.

4. Sgro C, Clinard F, Ouazir K, et al. Incidence of drug-induced hepatic injuries: a French population-based study. Hepatology. 2002;36:451-5.

5. Björnsson ES, Bergmann OM, Björnsson HK, Kvaran RB, Olafsson S. Incidence, presentation, and outcomes in patients with drug-induced liver injury in the general population of Iceland. Gastroenterology.2013;144(7):1419-25.

6. Squires RH Jr, Shneider BL, Bucuvalas J, Alonso E, Sokol RJ, Narkewicz MR, et al. Acute liver failure in children: the first 348 patients in the pediatric acute liver failure study group. J Pediatr. 2006;148(5):652-8.

7. Devarbhavi H, Karanth D, Prasanna KS, Adarsh CK, Patil M. Drug-Induced liver injury with hypersensitivity features has a better outcome: a single-center experience of 39 children and adolescents. Hepatology. 2011;54(4):1344-50.

8. Shin J, Hunt CM, Suzuki A, Papay JI, Beach KJ, Cheetham TC. Characterizing phenotypes and outcomes of drug-associated liver injury using electronic medical record data. Pharmacoepidemiol Drug Saf. 2013;22(2):190-8. doi: 10.1002/pds.3388. Epub 2012 Dec 19.

9. Molleston JP, Fontana RJ, Lopez MJ, Kleiner DE, Gu J, Chalasani N. Drug-induced Liver Injury Network. Characteristics of idiosyncratic drug-induced liver injury in children: results from the DILIN prospective study. J Pediatr Gastroenterol Nutr. 2011; 53(2):182-9.

10. Ferrajolo C, Capuano A, Verhamme KM, Schuemie M, Rossi F, Stricker BH, et al. Drug-induced hepatic injury in children:a case/noncase study of suspected adverse drug reactions in VigiBase. Br J Clin Pharmacol. 2010;70(5):721-8.

11. Wang SZ, Gao S, Liu YM, Huang YL, Chen YS, Wang XX, et al. Clinical characteristics of drug-induced liver injury in 31 pediatric cases. Zhonghua Gan Zang Bing Za Zhi. 2012;20(3):193-5.

12. Devarbhavi H, Dierkhising R, Kremers WK, Sandeep MS, Karanth D, Adarsh CK. Single-center experience with drug-induced liver injury from India: causes, outcome, prognosis, and predictors of mortality. Am J Gastroenterol. 2010;105:2396-2404.

13. Devarbhavi H, Singh R, Patil M, Sheth K, Adarsh CK, Balaraju G. Outcome and determinants of mortality in 269 patients with combination anti-tuberculosis drug-induced liver injury. J Gastroenterol Hepatol. 2013;28(1):161-7.

14. Faa G, Ekstrom J, Castagnola M, Gibo Y, Ottonello G, Fanos V. A developmental approach to drug-induced liver injury in newborns and children. Curr Med Chem. 2012;19(27):4581-94.

15. Russmann S, Kullak-Ublick GA, Grattagliano I. Current concepts of mechanisms in drug-induced hepatotoxicity. Curr Med Chem. 2009;16:3041-53.

16. Nguyen T, Sherratt PJ, Pickett CB. Regulatory mechanisms controlling gene expression mediated by the antioxidant response element. Annu Rev Pharmacol Toxicol. 2003;43:233-60.

17. Danan G, Benichou C. Causality assessment of adverse reactions to drugs-I. A novel method based on the conclusions of international consensus meetings: application to drug-induced liver injuries. J Clin Epidemiol. 1993;46(11):1323-30.

18. Maria VA, Victorino RM. Development and validation of a clinical scale for the diagnosis of drug-induced hepatitis. Hepatology. 1997;26(3):664-9.

19. Hanatani T, Sai K, Tohkin M, Segawa K, Kimura M, Hori K, et al. A detection algorithm for drug-induced liver injury in medical information databases using the Japanese diagnostic scale and its comparison with the Council for International Organizations of Medical Sciences/the Roussel Uclaf Causality Assessment Method scale. Pharmacoepidemiol Drug Saf. 2014 Mar 5. doi: 10.1002/pds.3603. [Epub ahead of print]

20. Suk KT, Kim DJ, Kim CH, Park SH, Yoon JH, Kim YS, et al. A prospective nationwide study of drug-induced liver injury in Korea. Am J Gastroenterol. 2012;107(9):1380-7. doi: 10.1038/ajg.2012.138. Epub 2012 Jun 26.

21. Wu SS, Chao CS, Vargas JH, Sharp HL, Martín MG, McDiarmid SV, et al. Isoniazid-related hepatic failure in children: a survey of liver transplantation centers. Transplantation. 2007;84(2):173-9.

22. Wu S, Xia Y, Lv X, Zhang Y, Tang S, Yang Z, et al. Effect of scheduled monitoring of liver function during anti-tuberculosis treatment in a retrospective cohort in China. BMC Public Health. 2012;12:454.

23. le Roux SM, Cotton MF, Myer L, le Roux DM, Schaaf HS, Lombard CJ, et al. Safety of long-term isoniazid preventive therapy in children with HIV: a comparison of two dosing schedules. Int J Tuberc Lung Dis. 2013;17(1):26-31.

24. Ohkawa K, Hashiguchi M, Ohno K, Kiuchi C, Takahashi S, Kondo S, et al. Risk factors for antituberculous chemotherapy-induced hepatotoxicity in Japanese pediatric patients. Clin Pharmacol Ther. 2002;72(2):220-6.

25. Wang PY, Xie SY, Hao Q, Zhang C, Jiang BF. NAT2 polymorphisms and susceptibility to anti-tuberculosis drug-induced liver injury: a meta-analysis. Int J Tuberc Lung Dis. 2012;16(5):589-95.

26. Hita EO, García JA, Gonzalez JC, Molina AA, Cordero MA, Escobar JS, et al. Amoxicillin-clavulanic acid hepatotoxicity in children. J Pediatr Gastroenterol Nutr. 2012;55(6):663-7.

27. Stewart JD, Horvath R, Baruffini E, Ferrero I, Bulst S, Watkins PB, et al. Polymerase-γ gene POLG determines the risk of sodium valproate-induced liver toxicity. Hepatology. 2010;52(5):1791-6.

28. Saneto RP, Lee IC, Koenig MK, Bao X, Weng SW, Naviaux RK, et al. POLG DNA testing as an emerging standard of care before instituting valproic acid therapy for pediatric seizure disorders. Seizure. 2010;19(3):140-6.

29. Ueda K, Ishitsu T, Seo T, Ueda N, Murata T, Hori M, et al. Glutathione S-transferase M1 null genotype as a risk factor for carbamazepine-induced mild hepatotoxicity. Pharmacogenomics. 2007;8(5):435-42.

30. Gulmez SE, Moore N, Pageaux GP, Lignot S, Horsmans Y, Stricker B, et al. Causality of Drugs Involved in Acute Liver Failure Leading to Transplantation: Results from the Study of AcuteLiver Transplant (SALT). Drug Saf. 2013Jun7. [Epub ahead of print]

31. Gulmez SE, Larrey D, Pageaux GP, Lignot S, Lassalle R, Jové J, et al. Transplantation for acute liver failure in patients exposed to NSAIDs or paracetamol (acetaminophen): the multinational case-population SALT study. Drug Saf. 2013;36(2):135-44.

32. Norris W, Paredes AH, Lewis JH. Drug-induced liver injury in 2007. Curr Opin Gastroenterol. 2008;24:287-97.

33. Larson AM. Acetaminophen hepatotoxicity. Clin Liver Dis. 2007;11:525-48.

34. Andrade RJ, Lucena MI, Fernández MC, Pelaez G, Pachkoria K, García-Ruiz E, et al. Drug-induced liver injury: an analysis of 461 incidences submitted to the Spanish registry over a 10-year period. Gastroenterology. 2005;129:512-21.

35. Liu CT, Chen TH, Cheng CY. Successful treatment of drug-induced acute liver failure with high-volume plasma exchange. J Clin Apher. 2013 Aug 7. doi: 10.1002/jca.21291. [Epub ahead of print]

36. Bunchorntavakul C, Reddy KR. Acetaminophen-related Hepatotoxicity. Clin Liver Dis. 2013;17(4):587-607. doi: 10.1016/j.cld.2013.07.005. Epub 2013 Sep 4.

37. Mindikoglu AL, King D, Magder LS, Ozolek JA, Mazariegos GV, Shneider BL. Valproic acid-associated acute liver failure in children: case report and analysis of liver transplantation outcomes in the United States. J Pediatr. 2011;158(5):802-7.

38. Idilman R, Ersoz S, Coban S, Kumbasar O, Bozkaya H. Antituberculous therapy-induced fulminant hepatic failure: successful treatment with liver transplantation and nonstandard antituberculous therapy. Liver Transpl. 2006;12(9):142730.

Chapter

33

Acute Liver Failure

Deirdre Kelly

INTRODUCTION

Acute liver failure (ALF) or fulminant hepatitis is a rare but potentially fatal disease. Mortality without supportive management and/or liver transplantation is in excess of 70%.

The definition of ALF is hepatic necrosis resulting in loss of liver function within weeks or a few months of the onset of clinical liver disease.[1]

This definition has been refined by the Pediatric Acute Liver Failure Study Group (PALF) to be more specific for children as follows:[2]

❑ The acute onset of liver disease with no known evidence of chronic liver disease.
❑ Biochemical and/or clinical evidence of severe liver dysfunction:
   • Hepatic-based coagulopathy [prothrombin time (PT) ≥20 sec or INR ≥2.0] that is not corrected by parenteral vitamin K
   • And/or hepatic encephalopathy [must be present if the (PT) 15–19.9 seconds or INR 1.5–1.9, but not if PT ≥20 sec or INR ≥2.0].

In the UK, the unique difficulty in detecting encephalopathy in infants means that this is no longer a criterion for super urgent listing for transplantation.

PATHOGENESIS

Acute liver failure (ALF) leads to multisystem organ failure, particularly affecting the brain and kidney. The process leading to hepatic injury is not known, but is multifactorial and dependent on the balance between the following factors.[3]

❑ Susceptibility of the host, e.g. neonate who develops fulminant HBV
❑ Severity and nature of hepatic injury, e.g. dose of acetaminophen
❑ The ability of the liver to regenerate.

Liver Regeneration

The ability of the liver to regenerate is the key to survival. Failure of regeneration may be due to prolonged viral injury and persistent viral replication with failure of eradication of the virus, as patients with ALF due to acetaminophen or other drug poisoning or hepatitis A have a better prognosis than those with indeterminate hepatitis.

Encephalopathy

Encephalopathy is a unique feature of ALF which occurs in most children with acute liver failure. It results from hepatocyte failure,[4] although the neuropharmacological events that lead to hepatic encephalopathy are complex and not completely understood. The liver either fails to produce neuroregulatory substances and/or fails to eliminate neurotoxins, which result in brain dysfunction. Potential neurotransmitters or neurotoxins include ammonia, glutamine, short-chain fatty acids, amino acids, mercaptans and octopamine, and more recently γ-aminobutyric acid (GABA). Acute hepatic encephalopathy is reversible. Cerebral edema complicates acute liver failure and may be reversible in the early stages.[5]

PATHOLOGY

The pathological features of acute liver failure differ according to etiology. There are three basic lesions.[6]

Hepatic necrosis: Severe hepatitis with loss of lobular architecture secondary to extensive hepatocyte necrosis with collapse of the reticulin framework is seen in either viral infection[3] or an idiosyncratic drug reaction. In viral hepatitis, necrosis tends to be panacinar in distribution while in toxic injury it is zonal. Most acute liver failure is associated with massive confluent necrosis. In indeterminate hepatitis, there may be lymphoid aggregates around bile ducts with congestion of centrilobular sinusoids while in hepatitis B there is a minimal inflammatory infiltrate. There may be evidence of regeneration.

Hepatocellular degeneration: In ALF due to metabolic or toxic injuries, there is hepatocellular degeneration with diffuse micro vesicular fatty infiltration of hepatocytes without hepatocyte necrosis or inflammatory infiltrate.[3]

Underlying cirrhosis: In acute liver failure due to either tyrosinemia type 1 or Wilson's disease, the pathological features will include pre-existing cirrhosis.

Recovery

Spontaneous recovery from acute liver failure is usually associated with complete histological recovery but if there has been severe necrosis, post-necrotic cirrhosis may develop.[7]

ETIOLOGY

The etiology of acute liver failure varies with the age of the child (Table 33.1). In neonates, infection or an inborn error of metabolism are common, while viral hepatitis, auto-immune hepatitis and drug induced liver failure are more likely in older children.

Table 33.1: Etiology of acute liver failure	
Neonate/Infant	
Infection	Septicemia
	Hepatitis B
	Adenovirus
	Echovirus
	Coxsackie
Metabolic	Galactosemia
	Neonatal hemochromatosis
	Tyrosinemia type I
	Mitochondrial disorders
	Fatty acid oxidation defects
Poisoning	Paracetamol/Acetaminophen

Older Children

- Viral hepatitis A, B, E
- Indeterminate hepatitis
- Drug induced
  - Paracetamol/Acetaminophen
  - Isoniazid
  - Antiepileptic
  - Sodium valproate
- Autoimmune hepatitis I or II
- Metabolic
  - Wilson's disease

ACUTE LIVER FAILURE IN INFANCY

Many neonates develop acute liver failure secondary to septicemia, due to *Streptococcus* or *Pnemococcus*. Specific causes of hepatitis include herpes simplex, hepatitis B, adenovirus, echovirus and coxsackievirus. Hepatitis A is rare in neonates.

Hepatitis B

Hepatitis B is vertically transmitted during pregnancy with an overall transmission rate of 70%, depending on the hepatitis B surface antigen or e-antigen status of the mother. Although the majority of infected infants become asymptomatic carriers, infants born to hepatitis e-antibody positive or hepatitis e-antigen negative and hepatitis e-antibody negative mothers may develop fulminant hepatitis within the first 12 weeks of life,[8] due to the transmission of a pre-core mutant virus from mother to child.[9]

Herpes Simplex

Herpes simplex virus (HSV) is a DNA virus that causes a generalized disease with associated hepatitis. The incubation period is 2–12 days and it is transmitted by close bodily contact, or perinatally by contact with maternal body fluids.

Neonatal HSV infection presents with a severe multisystem disorder with encephalitis, severe hepatitis, or acute liver failure[10] due to either type 1 or type 2 virus. infants have progressive jaundice, hepatosplenomegaly, raised hepatic transaminase levels and coagulopathy, during the second week of life.

Diagnosis is made by the isolation of virus or detection of HSV DNA from vesicle swabs or other tissue/aspirates Intranuclear inclusion bodies and multinucleate giant cells in scrapings or biopsy tissue are diagnostic as is a specific IgM response. Maternal first episode (primary) genital HSV infection within 6 weeks of delivery is a risk, although infection can occur in the absence of visible maternal lesions.

Aciclovir (neonatal dose is 20 mg/kg every 8 hours) is the drug of choice for disseminated HSV infection, with best results being obtained when treatment is started on the first day of illness. Liver transplantation may be indicated for acute liver failure without multiorgan failure.[11]

Echovirus

The enteroviruses (EV) are a rare cause of acute liver failure. Presentation is before 5 weeks with lethargy, jaundice, high levels of hepatic aminotransferases and severe coagulopathy. Meningitis may be present. Echovirus serotypes 3, 6, 7, 9, 11, 14, 19 and 21 have been reported in severe infections with hepatitis[12] although serotype 11 is the most virulent.

Coxsackievirus

Coxsackieviruses is a human enterovirus which causes a self-limiting gastrointestinal disease, but in neonates, coxsackie A and B may cause fulminant hepatitis, myocarditis or heart failure.[13] There is no specific treatment, but liver transplantation is effective for acute liver failure.

■ METABOLIC DISEASE

Acute liver failure secondary to metabolic disease usually presents with multisystem involvement. Infants are usually small for gestational dates, with hypotonia, severe coagulopathy, and encephalopathy. Neurologic problems such as nystagmus and convulsions may be secondary to cerebral disease or encephalopathy. Renal tubular acidosis is common. Investigations include a search for multiorgan disease.

Galactosemia

This rare autosomal disorder is secondary to a deficiency of galactose-1-phosphase uridyltransferase (GALT), essential for galactose metabolism, in the liver and red blood cells . It is inherited as an autosomal recessive with a frequency of between 1 in 10,000 and 1 in 60,000. There are more than 150 mutations reported in the GALT gene,[14] and this genetic heterogeneity contributes to the wide phenotypic heterogeneity. A significant reduction of the transferase is found in heterozygotes.

Clinical Picture

Acute illness results from the accumulation of the substrate galactose-1-phosphate (GAL-1-P) following the introduction of milk feeds.[15] Infants present with collapse, sepsis, hypoglycemia, and encephalopathy in the first few days of life or with progressive jaundice and liver failure. Ascites and hepatosplenomegaly may be noted. Cataracts are present. The disease may be complicated by gram-negative sepsis, which stimulates a life-threatening severe bleeding diathesis.

Hepatic Changes

Those dying in the first few weeks show diffuse hepato-cellular fatty change. In the next few months the liver shows pseudoglandular or ductular structures around the canaliculi which may contain bile. Regeneration is conspicuous, necrosis scanty and a macronodular cirrhosis results.

Diagnosis

The biochemical changes include galactosemia, galactosuria, hyperchloraemic acidosis, albuminuria and aminoaciduria. The diagnosis is established by the detection of urinary reducing substances in the absence of glycosuria, and confirmed by reduced GALT enzyme activity in erythrocytes. Hepatic pathology demonstrates fatty change, periportal bile duct proliferation, and iron deposition with extramedullary hematopoiesis. If galactose ingestion persists, hepatic fibrosis and cirrhosis may develop or be present at birth.[16]

Prognosis and Treatment

Liver function improves following exclusion of galactose from the diet unless liver failure or cirrhosis has developed. The long-term outcome is disappointing. Learning difficulties and growth disturbance are described and are more common in girls, 75% of whom also develop ovarian failure.

Neonatal Hemochromatosis (NNH)

This disease is the commonest cause of acute liver failure in the neonate. It is characterized by the prenatal accumulation of intrahepatic iron, due either to a primary disorder of fetoplacental iron handling, or a secondary manifestation of fetal liver disease.

There is no association with mutations in the genes for hereditary hemochromatosis or juvenile hemochromatosis.[17] NNH is extremely rare in first pregnancies, and once one affected child has been born the risk of recurrence in subsequent pregnancies is 80% but recurrence has never been reported in children born to the same father with different mothers. It is now thought to be a maternal alloimmune disorder.[18]

Clinical features include intrauterine growth retardation, premature delivery, hypoglycemia, jaundice, and coagulopathy within the first 2 weeks. The outcome is fatal without treatment.

Biochemical liver function tests demonstrate an elevated bilirubin, and reduced transaminases and albumin. Serum iron binding capacity is low and hypersaturated (90–100%), with a grossly elevated ferritin level [100 μg/dL (>1000 μg/L)]. Diagnostic liver biopsy is not feasible because of the coagulopathy, but extrahepatic siderosis is found in minor salivary glands obtained by lip biopsy. Magnetic resonance imaging may confirm excess hepatic or extrahepatic iron in pancreas and brain.

Liver histology demonstrates pericellular fibrosis, giant cell transformation, ductular proliferation, and regenerative nodules. The distribution of siderosis is within hepatocytes but there is extrahepatic parenchymal deposition, with sparing of the reticuloendothelial systems.

Medical management includes supportive therapy for acute liver failure and an 'antioxidant cocktail', which combines N-acetylcysteine (150 mg/kg/day), vitamin E (25 mg/kg/day), selenium (2–3 mg/kg/day), prostaglandin E1 (0.4–0.6 mg/kg/h), and desferrioxamine (30 mg/kg/day). Some children have responded to this regimen, but the majority require liver transplantation.

As the condition is considered an alloimmune disorder, the use of exchange transfusion seems logical. Beneficial results have been obtained using the combination of exchange transfusion and substituting intravenous immunoglobulin,[18a] but most infants require liver transplantation. Extrahepatic iron is mobilized following successful liver transplantation and does not recur.[19]

Antenatal diagnosis is not possible, but the diagnosis may be suspected by the detection of nonspecific abnormalities such as hydrops fetalis or intrauterine growth retardation. Prenatal iron accumulation may be detected by MRI, but the sensitivity is unknown. Maternal treatment with immunoglobulin infusion from 16 weeks gestation prevents recurrence in the majority.[20]

Disorders of Mitochondrial Energy Metabolism

This group of disorders include a wide range of clinical phenotypes with any mode of inheritance: autosomal recessive; autosomal dominant; or transmission through maternal DNA. Mutations in the gene encoding polymerase gamma, POLG1, cause mitochondrial DNA depletion or multiple mitochondrial DNA deletions resulting in highly heterogeneous group of mitochondrial diseases (see below).[21-23] The pathological effects are secondary to dysfunction of the electron transport chain resulting in cellular ATP deficiency, impaired fat oxidation and the generation of toxic free radicals. Clinical symptoms vary, depending on the nature of the primary defect, the tissue or organ distribution and abundance, and the importance of aerobic metabolism in the affected tissue. The constituent proteins of the electron transport chain are encoded in two genomes, either nuclear DNA or mitochondrial DNA (mitochondrial DNA) which is maternally inherited. In the context of liver failure, isolated deficiencies of the electron transport chain enzymes, mitochondrial DNA depletion syndromes and Alpers syndrome are relevant.

Deficiencies of the Electron Transport Chain Enzyme

Mitochondrial DNA depletions, induced by mutations of the nuclear genes POLG, DGUOK, and MPV17, are the major causes of these combined deficiencies.[22] The most common isolated defects are complexes 4 and 1. Infants present with multisystem involvement with hypotonia, cardiomyopathy, and proximal renal tubulopathy and a severe metabolic acidosis. Relevant diagnostic investigations include elevated blood lactate, lactate/pyruvate ratio >20, increased 3-OH-butyrate/acetoacetate ratio >2, or an increase in lactate, possible ketone bodies and, following a glucose load (2 g/kg), the detection of specific organic acids such as urinary 3-methyl-glutaconic acid or other Krebs cycle intermediates. Coagulopathy is usually extreme, and may prevent liver or muscle biopsy, or cerebrospinal fluid (CSF) examination. The diagnosis is based on demonstrating biochemical dysfunction of electron chain function in liver or muscle by histochemistry or enzyme analysis in fresh tissue. Demonstration of an elevated CSF lactate compared with plasma lactate indicates neurologic involvement.[24]

Supportive management is usually the only option. Liver transplantation is only successful if the defect is confined to the liver, but is contraindicated if multisystem involvement is obvious as neurologic deterioration persists or may develop post-transplant.[25]

Mitochondrial DNA Depletion Syndromes

Mitochondria normally contain more than one copy of mitochondrial DNA and replication is regulated by a number of factors encoded by nuclear genes. Mutations in these nuclear genes lead to a reduction in copy numbers of mitochondrial DNA resulting in mitochondrial depletion. Mutations have been found in genes encoding the mitochondrial enzymes DNA polymerase gamma, thymidine kinase, deoxyguanosine kinase, succinyl CoA-ligase and MPV.[21-23]

The clinical presentation and biochemical findings are similar to those of infants presenting with isolated electron transport chain deficiencies. Treatment is supportive as liver transplantation is contraindicated.[24] Antenatal diagnosis is possible if a mutation has been identified.

Alpers syndrome: This is an autosomal recessive, developmental mitochondrial DNA depletion disorder characterized by degenerative brain and liver disease which may be precipitated by valproate treatment.[22] Focal seizures usually precede liver disease. The clinical presentation is varied. Neurological features, lethargy and hypotonia are prominent. Hypertrophic cardiomyopathy and renal tubulopathy may develop. Hepatic involvement is unpredictable and includes isolated hepatomegaly; neonatal cholestasis; and acute liver failure with coagulopathy. The diagnosis is based on an elevated blood lactate, but this may be intermittent. Elevated cerebrospinal fluid (CSF)/plasma lactate ratio or elevated CSF protein suggests central nervous system involvement. Hepatic pathology is characterized by both micro- and macrovesicular steatosis, with hepatocyte degeneration and micronodular cirrhosis. Electron microscopy may reveal abnormal structure or number of mitochondria. Muscle histology may show increased lipid droplets. The presence of ragged red fibers on the Gomori stain are strongly suggestive of mitochondrial DNA abnormalities. The definitive diagnosis is based on identifying the genetic defect. Supportive management for acute liver failure is required with discontinuation of valproate. Transplantation is contraindicated if multisystem involvement is demonstrated.

Tyrosinemia Type I

Tyrosinemia type I is an autosomal recessive disorder due to a defect of fumaryl acetoacetase (FAA), which is the terminal enzyme in tyrosine degradation. The gene for FAA is on the short arm of chromosome 15. More than 40 mutations have been described to date,[26] although in some populations a single mutation may be prevalent. There is a high lifetime risk of developing hepatocellular carcinoma (HCC), which historically is 40%.[27]

Intermediate metabolites such as maleyl- and fumarylacetoacetate are highly reactive compounds that are locally toxic to the liver, while the secondary metabolite succinylacetone has both local and systemic effects, including cardiac, renal, and neurologic disease and inhibition of porphobilinogen synthase which is the cause of the neurological symptoms.

Clinical features are heterogeneous, even within the same family. Acute liver failure is a common presentation in infants between 1 and 6 months of age who present with mild jaundice, coagulopathy, encephalopathy, and ascites. Hypoglycemia is common, either due to liver dysfunction or hyperinsulinism from pancreatic islet cell hyperplasia.

In older infants, failure to thrive, coagulopathy, hepatosplenomegaly, hypotonia, and rickets are common. Biochemical liver function tests show an elevated bilirubin, transaminases, alkaline phosphatase, and a reduced albumin. Plasma amino acids indicate a three-fold increase in plasma tyrosine, phenylalanine, and methionine with grossly elevated α-fetoprotein levels. Urinary succinyl acetone is a pathognomonic but not an invariable finding. The diagnosis is confirmed by genetic analysis. Hepatic histology is nonspecific with steatosis, siderosis, and cirrhosis, which may be present in infancy.

Initial management is with a phenylalanine and tyrosine-restricted diet which may improve overall nutritional status and renal tubular function, but does not affect progression of liver disease. The discovery of 2(2-nitro-trifluoromethylbenzoyl)-1,3-cyclohexanedione (NTBC) or Nitisinone which prevents the formation of toxic metabolites, has altered the natural history of this disease in childhood and may reduce the need for liver transplantation in those who have acute liver failure.[28,29]

ACUTE LIVER FAILURE IN OLDER CHILDREN

Hepatitis A and B are the commonest causes of acute liver failure in the developing world.[8] However, in the UK and US as demonstrated by the PALF study, indeterminate hepatitis was the commonest cause (Table 33.2).

Virus Infection

Herpes simplex virus (HSV), varicella-zoster virus, cytomegalovirus, and Epstein–Barr virus (EBV) have been reported to cause acute liver failure, almost always in immunocompromised hosts, with EBV most frequently implicated.[30] Paramyxovirus, parvovirus B$_{19}$, and toga virus have been identified in some cases.

Hepatitis A Virus (HAV)

HAV has a worldwide distribution. It is endemic in early childhood in areas with poor living conditions and low socioeconomic status. The mean age of infection increases with improvement in sanitation. In the UK, an oral fluid based survey in 2001/2002 found only 4% of children aged 1–4 had serological evidence of past HAV infection, increasing to 26% in those aged 25–44.[30a] Transmission of the disease is by fecal contamination of drinking water or food and by person-to-person contact.

Acute HAV infection was a common cause of fulminant hepatic failure varying from 1.5% to 31% in both developing and developed countries.[30b,30c] Superinfection of chronic liver diseases leading to an acute on chronic

Table 33.2: Etiology of acute liver failure							
	n	Age (y)	HAV	HBV	Metab	Indet	AIH
PALF (2)	348	-	1%	-	10%	49%	6%
Phillipines (65)	26	17	19%	4%	-	-	-
Turkey (66)	74	-	18%	-	35%	21%	-
India (60)	130	7.5	53%	-	-	-	-
Argentina (67)	40	5.3	42%	-	-	35%	17%

hepatitis is also reported.[30d] In general the prognosis for recovery is better with HAV than other viruses, especially indeterminate hepatitis.

Hepatitis B (HBV)

Fulminant hepatic failure in acute HBV infection is about 1% in Western Europe and the USA. It is very rare in infants, though has been reported in babies born to HBsAg-positive, HBeAg-negative mothers who have viral mutants.[30e] The prognosis of HBV-related acute liver failure is generally worse than with other aetiologies, with spontaneous recovery occurring in fewer than 20% of cases.[31] Fortunately, universal hepatitis B vaccination in endemic areas of the world, such as Taiwan, has resulted in a significant decline in mortality associated with ALF secondary to HBV.[32]

Hepatitis C virus (HCV) is a rare cause for acute liver failure.[33]

Hepatitis E Virus (HEV)

HEV is due to an RNA virus with 4 genotypes, two of which are found in humans.[34] It is a water-borne infection in the developing world (HEV genotype 1, 2 or 4) while in developed countries, HEV infection occurs in returning travellers. The incubation period is 6 weeks (range 2–9 weeks) after primary exposure. Acute HEV is diagnosed by detecting HEV RNA, IgM and IgG antibody to recombinant HEV antigen.[34]

HEV infection is infrequent among children <10 years of age. In India, only 5 of 103 (5%) children were anti-HEV IgG-positive.[35] Acute liver failure does occur and is more common in pregnant women. There is no specific treatment

Nonviral Infectious Hepatitis

Other infections rarely lead to acute liver failure. These include: congenital syphilis, leptospirosis and, in endemic areas, *Coxiella burnetii* (Q fever), *Plasmodium falciparum* and *Entamoeba histolytica*. Systemic sepsis may occasionally present as acute liver failure.[36]

Indeterminate Hepatitis (Hepatitis non-A-E)

Hepatitis of indeterminate cause, formerly referred to as sporadic non-A-E hepatitis, is diagnosed when there is evidence of acute hepatitis in the absence of markers for hepatitis virus infection, the absence of clinical and/or serological evidence of systemic infection with other infectious agents, no exposure to drugs or toxins, and negative markers of autoimmune disease.[2] It is the most important cause of acute liver failure in children in developed countries.[37] The prognosis is poor, with a 5 to

43%) rate of spontaneous recovery indicating the need for early referral for liver transplantation. There is an association with aplastic anemia in 10–20% which may require bone marrow transplantation.

DRUG AND TOXIN-RELATED HEPATIC INJURY

Drug-induced acute liver failure (DALF) accounts for approximately 20% of pediatric acute liver failure (ALF). Although most patients experience milder drug hepatotoxic reactions such as hepatitis, cholestasis or asymptomatic enzyme elevation it is important to recognize the potential for progression to ALF. The commonest cause of DALF in children is acetaminophen (15% of all ALF in children in the UK and USA) while other drugs such as antituberculous and antiepileptic therapy account for 5%. The pathogenesis of the liver injury includes direct hepatotoxicity and idiosyncratic reactions for most drugs, although for others the mechanism of injury is assumed, based on clinical presentation and hepatic[38,39] (Table 33.3).

Acetaminophen (Paracetamol) Poisoning

Acetaminophen toxicity leads to a direct dose-dependent hepatotoxic effect. In childhood, acetaminophen toxicity may develop in children aged under 3 years of age, either by deliberate acetaminophen poisoning by carers, long-term chronic ingestion of acetaminophen, or deliberate overdose in adolescents.[42] Children have a lower incidence of liver failure with acetaminophen overdose than adults

Table 33.3: Drugs and toxins associated with acute liver failure
Hepatotoxic agents*
• Acetaminophen overdose
• *Amanita* species
• Salicylate (overdose)
• Iron (overdose)
Drugs associated with idiosyncratic reactions
• Isoniazid
• Propylthiouracil
• Sodium valproate
• Halothane
• Amiodarone
• Nonsteroidal anti-inflammatory agents
• Tetracycline
• Carbamazepine
• Lamotrigene
Recreational drugs associated with hepatic injury
• Cocaine
• Ecstasy

*Substances that are not hepatotoxic when used appropriately (unless taken with alcohol), perhaps because the rate of glutathione resynthesis is higher.

Excessive acetaminophen overwhelms the normal conjugation pathways of sulfation or glucuronidation, mandating that acetaminophen is metabolized by the alternate pathways through cytochrome P450. This produces NAPQI (N-acetyl-p-benzoqinoneimine) which is highly reactive and depletes glutathione. Accumulation of NAPQI leads to cell death and hence hepatocellular necrosis.[40]

Clinical features include anorexia, nausea and vomiting. In severe ingestion hypoglycemia and lactic acidosis are prominent early features. Hepatic enlargement and tenderness develop by the second day, while jaundice and encephalopathy typically develop between the third and fifth days associated with renal failure.[4,40]

Treatment with intravenous N-acetylcysteine 150 mg/kg in reducing dosages, if instituted early, is effective as it repletes glutathione thereby preventing injury, particularly if begun between 12–24 hours after ingestion. Children who develop severe hepatotoxicity need to be admitted to a specialist unit for management of acute liver and renal failure and consideration for liver transplantation.[43]

90% of children and adolescents recover with supportive measures but the prognosis is worse for those who have severe poisoning or have been taking acetaminophen in association with another drug.[41]

Sodium Valproate

Sodium valproate is associated with ALF especially in children aged less than 2 years. The risk is 1:8,000 if on sodium valproate monotherapy and 1:550 if on polytherapy. For children aged 3–10 years the risk of liver failure decreases to 1:6,000–12,000 and for children over 10 years of age decreases to less than 1:50,000.[44]

Clinical features include nausea, vomiting, increasing seizure frequency, jaundice, edema, and hypoglycemia leading to drowsiness and coma usually within the first 6 months of treatment. Biochemical investigations reveal moderate increases in hepatic transaminases and bilirubin, hypoaminemia, and severe coagulopathy. Hepatic histology demonstrates severe microvesicular fatty change with hepatocellular necrosis and occasionally cirrhosis.

Once liver disease is established, the outlook is poor unless valproate has been promptly discontinued. Carnitine is not effective in preventing or treating hepatotoxicity, but N-acetylcysteine may have a hepatoprotective role.[45] Liver transplantation is contraindicated as neurologic disease may progress.[46]

Autoimmune Hepatitis

Autoimmune hepatitis (both types I and II) cause liver failure in about 20% of patients[29] although it is more common in type II.[47,48] Many of these patients will respond to medical therapy (corticosteroid and azathioprine), avoiding the need for transplantation. Liver biopsy shows signs of chronic hepatitis (portal fibrosis and piecemeal necrosis) in addition to severe lobular hepatitis. The majority of patients have elevated IgG immunoglobulin and raised titers of antinuclear, anti-smooth muscle or anti-liver-kidney-microsomal antibodies.

Metabolic Diseases

The most common cause of metabolic disease leading to ALF in older children is Wilson's disease.

Clinical features include hepatic dysfunction (40%) and psychiatric symptoms (35%) and acute liver failure is a less common presentation.[49] Children may have a history of deteriorating school performance, abnormal behavior, lack of coordination, and dysarthria. Renal tubular abnormalities, renal calculi, and hemolytic anemia are associated features. The characteristic Kayser–Fleischer rings are rare before the age of 7 years and may be absent in up to 80% of older children.

Biochemical liver function tests indicate underlying chronic liver disease with low albumin (<35 g/L), minimal transaminitis, and a low alkaline phosphastase (<200 U/L). The diagnosis is established by detecting a low serum copper (<10 μmol/L), a low serum ceruloplasmin (<200 mg/L), excess urine copper (>1 μmol/24 h), particularly after penicillamine treatment (20 mg/kg/day), and an elevated hepatic copper (>250 mg/g dry weight of liver).

Histologic features of Wilson's disease depend on the clinical presentation. There may be microvesicular steatosis, chronic hepatitis, hepatocellular necrosis, multinucleated hepatocytes and Mallory's hyaline, hepatic fibrosis, and cirrhosis. In children who have fulminant hepatitis the histologic features are those of severe hepatocellular necrosis with cirrhosis.

Management is with a low copper diet and penicillamine, although children with ALF usually require liver transplantation.

Clinical Manifestations of Acute Liver Failure

The onset of liver disease varies according to etiology. There may be a prodromal illness with lethargy, fatigue, malaise, vomiting, diarrhea, and jaundice with the subsequent development of coagulopathy and encephalopathy. Encephalopathy is difficult to detect in infants and may present with drowsiness, irritability or day/night reversal of sleep rhythm. Older children become aggressive, which is misinterpreted as antisocial behavior.

Laboratory Investigations

- Marked conjugated hyperbilirubinemia in some cases of drug-induced hepatitis, fulminant hepatitis B and in idiopathic anicteric fulminant failure.[3,9,50]
- Aminotransferases (ALT, AST) may be very high (>1000 IU/L), or may be falling with a decreasing liver size, reflecting severe necrosis.
- Plasma ammonia is usually 2–8 times elevated (>100 µmol/L).
- Serum creatinine may be elevated secondary to renal complications, while the urea may be high (renal dysfunction, increased production from blood in the GI tract, dehydration) or low (failure of hepatic synthesis).
- Hypoglycemia may be present and difficult to correct.
- Arterial blood gas analysis may show a wide spectrum of abnormalities from respiratory alkalosis to mixed respiratory and metabolic acidosis, usually in association with hypoxemia.
- Electrolyte abnormalities are associated with vomiting and dehydration.
- Coagulation profiles demonstrate deficiencies of clotting factors and often evidence of consumptive coagulopathy.
- The platelet count is often reduced, due to consumption or reduced production (aplastic anemia occurs in10-20% of indeterminate hepatitis).
- The white blood cell count varies from high (stress response, secondary bacterial infection) to low (aplastic anemia).
- A baseline electroencephalogram (EEG) is helpful to stage coma and provide information on prognosis. Computed tomography (CT) scans are not useful early in encephalopathy, but may provide information on cerebral edema, hemorrhage, or irreversible brain damage.

Diagnosis

The diagnosis is established by the combination of clinical and biochemical features and specific diagnostic tests (Table 33.4). A histological diagnosis by liver biopsy may be contraindicated because of the abnormal coagulation. Transjugular biopsy to reduce the risk of bleeding is technically possible in children other than infants.

Table 33.4: Investigations in acute liver failure

Baseline essential investigations
Biochemistry
- Bilirubin, transaminases
- Alkaline phosphatase
- Albumin
- Urea and electrolytes
- Creatinine
- Calcium, phosphate
- Ammonia
- Acid–base, lactate
- Glucose
Hematology
- Full blood count, platelets
- PT, PTT
- Factors V or VII
- Blood group cross-match
Septic screen
- No lumbar puncture
Radiology
- Chest X-ray
- Abdominal ultrasound
- Head CT scan or MRI
Neurophysiology
- EEG
Diagnostic investigations
Serum
- Acetaminophen levels
- Cu, ceruloplasmin (>3 years)
- Autoantibodies
- Immunoglobulins
- Amino acids
- Hepatitis A, B, C, E
- EBV, CMV, HSV
- Leptospira (if clinically relevant)
- Other viruses
Urine
- Toxic metabolites
- Amino acids, succinylacetone
- Organic acids
- Reducing sugars

Abbreviations: CMV, cytomegalovirus; EBV, Epstein–Barr virus; HSV, herpes simplex virus; PT, prothrombin time; PTT, partial thromboplastin time.

Complications

The complications of acute liver failure are numerous and include: sepsis, gastrointestinal bleeding, cerebral edema, pancreatitis, renal and cardiac failure.

Management (Table 33.5)

The management of acute liver failure includes:
- Supportive management
- Prevention and treatment of complications while awaiting hepatic regeneration or a donor liver.

Table 33.5: Management of acute liver failure

No sedation except for procedures
Monitor:
- Heart and respiratory rate
- Arterial BP, CVP
- Core/toe temperature
- Neurological observations
- Gastric pH (>5.0)
- Blood glucose (>4 mmol/L)
- Acid–base
- Electrolytes
- PT, PTT

Fluid balance
- 75% maintenance
- Dextrose 10–50%
- Sodium (0.5–1 mmol/L)
- Potassium (2–4 mmol/L)

Maintain circulating volume with colloid/FFP
Coagulation support only if required

Drugs
- Vitamin K
- H$_2$-antagonist
- Antacids
- Lactulose/sodium benzoate
- N-acetylcysteine
- Broad-spectrum antibiotics
- Antifungals

Nutrition
- Enteral feeding (1–2 g protein/day)
- PN if ventilated

Abbreviations: BP, blood pressure; CVP, central venous pressure; FFP, fresh frozen plasma; PN, parenteral nutrition; PT, prothrombin time; PTT, partial thromboplastin time.

❑ Assessment of prognosis for liver transplantation
❑ Early consideration for transplantation

Supportive management for acute liver failure in childhood includes:

❑ Maintaining blood glucose levels greater than 4 mmol/L with 10–50% dextrose;
❑ Fluid restriction (50–75% of standard maintenance) using colloid to maintain circulating volume;
❑ Prevention of gastrointestinal hemorrhage from stress erosions using H$_2$ receptor antagonists (ranitidine 3 mg/kg q8h) and sucralfate (2–4 g/day) or proton pump inhibitors (Omeprazole 10–20 mg/day);
❑ Prevention of sepsis with broad-spectrum antibiotics (amoxicillin, cefuroxime, and metronidazole);
❑ Prophylactic antifungal therapy (fluconazole);
❑ In the early stages of establishing the prognosis and requirement for liver transplantation, coagulation support is not recommended. If coagulopathy is severe (prothrombin time > 60 seconds) and/or the decision for liver transplantation has been taken, then coagulation

support using fresh frozen plasma, cryoprecipitate and vitamin K (2–10 mg); is essential.

- Nutritional support—to reduce protein intake to 1–2 g/kg/day, either enterally or parenterally.
- To provide sufficient energy intake to reverse catabolism, either enterally or parenterally.
- Children who are mechanically ventilated should have parenteral nutrition, as it may be 7–10 days before full normal diet is resumed following transplantation.
- The use of N-acetylcysteine, which is particularly useful in paracetamol poisoning, has not been proven useful in the management of acute liver failure.[51]

Prevention and Treatment of Complications

Management of hepatic encephalopathy. In the early stages reduction of protein intake to 1–2 g/kg and provision of high calorie feeds using glucose polymer (8–10 g/kg) and oral lactulose may be sufficient. Addition of sodium benzoate[52] and or rifaxamine[53] may be helpful. Increasing encephalopathy unresponsive to conservative management requires elective ventilation

❑ The management of cerebral edema is critical for survival. Fluid restriction (50% maintenance), and the use of intravenous mannitol (0.5 g/kg over 4–6 hours) may be helpful in the short-term. Elective ventilation should be performed if Grade II or III hepatic coma develop or when cerebral edema is suspected. Convulsions should be promptly treated and may respond to thiopentone infusion. Monitoring of intracranial pressure is controversial, but may improve selection for liver transplantation.

❑ Electrolyte and acid–base disturbances include hyponatremia and/or hypernatremia, hypokalemia. Hypocalcemia and hypomagnesemia frequently occur and should be corrected.

❑ Acid–base disturbances are common and may be secondary to liver failure, sepsis, or the underlying disease. Severe metabolic acidosis requires intravenous sodium bicarbonate (8.4%), elective ventilation or bicarbonate dialysis. Respiratory failure and respiratory acidosis develop as coma deepens, requiring mechanical ventilation.

❑ Renal insufficiency occurs in 75% of children[50] and may be due to prerenal uremia, acute tubular necrosis, and functional renal failure. Functional renal failure (hepatorenal syndrome) is the commonest cause of renal insufficiency. Features include sodium retention (urinary sodium concentration <20 mmol/L), normal urinary sediment, and reduced urinary output (<1 mL/kg/h). The etiology is multifactorial, and electrolyte imbalance, sepsis, and hypovolemia all play a part. Endotoxemia may contribute to renal injury.

Management consists of maintaining circulating volume to prevent prerenal hypovolemia keeping the urine output >0.5 mL/kg/h. A fluid challenge (10 mL/kg) or frusemide (1–2 mg/kg IV or 0.25 mg/kg/h by infusion) may be effective. Established renal failure requires hemodialysis or filtration for fluid overload.

Hepatic Support

Attempts to remove potentially neuroactive toxins include double volume exchange transfusion, plasmapheresis, liver assist devices containing cultured hepatocytes and extracorporeal perfusion through a human or animal liver, have generally been ineffective.[54,55]

Molecular absorbent recirculating system (MARS) is an alternative form of hemodialysis which uses a specific filter to remove toxic products, but not albumin. Its use in the management of children is anecdotal, but it may have a role to play in creating a 'bridge to transplantation,[56] or in the setting of drug induced liver failure or toxic mushroom poisoning.

Hepatocyte transplantation as therapy for acute liver failure using cell suspensions or synthetic constructs is at an early stage of research, but show promise in animal models.[57,58]

SELECTION FOR LIVER TRANSPLANTATION

Selection for liver transplantation depends on the etiology of the disease, prognostic factors, the presence or absence of multisystem disease and/or reversible brain damage.[3,50,59-61]

In pediatric acute liver failure, patients with paracetamol poisoning or hepatitis A have the best prognosis for spontaneous recovery compared to infants or children with metabolic liver disease. Prognostic factors for survival are less well established in children than in adults, but children with metabolic liver disease or severe coagulopathy (prothrombin time >50 seconds) are less likely to recover.[37] In general, poor prognostic features indicating the immediate necessity for liver transplantation in infants include persistent prolonged coagulopathy (PT >50 seconds), rising bilirubin and falling transaminases. In older children, in whom encephalopathy is easier to detect, grade II or III hepatic coma indicates a poor prognosis.

It is important to exclude multisystem disease and to diagnose a mitochondrial disorder (plasma CSF, lactate, muscle biopsy). It is less easy to demonstrate irreversible cerebral damage because the cerebral sutures will not have fused in many neonates and infants and the classical signs of cerebral edema may not be present. The best guide to irreversible cerebral damage is the development of gray/white reversion on CT scan secondary to cerebral ischemia or the development of convulsions.

Liver Transplantation

Early consideration for liver transplantation is essential in order to expedite the search for a donor liver. Although age and size are no longer contraindications to liver transplantation the shortage of age and size matched organs for transplantation means that most children will receive a reduced or split liver graft.[62] Auxiliary liver transplantation, in which part of the recipient liver is left in situ to regenerate is still controversial treatment for fulminant hepatic failure, but recent studies have suggested that the graft may be removed if the original liver regenerates.[63] It is not suitable for transplantation for acute liver failure secondary to metabolic liver disease, as these livers are unlikely to recover and there may be a risk of hepatoma in the cirrhotic liver. Living related donation for acute liver failure is carried out by some centers, but has the disadvantage that families and potential donors have little time for preparation and counseling.[64]

Survival post-liver transplantation for acute liver failure has improved and most recipients can expect a 70% 5-year survival.[65] Survivors of liver transplantation for acute liver failure face psychological sequelae and thus preparation both of the family and the child (post-transplant) is mandatory.

SUMMARY

Acute liver failure in childhood is a rare but fatal disease which may develop secondary to metabolic liver disease or infection. The prognosis has been improved by the development of effective medical therapy for certain metabolic disorders and the success of liver transplantation, but is dependent on the presence of multisystem disease and reversible cerebral damage.[66,67]

REFERENCES

1. Williams R. Classification, etiology, and considerations of outcome in acute liver failure. Semin Liver Dis. 1996;16:343-8.
2. Squires RH Jr, Shneider BL, Bucuvalas J, Alonso E, Sokol RJ, Narkewicz MR, et al. Acute liver failure in children: the first 348 patients in the pediatric acute liver failure study group. J Pediatr. 2006;148(5):652-8.
3. Kelly DA. Fulminant hepatitis and acute liver failure. Management of Digestive and Liver Disorders in Infants and Children. Eds: JP Buts and EM Sokal. Elsevier Science 1993;577-93.

4. Ferenci P, Lockwood A, Mullen K, Tarter R, Weissenborn K, Blei AT. Hepatic encephalopathy—definition, nomenclature, diagnosis, and quantification: final report of the working party at the 11th World Congresses of Gastroenterology, Vienna. 1998. Hepatology. 2002;35(3):716-21.

5. Blei AT. Brain edema and portal-systemic encephalopathy. Liver Transpl. 2000;6(4 Suppl 1):S14-20.

6. Horney JT, Galambos JT. The liver during and after fulminant hepatitis. Gastroenterology. 1977;73:639-45.

7. Portmann B, Talbot IC, Day DW, Davidson AR, Murray-Lyon IM, Williams R. Histopathological changes in the liver following a paracetamol overdose: correlation with clinical and biochemical parameters. J Pathol. 1975;117:169-81.

8. Beath SV, Boxall EH, Watson RM, Tarlow MJ, Kelly D. Fulminant hepatitis B in infants born to anti-Hbe hepatitis B carrier mothers. Brit Med J. 1992;304:1169-70.

9. Chang MH. Hepatitis B virus mutation in children. Indian J Pediatr. 2006;73(9):803-7.

10. Benador N. Mannhardt W, Schranz D, et al. Three cases of neonatal herpes simplex infection presenting as fulminant hepatits. Eur J Pediatr. 1990;149:555-9.

11. de Ville de Goyet J, Kelly DA, Lee WS, McKiernan PJ, Ramani P, Tanner MS. Neonatal liver transplant for fulminant hepatitis caused by Herpes Simplex Virus Type 2. J Pediatr Gastroenterol Nutr. 2002;35:220-3.

12. Modlin JF, Kinney JS. Perinatal echovirus infection: insights from a literature review of 61 cases and 16 outbreaks in nurseries. Rev Infect Dis. 1986;8:918-26.

13. Chou LL, Chang P, Wu LC. Neonatal coxsackievirus B1 infection associated with severe hepatitis: report of three cases. Acta Paediatr Sin. 1995;36:296-9.

14. Tyfield L, Reichardt J, Fridovich-Keil J, Croke DT, Elsas LJ 2nd, Strobl W, et al. Classical galactosemia and mutations at the galactose-1-phosphate uridyl transferase (GALT) gene. Hum Mutat 1999;13:417-30.

15. Gitzelmann R. Galactose-1-phosphate in the pathogenesis of galactosemia. Eur J Paediatr. 1995;154(Suppl 2):S45.

16. Berry GT, Nissim I, Lin Z, Mazur AT, Gibson JB, Segal S. Endogenous synthesis of galactose in normal men and patients with hereditary galactosemia. Lancet 1995;346:1073-4.

17. Kelly AL, Lunt PW, Rodrigues F, Berry PJ, Flynn DM, McKiernan PJ, et al. Classification and genetic features of neonatal haemochromatosis: a study of 27 affected pedigrees and molecular analysis of genes implicated in iron metabolism. J Med Genet. 2001;38:599-610.

18. Whitington PF, Malladi P. Neonatal hemochromatosis: is it an alloimmune disease? J Pediatr Gastroenterol Nutr. 2005;40:544-9.

18a. Rand EB, Karpen SJ, Kelly S, Mack CL, Malatack JJ, Sokol RJ, Whitington PF. Treatment of neonatal hemochromatosis with exchange transfusion and intravenous immunoglobulin. J Pediatr. 2009;155(4):566-71.

19. Flynn DM, Mohan N, McKiernan P, Beath S, Buckels J, Mayer D, et al. Progress in treatment and outcome for children with neonatal haemochromatosis. Arch. Dis Child Fetal Neonatal Ed. 2003;88:F124-7.

20. Whitington PF, Hibbard JU. High-dose immunoglobulin during pregnancy for recurrent neonatal haemochromatosis. Lancet. 2004;364:1690-8.

21. Leonard JV, Schapira AH. Mitochondrial respiratory chain disorders II: neurodegenerative disorders and nuclear gene defects. Lancet. 2000;355:389-94.

22. Nguyen KV, Ostergaard E, Ravn SH, Balslev T, Danielsen ER, Vardag A, et al. POLG mutations in Alpers syndrome. Neurology 2005;65:1493-5.

23. Valnot I, Osmond S, Gigarel N, Mehaye B, Amiel J, Cormier-Daire V. et al. Mutations of the SCO1 gene in mitochondrial cytochrome c oxidase deficiency with neonatal-onset hepatic failure and encephalopathy. Am J Hum Genet. 2000;67:1104-9.

24. Thomson M, McKiernan P, Buckels J, Mayer D, Kelly D. Generalised mitochondrial cytopathy is an absolute contraindication to orthotopic liver transplant in childhood. J Pediatr Gastroenterol Nutr. 1998;26:478-81.

25. Iwama I, Baba Y, Kagimoto S, Kishimoto H, Kasahara M, Murayama K, Shimizu K. Case report of a successful liver transplantation for acute liver failure due to mitochondrial respiratory chain complex III deficiency. Transplant Proc. 2011;43(10):4025-8.

26. Heath SK, Gray RG, McKiernan P, Au KM, Walker E, Green A. Mutation screening for tyrosinaemia type I. J Inherit. Metab Dis. 2002;25:523-4.

27. Weinberg AG, Mize CE, Worthen HG. The occurrence of hepatoma in the chronic form of hereditary tyrosinemia. J Pediatr. 1976;88:434-8.

28. Lindstedt S, Holme E, Lock EA, Hjalmarson O, Strandvik B. Treatment of hereditary tyrosinaemia type I by inhibition of 4-hydroxyphenylpyruvate dioxygenase. Lancet. 1992;340:813-7.

29. McKiernan PJ. Nitisinone in the treatment of hereditary tyrosinaemia type 1. Drugs. 2006;66:743-50.

30. Feranchak AP, Tyson RW, Narkewicz MR, Karrer FM, Sokol RJ. Fulminant Epstein-Barr viral hepatitis: orthotopic liver transplantation and review of the literature. Liver Transpl Surg. 1998;4(6):469-76.

30a. Morris-Cunnington MC, Edmunds WJ, Miller E, Brown DW. A population-based seroprevalence study of hepatitis A virus using oral fluid in England and Wales. Am J Epidemiol. 2004;159(8):786-94.

30b. Bravo LC, Gregorio GV, Shafi F, Bock HL, Boudville I, Liu Y, Gatchalian SR. Etiology, incidence and outcomes of acute hepatic failure in 0-18 year old Filipino children. Southeast Asian J Trop Med Public Health. 2012;43(3):764-72.

30c. Bariş Z, Saltik Temızel IN, Uslu N, Usta Y, Demır H, Gürakan F, et al. Acute liver failure in children: 20-year experience. Turk J Gastroenterol. 2012;23(2):127-34.

30d. Lal J, Thapa BR, Rawal P, Ratho RK, Singh K. Predictors of outcome in acute-on-chronic liver failure in children. Hepatol Int. 2011;5(2):693-7.

30e. Hawkins AE, Gilson RJ, Beath. SV, et al. Novel application of a point mutation assay: evidence for transmission of hepatitis B viruses with precore mutations and their detection in infants with fulminant hepatitis B. J Med Virol. 1994;44(1):13-21.

31. Gimson AES, White YS, Eddleston WF, Williams R. Clinical and prognostic differences in fulminant hepatitis type A, B and non-A, non-B. Gut 1983;24:1194-8.

32. Kao J, Hsu H, Shau W, Chang M, Chen D. Universal hepatitis B vaccination and the decreased mortality from fulminant hepatitis in infants in Taiwan. J Pediatrics. 2001;139:349-52.

33. Farci P, Alter HJ, Shimoda A, Govindarajan S, Cheung LC, Melpolder JC, et al. Hepatitis C virus-associated fulminant hepatic failure. N Engl J Med. 1996;335:631-4.F.

34. Favorov MO, Fields HA, Purdy MA, et al. Serologic identification of hepatitis E virus infections in epidemic and endemic settings. J Med Virol. 1992;36:246-50.

35. Arkankalle VA, Tsarev SA, Shada MS, et al. Age-specific prevalence of antibodies to hepatitis A and E viruses in Pune, India, 1982 and 1992. J Infect Dis. 1995;171:447-50.

36. Dirix L, Polson RJ, Richardson A, Williams R. Primary sepsis presenting as fulminant hepatic failure. Quart J Med. 1989;271:1037-4.

37. Lee WS, McKiernan P, Kelly DA. Etiology, outcome and prognostic indicators of childhood fulminant hepatic failure in the United Kingdom. JPGN. 2005;40:575-81.

38. Arundel C, Lewis JH. Drug-induced liver disease in 2006. Curr Opin Gastroenterol. 2007;23(3):244-54.

39. Murray KF, Hadzic N, Wirth S, Bassett M, Kelly D. Drug-related hepatotoxicity and acute liver failure. J Pediatr Gastroenterol Nutr. 2008;47(4):395-405.

40. Bromer MW, Black M. Acetaminophen hepatoxicity. Clin Liver Dis. 2003;7:351-67.

41. Mahedevan SCBK, McKiernan PJ, Davies P, Kelly DA. Paracetomol-induced hepatotoxicity in children. Arch Dis in Children. 2006;91(7):598-603.

42. Rivera-Penera T, Gugig R, Davis J, et al. Outcome of acetaminophen overdose in pediatric patients and factors contributing to hepatotoxicity. J Pediatr. 1997;130(2):300-4.

43. Sztajnkerycer MJ, Bond GR. Chronic acetaminophen overdosing in children; risk assessment and management. Curr Opin Pediatr 2001;13(2):177-82.

44. Mindikoglu AL, King D, Magder LS, Ozolek JA, Mazariegos GV, Shneider BL. Valproic acid-associated acute liver failure in children: case report and analysis of liver transplantation outcomes in the United States. J Pediatr 2011;158(5):802-7. Epub 2010 Dec 16.

45. Lheureux PE, Hantson P. Carnitine in the treatment of valproic acid-induced toxicity. Clin Toxicol (Phila). 2009;47(2):101-11.

46. Thomson MA, Lynch S, Strong R, Shepherd RW, Marsh W. Orthotopic liver transplantation with poor neurologic outcome in valproate-associated liver failure; a need for critical risk-benefit appraisal in the use of valproate. Transplant Proc. 2000;32(1):200-3.

47. Reich DJ, Fiel I, Guarrera JV, Emre S, Guy SR, Schwartz ME. et al. Liver transplantation for autoimmune hepatitis. Hepatology. 2000;32(4 Pt 1):693-700.

48. Maggiore G, Porta G, Bernard O, Hadchouel M, Alvarez F, Homberg J-C, et al. Autoimmune hepatitis with initial presentation as acute hepatic failure in young children. J Pediatr. 1990;116:280-2.

49. Tanner S. Disorders of Copper Metabolism. In: Kelly DA (Ed) Diseases of the Liver and Biliary System in Children 3rd Ed. Wiley-Blackwell 2008,328-8.

50. Whitington P, Alonso E, Squires R. Acute Liver Failure. In: Kelly DA (Ed). Diseases of the Liver and Biliary System in Children. 3rd Ed. Wiley-Blackwell. 2008;169-88.

51. Squires RH, Dhawan A, Alonso E, Narkewicz MR, Shneider BL, Rodriguez-Baez N, et al. For the Pediatric Acute Liver Failure Study Group. Intravenous N-acetylcysteine in pediatric patients with non-acetaminophen acuteliver failure: A placebo-controlled clinical trial. Hepatology. 2013;57(4):1542-9.

52. Phongsamran PV, Kim JW, Cupo Abbott J, Rosenblatt A. Pharmacotherapy for hepatic encephalopathy. Drugs 2010;70(9):1131-48.

53. Sharma BC, Sharma P, Lunia MK, Srivastava S, Goyal R, Sarin SK. A Randomized, Double-Blind, Controlled Trial Comparing Rifaximin Plus Lactulose with Lactulose Alone in Treatment of Overt Hepatic Encephalopathy. Am J Gastroenterol. 2013 Jul 23. doi: 0.1038/ajg.2013.219. [Epub ahead of print]

54. Singer AL, Olthoff KM, Kim H, Rand E, Zamir G, Shaked A. Role of plasmapheresis in the management of acute hepatic failure in children. Ann Surg. 2001;234(3):418-24.

55. Hughes RD, Williams R. Use of bioartificial and artificial liver support devices. Semin Liver Dis. 1996;16:435-44.

56. Schaefer B, Schaefer F, Engelmann G, Meyburg J, Heckert KH, Zorn M, et al. Comparison of Molecular Adsorbents Recirculating System (MARS) dialysis with combined plasma exchange and haemodialysis in children with acute liver failure. Nephrol Dial Transplant 2011;26(11):3633-9. Epub 2011 Mar 18.

57. Devictor D, Tissieres P, Afanetti M, Debray D. Acute liver failure in children. Clin Res Hepatol Gastroenterol. 2011;35(6-7):430-7. Epub 2011 Apr 30.

58. Schneider A, Attaran M, Meier PN, Strassburg C, Manns MP, Ott M, et al. Hepatocyte transplantation in an acute liver failure due to mushroom poisoning. Transplantation. 2006;82(8):1115-6.

59. Sundaram V, Shneider BL, Dhawan A, Ng VL, Im K, Belle S, et al. King's College Hospital Criteria for Non-Acetaminophen Induced Acute Liver Failure in an International Cohort of Children. J Pediatr. 2012 Aug 18. [Epub ahead of print]

60. Srivastava A, Yachha SK, Poddar U. Predictors of outcome in children with acute viral hepatitis and coagulopathy. J Viral Hepat. 2012;19(2): Epub 2011 Aug 4.

61. Miloh T, Kerkar N, Parkar S, Emre S, Annunziato R, Mendez C, et al. Improved outcomes in pediatric liver transplantation for acute liver failure. Pediatr Transplant. 2010;14(7):863-9.

62. Faraj W, Dar F, Bartlett A, Melendez HV, Marangoni G, Mukherji D, et al. Auxiliary liver transplantation for acute liver failure in children. Ann Surg. 2010;251(2):351-6.

63. Mohamed El, Moghazy W, Ogura Y, Mutsuko M, Harada K, Koizumi A, et al. Pediatric living-donor liver transplantation for acute liver failure: analysis of 57 cases. Int. 2010;23(8):823-30. Epub 2010 Feb 16.

64. Chai PF, Lee WS, Brown RM, McPartland JL, Foster K, McKiernan PJ, et al. Childhood autoimmune liver disease: indications and outcome of liver transplantation. J Pediatr Gastroenterol Nutr. 2010;50(3):295-302.

65. Bravo LC, Gregorio GV, Shafi F, Bock HL, Boudville I, Liu Y, et al. Etiology, incidence and outcomes of acute hepatic failure in 0-18 year old Filipino children. Southeast Asian J Trop Med Public Health. 2012;43(3):764-772.

66. Bariş Z, Saltik Temızel IN, Uslu N, Usta Y, Demır H, Gürakan F, et al. Acute liver failure in children: 20-year experience. Turk J Gastroenterol. 2012;23(2):127-34.

67. D'Agostino D, Diaz S, Sanchez MC, Boldrini G. Management and prognosis of acute liver failure in children. Curr Gastroenterol Rep. 2012;14(3):262-9.

Chapter

34

Portal Hypertension

Sankaranarayanan VS, Srinivas S

DEFINITION

Portal hypertension is defined as an elevation of the portal venous pressure above 7–10 mm Hg (normal pressure is <7 mm Hg) or 30 cm of saline or intrasplenic pressure more than 17 mm Hg or wedged hepatic pressure more than 4 mm Hg above inferior venacaval pressure.[2,4,7-9,16]

The prevalence of portal hypertension in Indian children appears to be EHPVO (70%), cirrhosis (20%), NCPF (4%), Budd-Chiari syndrome (3%) and CHF (3%).[3] The article covers the definition, pathophysiology, classification, etiology, clinical profile, diagnosis and management of portal hypertension with more focus on extrahepatic type which is the predominant cause in India.

PATHOPHYSIOLOGY[3,5,6]

Portal vein is formed by the union of the superior mesenteric vein and splenic vein behind the head of pancreas and is about 6 mm long and 10–12 mm in older child. It is truncated and thick walled and so never becomes tortuous. It does not contain valves and so the pressure is more or less uniform in the entire spleno-portovenous axis. Functionally, it carries goodies (80% of arterial blood with 20% of oxygen) to the liver unlike other veins of the body. Both the mesenteric origin and intrahepatic termination of the portal vein (sinusoids) are only as capillaries. Left gastric (coronary vein) in lesser omentum, superior pancreaticoduodenal, pyloric and paraumbilical veins are the significant tributaries of the portal vein (Fig. 34.1). The portal vein divides into right and left branches which supply the respective lobes of the liver. The right branch receives the cystic vein and the left branch is joined by the umbilical vein. The terminal portion of the intrahepatic portal venules pierce the limiting plate of portal tract and forms the liver sinusoids.

Superior mesenteric vein is formed by the union of jejunal, ileal, middle colic veins. The two major tributaries are right gastroepiploic and pancreaticoduodenal veins.

Splenic vein is formed by confluence of tiny, around 5–12 channels at the splenic hilum. The major tributaries are the inferior mesenteric, short gastric and left gastroepiploic veins.

Inferior mesenteric vein is the continuation of the superior rectal/hemorrhoidal vein and is joined by the sigmoid and left colic vein.

In cirrhosis, increased hepatic vascular resistance occurs in hepatic microcirculation (sinusoidal portal hypertension) level due to the consequence of hepatic architectural disarray, active contraction of myofibroblasts, activated stellate cells and spasm of smooth muscle cells of intrahepatic veins. In addition endogenous and pharmacologic agents modify the dynamic component as found in Table 34.1.

- **Endothelin-1 (ET-1):[6]** It is a powerful vasoconstrictor synthesized by sinusoidal endothelial cells and they are implicated in increased HVR in cirrhosis liver and in development of liver fibrosis.
- **Nitric oxide (NO):[6]** It is a vasodilator substance synthesized by sinusoidal endothelial cells. In cirrhosis liver, the production of NO is decreased and endothelial NO synthetase activity and nitrite production by sinusoidal endothelial cells are reduced resulting in intrahepatic vasoconstriction (20–30%) and HVR.

In short, vascular resistance and portal blood flow in the portal venous system are the two important factors in the development of portal venous pressure (PVP) and PH.

PVP if >12 mm Hg will result in formation of variceal bleeding and ascites.

Table 34.1: Hepatic vasculature resistance (HVR)[6]

Factors that increases HVR	Factors that decreases HVR
Endothelin-1 (ET-1)	Nitric oxide (NO)
α-adrenergic stimulus	Prostacyclin
Angiotensin 11	Vasodilators, e.g. organic nitrates, adrenolytics, Ca channel blockers

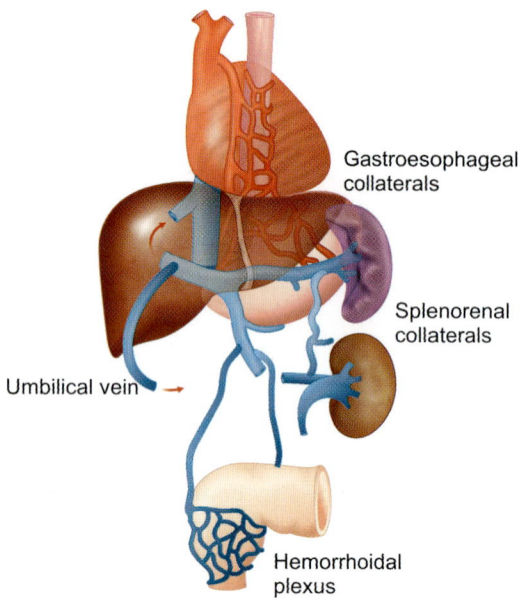

Gastroesophageal collaterals

Splenorenal collaterals

Umbilical vein

Hemorrhoidal plexus

Fig. 34.1: Major portocaval collaterals

Obstruction of portal vein, whatever the etiology, results in increased PVP, collateral circulation, diversion of obstructed blood flow by systemic veins and portosystemic collaterals opening up and dilatation of preexisting vascular channels connecting portal venous system and superior and inferior vena cava and active angiogenesis. Another major contribution is raised PVP due to concomitant splanchnic arteriolar vasodilatation causing increased portal venous inflow (Fig. 34.1)

Portal hypertension is always a pathological state, chronic and invariably a complication of underlying cirrhosis of liver manifesting as an increase in portal venous pressure where the pressure gradient between the portal vein and IVC (portal pressure gradient or PPG) is raised above the upper limit of normal (5 mm Hg). It is observed as an academic interest that esophageal varices are seen endoscopically when the PPG is >10 mm Hg, variceal bleeds and ascites is expected when PPG is >12 mm Hg and asymptomatic/subclinical when PPG is > 6–10 mm Hg above the IVC pressure (Normal 2 mm Hg).[12]

In clinical practice, it is to be remembered that variceal bleeding occurs invariably whenever the wedged hepatic venous pressure gradient (WHVPG) is >4 mm Hg above IVC pressure (in cirrhosis around 20 mm Hg). In both sinusoidal and postsinusoidal PH, WHVP is high whereas in EHPO and presinusoidal PH it is normal.

CLASSIFICATION[3]

❑ Extrahepatic (prehepatic): Portal vein obstruction (90%), splenorenal axis (10%) or long segment thrombus (10%)

❑ Intrahepatic: (i) presinusoidal, (ii) sinusoidal and (iii) postsinusoidal
❑ Posthepatic (rare).

ETIOLOGY[3,4,7-9,15]

Extrahepatic portal venous hypertension (EHPVO) is the most common cause of portal hypertension in children when compared to adults and invariably presents as recurrent upper gastrointestinal bleeding (GI bleeding). Nearly in 30% of index and 70% in recurrent bleeding it is fatal. Umbilical infection (10–20%), acute appendicitis, primary peritonitis, pyelonephritis, periportal inflammation, systemic sepsis, severe dehydration, abdominal Koch's and cholangitis are possible causes for thrombosis of portal vein resulting in EHPVO. Rare causes include hypercoagulable states such as polycythemia, protein C, protein S, antithrombin III deficiency may cause EHPVO. Celiac disease may be associated with protein C and protein S deficiency. Portal vein infiltration by tumor emboli or splenic vein thrombosis due to chronic pancreatitis is rare in children. Cirrhosis of liver and noncirrhotic portal hypertension may also be rarely associated with EHPVO. Portal vein may undergo cavernomatous malformation with leash of tiny vessels causing EHPVO. With high degree of suspicion and recent advances in investigations, the incidence of idiopathic portal hypertension is less.

The common causes of EHPVO (Fig. 34.2) are portal vein cavernoma, omphalitis/umbical sepsis/catheterization/infusion of soda bicarbonate, intrabdominal sepsis (appendicitis, necrotizing enterocolitis, peritonitis and

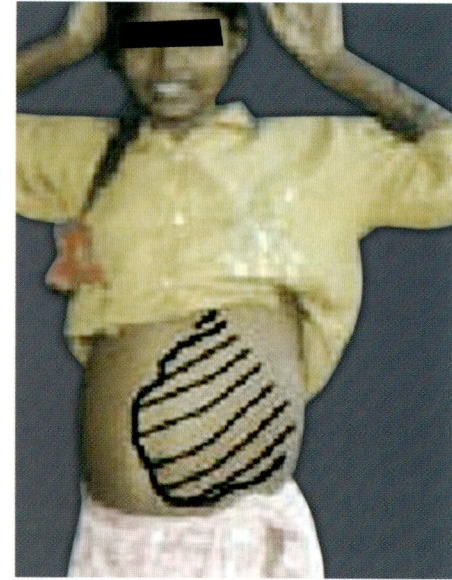

Fig. 34.2: Extrahepatic portal veous obstruction

distal pancreatitis causing splenic vein obstruction (sinistral/segmental PH), trauma or hypercoagulable states such as protein C or S or antithrombin III deficiency, polycythemia antiphospholipid Ab deficiency or idiopathic (around 50%).

Cirrhosis liver, noncirrhotic portal fibrosis, post-sinusoidal obstruction (e.g. veno-occlusive disease) and Budd-Chiari syndrome/inferior vena caval obstruction are of next to EHPVO only.

Presinusoidal PH

Congenital hepatic fibrosis (Fig. 34.3), noncirrhotic portal fibrosis, Caroli's disease, schistosomiasis.

Intrahepatic Sinusoidal PH[7-9]

Cirrhosis liver due to varied etiology (metabolic liver diseases like Wilson's disease, glycogen storage disorder (type IV, III), tyrosinemia (Fig. 34.4), galactosemia, hemochromatosis, alpha-1 antitrypsin deficiency), extrahepatic biliary atresia, drug-induced chronic hepatitis, autoimmune chronic hepatitis, hepatitis B and C infections, severe neonatal hepatitis, progressive familial intrahepatic cholestasis (Fig. 34.5), Alagille syndrome (Fig. 34.6),[10] histiocytosis, post-TPN, nodular regenerative hyperplasia, ICC and idiopathic.

Postsinusoidal PH

Veno-occlusive disease, Budd-Chiari syndrome.

CLINICAL FEATURES

Massive, often abrupt, painless, recurrent (even up to 5–6 episodes per patient) upper gastrointestinal bleeding with fairly well-tolerated liver function (with no ascites/peripheral edema/coagulopathy/encephalopathy until late stages) and firm moderate to massive splenomegaly with or without hypersplenism are the cardinal clinical features of EHPVO whereas in cirrhosis of liver (Figs 34.7 and 34.8), in addition, clinical picture of primary disease, liver cell failure, firm to hard nodular shrunken or

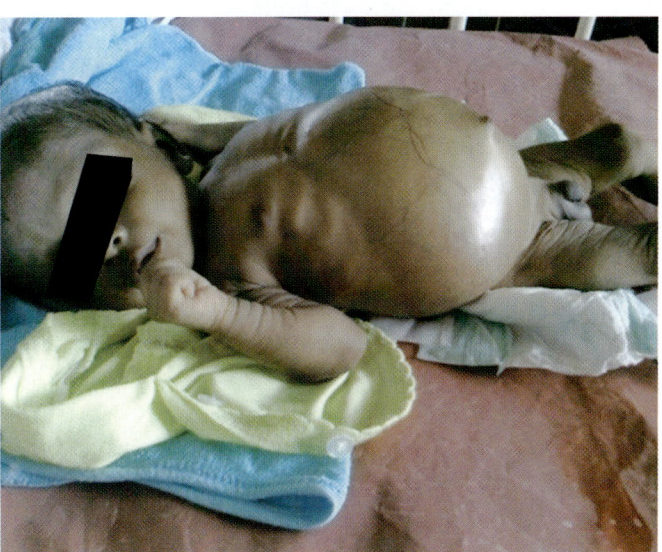

Fig. 34.4: Tyrosinemia

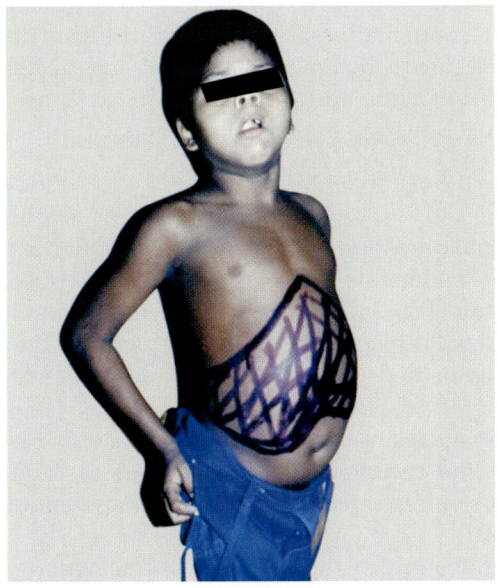

Fig. 34.3: Congenital hepatic fibrosis

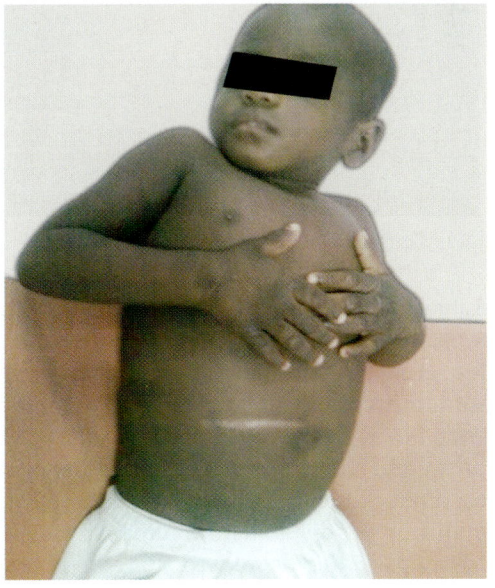

Fig. 34.5: Progressive familial intrahepatic cholestasis (PFIC)

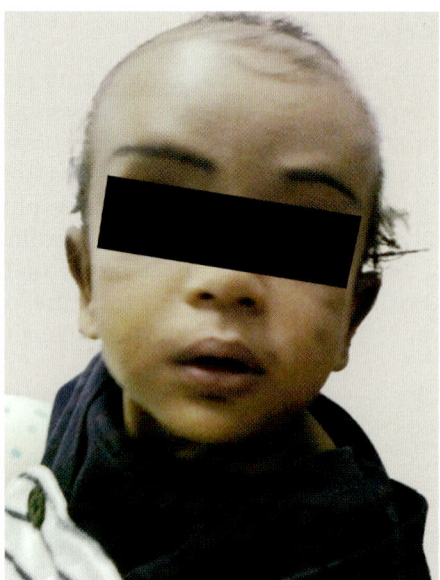

Fig. 34.6: Alagille syndrome

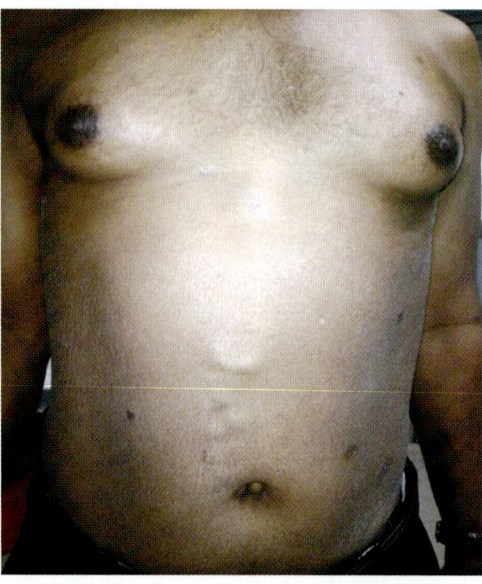

Fig. 34.7: Cirrhosis with gynecomastia and epigastric veins

enlarged liver and dilated anterior abdominal wall veins with flow away from umbilicus and ascites will be present. In addition, growth retardation, muscle wasting, reduction in sexual maturity rate will be present. The mean age of presentation is 5–6 years of age though no age is exempted in our set up and the severity and frequency of bleeding decreases after puberty. Pallor secondary to recurrent bleeding and or hypersplenism manifesting as the early fatigue, dyspepsia and decreased appetite to the effort intolerance of congestive failure are often seen especially in long standing cases.[3,4,12]

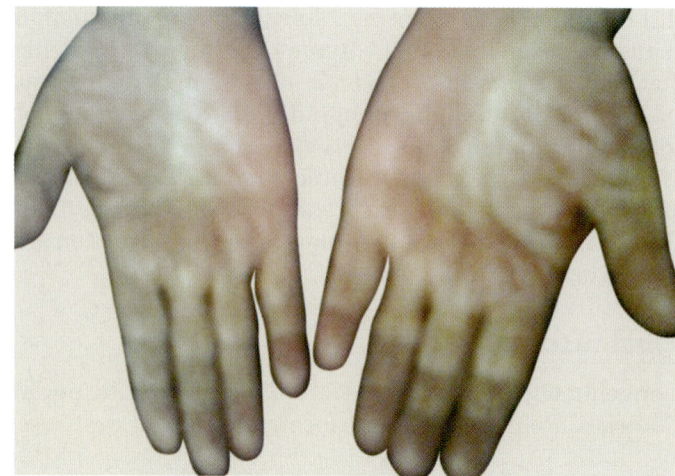

Fig. 34.8: Palmar erythema in cirrhosis liver

The predisposing causes of such hematemeses and melena are febrile upper respiratory infection (viral/ bacterial), use of nonsteroid anti-inflammatory drugs like aspirin, ibubrufen, etc. or ingestion of spicy or spiky food or improper introduction of nasogastric feeding tube or any endoscopic therapeutic procedures (variceal band ligation or sclerotherapy).

Splenomegaly especially firm is the most reliable sign of EHPVO and can be silently present as early as one month of age though usually seen before three years of age. The size of the spleen is not proportionate to the severity of portal hypertension and appears very small or not palpable during the episodes of massive upper gastrointestinal bleeding. Characteristically the epigastric veins and caput medussae seen in cirrhosis liver are absent in EHPVO due to the umbilical vein joining the left branch of portal vein at the hilum of the liver.[3,4] Rarely ascites may develope following a massive bleeding.

DIAGNOSIS[1-5,8,12]

Abdominal ultrasound will give details about the patency, size and collaterals of splenoportovenous axis, portal cavernoma (Fig. 34.9) presence of even minimal ascites, echotexture of liver, hepatic/intrahepatic portion of IVC block, right-sided pleural effusion and evidence of SOL liver.

Esophagogastroduodenoscopy not only helps to identify the esophageal, fundic varices and portal hypertensive gastropathy but also facilitates endotherapy. (Fig. 34.10)

Identification of the cause of portal hypertension is almost by laboratory etiological work up for CLD (cirrhosis, chronic hepatitis). Evaluation of hypercoagulable

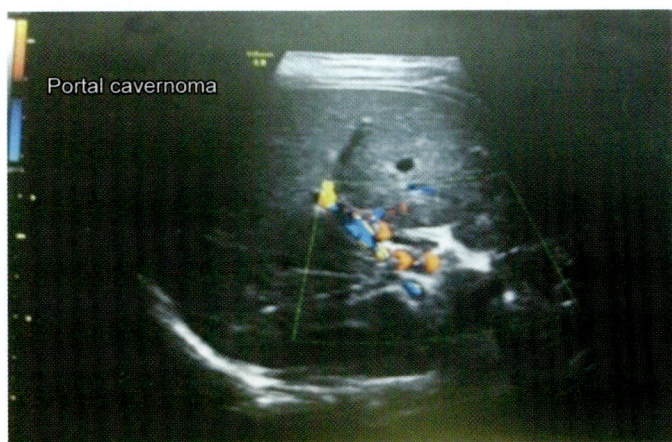

Fig. 34.9: USG abdomen—portal cavernoma

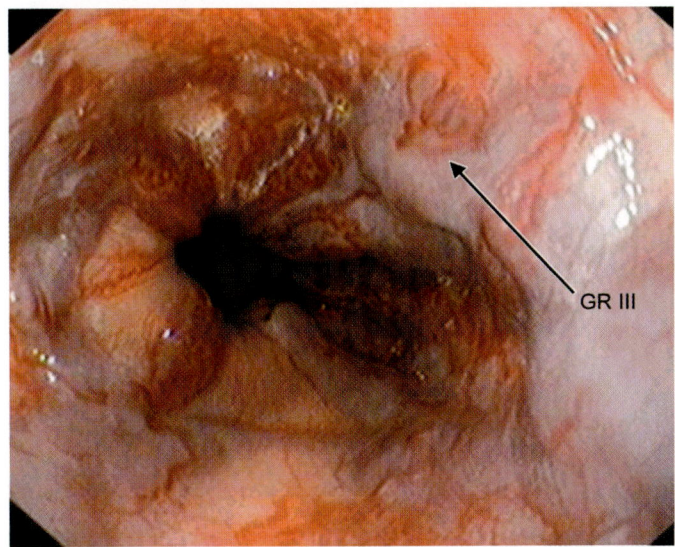

Fig. 34.10: Esophagogastroduodenoscopy—esophageal varices

states causing SPV axis thrombosis includes complete coagulation profile, protein C and S, antithrombin III, antiphospholipid antibody and fibrinogen estimation. Liver biopsy is diagnostic of cirrhosis, biliary atresia, NCPF, PFIC, etc. Work up for hypersplenism, post-transfusion complications and psychometry analysis of minimal hepatic encephalopathy is necessary.

Pressure criteria for portal hypertension: Portal venous pressure >10 mm of Hg (normal 10 mm of Hg).

Hepatic venous pressure gradient (HVPG): If >12 mm of Hg is a useful predictor of variceal bleed (Flow chart 34.1).

MANAGEMENT OF PORTAL HYPERTENSION IN CHILDREN[1-5,8,11-16,18] (FLOW CHART 34.1)

❑ Emergency resuscitation of upper GI bleeding, control of active bleeding with somatostatin and analogs or vasopressin and glypressin, emergency upper GI endoscopy (within 12 hours), control of immediate post-endoscopy procedure rebleed (continue somatostatin/analogs) and long-term prevention of late rebleeds with medical therapy (propranolol/isosorbide mononitrate or nadolol) or

❑ If bleeding is not controlled by above measures, emergency nonshunt surgery (devascularization/modified Tanner's procedure) or elective portovenous physiological REX shunt or TIPS or as a last resort liver transplantation needs to be the management protocol currently.

❑ Proper counseling of caregivers of the patient, for the need of long-term follow-up and natural course of the illness especially EHPVO with recurrent variceal bleeds is essential.

❑ The goal of treatment is as follows:
- To find out whether there is portal hypertension?
- What is the type (extrahepatic or cirrhotic or otherwise)?
- What is the status of liver function in long-standing cases (synthetic function of liver like S. albumin, A:G ratio and coagulation profile (prothrombin time/INR)?
- What is the likely cause?
- What are the complications and unsolved issues related to portal hypertension?
- What is the treatment protocol (medical and/or endoscopy or surgical)?

MANAGEMENT OF ESOPHAGEAL VARICES—ENDOSCOPIC THERAPY

Endoscopic examination is fundamental in order to classify the esophageal and gastric varices (Table 34.2) based on the size and presence of endoscopic features which have relavent implications in the management of patients,[32] source of bleeding and obtain homeostasis. After hemodynamic resuscitation all patients with suspected variceal bleed needs endotherapy (sclerotherapy (EST) or band ligation (EVBL) prevention of rebleeding can be achieved by chronic follow-up EST or EVBlL or shunt surgery.

Flow chart 34.1: Managent algorithm–variceal hemorrhage for older children[19]

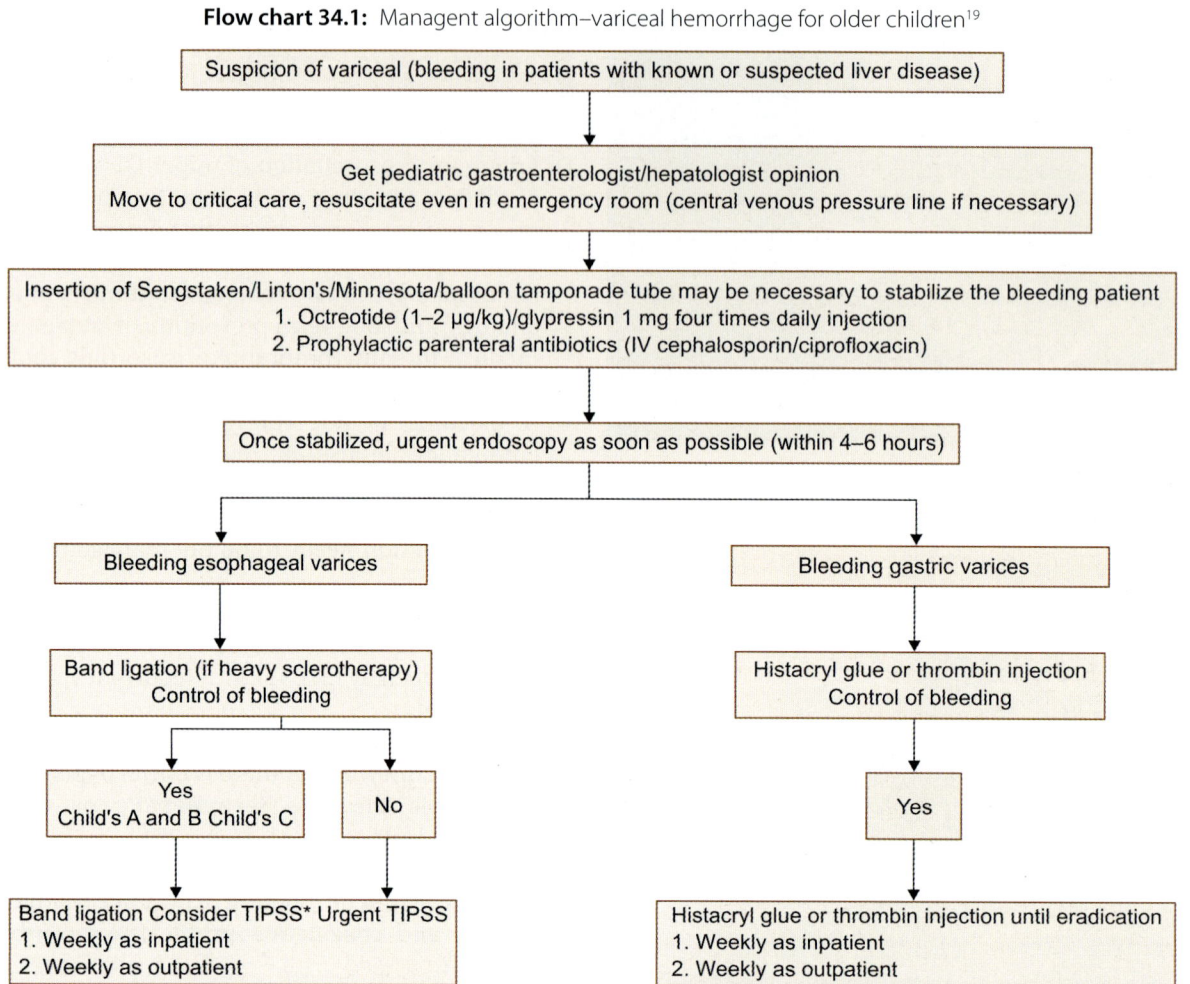

Table 34.2: Endoscopic classification of esophageal and gastric varices

Type	Size	Diameter	Charateristics
Esophageal			
F1	Small	<5 mm	Straight, minimally elevated
F2	Medium	>5 mm	Tortuous, occupying <1/3 of the lumen
F3	Large	>5 mm	Tortuous, occupying >1/3 of the lumen
Gastroesophageal			
GEV1		2–5 cm	Communicating with EVs, along with the gastric lesser curve
GE 2		2–3 mm	Along the gastric greater curve and fundus, more tortuous than GEV1
Isolated gastric varices			
IGV 1	Small	<5 mm	Fundal (rule out splenic vein thrombosis); may occur in the absence of EVs
IGV 2	Medium	5–10 mm	In the gastric corpus, antrum, or pylorus
	Large	>10 mm	

GEV1 indicates type 1 gastrointestinal varices; GEV2, type 2 gastrointestinal varices; IGV1, type1 isolated gastric varices; IGV2, isolated gastric varices

Endoscopic Sclerotherapy

Sclerotherapy agents: Fatty acid derivatives (sodium moruate and ethanolamine moruate) synthetic derivatives (3% sodium tetradecyl sulphate (STDS) and polidocanol ethoxysclerol/ethosuxerol)[13,20] and other agents (phenol and absolute alcohol) were used. No data to decide about an optimal sclerosing agent is available but currently STDS (diluted with saline/distilled water to 1–1.5%) and polidocanol are the most popular agents used in many centers.

Glue (N-butyl-2 cyanoacrylate) is used to obliterate the bleeding gastric fundal varices.

Clearing of stomach: A clearer vision during endoscopic viewing and quick procedure of endotherapy can be obtained by gastric lavages through nasogastric tube or intravenous infusion of low dose erythromycin 20 minutes before endoscopy especially in cirrhotic patients.[21]

Mode of action of endoscopic sclerotherapy: EST is based upon the principle of variceal thrombosis by injection of a sclerosing agent which later results in an ulcer and fibrosis.

Site and technique of sclerosing agents: Injections are directed at the bleeding sites in an acutely bleeding patient. Paravariceal "sand witch technique" injections are effective in decreasing blood oozing due to parietal edema and varix constriction which may fascilitate subsequent intravariceal injection of the sclerosant. Initial injection at gastroesophageal junction and subsequently in an ascending spiral fashion along the 5 cm of the esophagus.

Volume of sclerosant for injection: At each site around 1–2 mL and the total volume often required for each session is 6–10 mL although the practice of EST is still largely empiric and individualized.

Prevention of rebleeding and follow-up of patients: Once hemostasis has been achieved with emergency EST, it can be repeated within 1 week and later at intervals every 1–3 weeks until eradication of varices.[22]

Surveillance endoscopy: In view of variceal recurrence in up to 17–70% of patients after initial eradication, surveillance endoscopy should be performed at 6 months and 1 year and later at annual intervals.

Eradication rate of esophageal varices with EST is 80–100%.[23]

Complications of EST are fever, bacteremia, chest pain, dysphagia, rebleeding, superficial mucosal ulcerations (6–30%), esophageal perforation, pulmonary complications (mediastinitis, pleural effusion, ARDS), pericarditis, esophageal dysfunction and esophageal stricture and can occur within hours of the procedure or some even after 4 weeks such as stricture esophagus (6–20%).[23]

Choice of EST is preferred in children younger than 2 years of age due to insertion difficulty with a comparatively larger banding cylinder, those who cannot afford for EVB and active esophageal variceal bleed with pool of blood and the device at the tip of the endoscope may limit the field of vision.

Endoscopic variceal band ligation (EVBL): Strangulation of esophageal moderate to large variceal bleeding using multishoot band assembly especially in children above 2 years of age causes thrombosis of veins resulting in sloughing in 3–6 days resultins in shallow ulcers in a week and healing by 2–3 weeks. 3–6 bands are applied in each session to a maximum of 6 sessions before considering alternat therapy of bleeding varices. Administration of proton pump inhibitors results in the prevention of most of the above complications.

Limitatinos of EVBL: Not suitale in young children of less than 2 years of age, restricted fied of view, blood pooling within blood, inability to treat fundic varices, misfiring of bands, need for repeated intubations, overtube related complications.

Advantages of EVBL over EST: Fewer complications than EST (like esophageal strictures, EVBL induced bleeding ulcers, and systemic complications) and, if technically feasible, shold be preferred in terms of rebleeding rates and patient survival.[24,25]

EVBL followed by EST is a better modality of treatment in EHBVO and further studies to compare the superiority over EVBL or EST in children alone are welcome.[26]

Management of gastric varices and portal hypertensive gastropathy: Poddar et al. reported 70% of gastric varices, 90% of gastroesophageal varices in EHPVO (39% had isolated gastric varices).

Secondary gastric varices (varices appearing after eradication of esophageal varices), isolated gastric varices and gastroesophageal varices along the greater curve of the stomach are at greater risk of bleeding. Acute gastric variceal bleeding can be controlled with tissue glue (N-acetyl-2 butyl-cyanoacrylate) injection. Large fundal varices are considered for shunt surgery (cf. cirrhosis).

Mixing the cyanoacrylate glue with lipiodol decreases the the risk of premature polymerization and allows radiologic visualization of the injected vessel. Complications of glue injection include mediastinitis, pulmonary embolism, cerebral embolism, splenic infarction and endoscope damage.

Repeat of this glue injection if needed after 4 days is recommended.

TIPS can be used where endoscopic treatment is not feasible in refractory cases.[20,27]

Portal hypertensive gastropathy (PHG) bleeding is rare in children with EHPVO and empiric use of beta-blockers are recommended.

Colorectal variceal bleeding is rare in children and can be managed with sclerotherapy or band ligation.

In short, currently endoscopic band ligation is the primary choice for variceal bleeding in older children (above 2 years of age) and EST is still recommended as an alternate approach in these cases.

Primary prophylaxis is only indicated in some children and secondary prophylaxis is recommended for cirrhotic children where as meso-Rex shunt operation is the first choice for prophylaxis in children with EHPVO.[28]

Table 34.3 summariges the medications for portal hypertension, their mode of action and adverse side effects.

Drug Therapy of Portal Hypertension (Guidelines)

Acute bleeding episode includes antibiotics norfloxacin (10 mg/kg/12th hourly and in high risk patients, IV ceftriaxone preferred).

Recombinant activated factor VIIa corrects prothrombin time in patients with cirrhosis.

Drugs to Stop Bleeding[3,4,20]

The association of vasopressin infusion plus transdermal nitroglycerin remarkably reduces portal venous pressure.

Terlipressin 2 mg/4th hourly for first 48 hours and maintained up to 5 days at 1 mg/4th hourly to prevent rebleeding. Somatostatin: Initial bolus dose of 250 μg followed by 250 μg/hour, infusion till there is no bleed for 24 hours. Therapy to be continued for 5 more days to prevent early rebleed; negligible side effects.

Octreotide is a somtostatin analog with a longer half-life. The dose is given in the Table 34.3.[17]

Drug of choice depends on local resources. Terlipressin is preferred to be the first choice and somatostatin or octreotide are second choice and if these drugs are not available, vasopressin plus nitroglycerin can be the ultimate option.[19]

Combined Medical Therapy

Currently hemostatic treatment for variceal bleeding is to start on a vasoactive drug from admission, and to associate endoscopic therapy at the time of diagnostic endoscopy as early as 4 hours of admission after stabilizing the patient. Drug therapy may be started during transferral to hospital by medical/paramedical teams and maintained for up to 5 days to prevent early rebleeding.

Prevention of first bleeding and of rebleeding requires the use of orally active agents that reduce portal pressure. There appears to be no difference in the efficacy of propranolol and nadolol. Nadolol is administered once a day.[3,4,17]

Dose adjustment: The dose of beta-adrenergic blockers is determined by stepwise increases in dose until reaching

Table 34.3: Medications useful in portal hypertension, their mode of action and adverse side effects[17,20]			
Drug	Mode of action	Dose	Side effects
Propranolol	Reduces cardiac output, when sleeping pulse rate (55–60/min) drops to 25% causes vasoconstriction.	1 mg/kg/day	Low BP/bradycardia
Nadolol	Has long life. Beta blocker	Once daily	Headache, bradycardia
Somatostatin	Splanchnic vasoconstriction, short shelf life	25 μg/bolus then 250 μg/hourly infusion 2–5 days	Hyperglycemia GB stasis
Octreotide	Synthetic analog of somatostatin, long half life	1–2 μg/kg bolus, then 0.4–2 μg/kg 5 days	
Vasopressin	Splanchnic vasoconstriction. Reduces splanchnic blood flow	1 unit/3 kg body weight in 2 mL/kg of 5% dextrose infusion for 20 min can be repeated 2–3 times half hourly	Abd pain, myocardial infarct
Nitroglycerin	Vasodilatation, decrease venous return, reduces cardiac output	Combination with vasopressin useful	
Terlipressin	Vasoconstriction	2 mg 4th hourly for initial 48 hours; maintenance 1 mg/4 hr for 5 days	
Isosorbide mononitrate	Vasodilatation		

the maximum tolerated and this approach is probably more effective than titrating against heart rate to achieve a reduction of about 25%.

Prevention of Recurrent Variceal Bleeding

Because of high-risk of rebleeding in untreated patients, all patients surviving a variceal bleeding should receive urgent and active treatment for the prevention of rebleeding. In addition, those with poor liver function or other recurrent complications of portal hypertension should be considered for liver transplantation. The association of beta-blockers and variceal band ligation (EVBL) has been shown to be better than EVBL or drug therapy alone.

Prevention of Formation of Varices ("Preprimary" Prevention)[20]

Long-term administration of drugs (e.g. timolol) was unable to prevent the development of varices in patients with compensated cirrhosis.

TIPS and surgery are reserved as salvage therapy for patients who fail endoscopy therapy.

Survivors of variceal hemorrhage should be evaluated for liver transplantation. Specific treatment may be provided with EVBL while the patient awaits transplantation. Patient who failed endoscopic treatments may be treated by TIPS or surgery.

Newer drugs for treatment of portal hypertension: Prazosin, an alpha-1-adrenergic antagonist (0.05–0.1 mg/kg/day) markedly reduces HVPG in patients with cirrhosis, resulting in increased hepatic blood flow and reduction in hepatic vascular resistance. Probably the combination of prazosin and propranolol will be more effective than propranolol and isosorbide mononitrate.

Carvedilol, a nonselective beta-blocker with an alpha-1-adrenoreceptor blocking activity (0.1–0.2 mg/kg/day to a maximum dose of 12.5 mg/day) brings down portal pressure effectively but there is a risk of hypotension.[3,4,6,17]

Newer drugs appear safe and effective when their dose is carefully titrated.

MAIN INDICATIONS FOR SURGERY[3,4,11,12,18]

- ❑ Failure to arrest the bleeding in acute stage
- ❑ To prevent the recurrent bleeding
- ❑ Patients with bleed who cannot have access to tertiary care center
- ❑ Recurrent rebleeds even after 4 to 6 endotherapy sessions
- ❑ Intractable ascites
- ❑ Hypersplenism long-term bridge procedure before liver transplantation.

Emergency shunt surgeries are rarely done nowadays in the era of endoscopic management. Various emergency procedures done in severe variceal rebleeding even after repeat endotherapy are aimed to obliterate the varices surgically and to disconnect the vein between the portal system and the systemic vein (azygos) starting from Criles (Transthoracic ligation of varices) to combined thoracic and abdominal procedures (Sigiura and Futagawa). The most commonly used devascularization procedure is devascularization of lesser and greater curvature with or without splenectomy, skeletonization of lower 8 cm of esophagus and esophageal transection using stapling technique. Cirrhotics with splenic vein thrombosis are ideal for this procedure.

Types of shunt surgeries done are side-to-side lienorenal, proximal splenorenal, mesoportal bypass (Rex shunt), central splenorenal, mesocaval, portocaval and the overall results showed shunt patency in 85–98%.[29,30] and no report of post-shunt encephalopathy. Proximal splenorenal is the most commonly performed shunt along with a splenectomy and has the advantages of diversion of blood flow to decrease portal pressure, contol of bleeding, curing hypersplenism and 15-year survival of 95% with a rebleeding rate of 11% of EHPVO patients.[31]

Rex shunt (mesoportal bypass) is a new physiological shunt that restores mesenteric blood flow to the liver through Rex venous recessus (portion of left portal vein joining the umbilical vein) where the patient's own long vein is harvested (from internal jugular or long saphenous vein) to be used as a conduit to bypass from superior mesenteric vein to left branch of portal vein. As the Rex shunt provides complete cure of the patient with EHPVO it is the most preffered one currently though it is still not popular in our set up and developing countries.[23]

REFERENCES

1. Sarin SK, Sollano JD, Chawla YK, et al. Concensus on Extrahepatic Portal Vein Obstruction. Liver Int. 2006;26(5):512-9.
2. de Franchis R. Evolving Concensus in Portal hypertension; Report of the Baveno IV Concensus Workshop on methodology of diagnosis and therapy in portal hypertension. Journal of Hepatology. 2005;43:167-76.
3. Ganguly S. Portal hypertension. IAP Speciality Series on Pediatric Gastroenterology, 2nd edn, Jaypee Brothers. 2013;19:240-55.
4. Sankaranarayanan VS. Chronic liver disease and cirrhosis of liver in children—IAP Textbook of Pediatrics, Fifth edition, Jaypee Brothers. 2013;9(13):538-45.
5. Mihas AA, Sanyal AJ. Portal hypertension and gastrointestinal haemorrhage—Comprehensive Clinical Hepatology. 2nd edn, Mosby Elsevier; III—Clinical Manifestations of Liver Disease. 2010;9:137-53.
6. Grimaldi C, de Ville J, de Goyet, Nobili U. Portal Hypertension in Children—Clinics and Research—Hepatology and Gastroenterology. Elsevier. 2012;36(3):260-1.

7. Arora NK, Lodha R, Gulati S, et al. Portal hypertension in North Indian Children. Indian J Pediatrics. 1998;65:5855-91.

8. Shneider BL. Portal Hypertension—Liver Disease in Children. In: Suchy FJ, Sokol RJ, Balistreri WF (Eds). 3rd edn, Cambridge University Press. 2007;7:138-63.

9. Arora NK, Bhatia V. Chronic Liver Disease in India. Indian J Pediatr. 2008;75(Suppl):S69-73.

10. Alagille D, Odievre M, Gautier M, Dommergues JP. Hepatic ductular hypoplasia associated with characteristic facies, vertebral malformations, retarded physical, mental, and sexual development and cardiac murmur. J Pedtiatr. 1975;86(1):63-71.

11. Elena M, Puleo J, Grace ND. Portal hypertension and gastrointestinal bleeding—Handbook of Liver Disease. 2nd edn. In: Friedman LS, Keeffe EB (Eds). 2005;10:139-49.

12. Malathy S. Approach to a child with CLD. Indian J Pract Pediatr Hepatol. 2002;4(4):362-9.

13. Poddar U, Thappa BR, Puri P, et al. Non-cirrhotic portal fibrosis in children. Indian J Gastroenterology. 2000;19:12-3.

14. Poddar U, Thapa BR, Singh K. Band ligation plus sclerotherapy versus sclerotherapy alone in children with extrahepatic portal obstruction. J Clin Gastroenterol. 2005;2:286-9.

15. McClean P. Portal Hypertension: Spectrum and Medical Management in UK. The Indian J Pediatr. 2008;(Suppl 75):S93-6.

16. Javvaji S, Kumar A, Madan K, Garg PK, Acharya SK. Management of gastric variceal bleeding. Tropical Gastroenterol. 2007;28:51-7.

17. Garcia-Tsao G, Bosch J, Groszmann RJ. Portal hypertension and variceal bleeding—unsolved issues. Summary of an American Association for the Study of Liver Diseases and European Association for the Study of the Liver. Single-topic Conference Hepatology. 2008; 47(5):58-66.

18. Kamath PS. Portal Hypertension—Evidence-based Management—CME Proceedings of ISGCON. 2010;5:53-7.

19. McAvoy NC, Hayes PC. Portal Hypertension: A Management Problem—Problem-based Approach to Gastroenterology and Hepatology. In: Plevris JN, Howden CW, Blackwell W (Eds). 2012;15:189-201.

20. Mohan N, Kalra A. Gastrointestinal bleed in children. Indian J Pract Pediatr. 2011;13(2):157-70.

21. Zaman A. Managing the complications of cirrhosis—a practical approach. In: Frossard JL, Spahr L, Queneau PE, et al (Eds). Erythromycin intravenous bolus infusion in acute gastrointestinal bleeding: a randomized, controlled, double-blind trial. Gastroenterology. 2002;123:17-23.

22. Habib A, Sanyal AJ. Acute variceal hemorrhage. Gastrointest Endoscopy Clin N Am. 2007;17:223-52.

23. Poddar U, Borkar V. Management of extrahepatic portal venous obstruction (EHPVO): Current strategies. Tropical Gastroenterology. 2011;32(2):94-102.

24. Garcia-Pagan JC, Bosch J. Endoscopic band ligation in the treatment of portal hypertension. Nat Clin Pract Gastroenterol Hepatol. 2005;2:526-35.

25. Zargar SA, Javid G, Khan BA, Yattoo GN, Shah AH, Gulzar GM, et al. Endoscopic ligation compared with sclerotherapy for bleeding esophageal varices in children with extrahepatic portal venous obstruction. Hepatology. 2002;36:666-72.

26. Poddar U, Thappa BR, Singh K. Band ligation plus sclerotherapy versus sclerotherapy alone in children with extrahepatic portal vein obstruction. J Clin Gastroenterol. 2005;39:626-9.

27. Ryan BM, Stockbrugger RM, Ryan JM. A pathophysiologic, gastroenterologic, and radiologic approach to the management of gastric varices. Gastroenterology. 2004;126:1175-89.

28. Jin Kim S, Mo Kim K. Recent Trends in the Endoscopic Management of Variceal Bleeding in Children. Pediatr Gastroenterol Hepatol Nutr. 2013;16(1):1-90.

29. Mitra SK, Rao KLN, Narasimhan KL, Dilawari JB, Batra YK, Chawla Y, et al. Side-to-side lienorenal shunt without splectomy in noncirrhotic portal hypertension in children. J Pediatr Surg. 1993;28:398-401.

30. Prasad AS, Gupta S, Kohli V, Pande GK, Sahni P, Nundy S. Proximal splenorenal shunts for extrahepatic portal venous obstruction in children. Ann Surg. 1994;219:193-6.

31. Chaudhary N, Mehrotra S, Srivastava M, Nundy S. Review article. International Journal of Hepatology. 2013, Article ID 784842, 7 pages.

32. de Franchis R. Evolving Consensus in Portal Hyprtension. Report of the Baveno IV Consensus Workshop on methodology of diagnosis and therapy in portal hypertension. J Hepatol. 2005;99:1959-65.

Chapter

35

Liver Transplantation

Akshay Kapoor, Subash Gupta, Anupam Sibal, Vidyut Bhatia,
Neerav Goyal, Manav Wadhawan, Sarath Gopalan

INTRODUCTION

Pediatric liver transplantation (LT) has evolved over the last three decades and is now an established therapy for children with end-stage liver disease, acute liver failure and certain metabolic diseases. Refinement in surgical techniques, improvements in anesthesia, perioperative care and access to newer immunosuppressant drugs, have resulted in improved survival, with current 1 and 5 years survival rates greater than 90% and 85%, respectively.[1] The Japanese liver transplant society has reported excellent survival figures in 2,224 children who underwent living related liver transplant between 1989 and 2010. The 1, 5, 10 and 20 years patient survival rates were 88.3%, 85.4%, 82.8% and 79.6%, respectively.[2]

The first successful pediatric LT in India was performed at Indraprastha Apollo Hospital in 1998 in New Delhi.[3] Liver transplantation programs in India have developed over the last decade and with increasing expertise in pediatric transplant surgery, pediatric hepatology and intensive care, outcomes have improved. LT is now being offered to children less than 1 year of age and weighing less than 10 kg.[4] This subgroup of children was previously associated with increased risk of graft loss.[5]

INDICATIONS

The most commone indication for pediatric LT in the world and in India is extrahepatic biliary atresia (EHBA) followed by acute liver failure (ALF).[6] The indications are summarized in Table 35.1.

Table 35.1: Indications for pediatric liver transplantation		
Cholestatic indications	*Metabolic (primary hepatic) indications*	*Hepatocellular indications*
Biliary atresia	Alpha-1-antitrypsin deficiency*	Acute and subacute hepatic failure
Biliary hypoplasia (Alagille)	Tyrosinemia	Autoimmune liver disease (type I and II)
Nonsyndromic biliary paucity	Wilson's disease	Chronic hepatitis B or C
Progressive familial	Neonatal hemochromatosis	Polycystic liver disease
Giant cell hepatitis/neonatal hepatitis of unknown etiology	Glycogen storage disease type I, III,IV Cystic fibrosis*	
	Metabolic (primary nonhepatic) Crigler-Najjar-syndrome type I Ornithine transcarbamylase (OTC) deficiency Maple syrup urine disease (MSUD) Familial hypercholesterolemia Methylmalonic acidemia Propionic acidemia Citrin deficiency Hyperoxaluria (combined liver and kidney transplant) Atypical HUS (combined liver and kidney transplant)	
Non - resectable hepatic tumors		
Hepatoblastoma Hepatocellular carcinoma		

*Uncommon in India

Table 35.2: King's College criteria for LT in acute liver failure[12]	
Acetaminophen poisoning	*Other causes of ALF*
Arterial pH <7.3 or the following three factors:	PT >100 s/INR >6.5 or three of the following:
Prothrombin time >100 s/ INR >6.5	Age <10 years or >40
S. creatinine >3.5 mg/dL	Non-A, non-B hepatitis or drug induced disease
Encephalopathy grade III or IV	Duration of jaundice >7 days before encephalopathy INR >3.5
	S. bilirubin >17.6 mg/dL

Table 35.3: Indications for LT in end-stage chronic liver failure[13]	
Clinical parameters	*Laboratory parameteras*
1. Recurrent variceal bleeding	1. Prothrombin ratio (INR) >1.4
2. Refractory ascites	2. Indirect bilirubin >6 mg/dL
3. Intractable pruritus	3. Albumin <3.5 mg/dL
4. Growth retardation	4. Cholesterol <100 mg/day
5. Unacceptable quality of life	

Acute Liver Failure

LT is the only definitive treatment for ALF. Several prognostic scoring systems have been devised to predict mortality and to identify those requiring early LT. These include King's College Hospital (KCH) criteria,[7] MELD score, PELD score, APACHE II and Clichy criteria. The KCH criteria (Table 35.2) appear to have a higher specificity than sensitivity for acetaminophen induced ALF, while its negative predictive value for non-acetaminophen induced ALF is low.[8] Despite current therapeutic approaches, ALF results in death or liver transplantation (LT) in up to 45% of pediatric patients. The ability to predict ALF clinical outcomes and the need for LT, to stratify patients according to severity of illness is currently limited. Attempts have been made to use the MELD/PELD scoring system to assess prognosis in ALF with varying results. Both MELD and PELD were derived to predict the probability of mortality in patients who had chronic liver disease, which is an entity distinct from ALF. Although components of the MELD were thought to be a predictive factor in ALF (INR and bilirubin), the MELD score itself had poor specificity.[9] An INR >4 or factor V concentration of <25% are the best available criteria for listing for ALF.[10] A study of ALF from the SPLIT database suggested that grade IV encephalopathy, age less than 1 year and dialysis before transplantation were risk factors for poor outcomes.[11]

End-stage Chronic Liver Failure

As the natural history of EHBA is well known, patients with a failed Kasai procedure should be referred to a transplant center as soon as it is clear that the operation has failed. Failure to clear jaundice 3 months postprocedure is an indication for referral to a pediatric transplant unit. In other forms of chronic liver failure, precise prediction of need for liver replacement is difficult, as children with cirrhosis and portal hypertension can remain stable for months to years. The best guide is a fall in albumin, prolongation of prothrombin time, and persistent rise in bilirubin (Table 35.3).

Pediatric End-stage Liver (PELD) Disease Scoring System

PELD score was developed to predict death in children while waiting for transplant or the need for transfer to ICU, so as to prioritize donor liver allocation to children.[14]

It is calculated as 10*(0.480*In (bilirubin) + 1.857*In (INR) – 0.687*In (albumin) + 0.436 (if patient <1 year) + 0.667 (if growth failure <2 SD).

The PELD system confers special status and protection to pediatric organs and recipients but does not accurately predict outcomes post-transplantation. PELD has limited relevance in the Indian scenario and in the countries with limited cadaver donations as the vast majority of transplants are living related.

LT for Metabolic Disorders

LT is indicated for both primary metabolic liver disorders (Wilson's, tyrosinemia) and extrahepatic metabolic disorders due to enzyme deficiency (hyperoxaluria, MSUD). LT is performed in children with Wilson's disease (WD), who have developed decompensated cirrhosis refractory to medical therapy and for patients who present in ALF. A special prognostic score is available for children with WD and a score of 11 or more indicates high mortality, with 93% sensitivity and 98% specificity.[15] Neonatal hemochromatosis (NH) is a rare but still the most common cause of acute liver failure in the neonate. Antenatal treatment with intravenous immunoglobulins starting at 14 weeks' gestation has been shown to prevent the development of NH in subsequent pregnancies. Exchange transfusions and intravenous immunoglobulins form current therapy. The need for LT in this group of patients has decreased substantially.[16] In tyrosinemia, LT is indicated only if there is failure of NTBC therapy, ALF at presentation, hepatic dysplasia, or hepatocellular carcinoma. In progressive familial intrahepatic cholestasis (PFIC), decision to transplant is taken if there is established

Table 35.4: Contraindications to transplant[20]

Absolute contraindications
- Extrahepatic malignancy considered incurable by standard oncologic criteria
- Sepsis
  - Uncontrolled systemic infection
  - Acquired immunodeficiency syndrome
- Extrahepatic disease (incurable)
  - Irreversible massive brain injury
  - Uncorrectable congenital anomalies affecting major organs

Relative contraindications
- Malignancy that is considered cured or curable by standard oncologic criteria
- Sepsis
  - Treatable infection
  - Human immunodeficiency virus
- Extrahepatic disease
  - Progressive extrahepatic disease
  - Substance abuse

cirrhosis or intractable itching despite maximal medical therapy or surgical diversion. In glycogen storage disorders types I, III and IV, LT is indicated if there is poor metabolic control, decompensated cirrhosis or if multiple adenomas develop.[17] In cystic fibrosis LT, should be performed when the lung function is still preserved (FEV1 > 50%). Expanding indications of LT have revolutionized the management of metabolic disorders. In several metabolic conditions which do not result in liver failure, LT prevents the extrahepatic complications, such as kernicterus in Criggler-Najjar syndrome,[18] cardiac disease in hypercholesterolemia and metabolic decompensation (urea cycle defects, organic acidemias). Combined liver and kidney transplant (CLKT) is now the procedure of choice for patients with primary hyperoxaluria suffering from renal failure. CLKT has also offered new hope in patients with atypical HUS.[19]

There is a growing understanding on when not to transplant. Mitochondrial cytopathies, Niemann-Pick type A and B, organic acidemias with severe mental handicap and Crigler-Najjar disease with kernicterus are contraindications to transplantation (Table 35.4).

PRETRANSPLANT EVALUATION

Aim of assessment for LT are to confirm the diagnosis and severity of disease, to define the patient's general medical status, to determine eligibility and priority for transplant and to arrange interim supportive care.

Pretransplant Assessment Guidelines for Recipient

- Nutritional status
  - Height, weight, triceps skinfold, mid-arm muscle area

- Identification of hepatic complications
  - Ascites, varices
- Cardiac assessment
  - ECG, echo (contrast ECHO for HPS), chest X-ray
- Respiratory function
  - Oxygen saturation, ventilation perfusion scan, lung function tests (in cystic fibrosis)
- Neurological and developmental assessment
  - EEG, Development Assessment Scale for Indian Infants (DASII), Development Profile (DP- 2)
- Renal functions
  - Urea, creatinine, electrolytes
  - Urinary protein/creatinine ratio
  - 51 Cr-EDTA (if available)
- Dental assessment
- Radiology
  - Wrist X-ray for bone age and rickets
  - MRI/angiography (if portal vein anatomy equivocal)
- Serology
  - Cytomegalovirus
  - Epstein-Barr virus
  - Varicella zoster
  - Herpes simplex
  - Hepatitis A, B, C
  - HIV
- Hematology
  - Full blood count, platelets, blood group
- Immunization status.

Pretransplant Medical Management

Pretransplant management includes nutritional rehabilitation, immunization, and medical management of end-stage liver disease.

Nutritional Rehabilitation

Majority (70%) children presenting for LT to our center were malnourished.[21] Nutritional rehabilitation is necessary as optimizing nutrition improves postsurgical outcomes. Lower height Z-score has been associated with longer post-transplant hospital stay and increased hospitalization cost.[22-24] Nutritional support also provides the opportunity to lessen the technical difficulties seen in very small infants. Modular feeds allowing protein (3 g/kg), carbohydrate (using glucose polymers) and fat (50% medium and 50% long chain triglycerides) to provide calories up to 150 kcal/kg along with fat-soluble vitamins supplementation is recommended.

Immunization

It is essential to make sure that routine immunizations are complete. Children undergoing LT should be immunized against measles, mumps, rubella, varicella, diphtheria, tetanus, *Haemophilus influenzae* type-B, *Pneumococcus*, influenza, hepatitis A and B and polio. Vaccines should be given at least one month before LT to ensure seroconversion. After LT, vaccination with killed vaccines can be done provided the immunosuppression regimen has stabilized. Live vaccines should be avoided. Parents and other siblings should be advised to have annual influenza vaccines and pneumococcal vaccines should be repeated every five to six years.[6]

Management of Complications of Chronic Liver Disease

These include prevention and treatment of ascites, spontaneous bacterial peritonitis, hepatorenal syndrome, esophageal varices, hepatic encephalopathy, and pruritus.

Counseling

Counseling is a multidisciplinary process involving the transplant surgeon, the hepatologist, anesthetist, intensivist, dietician and a social worker. The family should be educated about the procedure, outcome and complications of the surgery and life-long immunosuppression. Children over 18 months may be prepared for the stressful procedure through innovative play therapy and books.

TRANSPLANT SURGERY

The transplant procedure involves excision of the diseased liver by division of the common bile duct (or Roux loop if there has been previous biliary surgery), hepatic artery, portal vein, and the inferior vena cava above and below the liver. The original surgery has undergone several modifications, but in general there are three phases:
1. Native liver dissection.
2. Anhepatic phase: In this phase the placement of the graft begins but the patient is functionally between livers. The vascular anastomoses are performed during this period.
3. Graft revascularization.

Reduction hepatectomy involves reducing the liver to transplantable portions comprising of segments 5–8 (right lobe, predominantly used in adolescents and adults), 2, 3 (left lateral segment) or 2–4 (left lobe) which by virtue of their independent vascular supply and venous drainage can function as complete and independent hepatic units. The left lateral segment or left lobe is most often used in pediatric LT. The use of sialistic mesh to close the abdominal cavity preserves graft perfusion and enables low tension abdominal closure when relatively large grafts

are used in small abdominal cavities. The liver shrinks over time and the abdomen can be closed later.[25]

Technical Variants

Living Related Liver Transplantation

Living related liver transplantation (LRLT) has immensely benefited the pediatric population, especially in India, where there is limited availability of deceased donor grafts. This is a procedure, in which a parent or a relative provides a part of their liver (commonly the left lateral segment). The major advantages of LRLT over a cadaveric LT for the recipient are:
- Elective procedure
- Healthy donor
- Short cold ischemia time which reduces possibility of graft non-function
- Possible immunological advantage due to a related donor.

The donor must be a relative of the child and preferably have a compatible blood group. ABO incompatible liver transplants have also been performed successfully by using pre-transplant conditioning with rituximab and/or plasmapheresis.[26] All donors undergo a comprehensive medical and psychological assessment. A government committee scrutinizes both donor and recipient in person and gives the final approval for surgery. No organ transplant can be performed without prior approval of this authorization committee. The objective of the committee is to ensure that living donor transplants are performed as per Transplantation of Human Organs Act and Rules 1994 and subsequent amendments made there under.

Split-liver Transplantation

Split-liver transplantation is an efficient transplant technique developed in response to donor graft shortage involves dividing a deceased donor graft into a left lateral segment (segments 2, 3) and a right trisegment which can then be transplanted to a child and an adult respectively.

Monosegmental Liver Transplantation

In this technique segment 2 or 3 is reduced from a lateral segment to make it suitable for possible for very small infants.[27]

Auxiliary Partial Liver Transplantation

This is a novel type of liver transplantation (the graft is placed with the diseased native liver in situ) that is performed where there is a possibility of native liver regeneration and immunosuppression withdrawal as

Table 35.5: Immunosuppressant drug toxicities

Cyclosporin A	Tacrolimus	MMF	Sirolimus
Nephrotoxicity	Nephrotoxicity	Cytopenias	Hyperlipidemia
Neurotoxicity	Neurotoxicity	Gastrointestinal toxicity	Gastrointestinal toxicity
Hypertension	Hypertension		Cytopenias
Hyperlipidemia	Hyperglycemia		
Hirsutism	Gastrointestinal toxicity		

Table 35.6: Dosage and monitoring

	Dosage*	Monitoring
Cyclosporin A	4–6 mg/kg/dose twice daily	Trough levels (C0) 2 hours post-dose (C2)
Tacrolimus	0.15 mg/kg/dose (within first 12 hours after abdominal closure), then 0.05 to 0.1 mg/kg/dose twice daily per oral	Trough level
Mycophenolate mofetil	15 mg/kg/dose twice daily or trough levels (C0) 600 mg/m^2 twice daily 1 hour post-dose(C1)	
Sirolimus	15 mg/m^2 once daily	After 4 days of therapy, then C0 twice weekly for 1st month, then weekly for 2nd month (Target: 5–15 µg/L)

* Recommended starting dose

in ALF. Careful, serial and meticulous follow-up with radiological screening and tapering of immunosuppression is required while the transplanted liver shrinks and degenerates and the native liver regenerates.[28]

Postoperative Course

Postoperative management is in the intensive care unit. The patient is monitored for early bile production, acid-base balance and coagulation. If the new graft is functioning well, the postoperative recovery may be straightforward, however, early-impaired graft function may rapidly result in a hemodynamically unstable patient with severe metabolic disturbances and multiorgan failure.

Immunosuppression

Apart from advances in surgical techniques, a huge contribution to successful LT is from the ongoing development in immunosuppressive therapy. Optimal immunosuppression aims prevention of rejection with least side effects and therefore demands a perfect balance of treatment during the vulnerable state after transplantation. While the initial treatment regimen of LT consisted of corticosteroids and azathioprine (AZT) with a graft survival of only 30%, the introduction of cyclosporine (CSA) in the early 1980s and tacrolimus (TAC) in the late 80s, revolutionized transplant medicine with 1-year

graft and patient survival rates as high as 90%.[29] The drug toxicities and doses are summarized in Tables 35.5 and 35.6, respectively.

The usual immunosuppressive regimen consists of TAC and prednisolone, with or without AZT or mycophenolate mofetil (MMF). Although cyclosporin has been successfully used safely and effectively in children, TAC based immunosuppression is preferred because it has been associated with less acute rejection, less estimated corticosteroid-resistant acute rejection rates and fewer cosmetic side effects, such as hirsutism. It also is associated with better long-term graft survival. There is no evidence for an increased risk of lymphoproliferative disease in children treated with TAC. However, TAC is associated with a greater incidence of de-novo diabetes and gastrointestinal side effects as compared to CSA.[30] T cells involved in acute rejection are characterized by the expression of activation markers such as the IL-2 R. Therefore, anti–IL-2 R target therapy appears to be a promising chance for specific immunosuppression. Two drugs Basiliximab (BAS) and Daclizumab (DAC) are available for use in this category although BAS has been used more extensively in children. Long-term use, including their incorporation into CNI sparing regimens in liver graft recipients with emerging nephrotoxicity or neurotoxicity has been validated.[31] The emphasis is now to minimize immunosuppression at the earliest. Most centers advocate early steroid withdrawal by 3–6 months. Many recipients more than 2 years after

LT maintain normal graft function (as determined by liver blood tests) on monotherapy with tacrolimus (levels <6 ng/mL) or cyclosporine (levels <100 ng/mL).

Complications

The main causes of graft loss in the first week include primary nonfunction, hepatic artery thrombosis (HAT) or portal vein thrombosis (PVT), systemic sepsis, and multiorgan failure (10%).[32]

Primary nonfunction of the graft (PNF) is a rare condition which requires immediate retransplantation. Signs of PNF include hemodynamic instability needing inotropic support, persistent and nonresolving metabolic acidosis, and coagulopathy. Possible factors include sub-optimal donor status, prolonged cold ischemia time and technical and immunological complications in the recipient.

HAT is a catastrophic complication and usually occurs due to arterial kinking, endothelial damage or due to liver edema (acute rejection). Hypotension, increased blood viscosity and sepsis may be additional factors. It manifests as graft dysfunction and needs immediate re-exploration. Late HAT is relatively rare due to the extensive development of collaterals and can be managed conservatively. PVT has an incidence of 5% and is common in children with small hypoplastic veins. It also presents as graft dysfunction and requires surgical intervention.

Infection in the immediate post-transplant period remains a major threat to the transplanted child. Poor graft function, ventilator dependence, gut perforation and re-transplantation are compounding factors. Gram-negative sepsis and fungal infections can be sinister and difficult to treat.

Other significant complications are acute rejection (AR), chronic rejection (CR), biliary leaks and strictures, viral infections [especially cytomegalovirus (CMV) and Epstein-Barr virus (EBV)], acute kidney injury, and fluid imbalance.[32]

AR is a common complication after LT and occurs within the first two–three weeks post-transplant. Up to 50% of children may develop AR at some point in time. Rising enzymes and flu like symptoms in the patient are characteristic. There is no serum or clinical marker that correlates with AR or clinically measured levels of immunosuppressants; histological proof is needed to diagnose AR because a clinical picture similar to AR can occur during infections. The Banff criteria have been formulated using a tripartite pathological focus on lymphocyte predominant portal infiltrates, cholangiolar damage and endothelitis on liver biopsy.[33] Most children respond to bolus doses of steroids, increased CNI levels, and/or immunosuppressants, such as mycophenolate and mTOR inhibitors.

CR may cause long-term graft dysfunction and fibrosis and eventual graft loss if not recognized and treated. The reported incidence of CR is 10%. Its presentation usually is associated with jaundice, pruritus, or biliary obstruction with elevated bilirubin, AST, ALT, alkaline phosphatase, and GGT levels. The Banff group defined the minimal histological features of CR as biliary epithelial changes affecting a majority of bile ducts with or without duct loss, foam cell obliterative arteriopathy, or bile duct loss affecting >50% of portal tracts. The treatment protocols are similar to those for AR and entail using a higher dose of the existing immunosuppressant; switching to a different immunosuppression regimen while keeping a backup for possible retransplantation.[33]

Biliary complications may be seen in 5–25% of children. They can be subtle when they present as fever and mild graft dysfunction or can cause biliary peritonitis. Anastomotic strictures can occur at the hepatico-jejunostomy site or at the ductal confluence. Gamma GT remains the most sensitive indicator of stricture formation and its elevation along with cholangitis are pointers to an obstructive pathology. Nonanastomotic/diffuse biliary strictures are relatively rare and present years later.[25]

CMV infection in a transplanted child can occur either as a de novo infection or due to reactivation of a previous infection secondary to immunosuppression. Primary CMV infection from a seropositive donor occurs early (1–3 months post-transplant) and is associated with invasive disease and increased mortality. Late CMV infections occur after withdrawal of chemoprophylaxis (ganciclovir). They are milder in their clinical course. CMV disease may manifest as a nonspecific viral syndrome or tissue-invasive disease. Nonspecific viral syndrome is characterized by fever and features of marrow depression (leukopenia, atypical lymphocytosis, and thrombocytopenia). Tissue-invasive CMV disease is manifested by visceral organ involvement (gastrointestinal tract, liver, and lungs). CMV has also been associated with rejection, fungal infection, and late patient and graft loss. Most of the centers give either intravenous ganciclovir or oral valganciclovir prophylaxis to CMV naïve recipients of CMV positive donors for a period ranging from 3–6 months. Established CMV disease characterized by pp65 antigenemia and a positive PCR needs to be treated with intravenous ganciclovir till complete clearance is established by two negative reports two weeks apart. Alternate drugs like foscarnet and cidofovir should be given only in cases of suspected non response to conventional therapy.[34]

EBV infection can be associated with an infectious mononucleosis like syndrome or with post-transplant lymphoproliferative disease (PTLD). PTLD tends to affect organs of the reticuloendothelial system and/or the transplanted liver. Therefore, it is important to classify the EBV status of both the donor and recipient. EBV infection should be suspected in post-transplant patients with prolonged fever and unexplained lymphadenopathy. A tissue biopsy should be performed for all cases in which the lesion can be identified on physical examination or CT/MRI scanning. EBV loads should also be monitored closely in such patients. Reducing immunosuppression is the first step in treating PTLD. Use of monoclonal antibodies like CD20 antibody Rituximab in conjuction with low dose corticosteroid therapy has been tried with variable success in EBV positive PTLD.[35]

The use of CNIs for preventing graft rejection predisposes the recipient to kidney dysfunction due to glomerular damage. Most of the pediatric studies show a progressive decrease in the eGFR during the first year post-LT.[36] Children with preexisting renal disease, e.g. those with Alagille syndrome, Caroli's syndrome and congenital hepatic fibrosis are more predisposed to renal dysfunction. Similarly children with hepatorenal syndrome in the pretransplant period have a greater chance of renal dysfunction. Use of IL 2R induction with lower doses of CNIs immediately after transplantation may be beneficial. Using ACE inhibitors and angiotensin II receptor blockers in children with concomitant hypertension and proteinuria has a protective effect on the eGFR. The list of complications is summarized in Table 35.7.

Retransplantation

On an average the rate of pediatric retransplantation is approximately 10%.[37,38] Retransplantation can be classified as occurring early (<30 days) or late (>30 days) from the original transplant. Early retransplantation is usually because of PNF of graft or hepatic artery thrombosis (HAT). Late retransplantation usually results from chronic rejection or biliary complications. Retransplantation is a higher-risk procedure than primary transplantation, with poorer results. Technically, it may be more difficult because recipient arterial structures, which were readily available for the first transplant, are lacking in subsequent procedures.

Novel Therapies

Looking beyond Immunosuppression: Tolerance

The ultimate goal of clinical transplantation is tolerance induction and acceptance of graft without need for life-long immunosuppression Tolerance (defined as the lack of an immune response to the foreign antigens expressed by an organ allograft in the absence of ongoing immunosuppressive therapy) is being researched as a means to eliminate the dependency on immunosuppressive agents and improve outcomes. Experience in LT recipients who have been poorly compliant with therapy or in whom immunosuppression has been withdrawn because of adverse effects suggests that it is possible in some cases to withdraw immunosuppression completely without precipitating graft rejection or loss. Because a signal through the T-cell receptor is required for tolerance and CNIs act early after alloantigen engagement to block this signal, they may prevent allorecognition and prevent the induction of tolerance. Therefore, to promote graft acceptance, a different immunosuppression approach is needed in which early allorecognition is encouraged and harmful effector responses, which result in graft rejection, are inhibited. Experimental strategies like mixed allogenic chimerism, co stimulation blockade and preconditioning are presently being developed.[39]

Liver-assist Devices

In liver failure since most of the toxins are albumin bound and non-filterable using conventional dialysis, different albumin dialysis systems have been developed (MARS, SPAD, Promethra). They are eventually nonbiological systems and may have a role in the treatment of specific

Table 35.7: Complications of pediatric liver transplantation		
Early (<1 month)	Intermediate (1–3 months)	Late (>3 months)
PNF	Late HAT, PVT	Late PVT, hepatic venous outflow obstruction
HAT, PVT	Biliary strictures	Chronic rejection
Acute rejection	Late acute rejection	Steatohepatitis, chronic fibrosis
Bile leak	Infections (Varicella, EBV, CMV)	Metabolic syndrome
Sepsis	PTLD	Infections (CMV, EBV)
Diarrhea	Decreasing GFR	Compliance and adherence issues
		Recurrence of disease activity
		De novo malignancies

forms of liver failure where the primary goal is to provide blood detoxification/purification. Biological systems are also being developed and appear to hold promise for treating liver failure where the primary objective is to provide whole liver functions which are impaired or lost. Experience of LAD in children is limited and restricted to small series. They are mainly research tools.[40]

Hepatocyte Transplantation

Hepatocyte transplantation (HT) is a potentially promising alternative to whole organ liver transplantation so as to overcome the imbalance between patients and available organs. Clinical observations have demonstrated the safety of the procedure and of patients who have undergone: HT. However, most publications refer to clinical cases with no unanimity of criteria as to indications, methodology, cellular cryopreservation or assessment of the response to HT. The indications for HT include ALF, Criggler Najjar syndrome, Urea cycle defects and other metabolic disorders. The technique involves infusing ABO compatible cryopreserved hepatocytes manually into the recipient. The portal vein is usually chosen for children with metabolic disorders. Between 5% and 10% of the recipient's estimated theoretical liver cell mass is transfused. The portal pressure needs to be monitored consistently to prevent side effects.[41] Alternatively, the hepatocytes can be transfused into the splenic artery or the peritoneum. Immunosuppression protocols are similar to the ones used for conventional LT. The infusion of hepatocytes into the liver or spleen is a safe procedure which patients tolerate well. It has the advantage of not being a major surgical procedure. It has lower morbidity, mortality and cost and is a far less invasive therapy than conventional transplant, offering the possibility of maximising resources because one single donor can be used for several recipients. Since the trials in HT are limited there are still unresolved issues regarding appropriate therapeutic mars of hepatocytes and engraftment parameters which have not been standardized. Therefore, HT is yet to establish itself as a therapeutic alternative of LT.

Life after Transplantation

Patients with growth failure secondary to liver disease resume growth with a general improvement in lifestyle. They can attend school and participate in age related activities. The majority of children resume normal growth within a year after LT but in an analysis of the SPLIT database more than 30% pediatric liver transplant recipients were less than the 10th percentile for height at 24 months

post-transplant.[43] Renal dysfunction has been noted in 30% long term survivors.[44] Current immunosuppressant drugs are associated with an increased risk for diabetes, dyslipidemia and obesity.[45-47]

Children who have received hepatic grafts enter puberty normally. Linear growth impairment and delayed puberty are common in pubertal liver transplant recipients, with pretransplant growth impairment identified as a potentially modifiable risk factor. Catch-up growth by the end of puberty may however be incomplete. Successful pregnancies have been reported with both CSA and TAC based immunosuppression. However, pediatric liver transplant recipients from 1988 to 1992 who survived into adulthood were found to have lower physical health related quality of life, measurable transplant related disability and lower health utility two decades later and a significant percentage had psychological issues.[48]

Special attention should be paid to the development of post-transplant metabolic syndrome (PTMS). The use of immunosuppressants, corticosteroids, calcineurin inhibitors, and the presence of risk factors, including nonalcoholic fatty liver disease (NAFLD), kidney and bone disease have been largely implicated in PTMS development. Strategies to reduce the progression of PMTS should include careful screening of patients for diabetes, dyslipidemia, and obesity, and to support weight reduction with a carefully constructed program, particularly based on diet modification and exercise.

Certain diseases are known to recur in the allograft post LT. Autoimmune hepatitis, PFIC type I and primary sclerosing cholangitis belong to this group.[32] Prolonged use of steroids can decrease the recurrence in children transplanted for autoimmune hepatitis. It is also important to note that patients who undergo LT for cystic fibrosis need continuous monitoring of other systems, including the lung and heart.

Registries and Databases

Large, multi-institutional registry databases like the SPLIT registry are used to monitor trends in transplantation and planning clinical trials. In India, published data are currently available from individual centers and there is an urgent need to set up such a transplant registry.

■ LIVER TRANSPLANTATION IN INDIA

In the West, approximately 2–3 pediatric liver transplants per million population are performed annually. At that rate, around 2–3000 children will need liver transplants in India every year. This estimate is likely to be representative, since the incidence of EHBA (1/12,000 to 1/18,000), which is the most commone indication for LT, is similar throughout the world.

Mehrotra et al.[49] reported that 79% of babies with EHBA in their center from north India required transplantation. Sixty one percent of older children with cirrhosis and 67% with fulminant hepatic failure fulfill criteria for liver transplantation. EHBA was the most common indication, followed by metabolic liver disease in a series of 28 children transplanted in South India.[50]

Selection of patients for transplantation requires consideration of not only medical criteria, but also the socioeconomic and educational background of the family. This is of paramount importance, because in addition to the initial expenditure, receiving a transplant also involves a lifelong commitment on the part of the patient and family to spend on immunosuppression and to adhere strictly to the postoperative care protocol, including anti-infection precautions and long-term medication. If a graft is lost due to poor patient compliance, it is a colossal waste of efforts of the treating team, of the donor resources and the expenses incurred on the procedure.

The first successful pediatric liver transplant was carried out in November 1998 at our center in India.[3] He is leading a normal life, attending regular school and has been on follow up for 15 years. With increasing experience, LT is now offered for complicated cases, for metabolic diseases and other rare disorders. The first successful transplant for ALF in India, a transplant in the youngest child in India and the first successful transplant of a child with Crigler-Najjar syndrome were all reported from our center.[18,51,52] With growing expertise, LT has also been successful in small infants. Patient and graft survival of 100% at 11 months were reported in our series of 5 children transplanted at weight below 7.5 kg.[4] Successful transplants for MSUD, hyperoxaluria and factor VII deficiency have been reported by other centers. The success of both pediatric liver and kidney transplant programs in the country has spurred the development of programs for combined liver and kidney transplants. Combined liver and kidney transplants are now being performed in increasing numbers. Another achievement from India is the world's youngest domino liver transplant. More than 450 pediatric liver transplants have now been performed in India.

Although, the cost of LT in India is less than one tenth of that in the West, this is at times prohibitive factor for some families. Constant effort must be made towards decreasing the cost of transplantation (currently Rs. 12–15 lakhs for children at our center). With increasing acceptance of LT amongst the medical community and the public at large, there is now the potential for the number of liver transplants to increase many fold so as to offer hope to the thousands of children who suffer from liver failure.[53] Current concerns are now shifting from an initial aim of early post-transplant survival to long-term survival and quality of life. The other challenge is to improve the number of cadaveric donations in our country.[54]

SUMMARY

LT is now a well-established lifesaving surgery for children with liver failure. Graft and patient survival have continued to improve as a result of improvements in medical, surgical, anesthetic management, organ availability and early identification and treatment of postoperative complications. The utilization of living-related donors and split-liver grafts has provided more organs for pediatric patients. Newer immunosuppression regimens, including induction therapy, have had a significant impact on graft and patient survival. The future entails identification of risk factors associated with long-term immunosuppression; development of tolerance-inducing regimens and definition of biomarkers that reflect the level of clinical immunosuppression. Other aspects of liver transplantation like development of instruments for the measurement of health wellness; identification of risk factors that impede growth and intellectual development before and after the surgery and transition of care for adolescents will require attention in the future.

REFERENCES

1. Rook M, Rand E. Predictors of long-term outcome after liver transplant. Curr Opin Organ Transplant. 2011;16(5):499-504.
2. Kasahara M, Umeshita K, Inomata Y, Uemoto S, Japanese Liver Transplantation S. Long-term outcomes of pediatric living donor liver transplantation in Japan: an analysis of more than 2200 cases listed in the registry of the Japanese Liver Transplantation Society. Am J Transplant. 2013;13(7):1830-9.
3. Poonacha P, Sibal A, Soin AS, Rajashekar MR, Rajakumari DV. India's first successful pediatric liver transplant. Indian Pediatr. 2001;38(3):287-91.
4. Kaur S, Wadhwa N, Sibal A, Jerath N, Sasturkar S. Outcome of live donor liver transplantation in Indian children with bodyweight <7.5 kg. Indian Pediatr. 2011;48(1):51-4.
5. Cacciarelli TV, Dvorchik I, Mazariegos GV, Gerber D, Jain AB, Fung JJ, et al. An analysis of pretransplantation variables associated with long-term allograft outcome in pediatric liver transplant recipients receiving primary tacrolimus (FK506) therapy. Transplantation. 1999;68(5):650-5.
6. Taylor RM, Franck LS, Gibson F, Dhawan A. Liver transplantation in children: part 1--peri-operative issues. J Child Health Care. 2005;9(4):256-73.
7. O'Grady JG, Alexander GJ, Hayllar KM, Williams R. Early indicators of prognosis in fulminant hepatic failure. Gastroenterology. 1989;97(2):439-45.

8. Blei AT. Selection for acute liver failure: have we got it right? Liver Transpl. 2005(11 Suppl 2):S30-4.

9. Polson J. Assessment of prognosis in acute liver failure. Semin Liver Dis. 2008;28(2):218-25.

10. Shanmugam NP, Dhawan A. Selection criteria for liver transplantation in paediatric acute liver failure: the saga continues. Pediatr Transplant. 2011;15(1):5-6.

11. Baliga P, Alvarez S, Lindblad A, Zeng L, Studies of Pediatric Liver Transplantation Research G. Posttransplant survival in pediatric fulminant hepatic failure: the SPLIT experience. Liver Transpl. 2004;10(11):1364-71.

12. Sundaram V, Shneider BL, Dhawan A, Ng VL, Im K, Belle S, et al. King's College Hospital Criteria for non-acetaminophen induced acute liver failure in an international cohort of children. J Pediatr. 2013;162(2):319-23 e1.

13. Debray D, Bernard O, Gauthier F. [Pediatric liver transplantation]. Presse Med. 2009;38(9):1299-306. Transplantation hepatique chez l'enfant.

14. McDiarmid SV, Anand R, Lindblad AS. Development of a pediatric end-stage liver disease score to predict poor outcome in children awaiting liver transplantation. Transplantation. 2002;74(2):173-81.

15. Dhawan A, Taylor RM, Cheeseman P, De Silva P, Katsiyiannakis L, Mieli-Vergani G. Wilson's disease in children: 37-year experience and revised King's score for liver transplantation. Liver Transpl. 2005;11(4):441-8.

16. Rodrigues F, Kallas M, Nash R, Cheeseman P, D'Antiga L, Rela M, et al. Neonatal hemochromatosis--medical treatment vs. transplantation: the king's experience. Liver Transpl. 2005;11(11):1417-24.

17. Bahador A, Dehghani SM, Geramizadeh B, Nikeghbalian S, Bahador M, Malekhosseini SA, et al. Liver Transplant for Children With Hepatocellular Carcinoma and Hereditary Tyrosinemia Type 1. Exp Clin Transplant. 2014.

18. Guru FR, Sibal A. Liver transplant for Crigler-Najjar syndrome. Indian Pediatr. 2010;47(3):285-6.

19. Saland JM, Emre SH, Shneider BL, Benchimol C, Ames S, Bromberg JS, et al. Favorable long-term outcome after liver-kidney transplant for recurrent hemolytic uremic syndrome associated with a factor H mutation. Am J Transplant. 2006;6(8):1948-52.

20. Scatton O, Sepulveda A, Soubrane O. [Living donor liver transplantation]. Presse Med. 2009;38(9):1266-71. Transplantation hepatique a partir d'un donneur vivant.

21. Sibal A, Pao M, Sharma S, Rajakumari DV, Rajasekar MR. Liver Transplantation. Apollo Medicine. 2005;2(4):324-7.

22. Huisman EJ, Trip EJ, Siersema PD, van Hoek B, van Erpecum KJ. Protein energy malnutrition predicts complications in liver cirrhosis. Eur J Gastroenterol Hepatol. 2011;23(11):982-9.

23. Shepherd RW, Chin SE, Cleghorn GJ, Patrick M, Ong TH, Lynch SV, et al. Malnutrition in children with chronic liver disease accepted for liver transplantation: clinical profile and effect on outcome. J Paediatr Child Health. 1991;27(5):295-9.

24. Tsiaousi ET, Hatzitolios AI, Trygonis SK, Savopoulos CG. Malnutrition in end stage liver disease: recommendations and nutritional support. J Gastroenterol Hepatol. 2008;23(4):527-33.

25. Ciria R, Davila D, Khorsandi SE, Dar F, Valente R, Briceno J, et al. Predictors of early graft survival after pediatric liver transplantation. Liver Transpl. 2012;18(11):1324-32.

26. Soin AS, Raut V, Mohanka R, Rastogi A, Goja S, Balachandran M, et al. The use of ABO-incompatible grafts in living donor liver transplantation--first report from India. Indian J Gastroenterol. 2014;33(1):72-6.

27. Mentha G, Belli D, Berner M, Rouge JC, Bugmann P, Morel P, et al. Monosegmental liver transplantation from an adult to an infant. Transplantation. 1996;62(8):1176-8.

28. Faraj W, Dar F, Bartlett A, Melendez HV, Marangoni G, Mukherji D, et al. Auxiliary liver transplantation for acute liver failure in children. Ann Surg. 2010;251(2):351-6.

29. Al-Hussaini A, Tredger JM, Dhawan A. Immunosuppression in pediatric liver and intestinal transplantation: a closer look at the arsenal. J Pediatr Gastroenterol Nutr. 2005;41(2):152-65.

30. Kelly D, Jara P, Rodeck B, Lykavieris P, Burdelski M, Becker M, et al. Tacrolimus and steroids versus ciclosporin microemulsion, steroids, and azathioprine in children undergoing liver transplantation: randomised European multicentre trial. Lancet. 2004;364(9439):1054-61.

31. Nobili V, Comparcola D, Sartorelli MR, Diciommo V, Marcellini M. Mycophenolate mofetil in pediatric liver transplant patients with renal dysfunction: preliminary data. Pediatr Transplant. 2003;7(6):454-7.

32. Kelly DA, Bucuvalas JC, Alonso EM, Karpen SJ, Allen U, Green M, et al. Long-term medical management of the pediatric patient after liver transplantation: 2013 practice guideline by the American Association for the Study of Liver Diseases and the American Society of Transplantation. Liver Transpl. 2013;19(8):798-825.

33. Banff schema for grading liver allograft rejection: an international consensus document. Hepatology. 1997;25(3):658-63.

34. Wadhawan M, Gupta S, Goyal N, Vasudevan KR, Makki K, Dawar R, et al. Cytomegalovirus infection: its incidence and management in cytomegalovirus-seropositive living related liver transplant recipients: a single-center experience. Liver Transpl. 2012;18(12):1448-55.

35. Lu BR, Park KT, Hurwitz M, Cox KL, Berquist WE. Impact of immunosuppression on the development of Epstein-Barr virus (EBV) viremia after pediatric liver transplantation. Transplant Proc. 2013;45(1):301-4.

36. Bishop JR, Burniston MT, Barnfield MC, Stringer MD, Prasad R, Davison SM, et al. Renal function evaluated by measured GFR during follow-up in pediatric liver transplant recipients. Pediatr Transplant. 2009;13(1):96-103.

37. Bourdeaux C, Brunati A, Janssen M, de Magnee C, Otte JB, Sokal E, et al. Liver retransplantation in children. A 21-year single-center experience. Transpl Int. 2009;22(4):416-22.

38. Ng V, Anand R, Martz K, Fecteau A. Liver retransplantation in children: a SPLIT database analysis of outcome and predictive factors for survival. Am J Transplant. 2008;8(2):386-95.

39. Liu XQ, Hu ZQ, Pei YF, Tao R. Clinical operational tolerance in liver transplantation: state-of-the-art perspective and future prospects. Hepatobiliary Pancreat Dis Int. 2013;12(1):12-33.

40. Chamuleau RA. Future of bioartificial liver support. World J Gastrointest Surg. 2009;1(1):21-5.

41. Pareja E, Cortes M, Gomez-Lechon MJ, Maupoey J, San Juan F, Lopez R, et al. [Current status and future perspectives of

hepatocyte transplantation]. Cir Esp. 2014;92(2):74-81. Estado actual y perspectivas futuras del trasplante de hepatocitos.

42. Dhawan A, Strom SC, Sokal E, Fox IJ. Human hepatocyte transplantation. Methods Mol Biol. 2010;640:525-34.

43. Ng VL, Fecteau A, Shepherd R, Magee J, Bucuvalas J, Alonso E, et al. Outcomes of 5-year survivors of pediatric liver transplantation: report on 461 children from a north american multicenter registry. Pediatrics. 2008;122(6):e1128-35.

44. Campbell KM, Yazigi N, Ryckman FC, Alonso M, Tiao G, Balistreri WF, et al. High prevalence of renal dysfunction in long-term survivors after pediatric liver transplantation. J Pediatr. 2006;148(4):475-80.

45. Everhart JE, Lombardero M, Lake JR, Wiesner RH, Zetterman RK, Hoofnagle JH. Weight change and obesity after liver transplantation: incidence and risk factors. Liver Transpl Surg. 1998;4(4):285-96.

46. Varo E, Padin E, Otero E, Tome S, Castroagudin JF, Delgado M, et al. Cardiovascular risk factors in liver allograft recipients: relationship with immunosuppressive therapy. Transplant Proc. 2002;34(5):1553-4.

47. Hathout E, Alonso E, Anand R, Martz K, Imseis E, Johnston J, et al. Post-transplant diabetes mellitus in pediatric liver transplantation. Pediatr Transplant. 2009;13(5):599-605.

48. Mohammad S, Hormaza L, Neighbors K, Boone P, Tierney M, Azzam RK, et al. Health status in young adults two decades after pediatric liver transplantation. Am J Transplant. 2012;12(6):1486-95.

49. Mehrotra P, Yachha SK. Need for liver transplantation in Indian children. Indian Pediatr. 1999;36(4):356-61.

50. D'Cruz AL. Pediatric liver transplantation in India: Its time has come. J Indian Assoc Pediatr Surg. 2011;16(1):1.

51. Mishra D, Singh R, Sibal A. Liver transplantation for fulminant hepatitis A infection. Indian Pediatr. 2002;39(2):189-92.

52. Sibal A, Shah UH. The youngest successful pediatric liver transplant in India. Indian Pediatr. 2009;46(5):446.

53. Sibal A, Bhatia V, Gupta S. Fifteen years of liver transplantation in India. Indian Pediatr. 2013;50(11):999-1000.

54. Bhatia V, Sibal A. Are fathers catching up with mothers in liver donation? Indian Pediatr. 2013;50(1):158.

Chapter

36

Liver Tumors

Huma Cheema, Manas Kalra, Amita Mahajan

INTRODUCTION

Liver tumors account for 1–2% of pediatric malignancies. Hepatoblastoma is the most common malignant pediatric neoplasm (2/3rd of liver tumors) and is diagnosed in the first 3 years of life. The other liver tumors in children are hepatocellular carcinoma (HCC), germ cell tumors, rhabdoid tumors, and sarcomas. HCC, which is the most common neoplasm of liver in adults, is rare in children especially under the age of 10 years. Benign liver lesions in children comprise of hemangiomas, hemangioendotheliomas, hepatic adenomas, focal nodular hyperplasia and hamartomas.[1,2] There has been a marked improvement in overall survival (OS) of children with hepatoblastoma (> 80%). This is largely attributable to highly effective neoadjuvant and adjuvant chemotherapy, international collaborative trials and improvement in surgical techniques.[3] In this chapter we describe the epidemiology, clinical presentation and management of liver tumors in children with main emphasis on the hepatoblastoma.

HEPATOBLASTOMA

Etiology and Epidemiology

A rising incidence of hepatoblastoma has been documented in the recent years owing to better survival of premature infants and low birth weight babies with improvements in supportive care. Free radical-mediated damage from oxygen administration and total parenteral nutrition have been postulated as the causes for liver damage in preterm babies leading to hepatoblastoma in the later age. Also, like other pediatric liver tumors, hepatoblastoma at a also associated with certain tumor predisposition syndromes listed in Table 36.1.

Hepatoblastoma has also been linked to parental smoking and parental exposure to heavy metals during

Table 36.1: Common liver tumor predisposing syndromes

Tumor predisposing syndrome	Liver tumor
Beckwith Wiedemann syndrome	HB, HE
Familial adenomatous polyposis	HB, HCC, adenomas
Li-Fraumeni syndrome	HB, sarcoma
Edwards' syndrome	HB
Alagille syndrome	HCC
Hereditary tyrosinemia	HCC
Glycogen storage disease I	HB, HCC, adenoma
Fanconi anemia, ataxia, telangiectasia	HCC

HB, hepatoblastoma; HCC, hepatocellular carcinoma; HE, hemangioendothelioma

welding, painting, soldering, and handling petroleum products.[4,5]

Clinical Features

The usual clinical presentation is a firm mass palpable in the abdomen. The child is usually anicteric. Dysmorphology related to an underlying syndrome may be present in a few. Some may have development of secondary sexual characters owing to a beta-hCG secreting component in their tumor.

Investigations

Ultrasound of the abdomen is a good screening test. This should be followed by serum Alpha fetoprotein (AFP) levels which is raised in >90% of children with hepatoblastoma. AFP levels must be interpreted with caution as the levels are normally raised in young infants. A contrast enhanced CT scan abdomen or a MRI is mandatory along with a HRCT of chest to look for metastatic disease. The role of

PET scan in initial assessment of hepatoblastoma is still unclear as some of the favorable variants with low mitotic activity may not show FDG uptake. However, most patients with hepatoblastoma show FDG avidity and it may help in detecting clinically silent bony metastases.[6]

Histology

Weinberg et al. in 1983 for the first time described that hepatoblastoma comprised of a mixed bag of histopathological variants, including an epithelial variety with a combination of mixed embryonal and fetal components, a mesenchymal variant, a well differentiated fetal and a small cell undifferentiated variant. It is now well known that the well-differentiated fetal pattern has an excellent prognosis with surgical resection alone and the small cell undifferentiated pattern does uniformly poorly as compared to the other variants. The latter is often associated with low AFP levels and has a loss of INI 1 expression like rhabdoid tumors. Loper terrada D et al.[7] recently published the proceedings of the Los Angeles children's oncology group (COG) international pathology pediatric liver symposium in which the current International Pediatric Liver Tumor Consensus Classification has been described (Table 36.2). This classification takes into account the prognostically different variants of hepatoblastoma and identifies the difficulty in classifying some of the mixed/pleomorphic variants. International collaboration and biological sample collection is critical to develop an appropriate classification of these rare tumors, and it is vital to clinically correlate some of the histologic subtypes with their outcomes. It is anticipated that in the future will see the incorporation of molecular biomarkers into diagnostic and therapeutic algorithms.[8]

Staging and Risk Stratification

Pretreatment extent of disease (PRETEXT) devised by the International Childhood Liver Tumors Strategy Group (SIOPEL) is the standard method of risk stratification for most of the international trials in hepatoblastoma. PRETEXT describes the extent of tumor involvement of the four main sections of the liver: right posterior section (Couinaud 6, 7); right anterior section (Couinaud 5, 8); left medial section (Couinaud 4a, 4b) and left lateral section (Couinaud 2, 3). The PRETEXT number is assigned based on the highest number of contiguous liver sections free of tumor, subtracted from four. PRETEXT is further annotated depending upon extension of tumor beyond the hepatic parenchyma of the major sections (Table 36.3 and Fig. 36.1).

The COG system stages hepatoblastoma from stage I to IV after initial surgery (prior to starting chemotherapy). It has been reported that PRETEXT stage in comparison to COG staging identifies patients who are good candidates for upfront surgical resection (PRETEXT I and II) and those who are good candidates for early referral for liver transplant (PRETEXT IV).[6,9-11] COG is currently trying to evaluate the feasibility and interobserver variability in reporting PRETEXT staging and its ability for a correct

Table 36.2: International consensus classification of hepatoblastoma

Epithelial
- Fetal
- Embryonal
- Macrotrabecular
- Small cell undifferentiated (SCU)
- Cholangioblastic

Mixed
- Stromal derivatives
- Teratoid

Table 36.3: Pretreatment extent of disease (1/4 before chemotherapy)/post-treatment extent of disease (1/4 after chemotherapy) I, II, III, IV; and annotation (V, P, E, M, C, F, and R) definitions[11]

Pretext/post-text	Definition
I	One section involved
	Three adjoining sections are tumor free
II	One or two sections are involved
	Two adjoining sections are tumor free
III	Two or three sections involved
	One adjoining section is tumor free
IV	Four sections involved
Annotation	
V	Venous involvement, V, denotes vascular involvement of the retrochepatic vena cava or involvement of all three majorhepatic veins (right, middle and left)
P	Portal involvement, P, denotes vascular involvement of the main portal vein and/ or both right and left portal veins
E	Extrahepatic involvement of a contiguous structure such as the diaphragm, abdominal wall, stomach, colon and so on
M	Distant metastatic disease (usually lungs, very rarely bone, or brain)
C	Caudate lobe
F	Multifocal tumor nodules
R	Tumor rupture prior to diagnosis

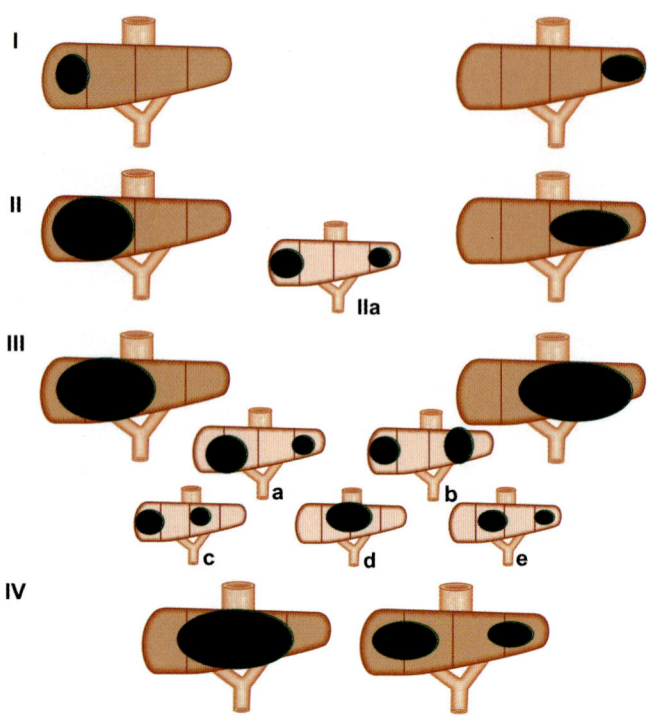

Fig. 36.1: Pretext classification system[11]

Table 36.4: Adverse prognostic factors in children with hepatoblastoma
• Poor prognostic indicators • Metastatic disease (M+) • AFP <100 or >1 million • Age > 6 years • Small cell undifferentiated histology • PRETEXT IV • Unresectable vessel involvement (V+, P+) • Extrahepatic tumor extension (E+) • Positive surgical margins • Poor response to chemotherapy

early transplant referral. Other factors associated with a worse outcome are enlisted in Table 36.4.

Treatment

Hepatoblastoma therapy has evolved from surgery only to modern day treatment comprising of neoadjuvant chemotherapy followed by surgery and adjuvant chemotherapy. There has been a divide across the Atlantic as to the timing of surgery with European groups giving pre operative chemotherapy to all patients (SIOPEL studies) and American groups opting for an upfront surgical resection in most cases (INT, CCG, POG and now COG studies). In developing world where the presentation is often delayed, the SIOPEL approach is the preferred

modality. Upfront surgery may still be a good option in children with PRETEXT stage I and II.

Chemotherapy

Marked progress has been made in the survival of patients with standard and high-risk hepatoblastoma due to cooperative multicentric trials done by the European (SIOPEL), American (COG), German, Italian and Japanese groups. Also improvement in surgical techniques and supportive care has led to excellent outcomes of this malignant disorder.

SIOPEL Studies

In SIOPEL 1 study, cisplatin plus doxorubicin (PLADO) was used as neoadjuvant chemotherapy. This resulted in a 5-year event-free survival (EFS) of 66% and an OS of 75%. Those with metastatic disease or involvement of all 4 sections of liver had 5-year EFS 28% and 46% respectively.[9,12,13]

In SIOPEL 2 study, standard risk patients received 6 courses of only cisplatin chemotherapy. Their 3-year OS and EFS were 91% (+/-7%) and 89% (+/-7%). The high risk patients were treated with addition of a novel agent carboplatin. They were given cisplatin alternating every 2 weeks with carboplatin and doxorubicin. For the High risk group OS and EFS were 53% (+/-13%) and 48% (+/-13%), respectively.[14]

To validate the efficacy of single agent cisplatin in standard risk patients SIOPEL 3 tested in a randomised way the use of cisplatin monotherapy versus PLADO regimen every 2 weekly. In the cisplatin only arm, the 3-year EFS and OS were 83% and 95% respectively, and in the arm treated with PLADO these figures were 85% and 93% respectively, indicating that there is no advantage of adding doxorubicin to standard risk patients. Also, children receiving PLADO suffered more acute grade 3 or 4 side effects (74.4% vs. 20.6%). SIOPEL 3 high-risk study treated children with alternating cycles of cisplatin and carboplatin plus doxorubicin similar to SIOPEL 2 high-risk arm but the order of medications was in a different fashion for some practical reasons. The study resulted in a 3 year EFS and OS of 65% and 69%.[15,16]

SIOPEL 4 tried to evaluate the usage of dose dense cisplatin, administered in a weekly manner along with 3 weekly doxorubicin in high-risk hepatoblastoma patients followed by radical surgery or liver transplant. They used carboplatin and doxorubicin to eradicate postoperative residual disease. Almost 79% children were in complete remission at the end of therapy. EFS at 3 years was 76% and OS was 83%. Most common serious adverse effect was ototoxicity with a moderate-to-severe ototoxicity being documented in 50% patients.[17]

SIOPEL 6 study is trying to evaluate if ototoxicity due to cisplatin can be minimized by addition of sodium thiosulfate in standard risk hepatoblastoma patients.

Other approaches: The American colleagues have traditionally used 5 fluorouracil and vincristine in addition to the conventional agents and have found similar results with standard and high risk patients. The current COG study AHEP0731 is trying to test the role of upfront vincristine-irinotecan (VI) window in high-risk patients and those who show a good response will receive a total of 6 cycles of C5VD (cisplatin, 5 fluorouracil, vincristine, doxorubicin) therapy with 2 more cycles of VI. Non-responder patients get only conventional C5VD therapy. Stage I pure fetal histology hepatoblastoma will be treated with surgery only. Other patients with stage I or with stage II disease will be treated with 2 adjuvant cycles of C5V. Patients with stage I/II SCU or any stage III hepatoblastoma will be administered 6 cycles of C5VD therapy along with surgical resection of the tumor. Attempts to improve survival with usage of high dose chemotherapy followed by stem cell rescue have not been very helpful in children with advance or relapsed disease.[18]

Surgery

A good surgical resection remains the corner stone of hepatoblastoma management. It is important to meticulously study the surrounding anatomy with MRI, CT, and/or a hepatic angiogram and assess the surgical resectability. Draining lymph nodes are sampled and pulmonary nodules if presented are resected. Novel techniques like liver transplant, hepatic exclusion and Pringle ultrasonic dissection have played a major role. The american strategy has traditionally pushed for an upfront surgical removal. In their latest trial they have recommended upfront surgery only for PRETEXT I and II tumors, when the diagnostic imaging shows clear radiographic margins on the contralateral portal vein, the middle hepatic vein, and the retrohepatic inferior vena cava.[11]

Liver Transplant

Liver transplant can be considered for any patient with hepatoblastoma where a complete surgical clearance of disease is deemed difficult. This can happen in PRETEXT III and IV disease, multifocal tumor and where the tumor is deeply invading vascular structures. Upfront liver transplant after no adjuvant chemotherapy has much better outcome than a rescue transplant after a recurrence post chemotherapy and surgery. The role for chemotherapy post liver transplant is controversial especially in cases with excellent response to neoadjuvant chemotherapy. An early referral to a center with expertise in liver surgery and transplant is vital to plan a timely therapy.

Unnecessary delay and continued chemotherapy leads to bad outcomes secondary to development of resistance to chemotherapeutic agents. It is a must to ensure that metastatic sites are clear prior to liver transplant either with chemotherapy alone or with the help of surgery. The current COG trail and the Pediatric Liver Unresectable Tumor Observatory (PLUTO) registry are prospectively looking at the role of liver transplant in patients with high-risk hepatoblastoma.[11,19,20,21]

HEPATOCELLULAR CARCINOMA

Hepatocellular carcinoma is a rare liver tumor mainly presenting after the age of 10 years. It is more commonly seen in children suffering from hepatitis B or C infection (active disease or carrier state) and having cirrhosis secondary to it. Screened blood products and vaccination against hepatitis B is important to prevent the occurrence of this rather chemoresistant disease to some extent. Surgery is the mainstay of treatment. Some centers use hepatoblastoma like chemotherapy for these patients with success seen in less than 30% of patients. Sorafenib has been used with some success in adults with this disorder. In a study by Schmid et al on 12 children with HCC, sorafenib was combined with conventional PLADO. Almost 50% patients were in CR after a period of 20 months. Hand foot skin reaction was the main toxicity associated with sorafenib.[5,22]

Benign Liver Tumors

These comprise around 30% of the total liver tumors seen in childhood with hemangiomas being the most common. Hemangioendothelioma is a type of hemangioma that usually presents in infancy and is more common in girls. Children can present with asymptomatic abdominal mass or with high output failure due to arteriovenous shunting. Some can present with features suggestive of consumptive coagulopathy (Kasabach Merritt syndrome) or hypothyroidism secondary to antibodies to TSH. Many of these lesions subside spontaneously by 24 months of life. Some may need steroid, propranolol or surgical intervention to control symptoms.[23,24] Mesenchymal hamartomas are most likely true neoplasm rather than a hamartoma that present as large benign multicystic liver mass in young children. MRI or CT of the abdomen shows cystic lesions or solid mass lesion in one or both lobes. Malignant transformation has been rarely reported.[25] Focal nodular hyperplasia, a rare entity in children is a mass lesion with hepatocytic nodules separated with fibrous bands with a central fibrous core that contains malformed vessels but no portal vein along with bile duct reaction. This is seen in children treated with chemotherapy especially post-stem cell transplant and in children with congenital or surgical porta systemic shunts, indicating that an abnormal vascular supply is key to their pathogenesis. If the characteristic central scar is seen on imaging and the lesion is small, they can be conservatively managed with serial monitoring. Surgical excision may be needed in case of large lesions. Hepatic adenomas are either seen sporadically or associated with glycogen storage disorder or therapy with anabolic steroids in children having fanconi anemia. Children with surgical shunts can also develop adenomas. Management mainly comprises of withdrawal of predisposing factors if possible and surgical excision in case of large tumors.[26] Hepatic adenomas can be seen sporadically or in association with glycogen storage disorders.

REFERENCES

1. Darbari A, Sabin KM, Shapiro CN, et al. Epidemiology of primary hepatic malignancies in US. children. Hepatology. 2003;38:560-6.
2. Finegold MJ. Hepatic tumors in childhood. In: Russo P, Ruchelli E, Piccoli DA (Eds). Pathology of pediatric gastrointestinal and liver disease. New York: Springer Verlag; 2004.
3. Czauderna P, Lopez-Terrada D, Hiyama E, et al. Hepatoblastoma state of the art: pathology, genetics, risk stratification, and chemotherapy. Curr Opin Pediatr. 2014;26(1):19-28.
4. Hecka JE, Meyersa TJ, Lombardia C, et al. Case-control study of birth characteristics and the risk of hepatoblastoma Cancer Epidemiol. 2013;37(4):390-5.
5. Litten JB, Tomlinson GE. Liver Tumors in Children. The Oncologist. 2008;13:812-20.
6. McCarville MB, Roebuck DJ. Diagnosis and Staging of Hepatoblastoma: Imaging Aspects. Pediatr Blood Cancer. 2012;59:793-9.
7. Lopez-Terrada D, Zimmermann A. Current Issues and Controversies in the Classification of Pediatric Hepatocellular Tumors. Pediatr Blood Cancer. 2012;59:780-4.
8. Lopez-Terrada D, Alaggio R, De Davila MT, et al. Towards an international pediatric liver tumor consensus classification: proceedings of the Los Angeles COG International Pathology Pediatric Liver Tumors Symposium. Mod Pathol. 2014;27(3):472-91.
9. Brown J, Perilongo G, Shafford E, et al. Pretreatment prognostic factors for children with hepatoblastoma: results from the International Society of Paedia-tric Oncology (SIOP) study SIOPEL 1. Eur J Cancer. 2000;36:1418-25.
10. Roebuck DJ, Aronson D, Clapuyt P, et al. 2005 PRETEXT: a revised staging system for primary malignant liver tumours of childhood developed by the SIOPEL group. Pediatr Radiol. 2007; 37:123-32.
11. Meyers RL, Tiao G, Goyet J, et al. Hepatoblastoma state of the art: pre-treatment extent of disease, surgical resection guidelines and the role of liver transplantation. Curr Opin Pediatr. 2014-26:29-36.
12. Aronson DC, Schnater JM, Staalman CR, et al. Predictive value of the pretreatment extent of disease system in hepatoblastoma: results from the international society of pediatric oncology liver tumor study group SIOPEL-1 study. J Clin Oncol. 2005;23:1245-2.
13. Pritchard J, Brown J, Shafford E, et al. Cisplatin, doxorubicin, and delayed surgery for childhood hepatoblastoma: a successful approach— results of the first prospective study of the International Society of Pediatric Oncology. J Clin Oncol. 2000;18(22):3819-28.
14. Perilongo G, Shafford E, Maibach R, et al. Risk-adapted treatment for childhood hepatoblastoma. final report of the second study of the International Society of Paediatric Oncology--SIOPEL 2. Eur J Cancer. 2004;40(3):411-21.
15. Perilongo G, Maibach R, Shafford E, et al. Cisplatin versus cisplatin plus doxorubicin for standard risk hepatoblastoma. N Engl J Med. 2009;361:1662-70.
16. Zsiros J, Maibach R, Shafford E, et al. Successful treatment of childhood high- risk hepatoblastoma with dose-intensive multiagent chemotherapy and sur- gery: final results of the SIOPEL-3HR study. J Clin Oncol. 2010;28:2584-90.
17. Zsiros J, Brugieres L, Brock P, et al. Dose-dense cisplatin-based chemotherapy and surgery for children with high risk hepatoblastoma (SIOPEL 4): a prospective, single-arm, feasibility study. Lancet Oncol. 2013;14:834-42.
18. Perilongo G, Otte JB. Autologous peripheral blood stem-cell transplantation with a double-conditioning regimen for recurrent hepatoblastoma after liver transplantation: a valid therapeutic option or just too much? Pediatr Transplant. 2009;13:148-9.
19. Otte JB, Meyers RL, de Ville de Goyet J. Transplantation for liver tumors in children: time to (re)set the guidelines? Pediatr Transplant. 2013;17:710-2.
20. McAteer JP, Goldin AB, Healy PJ, Gow KW. Surgical treatment of primary liver tumors in children: time to reconsider the role of liver transplantation? Pediatr Transplant. 2013;17:744-50.
21. Otte JB, Meyers R. PLUTO first report. Pediatr Transplant. 2010;14:830-5.
22. Schmid I, Häberle B, Albert MH, et al. Sorafenib and cisplatin/doxorubicin (PLADO) in pediatric hepatocellular carcinoma. Pediatr Blood Cancer. 2012;58(4):539.
23. Meyers RL. Tumors of the liver in children. Surg Oncol. 2007;16(3):195-203.
24. Kochin IN, Miloh TA, Arnon R, Iyer KR, Suchy FJ, Kerkar N. Benign liver masses and lesions in children: 53 cases over 12 years. Isr Med Assoc J. 2011;13(9):542-7.
25. Stringer MD, Alizai NK. Mesenchymal hamartoma of the liver: a systematic review. J Pediatr Surg. 2005;40(11):1681-90.
26. Balabaud C, Al-Rabih WR, Chen PJ, et al. Focal Nodular Hyperplasia and Hepatocellular Adenoma around the World viewed through the Scope of theImmunopathological Classification. Int J Hepatol. 2013;1-12.

BIBLIOGRAPHY

1. Abenoza P, et al. Hepatoblastoma: an immunohistochemical and ultrastructural study. Hum Pathol. 1987;18:1025-35.

2. Aronson DC, Schnater JM, Staalman CR, et al. Predictive value of the pretreatment extent of disease system in hepatoblastoma: results from the International Society of Pediatric Oncology Liver Tumor Study Group SIOPEL-1 study. J Clin Oncol. 2005;23(6): 1245-52.

3. De Ioris M1, Brugieres L, Zimmermann A, et al. Hepatoblastoma with a low serum alpha-fetoprotein level at diagnosis: the SIOPEL group experience. Eur J Cancer. 2008;44(4):545-5.

4. Zynger DL, Gupta A, et al. Expression of glypican 3 in hepatoblastoma: an immunohistochemical study of 65 cases. Human Pathology. 2008:39(5):224-30.

5. Emre S, McKenna GJ. Liver tumors in children. Pediatric transplantation. 2004;8(6):632-8.

6. Evans AE, Land VJ, Newton WA, et al. Combination chemotherapy (vincristine, Adriamycin, cyclophosphamide, and 5-fluorouracil) in the treatment of children with malignant hepatoma. Cancer. 1982;50:821-6.

7. Faraj W, Dar F, Marangoni G, Bartlett A, Melendez HV, Hadzic D, et al. liver transplant for hepatoblastoma. Liver Transpl. 2008;14(11):1

8. Filler RM, Ehrlich PF, Greenberg ML, et al. Preoperative chemotherapy in hepatoblastoma. Surgery. 1991;110:591-6.

9. Haas JE, Muczynski KA, Krailo M, et al. Histopathology and prognosis in childhood hepatoblastoma and hepatocarcinoma. Cancer. 1989;64:1082-95.

10. Habrand JL, Nehme D, Kalifa C, et al. Is there a place for radiation therapy in the management of hepatoblastomas and hepatocellular carcinomas in children? Int J Radiat Oncol Biol Phys. 1992;23(3):525-31.

11. Hamada Y, Takada K, Fukunaga S, Hioki K.Hepatoblastoma associated with Beckwith-Wiedemann syndrome and hemihypertrophy Pediatr Surg Int. 2003;19(1-2):112-4.

12. Heimann A, et al. Hepatoblastoma presenting as isosexual precocity. The clinical importance of histologic and serologic parameters. J Clin Gastroenterol. 1987;9:105-10.

13. Hirschman BA, Pollock BH, Tomlinson GE. The spectrum of APC mutations in children with hepatoblastoma from familial adenomatous polyposis kindreds. J. Pediatr. 2005;147(2):263-6.

14. Ishak K, Goodman Z, Stocker J. Tumors of the liver and intrahepatic bile ducts. In: Rosai J, Sobin L (Eds): Atlas of tumor pathology. 3rd Series edition. Washington, DC: Armed Forces Institute of Pathology; 2000.

15. Koh KN1, Park M, Kim BE, et al. Prognostic implications of serum alpha-fetoprotein response during treatment of hepatoblastoma. Pediatr Blood Cancer. 2011;57(4):554-60.

16. Lack EE, Neave C, Vawter GF. Hepatoblastoma. A clinical and pathologic study of 54 cases. Am J Surg Pathol. 1982:6:693-705.

17. Novak D, Suchy E Balistreri W. Disorders of the liver and biliary system relevent to clinical practice. In: Oski F (Ed): Principles and practice of pediatrics. Philadelphia: JB Lippincott. 1990;1746-77.

18. O'Brien W, Finlay JL, Giibert-Barness EF. Patterns or antigen expression in Hepatoblastoma and hepatocellular carcinoma in childhood. Pediatr Hematol Oncol. 1989;6:361-5.

19. Ortega JA, Douglass EC, Feusner JH, et al. Randomized comparison of cisplatin/vincristine/fluorouracil and cisplatin/continuous infusion doxorubicin for treatment of pediatric hepatoblastoma: A report from the Children's Cancer Group and the Pediatric Oncology Group. J Clin Oncol. 2000;18(14):2665-75.

20. Powers C, et al. Primary liver neoplasms: MR imaging pathologic correlation. Radiographics. 1994;14:459-82.

21. Pritchard J, Brown J, Shafford E, et al. Cisplatin, doxorubicin, and delayed surgery for childhood hepatoblastoma: a successful approach--results of the first prospective study of the International Society of Pediatric Oncology. J Clin Oncol. 2000;18(22):3819-28.

22. Ramsay AD1, Bates AW, et al. Variable antigen expression in hepatoblastomas. Immunohistochem Mol Morphol. 2008;16(2):140-7. doi: 10.1097/PAI.0b013e318032cf72

23. Rowland JM. Hepatoblastoma: assessment of criteria for histologic classification. Med Pediatr Oncol. 2002;39(5):478-83.

24. Sanders RP, Furman WL. "Familial adenomatous polyposis in two brothers with hepatoblastoma: implications for diagnosis and screening". Pediatr Blood Cancer. 2006;47(6):851-4.

25. Selby DM, Stocker JT Waclawiw MA, et al. Hemangioendothelioma of the liver. Hepatology. 1994;20(pan 1):39-45.

26. Srocker J. An approach to handling pediatric liver tumors. Am j Clin Pathol. 1998;109(suppl 1):68-73.

27. Stocker J, Conran R, Selby D. Tumor and of pseudotumors of the liver. In: Stocker J, Askin F, eds. Pathology of solid tumor in children. London: Chapman & Hall. 1998;83-110.

28. Stringer MD, et al. Improved ouccome for children with hepatoblastoma. Br J Surg. 1995;82:386-91.

29. Tanaka K, et al. Hepatoblastoma in a 2-year-old girl with trisomy 18. Eur J Pediatr Surg. 1992;2:298-300.

30. Tanimura M, Matsui I, Abe J, et al. Increased risk of hepatoblastoma among immature children with a lower birth weight. Cancer Res. 1998;58(14):3032-5.

31. Van Eyken P, et al. A cytokeratin-immunohisrochemical study of hepatoblastoma. Hum Pathol. 1990;21:302-8.

32. von Schweinitz D, Hecker H, Schmidt-von-Arndt G, Harms D. Prognostic factors and staging systems in childhood hepatoblastoma. Int J Cancer. 1997;74(6):593-9.

33. Watanabe I, Yamaguchi M, Kasai M. Histologic characreristics of gonadotropin-producing hepatoblastoma: a survey of seven cases from Japan. J Pediatr Surg. 1987;22:406-11.

34. Zsíros J, Maibach R, Shafford E, et al. Successful treatment of childhood high-risk hepatoblastoma with dose-intensive multiagent chemotherapy and surgery: final results of the SIOPEL-3HR study. J Clin Oncol. 2010;28(15):2584-90.

Chapter

37

Liver in Systemic Illness

Hanifah Oswari

INTRODUCTION

The liver has dual blood supply from systemic and portal veins. It is the largest parenchymal organ in the body and receives 25% of the resting cardiac output.[1] The liver plays a central role in the metabolism of proteins, carbohydrates, fats and many drugs. It has an important role in induction of immune tolerance and can be a target for immune-mediated damage. All these make it prone to injury by various systemic conditions.

Clinicians should be aware that the liver does not only present as a victim, but can trigger and/or sustain multiorgan failure. Awareness of such complications are of central clinical importance. It is critical for clinicians to predominantly identify the underlying risk factors that contribute to the hepatic involvement so as to initiate curative measures as early as possible and avoid unnecessary or inappropriate treatments. This chapter reviews liver injury and common systemic illnesses in children.

CRITICALLY ILL PATIENT

Critically ill patients may exhibit liver dysfunction. Liver dysfunction can be divided into two major patterns: (1) cholestatic and (2) hypoxic liver injury (HLI). About 20% of the critically ill patients develop cholestasis and 10% suffer from HLI during their stay at the intensive care unit (ICU). Cholestasis is the most common feature of liver dysfunction at the intensive care unit. The prevalence of cholestasis ranges from 0.6 to 54%.[2]

Dramatic increase in the aminotransferase levels can be due to HLI.[3] It can occur in up to 10% of critically ill patients in the ICU. HLI is usually defined by 3 clinical conditions: (1) acute cardiac, circulatory, or respiratory failure, (2) an abrupt and transient increase in serum aminotransferase levels to at least 20 times the upper limit of normal, and (3) exclusion of other causes for increased aminotransferase levels such as viral or drug-induced hepatitis.[4,5] Recovery from liver dysfunction may improve if the primary disorder treatment is satisfactory, but inadequate or unsuccessful treatment may result in progressive liver dysfunction.

INFECTION

Sepsis

In severe sepsis, especially in neonates with sepsis, patients may develop cholestasis. It is known as sepsis-associated cholestasis. The liver plays a major role in bacterial scavenging and inactivation of bacterial products, including the production and clearance of inflammatory mediators.[6] Cholestasis in sepsis develops from either a functional defect in bile formation at the hepatocellular level, or impairment in bile secretion or bile flow at the level of the small or large bile ducts.[7-9]

The majority of patients with sepsis will present with functional hepatocellular cholestasis; however, patient with septic shock may show an increase of aminotransferases. Besides jaundice and conjugated hyperbilirubinemia, patients may show acholic stool and hepatomegaly, and increase of serum aminotransferases or alkaline phosphatase (ALP).[10] In neonates with sepsis who develop cholestasis, the length of hospital stay is 1.5 times longer and mortality is 2.25 times higher than with sepsis only.[10] The level of gamma-glutamyl transpeptidase (GGT) less than 85.5 IU/L and serum aspartate aminotransferase (AST) more than 51.0 IU/L may predict poor prognostic value of biochemical liver parameters in neonates with sepsis-associated cholestasis.[11]

Differential diagnosis of sepsis-associated cholestasis is ischemic hepatitis, total parenteral nutrition (TPN)-related cholestasis, and drug-induced cholestasis. Treatment for sepsis-associated cholestasis is mainly focused on eradicating the underlying infection and management for sepsis.

Dengue Hemorrhagic Fever

Hepatomegaly is a common finding in dengue infection. It has been reported that hepatomegaly was found in 74% and jaundice in 25% of the patients with dengue infection.[12]

Manifestations of dengue fever such as hepatitis, fulminant hepatic failure, and acalculous cholecystitis have been reported.[13-17] Hepatic manifestations can be characterized by symptoms of acute hepatitis with pain in the hypochondrium, hepatomegaly, jaundice and raised aminotransferase levels. AST levels are usually on the higher side in children with dengue infection and the elevations are usually modest (2–5 times the upper limit of normal values), but marked elevations (5–15 times the upper limit of normal) are occasionally found.[18,19] In hepatitis, the levels of these enzymes peak on the ninth day after the onset of symptoms and gradually return to normal levels within 2–3 weeks.[12] In most cases, hepatic involvement prolongs the clinical course of this self-limiting viral infection but it does not constitute a sign of worse prognosis.[12,20]

Typhoid Fever

Typhoid fever is characterized by severe systemic illness with fever and abdominal pain. The liver is commonly involved in patients with typhoid fever. Approximately 27% of patients have hepatomegaly, and 5–10% of patients will have clinical jaundice.[21]

Abnormal aminotransferase tests are frequently observed.[22,23] The clinical and laboratory picture although rare may be suggestive of acute viral hepatitis.[24] With typhoid hepatitis compared to viral hepatitis, a higher proportion of patients develop fever above 40°C (44% versus 4%, respectively) and have relative bradycardia (42% vs. 4%). Besides these, *Salmonella* hepatitis was associated with low-peak serum alanine aminotransferase (ALT), low-peak serum aspartate aminotransferase, and high-peak serum ALP (296 versus 3,234 U/L, 535 versus 2,844 U/L, and 500 versus 228 U/dL, respectively).[24]

LIVER IN THE PRESENCE OF ALTERED SYSTEMIC CIRCULATION

Children with circulatory disturbances may develop liver dysfunction. About 25% of cardiac output is targeted to the liver. The liver dysfunction is related to ischemic condition and liver congestion.

Ischemic Hepatitis

Acute hypoperfusion of the liver may cause a diffuse hepatic injury that is known as an ischemic hepatitis, shock liver or hypoxic hepatitis. Shock may cause ischemic hepatitis; however, ischemic hepatitis may develop even if the patient has not experienced shock. Ischemic hepatitis has also been reported in hepatic artery thrombosis after liver transplantation, severe respiratory failure and systemic hypoxia.[4]

Patients with ischemic hepatitis may typically present with a marked and rapid increase in serum aminotransferases, massive increase of lactate dehydrogenase (LDH) levels and bilirubin after hemodynamic instability or hypoxia. Aminotransferases may rise up to 5,000–10,000 IU/L in 24–48 hours after an ischemic insult but usually return to normal within 7–10 days after the initial ischemic insult.[25] The serum bilirubin level then begins to increase after the aminotransferase levels have begun to decrease. Serum ALP is usually normal or mildly increased to less than twice the upper limit of normal. Cholestasis may occur in bypass surgery if the bypass time exceeds 2 hours.[26]

The etiopathogenetic mechanisms in ischemic hepatitis are left cardiac failure (cardiac arrhythmia, cardiomyopathy, pericardial tamponade, acute myocardial infarction), trauma, burns, severe dehydration and hemorrhage.[25]

There are three characteristics that differentiate ischemic hepatitis from acute viral hepatitis: (1) serum aminotransferases levels are rapidly returned to normal in ischemic hepatitis, it usually returns to normal in 7–10 days, (2) LDH elevation is more marked in ischemic hepatitis than acute viral hepatitis, (3) renal damage occurs more frequently in ischemic hepatitis than acute viral hepatitis.[25]

The main treatment for ischemic hepatitis is to correct the circulatory disturbance. There is no specific therapy for ischemic hepatitis. To improve hepatosplanchnic blood flow, infusion of renal-dose dopamine has been suggested.[27] The prognosis of ischemic hepatitis is usually good and self-limiting.

Congestive Hepatopathy

Congestive hepatopathy or liver congestion is caused by right-sided heart failure. The causes of right-sided heart failure include mitral stenosis, tricuspid regurgitation, constrictive pericarditis, pulmonary atresia, tetralogy of Fallot and cardiomyopathy. Patients with congestive changes are typically asymptomatic and frequently identified only when routine laboratory analysis shows subtle abnormalities in liver function tests.[28]

The clinical picture for liver congestion is hepatomegaly (95–99%), ascites (7–49%), splenomegaly (12–25%), and/or jaundice (less than 20%).[29] Laboratory findings typically reveals mild, nonspecific increase in the serum aminotransferase levels, usually less than 2–3 times the upper limit of normal.[30] The total bilirubin level is only mildly increased (less than 3 mg/dL) and predominantly unconjugated. Increases in bilirubin level have been shown to correlate with the severity of right atrial pressure and passive congestion, and patients with severe right ventricular failure can become jaundiced.[30]

A diagnosis of liver congestion should be suspected in any patient with abnormal liver tests and, a clinical picture of congestive heart failure or increased central venous pressure (CVP). Serologic evaluation for other causes of viral and metabolic liver disease should be performed to exclude primary liver disease. The best support for the diagnosis is the improvement of liver function with treatment of the underlying cardiac condition.[30] The primary approach for restoring normal liver functions in liver congestion is to treat the underlying cardiac disease and improve forward cardiac output this will improve liver function tests and reduce ascites.

HEMATOLOGIC DISORDERS

Hemolytic Anemia

Hemolysis can be caused by abnormality of erythrocyte, its membranes or other extrinsic factors. In sickle cell anemia, the erythrocytes are prone to hemolysis and this will disrupt the blood flow causing vaso-occlusive crisis and organ injury. The hepatic complication in sickle cell include secondary iron overload from multiple blood transfusions and pigment cholelithiasis caused by red cell breakdown.[31] Hyperbilirubinemia may be caused by hemolysis, infection, or intrahepatic sickling (sickle cell hepatopathy), and this finding may be associated with mild to severe liver dysfunction.[32]

The symptoms of liver dysfunction may be found as right upper quadrant pain, jaundice, hepatomegaly and fever. These symptoms are typical of both cholangitis and cholecystitis and difficult to distinguish.[33]

In thalassemia, the major cause of liver injury is hemochromatosis because of massive iron deposition in the liver related to multiple blood transfusions. The other possibility of liver disease in thalassemia is viral hepatitis B or C, which is acquired from blood transfusion. Gallstones are common in thalassemia, but usually asymptomatic unless the stones are impacted in the common bile duct.[34]

Leukemia

Liver involvement in leukemia is usually asymptomatic at the time of diagnosis, but liver infiltration at autopsy was found in 95% of patient with acute lymphocytic leukemia (ALL) and 75% of patient with acute myeloid leukemia (AML).[35,36] Liver infiltration in ALL is in the portal tracts, and in AML it is in the portal tracts and sinusoids.[31]

The majority of patients with ALL and some of patients with AML are found with hepatomegaly. Liver involvement in leukemia is more common in advance stages of the disease. Children with ALL may present as fulminant hepatic failure. The pathogenesis is not clear and may be related to viral infections, sepsis, or ischemic hepatopathy with submassive necrosis that is caused by infiltrating leukemic cells that obstruct the hepatic blood flow.[37]

Acute myeloid leukemia does not usually cause liver injury, but obstructive jaundice and cholestatic hepatitis secondary to sinusoidal infiltration have been reported, and improved with chemotherapy.[38] Chemotherapy treatment for leukemia may affect the liver. Hepatic damage is more likely in children receiving prolonged treatment.[39] Methotrexate, one of the chemotherapeutic agents used in ALL, can cause hepatotoxicy and is usually dose-related. 6-mercaptopurine, another chemotherapeutic agent used in maintenance therapy for ALL, is also hepatotoxic and may cause hepatic necrosis and cholestasis that may be fatal.[40] Chemotherapies that may induce hepatotoxicity are listed in Table 37.1.

Lymphoma

Patients with non-Hodgkin's lymphoma (NHL) have more liver involvement such as lymphomatous infiltration and extrahepatic obstruction than Hodgkin's lymphoma (HL). 16–43% of patients with NHL having liver involvement.[51] The clinical symptoms of hepatic infiltration in NHL are similar to those of HL. Patients with extensive hepatic infiltration may be asymptomatic, although patients with NHL are more likely to have jaundice as a result of extrahepatic obstruction.

Liver involvement in HL is present in 5% of cases, and it increases to 30% during the course of the disease, and up to 50% at autopsy.[52] Cholestasis can occur as a result of direct infiltration, extrahepatic biliary obstruction, hemolysis, viral hepatitis, or drug-induced liver disease. Liver infiltration may cause acute hepatic failure.[53] Cholestasis may be associated with vanishing bile duct syndrome.[54]

COLLAGEN VASCULAR DISEASE

Systemic Lupus Erythematosus

Systemic lupus erythematosus (SLE) patients have a 25–50% chance of developing abnormal liver function in their lifetime. Hepatomegaly is a common finding in SLE. Up to 70% of children and adults with SLE were detected with hepatomegaly without hepatic symptoms. Splenomegaly is a feature of active disease.[55]

Table 37.1: Liver disease induced by chemotherapy			
Chemotherapy	Type of liver disease	Clinical features	Risk factors
Methotrexate[41,42]	Acute hepatitis, steatosis (macrovesicular) and presinusoidal portal tract fibrosis	Increase ALT, AST and ALP	Dose-dependent
Doxorubicin[43]	Acute hepatitis, chronic active hepatitis	Increased aminotransferases, LDH and ALP	Acute hepatitis: dose-dependent
6-Mercaptopurine[44]	Acute zonal necrosis, macrovesicular steatosis, cholestatic hepatitis, veno-occlusive disease	Elevated aminotransferase levels	Rare association
L-asparaginase[42,45]	Microvesicular steatosis	• Elevations of aminotransferase, bilirubin, and ALP • Decreased serum albumin, ceruloplasmin, haptoglobin, transferrin, and γ-globulins • Coagulopathy (decreased levels of coagulation factors II, VII, IX, X, and fibrinogen; increase partial thromboplastin time • Hyperammonemia	Partly dose-dependent
Cyclophosphamide[42,46]	Acute hepatitis	Elevations of aminotransferase, bilirubin, and ALP	Dose-dependent
6-Thiguanine[42,47]	Acute hepatitis, Budd-Chiari syndrome, veno-occlusive disease	Elevations of aminotransferase, bilirubin, and ALP	Dose-dependent
Azathioprine[48]	Cholestasis hepatitis, Budd-Chiari syndrome, veno-occlusive disease, nodular regenerative hyperplasia	Nonspecific liver test abnormalities, cholestasis with or without hepatitis, bile duct injury and vascular injury	
Cisplatin[42,49]	Microvesicular steatosis	Liver failure, steatosis, cholestasis, elevation of AST, ALT, ALP, LDH, bilirubin	Rare association
Bleomycin[42]	Microvesicular steatosis	Increases of AST, ALT, and bilirubin (low incidence)	
Busulphan[50]	Budd-Chiari syndrome, veno-occlusive disease	Hepatomegaly, jaundice or hyperbilirubinemia, and ascites and/or a weight gain of >5%. Elevated levels AST and/or ALT	
Dactinomycin[42]	Budd-Chiari syndrome, veno-occlusive disease, nodular regenerative hyperplasia	Transient AST elevation	

Abbreviations: ALP, alkaline phosphatase; ALT, alanine aminotransferase; AST, serum aspartate aminotransferase; LDH, lactate dehydrogenase.

Aminotransferases may be abnormal in 25–40% of adult patients with SLE,[33] however, liver abnormalities are not a significant cause of morbidity and mortality.[55]

Spectrum of hepatic disorders that has been associated with SLE are Budd-Chiari syndrome, veno-occlusive disease, obstructive jaundice, autoimmune hepatitis, primary biliary cirrhosis, granulomatous hepatitis, chronic hepatitis with immunoglobulin A (IgA) or immunoglobulin D (IgD) deficiency, idiopathic portal hypertension coexisting with SLE.[56]

Hepatic manifestations in neonatal lupus erythematosus include asymptomatic elevated liver function tests, mild hepatosplenomegaly, cholestasis, and hepatitis.[57-59]

In one report, hepatobiliary disease occurred in 19 of 219 infants (9%) with neonatal lupus, usually in conjunction with either cardiac or cutaneous involvement.[60]

Serum aspartate aminotransferase, ALT, ALP may also be abnormal in patients receiving NSAIDs. Salicylate therapy used in adult patients with SLE may affect the liver by dose dependent mechanism.[61] However, doses less than 2.5 g/day or blood salicylate level less than 25 mg/dL will not affect the liver.

Juvenile Rheumatoid Arthritis

Hepatomegaly is a common finding in juvenile rheumatoid arthritis (JRA) patients, although it is more common to detect splenomegaly.[55] Hepatomegaly usually decreases with time. Progressive and persistent hepatomegaly may be related to secondary amyloidosis.[62]

Abnormality in biochemical liver tests is present in 18–50% of cases. Serum aminotransferase levels are usually normal, and ALP levels may increase in up to 50% of patients.[63] The source of the elevated ALP is unclear. In one-third of patients with rheumatoid arthritis who were found with raised ALP levels, GGT and 5'-nucleotidase were frequently found to be at normal levels. Liver dysfunction may be caused by medication such as aspirin or other NSAIDs. Serum aminotransferase is mildly elevated in 60% of pediatric patient receiving salicylate therapy.[64,65]

■ NUTRITIONAL DISORDERS

Celiac Disease

About 30–50% of children with celiac disease have elevated aminotransferases, particularly in patients presenting with the classical symptoms of the disease,[66-68] however, aminotransferases in most patients will be normalized with a gluten-free diet.

Patients with celiac disease have increased risks for developing a variety of liver disease, including acute hepatitis, chronic hepatitis with autoimmune hepatitis, primary sclerosing cholangitis (SC) primary biliary cirrhosis, and liver cirrhosis.[68,69] The cause of the hepatic injury remains uncertain but most likely related to the passage of antigens through the injured intestinal mucosa because there is a prompt response to a gluten-free diet.[55]

Obesity

Obesity is associated with fatty liver or nonalcoholic fatty liver disease (NAFLD), which may have a clinical spectrum of liver abnormalities.[70,71] The spectrum of abnormalities includes steatosis (increased liver fat without inflammation) and nonalcoholic steatohepatitis (NASH, fatty liver with inflammation). NASH may lead to fibrosis, cirrhosis, and ultimately to liver failure if not treated.[72] As the prevalence of obesity in children is increasing, NAFLD is also seen increasing among children.[73,74] This rise is alarming because of its close association with the development of metabolic syndrome.[75] There are clinical associations between NAFLD and metabolic syndrome, including insulin resistance, dyslipidemia, and hypertension, independent of the degree of obesity.[76] The pathogenesis of NAFLD has not been fully understood. The most widely supported theory implicates insulin resistance as the key mechanism leading to hepatic steatosis, and perhaps also to steatohepatitis. A "second hit", or additional oxidative injury, is required to manifest the necroinflammatory component of steatohepatitis.[77,78]

In initial assessments of children with suspicion of fatty liver, pediatricians should take detailed clinical histories with special attention to information regarding nutritional intake and drug consumption.[75] Obese children with hepatic dysfunction are usually asymptomatic. However, they may have right upper quadrant pain, hepatomegaly or nonspecific symptoms such as abdominal discomfort, weakness, fatigue or malaise. Clinical symptoms such as jaundice, palmar erythema, spider angiomata or encephalopathy are uncommon. Laboratory abnormalities include elevations in liver aminotransferases (ALT and AST), ALP, and GGT.[71,79-81] Serum levels of aminotransferases may be reduced even in the presence of NASH and fibrosis, liver function test cannot represent the severity of NAFLD.[82]

Liver ultrasonography can detect fatty liver when steatosis involves more than 30% of hepatocytes.[83] A large prospective pediatric cohort study has shown good correlation between liver steatosis score by ultrasonography and the severity of hepatic steatosis on liver biopsy.[84]

Liver biopsy is the only way to differentiate between simple steatosis, steatohepatitis and fibrosis, and can be helpful in excluding other causes of elevated serum aminotransferases. However, the results of a liver biopsy are not likely to provide clinical benefit because there is currently no specific treatment for NAFLD other than weight management. The indications for liver biopsy for suspected NAFLD have not been established in children.[81] Liver biopsy may be required if the liver dysfunction suggest more severe or progressive liver disease or raises concerns about the cause of the liver disease which requires evaluation by liver biopsy.

Weight management is still the only established treatment for NAFLD, with emphasis on physical activity because of its utility in improving insulin sensitivity, which appears to be an important pathway for the development of NAFLD. There is improvement in liver histology or aminotransferase activity after weight loss.[85-88]

Total Parenteral Nutrition

Infants with a history of prematurity and/or short bowel syndrome are prone to develop cholestatic liver disease attributable to total parenteral nutrition, when other specific causes of liver injury are ruled out. This is recognized as parenteral nutrition-associated liver disease (PNALD), also known as parenteral nutrition-associated cholestasis (PNAC). All infants with cholestasis should be evaluated for biliary obstruction (e.g. biliary atresia), infection, metabolic and genetic liver diseases that need specific therapy. PNALD develops in 40–60% of infants who need long-term TPN for intestinal failure.[89] The clinical spectrum includes cholestasis, cholelithiasis, hepatic fibrosis with progression to biliary cirrhosis and the development of portal hypertension and liver failure in a significant number of children who are totally parenterally fed.[89] PNALD is less common and generally less severe among older children and adults, but may occur in those undergoing long-term treatment with parenteral nutrition. Cholestasis predominates in infants while older children and adults develop steatosis and steatohepatitis.

Risk factors for developing PNALD are young age, short bowel syndrome, inter current infections, lack of enteral feedings, and duration of parenteral nutrition. Emerging evidence suggests that soybean oils that are used in conventional intravenous lipid emulsions may contribute to the risk for developing PNALD. Risk factors for PNALD include prematurity, low birthweight, and intrauterine growth restriction, suggesting that immaturity of the liver is a predisposing factor.

Infants with PNALD typically develop cholestasis about 2 weeks after commencing parenteral nutrition, but the onset may be later. The laboratory findings are not specific; in addition to conjugated bilirubin, AST, ALT, and GGT may be mildly elevated.[90,91]

The principal step in the management of PNALD is to start enteral feedings to reduce the need for parenteral nutrition. Enteral feeding exposes the gastrointestinal tract to nutrient and hormonal stimuli, which are not present when the bowel is kept empty.[92]

■ IMMUNODEFICIENCY

Defects in the defense mechanism can be divided in primary and secondary immunodeficiencies. Primary immunodeficiencies (PIDs) are genetic disorders of the innate, cellular and/or humoral immune system. Secondary immunodefiencies also known as acquired immunodeficiencies can result from HIV infection, various immunosuppressive agents, such as particular medications (e.g. chemotherapy, immunosuppressive drugs or after organ transplants). Hepatic complications in children with immune deficiencies can be related to chronic infections or the side effect of drugs used to control infection (antibiotic or antifungal prophylaxis such as for

crytosporidium parvum). *Crytosporidium parvum* has been implicated in development of SC in HIV infection.[93]

Primary Immunodeficiencies

The most common hepatic complication of the PIDs is SC. Around 24% of children with PIDs are estimated to have some form of liver involvement.[94] The most frequent causes of PIDs are combined immunodeficiency (CID), hyper-immunoglobulin M (IgM) syndrome and common variable immunodeficiency.[94] Patients may be referred because of acute liver decompensation, clinical and/or biochemical abnormalities suggesting liver disease.[94] Clinical features of children with PIDs are hepatomegaly or hepatosplenomegaly with abnormal AST and/or GGT. The abnormal AST and GGT may be only trivial or transient. These clinical features of SC in PIDs are different from classical symptoms of cholangiopathy such as jaundice, fatigue, or pruritus. Ultrasonography is a useful screening tool for children with PIDs that may detect bile duct extrahepatic or intrahepatic mild dilatation and splenomegaly. Evaluation with liver biopsy and cholangiography may be indicated after ultrasonography screening.[94]

Hyper-immunoglobulin M Syndrome

Children with hyper-IgM syndrome suffer from neutropenia, opportunistic infections, chronic mouth ulcers, chronic diarrhea, failure to thrive and poorly defined chronic encephalopathy.[95] Hyper-IgM syndrome is caused by absence of CD40 ligand (CD40L) on activated lymphocytes and lack of interaction with CD40 molecules from B cells in the X-linked form (CD40L deficiency), or defective expression of activation-induced cytidine deaminase (AID) on B cells in the autosomal recessive form of the disease.[96]

This condition is a paradigm for immune deficiency-associated SC, If the patient having SC is not treated and cured it may progress to chronic biliary disease and cirrhosis in the majority of cases. Liver disease in patients with CD40L deficiency may also be secondary to cytomegalovirus (CMV) infection. However, many children with hyper-IgM syndrome may remain clinically asymptomatic well into the second decade of life, when progression of the liver disease typically occurs. Liver transplantation has been attempted for end-stage biliary disease, but fatal cholangiopathy recurs within months after transplantation. It has become clear that correction of the immune defect is essential for patient and graft survival. Hematopoietic stem cell transplantation is able to correct the immune deficiency.[97,98]

Secondary Immunodeficiencies

HIV Infection

The majority of children with HIV acquired the infection vertically from HIV-infected mothers. Clinical symptoms of liver disease in HIV patients include jaundice, hepatomegaly, and mild to moderate elevation of ALP, increase of GGT, AST, and bilirubin level. Abdominal ultrasonography may find mild dilatation of the bile ducts, enlarged gallbladder, and abnormal echo pattern of the liver with mild splenomegaly.[99]

HIV-related cholangiopathy associated with infections such as *Cryptosporidia, Microsporidia* and CMV were frequently reported in children and adults.[100] Although Kupffer cells and endothelial cells are potential sites of human immunodeficiency virus 1 (HIV-1) infection, current studies do not indicate that the liver is a major reservoir for this virus. Drug hepatotoxicity, multimicrobial infections of the biliary tree resembling SC and a variety of nonspecific hepatic changes should be considered in evaluating AIDS patients or HIV-infected patients with evidence of liver dysfunction.[101] Liver disorders caused by viral hepatitis (chronic hepatitis B and C, adenovirus, CMV, and Epstein-Barr virus) have also been described.

REFERENCES

1. Lautt WW. Hepatic vasculature: a conceptual review. Gastroenterology. 1977;73:1163-9.
2. Chand N, Sanyal AJ. Sepsis-induced cholestasis. Hepatology. 2007;45:230-41.
3. Whitehead MW, Hawkes ND, Hainsworth I, Kingham JG. A prospective study of the causes of notably raised aspartate aminotransferase of liver origin. Gut. 1999;45:129-33.
4. Henrion J, Schapira M, Luwaert R, et al. Hypoxic hepatitis: clinical and hemodynamic study in 142 consecutive cases. Medicine (Baltimore). 2003;82:392-406.
5. Fuhrmann V, Kneidinger N, Herkner H, et al. Hypoxic hepatitis: underlying conditions and risk factors for mortality in critically ill patients. Intensive Care Med. 2009;35:1397-405.
6. Dhainaut JF, Marin N, Mignon A, Vinsonneau C. Hepatic response to sepsis: interaction between coagulation and inflammatory processes. Crit Care Med. 2001;29:S42-7.
7. Trauner M, Meier PJ, Boyer JL. Molecular pathogenesis of cholestasis. N Engl J Med. 1998;339:1217-27.
8. Arrese M, Trauner M. Molecular aspects of bile formation and cholestasis. Trends Mol Med. 2003;9:558-64.
9. Trauner M, Meier PJ, Boyer JL. Molecular regulation of hepatocellular transport systems in cholestasis. J Hepatol. 1999;31:165-78.
10. Bachtiar KS, Oswari H, Batubara JRL, et al. Cholestasis sepsis at neonatology ward and neonatal Intensive Care Unit Cipto Mangunkusumo Hospital 2007 : incidence, mortality rate and associated risk factors. Med J Indones. 2008;17:107-13.
11. Oswari H, Widjaja RK, Rohsiswatmo R, Cleghorn G. Prognostic value of biochemical liver parameters in neonatal sepsis-associated cholestasis. J Paediatr Child Health. 2013;49:E6-11.
12. Mohan B, Patwari AK, Anand VK. Hepatic dysfunction in childhood dengue infection. J Trop Pediatr. 2000;46:40-3.
13. Sedhain A, Adhikari S, Regmi S, et al. Fulminant hepatic failure due to dengue. Kathmandu Univ Med J (KUMJ). 2011;9:73-5.
14. Vijayalakshmi AM, Devaprasath S. Fulminant hepatic failure in primary dengue infection. Indian Pediatr. 2010;47:280.
15. Soundravally R, Narayanan P, Bhat BV, et al. Fulminant hepatic failure in an infant with severe dengue infection. Indian J Pediatr. 2010;77:435-7.
16. Subramanian V, Shenoy S, Joseph AJ. Dengue hemorrhagic fever and fulminant hepatic failure. Dig Dis Sci. 2005;50:1146-7.
17. Karunatilake H, Vithiya K, Arasalingam A, et al. Acalculous cholecystitis and dengue fever. Ceylon Med J. 2008;53:30.
18. Kalayanarooj S, Vaughn DW, Nimmannitya S, et al. Early clinical and laboratory indicators of acute dengue illness. J Infect Dis. 1997;176:313-21.
19. Schwartz E, Mendelson E, Sidi Y. Dengue fever among travelers. Am J Med. 1996;101:516-20.
20. Aneja VK, Kochar G, Neelam B. Unusual manifestations of dengue fever. Apollo Medicine. 2010;7:69-76.
21. Novak DA, Lauwers GY, Kradin RL. Bacterial, parasitic, and fungal infections of the liver. In: Suchy FJ, Sokol RJ, Balistreri WF (Eds). Liver Disease In Children. Cambridge: Cambridge University Press; 2007. pp. 871-98.
22. Stuart BM, Pullen RL. Typhoid; clinical analysis of 360 cases. Arch Intern Med (Chic). 1946;78:629-61.
23. Wang JL, Kao JH, Tseng SP, et al. Typhoid fever and typhoid hepatitis in Taiwan. Epidemiol Infect. 2005;133:1073-9.
24. El-Newihi HM, Alamy ME, Reynolds TB. Salmonella hepatitis: analysis of 27 cases and comparison with acute viral hepatitis. Hepatology. 1996;24:516-9.
25. Gitlin N, Serio KM. Ischemic hepatitis: widening horizons. Am J Gastroenterol. 1992;87:831-6.
26. Michalopoulos A, Alivizatos P, Geroulanos S. Hepatic dysfunction following cardiac surgery: determinants and consequences. Hepatogastroenterology. 1997;44:779-83.
27. Angehrn W, Schmid E, Althaus F, et al. Effect of dopamine on hepatosplanchnic blood flow. J Cardiovasc Pharmacol. 1980;2:257-65.
28. Giallourakis CC, Rosenberg PM, Friedman LS. The liver in heart failure. Clin Liver Dis. 2002;6:947-67, viii-ix.
29. Richman SM, Delman AJ, Grob D. Alterations in indices of liver function in congestive heart failure with particular reference to serum enzymes. Am J Med. 1961;30:211-25.
30. Weisberg IS, Jacobson IM. Cardiovascular diseases and the liver. Clin Liver Dis. 2011;15:1-20.
31. Shimizu Y. Liver in systemic disease. World J Gastroenterol. 2008;14:4111-9.
32. Bandyopadhyay R, Bandyopadhyay SK, Dutta A. Sickle cell hepatopathy. Indian J Pathol Microbiol. 2008;51:284-5.

33. Malnick S, Melzer E, Sokolowski N, Basevitz A. The involvement of the liver in systemic diseases. J Clin Gastroenterol. 2008;42:69-80.

34. Beath SV. The liver in systemic illness. In: Kelly D (Ed). Disease of the liver and biliary system in children, 3rd edition. Singapore: Blackwell's publishing; 2008. pp. 381-403.

35. Sharma Poudel B, Karki L. Abnormal hepatic function and splenomegaly on the newly diagnosed acute leukemia patients. JNMA J Nepal Med Assoc. 2007;46:165-9.

36. Roldberg GM, Rubenstone AI, Saphir O. A study of malignant lymphomas and leukemias. IV. Diagnosis of controversial cases of leukemia (with reference to histological criteria). Cancer. 1961;14:30-5.

37. Litten JB, Rodriguez MM, Maniaci V. Acute lymphoblastic leukemia presenting in fulminant hepatic failure. Pediatr Blood Cancer. 2006;47:842-5.

38. Wandroo FA, Murray J, Mutimer D, Hubscher S. Acute myeloid leukaemia presenting as cholestatic hepatitis. J Clin Pathol. 2004;57:544-5.

39. Tang H, Neuberger J. Review article: methotrexate in gastroenterology--dangerous villain or simply misunderstood? Aliment Pharmacol Ther. 1996;10:851-8.

40. Laidlaw ST, Reilly JT, Suvarna SK. Fatal hepatotoxicity associated with 6-mercaptopurine therapy. Postgrad Med J. 1995;71:639.

41. Chen Z, Li XP, Li ZJ, et al. Reduced hepatotoxicity by total glucosides of paeony in combination treatment with leflunomide and methotrexate for patients with active rheumatoid arthritis. Int Immunopharmacol. 2013;15:474-7.

42. King PD, Perry MC. Hepatotoxicity of chemotherapy. Oncologist. 2001;6:162-76.

43. El-Sayyad HI, Ismail MF, Shalaby FM, et al. Histopathological effects of cisplatin, doxorubicin and 5-flurouracil (5-FU) on the liver of male albino rats. Int J Biol Sci. 2009;5:466-73.

44. Masia R, Pratt DS, Misdraji J. A histopathologic pattern of centrilobular hepatocyte injury suggests 6-mercaptopurine-induced hepatotoxicity in patients with inflammatory bowel disease. Arch Pathol Lab Med. 2012;136:618-22.

45. Muss HB, Spell N, Scudiery D, et al. A phase II trial of PEG-L-asparaginase in the treatment of non-Hodgkins lymphoma. Invest New Drugs. 1990;8:125-30.

46. Goldberg JW, Lidsky MD. Cyclophosphamide-associated hepatotoxicity. South Med J. 1985;78:222-3.

47. Larrey D, Freneaux E, Berson A, et al. Peliosis hepatis induced by 6-thioguanine administration. Gut. 1988;29:1265-9.

48. Farrell GC. Drug-induced hepatic injury. J Gastroenterol Hepatol. 1997;12:S242-50.

49. Pollera CF, Ameglio F, Nardi M, et al. Cisplatin-induced hepatic toxicity. J Clin Oncol. 1987;5:318-9.

50. Vassal G, Hartmann O, Benhamou E. Busulfan and veno-occlusive disease of the liver. Ann Intern Med. 1990;112:881.

51. Singh MM, Pockros PJ. Hematologic and oncologic diseases and the liver. Clin Liver Dis. 2011;15:69-87.

52. Birrer MJ, Young RC. Differential diagnosis of jaundice in lymphoma patients. Semin Liver Dis. 1987;7:269-77.

53. Rowbotham D, Wendon J, Williams R. Acute liver failure secondary to hepatic infiltration: a single centre experience of 18 cases. Gut. 1998;42:576-80.

54. Hubscher SG, Lumley MA, Elias E. Vanishing bile duct syndrome: a possible mechanism for intrahepatic cholestasis in Hodgkin's lymphoma. Hepatology. 1993;17:70-7.

55. Farrell MK, Bucuvalas JC. Systemic disease and the liver. In: Suchy FJ, Sokol RJ, Balistreri WF (Eds). Liver disease in children, 3rd edition. Cambridge: Cambridge university press; 2007. p. 897-927.

56. van Hoek B. The spectrum of liver disease in systemic lupus erythematosus. Neth J Med. 1996;48:244-53.

57. Silverman E, Jaeggi E. Non-cardiac manifestations of neonatal lupus erythematosus. Scand J Immunol. 2010;72:223-5.

58. Kim KR, Yoon TY. A case of neonatal lupus erythematosus showing transient anemia and hepatitis. Ann Dermatol. 2009;21:315-8.

59. Lynn Cheng C, Galbraith S, Holland K. Congenital lupus erythematosus presenting at birth with widespread erosions, pancytopenia, and subsequent hepatobiliary disease. Pediatr Dermatol. 2010;27:109-11.

60. Lee LA, Sokol RJ, Buyon JP. Hepatobiliary disease in neonatal lupus: prevalence and clinical characteristics in cases enrolled in a national registry. Pediatrics. 2002;109:E11.

61. Seaman WE, Ishak KG, Plotz PH. Aspirin-induced hepatotoxicity in patients with systemic lupus erythematosus. Ann Intern Med. 1974;80:1-8.

62. David J, Vouyiouka O, Ansell BM, et al. Amyloidosis in juvenile chronic arthritis: a morbidity and mortality study. Clin Exp Rheumatol. 1993;11:85-90.

63. Thompson PW, Houghton BJ, Clifford C, et al. The source and significance of raised serum enzymes in rheumatoid arthritis. Q J Med. 1990;76:869-79.

64. Bernstein BH, Singsen BH, King KK, Hanson V. Aspirin-induced hepatotoxicity and its effect on juvenile rheumatoid arthritis. Am J Dis Child. 1977;131:659-63.

65. Rich RR, Johnson JS. Salicylate hepatotoxicity in patients with juvenile rheumatoid arthritis. Arthritis Rheum. 1973;16:1-9.

66. Farre C, Esteve M, Curcoy A, et al. Hypertransaminasemia in pediatric celiac disease patients and its prevalence as a diagnostic clue. Am J Gastroenterol. 2002;97:3176-81.

67. Bonamico M, Pitzalis G, Culasso F, et al. [Hepatic damage in celiac disease in children]. Minerva Pediatr. 1986;38:959-62.

68. Vajro P, Paolella G, Maggiore G, Giordano G. Pediatric celiac disease, cryptogenic hypertransaminasemia, and autoimmune hepatitis. J Pediatr Gastroenterol Nutr. 2013;56:663-70.

69. Ludvigsson JF, Elfstrom P, Broome U, et al. Celiac disease and risk of liver disease: a general population-based study. Clin Gastroenterol Hepatol. 2007;5:63-9 e1.

70. Matteoni CA, Younossi ZM, Gramlich T, et al. Nonalcoholic fatty liver disease: a spectrum of clinical and pathological severity. Gastroenterology. 1999;116:1413-9.

71. Speiser PW, Rudolf MC, Anhalt H, et al. Childhood obesity. J Clin Endocrinol Metab. 2005;90:1871-87.

72. Feldstein AE, Charatcharoenwitthaya P, Treeprasertsuk S, et al. The natural history of non-alcoholic fatty liver disease in children: a follow-up study for up to 20 years. Gut. 2009;58:1538-44.

73. Schwimmer JB, McGreal N, Deutsch R, et al. Influence of gender, race, and ethnicity on suspected fatty liver in obese adolescents. Pediatrics. 2005;115:e561-5.

74. Welsh JA, Karpen S, Vos MB. Increasing prevalence of nonalcoholic fatty liver disease among United States adolescents, 1988-1994 to 2007-2010. J Pediatr. 2013;162:496-500 e1.

75. Nobili V, Svegliati-Baroni G, Alisi A, et al. A 360-degree overview of paediatric NAFLD: recent insights. J Hepatol. 2013;58:1218-29.

76. Strauss RS, Barlow SE, Dietz WH. Prevalence of abnormal serum aminotransferase values in overweight and obese adolescents. J Pediatr. 2000;136:727-33.

77. Pagano G, Pacini G, Musso G, et al. Nonalcoholic steatohepatitis, insulin resistance, and metabolic syndrome: further evidence for an etiologic association. Hepatology. 2002;35:367-72.

78. Sanyal AJ, Campbell-Sargent C, Mirshahi F, et al. Nonalcoholic steatohepatitis: association of insulin resistance and mitochondrial abnormalities. Gastroenterology. 2001;120:1183-92.

79. Franzese A, Vajro P, Argenziano A, et al. Liver involvement in obese children. Ultrasonography and liver enzyme levels at diagnosis and during follow-up in an Italian population. Dig Dis Sci. 1997;42:1428-32.

80. Tazawa Y, Noguchi H, Nishinomiya F, Takada G. Serum alanine aminotransferase activity in obese children. Acta Paediatr. 1997;86:238-41.

81. Huang JS, Barlow SE, Quiros-Tejeira RE, et al. Consensus Statement: Childhood Obesity for Pediatric Gastroenterologists. J Pediatr Gastroenterol Nutr. 2012.

82. Mofrad P, Contos MJ, Haque M, et al. Clinical and histologic spectrum of nonalcoholic fatty liver disease associated with normal ALT values. Hepatology. 2003;37:1286-92.

83. Saadeh S, Younossi ZM, Remer EM, et al. The utility of radiological imaging in nonalcoholic fatty liver disease. Gastroenterology. 2002;123:745-50.

84. Shannon A, Alkhouri N, Carter-Kent C, et al. Ultrasonographic quantitative estimation of hepatic steatosis in children With NAFLD. J Pediatr Gastroenterol Nutr. 2011;53:190-5.

85. Huang MA, Greenson JK, Chao C, et al. One-year intense nutritional counseling results in histological improvement in patients with non-alcoholic steatohepatitis: a pilot study. Am J Gastroenterol. 2005;100:1072-81.

86. Reinehr T, Schmidt C, Toschke AM, Andler W. Lifestyle intervention in obese children with non-alcoholic fatty liver disease: 2-year follow-up study. Arch Dis Child. 2009;94:437-42.

87. Pozzato C, Verduci E, Scaglioni S, et al. Liver fat change in obese children after a 1-year nutrition-behavior intervention. J Pediatr Gastroenterol Nutr. 2010;51:331-5.

88. Nobili V, Marcellini M, Devito R, et al. NAFLD in children: a prospective clinical-pathological study and effect of lifestyle advice. Hepatology. 2006;44:458-65.

89. Kelly DA. Liver complications of pediatric parenteral nutrition--epidemiology. Nutrition. 1998;14:153-7.

90. Teitelbaum DH. Parenteral nutrition-associated cholestasis. Curr Opin Pediatr. 1997;9:270-5.

91. Hofmann AF. Defective biliary secretion during total parenteral nutrition: probable mechanisms and possible solutions. J Pediatr Gastroenterol Nutr. 1995;20:376-90.

92. Jeejeebhoy KN. Management of short bowel syndrome: avoidance of total parenteral nutrition. Gastroenterology. 2006;130:S60-6.

93. Petersen C. Cryptosporidiosis in patients infected with the human immunodeficiency virus. Clin Infect Dis. 1992;15:903-9.

94. Rodrigues F, Davies EG, Harrison P, et al. Liver disease in children with primary immunodeficiencies. J Pediatr. 2004;145:333-9.

95. Winkelstein JA, Marino MC, Ochs H, et al. The X-linked hyper-IgM syndrome: clinical and immunologic features of 79 patients. Medicine (Baltimore). 2003;82:373-84.

96. Durandy A, Honjo T. Human genetic defects in class-switch recombination (hyper-IgM syndromes). Curr Opin Immunol. 2001;13:543-8.

97. Horwitz ME. Stem-cell transplantation for inherited immunodeficiency disorders. Pediatr Clin North Am. 2000;47:1371-87.

98. Thomas C, de Saint Basile G, Le Deist F, et al. Brief report: correction of X-linked hyper-IgM syndrome by allogeneic bone marrow transplantation. N Engl J Med. 1995;333:426-9.

99. Chung CJ, Sivit CJ, Rakusan TA, et al. Hepatobiliary abnormalities on sonography in children with HIV infection. J Ultrasound Med. 1994;13:205-10.

100. Bouche H, Housset C, Dumont JL, et al. AIDS-related cholangitis: diagnostic features and course in 15 patients. J Hepatol. 1993;17:34-9.

101. Lefkowitch JH. Pathology of AIDS-related liver disease. Dig Dis. 1994;12:321-30.

Index

Page numbers followed by *t* refer to table, *f* refer to figure, *fc* refer to flow chart and *b* refer to box.